Traumatic Brain Injury (TBI)

Traumatic Brain Injury (TBI): Interventions to Support Occupational Performance

Neurorehabilitation in Occupational Therapy Series, Volume 3

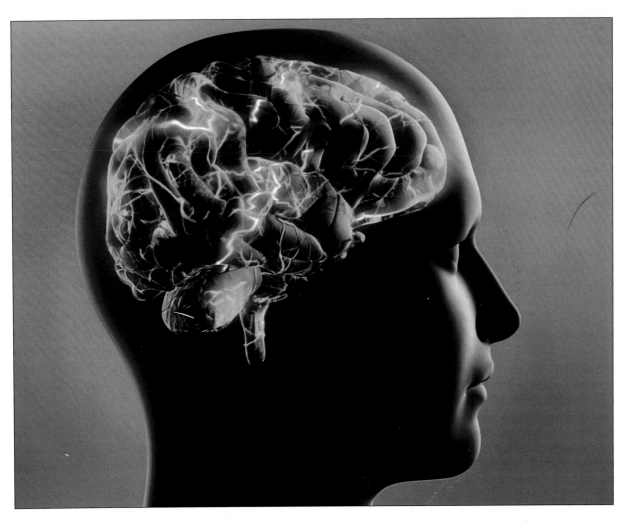

Edited by Kathleen M. Golisz, OTD, OTR/L, and
Mary Vining Radomski, PhD, OTR/L, FAOTA
Series Senior Editor: Gordon Muir Giles, PhD, OTR/L, FAOTA

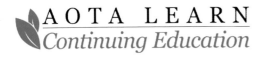

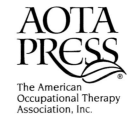

The American
Occupational Therapy
Association, Inc.

AOTA Centennial Vision
We envision that occupational therapy is a powerful, widely recognized, science-driven, and evidence-based profession with a globally connected and diverse workforce meeting society's occupational needs.

Mission Statement
The American Occupational Therapy Association advances the quality, availability, use, and support of occupational therapy through standard-setting, advocacy, education, and research on behalf of its members and the public.

AOTA Staff
Frederick P. Somers, *Executive Director*
Christopher M. Bluhm, *Chief Operating Officer*
Maureen Peterson, *Chief Professional Affairs Officer*

Chris Davis, *Director, AOTA Press*
Caroline Polk, *Digital Publishing Manager*
Ashley Hofmann, *Development/Production Editor*
Barbara Dickson, *Production Editor*

Debbie Amini, *Director, Professional Development*
Sarah Hertfelder, *Continuing Education Consultant*

Rebecca Rutberg, *Director, Marketing*
Jennifer Folden, *Marketing Specialist*
Amanda Goldman, *Marketing Specialist*

American Occupational Therapy Association, Inc.
4720 Montgomery Lane
Bethesda, MD 20814
301-652-AOTA (2682)
TDD: 800-377-8555
Fax: 301-652-7711
www.aota.org
To order: 1-877-404-AOTA or store.aota.org

Disclaimers
This publication is designed to provide accurate and authoritative information in regard to the subject matter covered. It is sold or distributed with the understanding that the publisher is not engaged in rendering legal, accounting, or other professional service. If legal advice or other expert assistance is required, the services of a competent professional person should be sought.

—From the Declaration of Principles jointly adopted by the
American Bar Association and a Committee of Publishers and Associations

It is the objective of the American Occupational Therapy Association to be a forum for free expression and interchange of ideas. The opinions expressed by the contributors to this work are their own and not necessarily those of the American Occupational Therapy Association/AOTA Press.

ISBN: 978-1-56900-377-0

Library of Congress Control Number: 2015952878

Cover design by Debra Naylor, Naylor Design, Inc., Washington, DC
Composition and printing by Automated Graphic Systems, Inc., White Plains, MD
Publication management by Steve Pazdan, College Park, MD

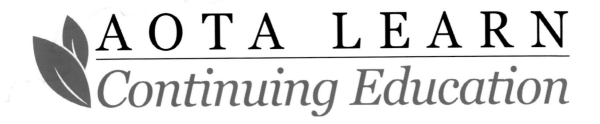

Make Your Learning Count!

Earn Continuing Education Credit (AOTA CEUs/Contact Hours/NBCOT® PDUs) With This Publication.

SPCC Purchase: If you purchased *Traumatic Brain Injury (TBI): Interventions to Support Occupational Performance, Neurorehabilitation in Occupational Therapy Series, Volume 3,* as an AOTA Self-Paced Clinical Course (SPCC), you are enrolled in the continuing education (CE) activity for this publication. After placing your order, you received information via e-mail to complete the CE activity (exam) for this course at AOTA LEARN (**www.aota.org/learn**), AOTA's online center for professional development.

- The CE exam is available on AOTA LEARN to print and review as you read the SPCC.
- When you finish reading, complete the CE exam on AOTA LEARN.
- Successful completion of the exam requires a minimum passing score of 75%. You are provided with two attempts to pass the exam. If required, additional attempts to pass the exam can be purchased by calling 877-404-AOTA (2682).
- With successful course completion, you will instantly receive a certificate and transcript to download or print to verify your learning for state licensure, certification, employers, or your own professional development.

Publication Purchase: If you purchased the textbook only of *Traumatic Brain Injury (TBI): Interventions to Support Occupational Performance, Neurorehabilitation in Occupational Therapy Series, Volume 3,* you can formally recognize your learning from topic experts and receive CE credit. You may enroll for 20 contact hours (2 AOTA CEUs/25 NBCOT PDUs) addressing the learning objectives listed when you order your CE exam.

Ordering is easy! As a purchaser of this publication, order the SPCC exam only (price will reflect exam only):

- Enter **Order #3033OLE** online at **http://store.aota.org**, or by phone at 877-404-AOTA (2682).
- Once you place an order, you will immediately receive an e-mail with your CE exam access information.

There are even more reasons to learn with an AOTA SPCC:

- Upon successful completion of the SPCC exam, earn **nondegree graduate credits from Colorado State University.** Learn more on the next page.
- This publication may be used to support one of the Knowledge Criteria for appropriate **AOTA Board or Specialty Certifications.** Learn more at **aota.org/certification.**
- Learning with AOTA SPCCs provides a **depth of knowledge from experts** that can assist in achieving clinical excellence. Your colleagues and clients benefit when you apply your enhanced expertise.

Discontinuation: When an AOTA SPCC is discontinued, notification is provided at **aota.org/ce** and in AOTA periodicals. SPCC learners have 1 year from first notification of discontinuation to complete the SPCC exam and receive CE credit.

Colorado State University (CSU) Nondegree Graduate Credit

To obtain nondegree graduate credit from CSU, do the following:

Contact CSU at the following address to obtain the most current registration form and tuition rate; refer to *OT 590 735 Workshop: Traumatic Brain Injury (TBI): Interventions to Support Occupational Performance, Neurorehabilitation in Occupational Therapy Series, Volume 3.*

Colorado State University Online
Division of Continuing Education
1040 Campus Delivery
Fort Collins, CO 80523-1040
Attn: Contract Courses

Phone 970-491-5288
E-mail: onlineplus_questions@colostate.edu

You may obtain 2 CSU nondegree graduate credits for completing this course.

The following terms and conditions apply:

1. SPCC learners have 2 years from the time of purchase to complete the AOTA SPCC for optional, nondegree graduate credit from CSU.
2. AOTA allows learners to retake the SPCC exam 2 times. After 2 attempts, learners can purchase additional attempts.
3. When learners pass an exam, AOTA issues them a continuing education certificate of completion and informs CSU of their course grade.
4. Learners who have not obtained a satisfactory grade on their exam and have applied for CSU nondegree graduate credit should contact CSU directly, at the address above, to discuss the timeline for keeping the CSU registration process active.
5. CSU tuition and fees are subject to change.

Contents

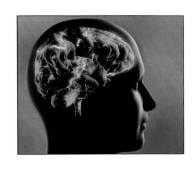

Boxes, Exhibits, Figures, and Tables

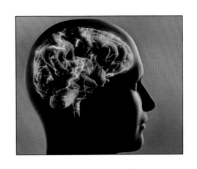

Boxes

Exhibits

Figures

Tables

Foreword

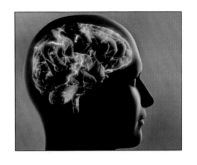

Traumatic brain injury (TBI) is a widespread public health issue that can occur at any age. Approximately every 23 seconds, someone in the United States sustains a TBI. It can be the result of a car or bicycle accident, a fall, a sports or recreational injury, an assault, or military combat. Whatever the cause, TBI can dramatically and suddenly change a person's life—working and juggling multiple responsibilities one day and in a coma or unable to perform basic self-care activities the next.

Even a TBI classified as mild can result in a devastating disruption to every aspect of a person's life, despite the absence of outward signs of disability. Brain injuries can alter personality; disrupt interpersonal relationships; cause emotional changes; shake a person's sense of self-confidence and self-identity; and have a significant impact on the person's roles, lifestyle, and responsibilities, as well as on those of significant others.

The complexity of brain injury, and the rapid and continual growth of knowledge in the field, cannot be overstated. *Traumatic Brain Injury (TBI): Interventions to Support Occupational Performance* provides a comprehensive synthesis of a vast amount of up-to-date literature while simultaneously providing practical information on TBI that will guide occupational therapy practitioners in clinical practice. Topics range from prevention, mechanisms of injury, and advances in neuroscience and plasticity through the continuum of care from coma to acute care to community integration and participation. A chapter on special considerations for TBI in military personnel further complements the compendium of topics. The chapters integrate science and evidence-based literature with practical occupational therapy applications.

Assessment and treatment of clients with TBI present special challenges because each injury and course of recovery is different, and the person may not be fully aware of the changes that have occurred. The use of a hypothetical clinical case interwoven throughout several chapters takes readers through the occupational therapy process across settings, reflecting the multistage nature of recovery. The case of Diane Archer illustrates how occupational therapy assessment and intervention change as the person progresses through the continuum of recovery. A close-up view of the complex issues, challenges, and decisions faced by the therapist, as well as by the client and family, across different points of recovery is demonstrated in a clear and easily readable style through the case format.

This Self-Paced Clinical Course and textbook highlight the significant and unique contributions that occupational therapists make to the health care team in rehabilitation of people with TBI. The holistic perspective of occupational therapy is demonstrated across several chapters that discuss the importance of the context of the person's life, including consideration of lifestyle, family support, psychosocial, emotional, and cultural factors. In addition to analyzing the factors that are interfering with occupational performance, many of the chapters reflect occupational therapy's expertise and unique focus on occupation, meaningful activities, and helping people get back to living their lives.

In summary, *Traumatic Brain Injury (TBI): Interventions to Support Occupational Performance* provides a synthesis of the current state of knowledge needed to successfully manage the full spectrum of issues, challenges, and complex occupational performance needs of people with TBI. Tables on outcome assessments, websites, and extensive references throughout the book provide readers with valuable resources. This publication will serve as a premier guide to effective delivery of evidence-based interventions for people with TBI and will be valuable for occupational therapy practitioners, educators, and students.

—Joan P. Toglia, PhD, OTR/L, FAOTA
Dean, School of Health and Natural Sciences
Professor, Occupational Therapy
Mercy College
Dobbs Ferry, NY

Note From the Series Senior Editor

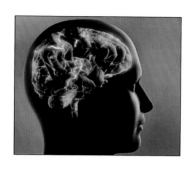

I am grateful to have been asked again by the American Occupational Therapy Association (AOTA) to be senior editor for the Neurorehabilitation Self-Paced Clinical Course (SPCC) and publication series. Titles in this series are intended to serve as textbooks for advanced-level occupational therapy students and to enhance the skills of practicing clinicians. The series also offers excellent continuing education opportunities with the ability to earn AOTA CEUs, contact hours, and National Board for Certification in Occupational Therapy (NBCOT®) professional development units, in addition to nondegree graduate credit through Colorado State University.

Traumatic Brain Injury (TBI): Interventions to Support Occupational Performance is the third in this series to be issued in a new edition; new editions of *Stroke: Interventions to Support Occupational Performance* and *Neurocognitive Disorder (NCD): Interventions to Support Occupational Performance* are already available.

Several factors make the publication of this SPCC and text timely. More than 25% of occupational therapists currently report working with clients with TBI, so the development of advanced skills in this area is important for many occupational therapists (NBCOT, 2013). Since the previous edition of this SPCC was published, there has been increased understanding of both the short- and long-term effects of repeated mild TBI (mTBI). The difficulties experienced by U.S. service members after exposure to blast-related mTBI have highlighted for the general public the aftereffects of TBI and put a spotlight on the limited services available for many people who retain problems in community living long after the acute recovery period.

Similarly, evidence of the important role of functional occupational-based interventions in rehabilitation after TBI has been increasing (Clark-Wilson, Giles, & Baxter, 2014; Giles, 2010; Vanderploeg et al., 2006, 2008)—evidence that presents a challenge and an opportunity for occupational therapists (AOTA, 2013).

This SPCC and publication reflect the significant advances made in our understanding of TBI and its treatment over the past decade and provide readers with the information that they need to be current and evidence based in their interventions. Dr. Kathleen M. Golisz and Dr. Mary Vining Radomski—both recognized experts in TBI rehabilitation—have gathered an outstanding group of researchers and clinicians to write the chapters. We expect that use of this text and SPCC will advance the clinical practice skills of occupational therapists working with this often demanding population.

—Gordon Muir Giles, PhD, OTR/L, FAOTA

References

American Occupational Therapy Association. (2013). Cognition, cognitive rehabilitation, and occupational performance. *American Journal of Occupational Therapy, 67*(Suppl.), S9–S31. http://dx.doi.org/10.5014/ajot.2013.6789

Clark-Wilson, J., Giles, G. M., & Baxter, D. (2014). Revisiting the neurofunctional approach: Conceptualizing the core components for the rehabilitation of everyday living skills. *Brain Injury, 28,* 1646–1656. http://dx.doi.org/10.3109/02699052.2014.946449

Giles, G. M. (2010). Cognitive versus functional approaches to rehabilitation after traumatic brain injury: Commentary on a randomized controlled trial. *American Journal of Occupational Therapy, 64,* 182–185. http://dx.doi.org/10.5014/ajot.64.1.182

National Board for Certification in Occupational Therapy. (2013). *2012 practice analysis of the Occupational Therapist Registered: Executive summary.* Gaithersburg, MD: Author.

Vanderploeg, R. D., Collins, R. C., Sigford, B. J., Date, E., Schwab, K., & Warden, D.; Defense and Veterans Brain Injury Center Veterans Health Administration, Study Planning Group. (2006). Practical and theoretical considerations in designing rehabilitation trials: The DVBIC cognitive–didactic versus functional–experiential treatment study experience. *Journal of Head Trauma Rehabilitation, 21,* 179–193.

Vanderploeg, R. D., Schwab, K., Walker, W. C., Fraser, J. A., Sigford, B. J., Date, E. S., . . . Warden, D. L.; Defense and Veterans Brain Injury Center Study Group. (2008). Rehabilitation of traumatic brain injury in active duty military personnel and veterans: Defense and Veterans Brain Injury Center randomized controlled trial of two rehabilitation approaches. *Archives of Physical Medicine and Rehabilitation, 89,* 2227–2238. http://dx.doi.org/10.1016/j.apmr.2008.06.015

Acknowledgments

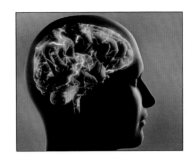

We would like to thank the authors who contributed to this new edition of the Self-Paced Clinical Course and publication *Traumatic Brain Injury (TBI): Interventions to Support Occupational Performance,* some of whom worked on the previous edition and some of whom have provided new chapters for this book. Their work, expertise, and writing in the area of rehabilitation with people with TBI contribute to the knowledge and practice of occupational therapy colleagues and students.

We thank our most memorable teachers: our patients with TBI and their families. They instilled curiosity to research the literature and encouraged us to think outside of the box, listen empathetically, and collaborate with them to achieve quality of life as they worked to reengage in their meaningful occupations.

We thank Gordon Muir Giles, our series senior editor, who focused the work and encouraged the process, and Sarah Hertfelder, who saw this project through to the end even though she officially retired during its production. We hope she is enjoying new meaningful occupations in this life transition. Our thanks also to the editorial staff at AOTA Press who put the finishing touches on the work.

Kathleen would like to express her gratitude to Mary Vining Radomski, who joined this project, giving Kathleen the gift of time to focus on her role as a daughter to aging parents with health challenges.

**—Kathleen M. Golisz, OTD, OTR/L, and
Mary Vining Radomski, PhD, OTR/L, FAOTA**

We appreciate the time and thoughtful comments of our reviewers, who helped us reflect on and improve our work:

- **Michele Darger, MOTR/L, CBIS**
  Lead Occupational Therapist
  Inpatient Rehabilitation/Brain Recovery Team
  Courage Kenny Rehabilitation Institute
  Abbott Northwestern Hospital
  Minneapolis

- **Leslie Davidson, PhD, OT/L, FAOTA**
  Director of Occupational Therapy
  Shenandoah University
  Winchester, VA

- **Clare Giuffrida, PhD, OTR/L, FAOTA**
  Occupational Therapist and Clinical Assistant Professor
  Department of Physical Medicine and Rehabilitation
  College of Medicine
  Rush University
  Chicago

About the Editors and Authors

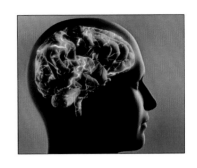

About the Volume Editors

Kathleen M. Golisz, OTD, OTR/L, is the associate dean for the Mercy College School of Health and Natural Sciences in Dobbs Ferry, New York, and a professor in the Occupational Therapy Graduate Program. Dr. Golisz has extensive experience working with adults with TBI in rehabilitation and community settings. She has presented lectures and workshops on the topics of occupational therapy with 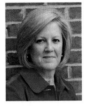 clients with brain trauma and cognitive rehabilitation both nationally and internationally. Dr. Golisz authored *Occupational Therapy Practice Guidelines for Adults With Traumatic Brain Injury* (American Occupational Therapy Association, 2009), which was included in the National Guideline Clearinghouse of the Agency for Healthcare Research and Quality. In 2013, she coauthored, with Joan P. Toglia, a chapter for the second edition of *Brain Injury Medicine: Principles and Practice* titled "Therapy for Activities of Daily Living: Theoretical and Practical Perspectives." She has also coauthored the cognitive rehabilitation chapter in the past three editions of *Willard and Spackman's Occupational Therapy.*

Mary Vining Radomski, PhD, OTR/L, FAOTA, is an occupational therapist and clinical scientist at the Courage Kenny Research Center in Minneapolis. She received her BS in occupational therapy and her MA and PhD in educational psychology from the University of Minnesota. Her clinical work and writing of the past 2 decades have 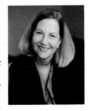 centered on cognitive assessment and intervention for adults with mild cognitive impairment. These interests inform her two primary programs of research: cognitive assessment and treatment of soldiers with mTBI and assessment and treatment of people with cognitive dysfunction associated with treatment for cancer. Between 2009 and 2013, she was an Oak Ridge Institute for Science and Education

Fellow with the Rehabilitation and Reintegration Division (Health Policy and Services, Army Medical Department, Office of the Surgeon General) and was involved in supporting the development and implementation of evidence-based guidance for military occupational and physical therapists specific to soldiers with mTBI. She is currently funded by the U.S. Army Medical Research and Materiel Command as part of an interdisciplinary military–civilian research team that is developing a functional assessment to inform return to duty after concussion and as principal investigator of a study examining the impact of training soldiers to use implementation intentions as part of cognitive rehabilitation. Along with Catherine A. Trombly Latham, she has coedited three editions of *Occupational Therapy for Physical Dysfunction*.

About the Series Senior Editor

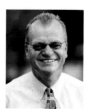

Gordon Muir Giles, PhD, OTR/L, FAOTA, was senior occupational therapist at the first program in the world for behavior disorder after brain injury. He was responsible for developing the clinical program in the first publicly funded neurobehavioral program in the western United States in 1993. Professor Giles is clinically responsible for a 65-bed neurobehavioral program in Fremont, California, and a 165-bed program in Sunnyvale for people whose psychiatric condition complicates the management of their medical condition. In the early 1990s, Professor Giles (in association with Jo Clark-Wilson) developed the Neurofunctional Approach to brain injury rehabilitation, which was demonstrated to be effective in the largest randomized comparison trial of brain injury rehabilitation ever conducted. The Neurofunctional Approach is the only functional approach shown to be effective in people who have had a TBI over 10 years previously. His most recent publications and research interests are centered on the role of relationships and on nonaversive intervention in rehabilitation of people with brain injury and behavior disorder. In addition to his clinical responsibilities, Professor Giles teaches at Samuel Merritt University, a health sciences university located in Oakland, California.

About the Authors

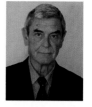

Fred Feuchter, PhD, received his doctorate in human anatomy from the University of Iowa School of Medicine in 1979. He has held several faculty positions in anatomy, including postdoctoral fellow at the University of Washington School of Medicine (1979–1982), assistant professor of anatomy at the University of New Mexico School of Medicine (1982–1989), director of morphological programs at the University of New Mexico Allied Health Division (1989–1994), and visiting associate professor of anatomy at the University of California, San Francisco, School of Medicine (1995–2005). He has been at Samuel Merritt University in Oakland, California, since 1994, where he currently serves as professor and chair of the basic sciences department. He has served two terms as president of the faculty organization. Professor Feuchter teaches human anatomy and physiology and functional neurosciences and directs students in research projects. His current research interests include development of interactive media for use in his courses and three-dimensional computer reconstruction of parts of the human brain and spinal cord.

Christina C. Lewis, PhD, received her doctorate in physiology from Colorado State University in 2002. Her doctoral research investigated the mechanisms of airway remodeling in asthma and was conducted at National Jewish Medical and Research Center in Denver. Dr. Lewis conducted her postdoctoral fellowship at the Lung Biology Center at the University of California, San Francisco, where her 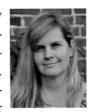 work focused on using gene expression studies to characterize molecular signatures associated with multiple mouse models of lung disease. Dr. Lewis's current research seeks to understand how airway epithelial biology mediates and regulates the susceptibility and pathogenesis of asthma. Her research has used both human disease studies and murine model systems of asthma and has used genomic approaches to describe the underlying cellular and molecular events of the inflammatory process in allergic airway disease. Previously, she taught courses in anatomy, physiology, genetics and genomics, cellular physiology, and pathology at Earlham College, Richmond, Indiana; the University of California, San Francisco; and the University of California, Berkeley. She is currently on the faculty at Samuel Merritt University in Oakland, California, where she teaches anatomy, physiology, and pathophysiology in the nurse anesthesia, occupational therapy, and physician assistant programs.

Robin McNeny, OTR/L, graduated from Virginia Commonwealth University (VCU) in Richmond, Virginia, in 1977 with a degree in occupational therapy. When she began her career at the VCU Health System, then the Medical College of Virginia Hospitals, brain injury rehabilitation was in its infancy, with few people surviving severe trauma to the brain. In the late 1970s, progress in emergency medicine, particularly 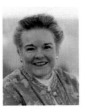 the management of intracranial pressure, coupled with improved management of postinjury complications, resulted in an increased number of survivors of severe TBI. The Medical College of Virginia was on the cutting edge of this life-saving research. McNeny worked with her first patient with a severe brain injury in 1978 and subsequently found herself on the ground floor of program development for and service provision to survivors of severe head trauma in need of rehabilitation. McNeny was selected as the occupational therapist to serve on the interdisciplinary team of professionals, led by physiatrist Dr. Henry Stonnington, who established the first comprehensive brain injury rehabilitation program in Richmond. The Brain Injury Rehab Unit at the Medical College of Virginia Hospitals soon expanded from the initial 8 beds to 15 beds to meet the burgeoning demand for brain injury rehabilitation services. In addition to her clinical practice in brain injury rehabilitation, McNeny served for 25 years on the planning committee for the VCU Brain Injury Conference held annually in Williamsburg. The Williamsburg Conference was the first interdisciplinary conference on brain injury rehabilitation in the United States and is still held every summer. She has contributed chapters to several texts on brain injury rehabilitation; authored articles for scholarly, peer-reviewed journals; mentored new occupational therapists in the practice of brain injury rehabilitation; lectured on brain injury rehabilitation at the VCU School of Occupational Therapy and at conferences; provided clinical education to countless occupational therapy students; and engaged in considerable program development. McNeny is now largely retired from clinical practice. She was recognized in 2014 by her alma mater with its Making a Difference Alumni Award.

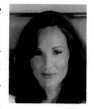

M. Tracy Morrison, OTD, OTR/L, is the chairperson of the program in occupational therapy at Arkansas State University. Dr. Morrison previously served as a faculty member at Washington University School of Medicine and the University of Kansas Medical Center. Dr. Morrison's research focuses on the measurement of executive processing and the relationship between executive dysfunction and occupational performance. Dr. Morrison's doctoral and postdoctoral training took place at Washington University School of Medicine. She currently leads three research studies focused on the recovery of executive abilities after brain injury.

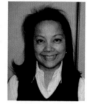

Marianne H. Mortera, PhD, OTR/L, received her MA and PhD in occupational therapy from New York University. She is conducting research examining the determinants of return to productivity among Operation Enduring Freedom and Operation Iraqi Freedom veterans who have sustained mTBI with concomitant PTSD at the James J. Peters Veterans Affairs Medical Center in the Bronx, New York. She has also developed and initially tested the Mortera Cognitive Screening Measure and the Cognitive Screen for Grooming. As an occupational therapy faculty member in entry-level and postprofessional programs for 26 years, she has taught courses in neuroscience, neurorehabilitation, physical disabilities, medical conditions, the development of frames of reference, theory, research methods and proposal writing, and applied scientific inquiry at New York University, Long Island University, Columbia University, Mercy College (Dobbs Ferry, New York), and A. T. Still University (Kirksville, Missouri). She has also presented extensively on cognitive assessment and the development and testing of the Structured Functional Cognitive Assessment method.

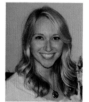

Jenny Owens, OTD, OTR/L, has worked with veterans with mTBI and PTSD since 2007, when awareness of this growing population was heightened among military and medical communities. Through her experience working at the Warrior Resiliency and Recovery Center at Fort Campbell, Kentucky, she developed an expertise in the treatment of cognitive, visual, and psychosocial sequelae of mTBI. Dr. Owens instituted functionally relevant evaluation and treatment protocols geared toward identifying and treating the subtle but functionally limiting cognitive and visual deficits associated with mTBI. With the input of her soldier patients, she developed community-based interventions to simulate the challenges of Army life (such as convoy operations and scouting missions) with the goal of assisting service members in meeting their goal of returning to duty. In doing so, she observed a gap in the system concerning the method used to determine a service member's readiness to return to duty. She, along with members of a multidisciplinary team, developed Fort Campbell's Military Functional Assessment Program, the first of its kind in the nation, to collectively assess service members' ability to perform key job requirements before returning them to the front lines. In 2013, Dr. Owens shifted her focus from clinical work to engage in a research project exploring cognitive rehabilitation for executive dysfunction among a military mTBI population. Additionally, she and her husband founded and currently direct a nonprofit organization, REBOOT Combat Recovery, that provides free face-to-face programs to help service members and their families heal from the spiritual wounds of war.

Steven Wheeler, PhD, OTR/L, CBIS, is associate professor of occupational therapy at the West Virginia University School of Medicine and a Certified Brain Injury Specialist. Dr. Wheeler has published and presented on community reentry issues after TBI both nationally and internationally. He received his occupational therapy training at the University of Western Ontario and his PhD 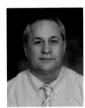 in health-related sciences with a specialty in occupational therapy from Virginia Commonwealth University. His dissertation topic was community participation and life satisfaction after intensive community-based rehabilitation using a Life Skills Training approach. Dr. Wheeler serves as a consultant with NeuroRestorative, a community-based brain injury rehabilitation program in Ashland, Lexington, and Louisville, Kentucky. He is also a Governor's Appointee on the West Virginia TBI/SCI Rehabilitation Fund Board.

Introduction

Kathleen M. Golisz, OTD, OTR/L, and
Mary Vining Radomski, PhD, OTR/L, FAOTA

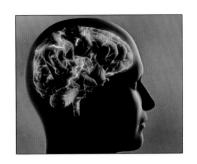

Overall Learning Objectives

After completing this Self-Paced Clinical Course (SPCC) and reading this publication, learners and readers will be able to

- Identify prevention strategies to reduce the risk of **traumatic brain injury** (TBI);
- Explain the pathophysiology of primary and secondary brain injuries;
- Discuss the continuum of care and natural recovery from TBI;
- Describe the clinical presentation of people with TBI across the continuum of care;
- Identify assessments to evaluate physical, cognitive, and psychosocial **impairments** and their functional implications for clients with TBI;
- Describe evidence-based occupational therapy interventions for people with TBI across the continuum of care;
- Identify special considerations for evaluating and treating military personnel who experience TBI;
- Identify methods for measuring recovery from TBI; and
- Appreciate the challenges experienced by family members of people with TBI and determine how to address their needs as part of a comprehensive occupational therapy intervention plan.

About This Work

This work is the second edition of the SPCC on traumatic brain injury (TBI) first published in 2006 by the American Occupational Therapy Association (AOTA; Golisz, 2006). Even a large project such as this one is selective, and not every topic can be covered. This highly successful SPCC has benefited from extensive user feedback but retains many of the innovative features that made the first edition so successful.

This SPCC on TBI is also being produced as a text. Both SPCC and text are designed for advanced-level students or practicing occupational therapists who want to further explore this important area of competence. For licensed occupational therapists, it can be used to provide either continuing education units or college credit. This text on TBI is part of a series of works on neurorehabilitation produced by AOTA Press and AOTA CE with Gordon Muir Giles as senior editor. Texts in the series also include *Neurocognitive Disorder (NCD)* and *Stroke*.

It is hard to imagine a population more in need of the knowledge and skills of occupational therapists than people with TBI. The complex and interrelated physical (Walker & Pickett, 2007), cognitive (Wortzel & Arciniegas, 2012), and psychiatric and emotional (Schwarzbold et al., 2008) sequelae of TBI that begin at point of injury have the potential to influence the client's capacities, activities, relationships, and roles (Rabinowitz & Levin, 2014) for months and years to come (Bazarian, Cernak, Noble-Haeusslein, Potolicchio, & Temkin, 2009). Beginning with acute medical care and through inpatient, outpatient, home, and community settings, expert occupational therapists enable clients with TBI to live out their full potential.

The superordinate goal of this work is to ensure that occupational therapists have the requisite high level of expertise to both meet the needs of the population with TBI and provide leadership toward function-oriented **rehabilitation** for the field. To that end, chapters were written by practicing clinicians, educators, and researchers, and the topics are intended to reflect the leading edge of current clinical practice and theory in occupational therapy.

This work has two main sections. Section I comprises Chapters 1, 2, and 3, which provide the core concepts and theoretical foundations that inform occupational therapy across the continuum of recovery and reintegration for people with TBI. In Chapter 1, Kathleen M. Golisz outlines key concepts related to incidence, classification, and pathology of TBI along with relevant contextual issues across the recovery trajectory; in Chapter 2, Fred Feuchter, Gordon Muir Giles, and Christina C. Lewis summarize neuroanatomy relative to TBI; and in Chapter 3, Gordon Muir Giles and M. Tracy Morrison discuss **cognition**, cognitive assessment, and rehabilitation as related to TBI. Information in these chapters will be particularly valuable to those who are looking to further their knowledge in one particular facet of TBI rehabilitation or those who are looking for the foundational knowledge necessary to work with clients with TBI.

The five chapters in Section II provide detailed discussions of occupational therapy assessment and intervention at each phase of the recovery, rehabilitation, and community and social reintegration continuum. In Chapter 4, Kathleen M. Golisz introduces the case of hypothetical client Diane Archer, which is further developed in Chapters 5, 6, and 7. The case emphasizes the personal, social, and medical contexts of occupational therapy across the rehabilitation and recovery continuum to facilitate practice-relevant learning. However, it is not intended to replicate specific details of the typical medical record.

In Chapter 5, Robin McNeny presents evidence-based approaches to early rehabilitation during and after **coma.** In Chapter 6, Marianne H. Mortera examines occupational therapy during acute, inpatient, and subacute rehabilitation phases of recovery, and in Chapter 7, Steven Wheeler extends that explication into the community-level phase, focusing on resumption of work, **leisure,** and social roles.

In Chapter 8, Jenny Owens discusses how occupational therapists may adapt these approaches to meet the unique needs of service members with TBI. Finally, just like the first two volumes in this series, this third and final volume concludes with a detailed glossary that corresponds to boldfaced terms in the text, as well as comprehensive subject and citation indexes.

Just as in the first edition, we welcome feedback so as to improve future editions of this work.

References

Bazarian, J. J., Cernak, I., Noble-Haeusslein, L., Potolicchio, S., & Temkin, N. (2009). Long-term neurologic outcomes after traumatic brain injury. *Journal of Head Trauma Rehabilitation, 24,* 439–451. http//dx.doi.org/10.1097/HTR.0b013e3181c15600

Golisz, K. M. (Ed.). (2006). *Neurorehabilitation of the client with traumatic brain injury* (Neurorehabilitation Self-Paced Clinical Course Series). Bethesda, MD: American Occupational Therapy Association.

Rabinowitz, A. R., & Levin, H. S. (2014). Cognitive sequelae of traumatic brain injury. *Psychiatric Clinics of North America, 37,* 1–11. http//dx.doi.org/10.1016/j.psc.2013.11.004

Schwarzbold, M., Diaz, A., Martins, E. T., Rufino, A., Amante, L. N., Thais, M. E., . . . Walz, R. (2008). Psychiatric disorders and traumatic brain injury. *Neuropsychiatric Disease and Treatment, 4,* 797–816.

Walker, W. C., & Pickett, T. C. (2007). Motor impairment after severe traumatic brain injury: A longitudinal multicenter study. *Journal of Rehabilitation Research and Development, 44,* 975–982. http//dx.doi.org/10.1682/JRRD.2006.12.0158

Wortzel, H. S., & Arciniegas, D. B. (2012). Treatment of post-traumatic cognitive impairments. *Current Treatment Options in Neurology, 14,* 493–508. http//dx.doi.org/10.1007/s11940-012-0193-6

Section I: Core Concepts

CHAPTER 1
Overview

Kathleen M. Golisz, OTD, OTR/L

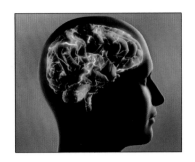

Learning Objectives

After completion of this chapter, readers will be able to
- Identify the risk factors for **traumatic brain injury** (TBI);
- Identify prevention strategies to decrease the incidence of TBI;
- Differentiate the different types of TBI;
- Recognize the clinical significance of underlying brain pathology caused by TBI; and
- Identify appropriate methods for measuring recovery from TBI.

Incidence and Definition of *Traumatic Brain Injury*

Each year, approximately 1.7 million people in the United States sustain a traumatic brain injury (TBI), with 275,000 people requiring hospitalization and approximately 1.4 million people being released from the emergency department (ED) with a diagnosis of mild TBI (mTBI; Faul, Xu, Wald, & Coronado, 2010). Approximately 52,000 people annually die as a result of TBI, representing approximately one-third of all injury-related deaths in the United States. Centers for Disease Control and Prevention (CDC) statistics have shown that TBI-related deaths decreased 8.2% in the overall population between 1997 and 2007 (Coronado et al., 2011). Death rates for older adults (i.e., adults ages 75 or older), however, increased, typically as a result of falls, continuing to make TBI a major public health issue (Coronado et al., 2011). As the Baby Boomers enter this age category, the TBI-related death rate for older adults, who typically have poorer outcomes from TBI, may continue to increase (Hukkelhoven et al., 2003).

Approximately 1% to 2% of the U.S. civilian population, or 3.2 to 5.3 million people, are estimated to be living with a long-term disability (e.g., loss of physical or mental function) as a result of TBI (Coronado et al., 2011; Selassie et al., 2008;

Key Words

- brain concussion
- classification
- coma
- complications
- etiology
- occupational therapy
- outcome measures
- pathology
- prevention
- rehabilitation
- risk factors
- traumatic brain injury

Zaloshnja, Miller, Langlois, & Selassie, 2008). This estimate does not include the more than 244,000 military personnel diagnosed with TBI (Defense and Veterans Brain Injury Center, 2012) or the unknown number of people who sustained TBIs and were not seen in EDs or hospitalized.

The term *TBI* encompasses a wide spectrum of causes of brain damage with a variety of clinical presentations. The International and Interagency Initiative Toward Common Data Elements for Research on Traumatic Brain Injury and Psychological Health (Menon, Schwab, Wright, & Maas, 2010) has defined *TBI* as "an alteration in brain function, or other evidence of brain pathology, caused by an external force" (p. 1637). This definition has also been accepted by the Brain Injury Association of America (n.d.).

The long-term **impairments** and disabilities associated with living with TBI are serious, and the full costs, both human and economic, are difficult to measure. In 2010, the direct costs (i.e., acute and **rehabilitation** medical care) and indirect or socioeconomic costs (i.e., loss of productivity) of TBI were estimated to be more than $76.5 billion annually (Coronado, McGuire, Faul, Sugerman, & Pearson, 2012). Early and aggressive treatment of people with TBI is cost-effective and results in better outcomes regardless of the person's age (Whitmore et al., 2012).

The Traumatic Brain Injury Model Systems National Data and Statistical Center (2010), established in 1987 with funding from the National Institute on Disability and Rehabilitation Research, has as its central mission the goal to improve care and outcomes for people with TBI. The data generated by the 16 TBI Model Systems program have helped build both research and practice guidelines for the provision of care to clients with TBI and their families. Data from both the current and the past TBI Model Systems program centers have contributed to a national database of people with TBI that provides information on the demographics of those who have sustained TBI and has enabled long-term follow-up on their recovery.

Primary Prevention Programs

Nationally, a greater emphasis has been placed on education-based prevention programs focused on decreasing the incidence of TBI resulting from several specific causes. The CDC Heads Up program (CDC, 2007) focuses on the prevention of **concussion** in sports. The program provides guidelines to assist coaches in identifying athletes who may be experiencing concussive symptoms and recommends actions to take to reduce athletes' potential for repeat injury or second-impact syndrome (Herring et al., 2011; McCrory, Davis, & Makdissi, 2012). Between 2009 and 2013, all 50 U.S. states enacted return-to-play laws to protect young athletes and aid their recovery from concussions (National Conference of State Legislatures, 2014). These laws, often named after a young athlete who sustained a brain injury in a sport, require that an athlete receive clearance from a medical professional before returning to play. Modification to some sporting equipment (e.g., helmets or protective headgear for sports such as cycling, baseball, hockey, skiing, horseback riding, skateboarding) and to the actions athletes engage in during their sport (e.g., decreased use of head shots in soccer) may also lead to decreased rates of sports-related TBI.

Prevention initiatives focused on the older population, such as the CDC's (2012) Help Seniors Live Better Longer: Prevent Brain Injury, focus on reducing falls, the most common cause of TBI in older adults. The CDC has compiled a review of effective fall interventions (e.g., education and exercise) that addresses the various factors contributing to falls among older adults (e.g., medications, vision changes, home hazards; National Center for Injury Prevention and Control, 2008). Occupational therapists practicing in community settings should incorporate these prevention strategies into their work with the older population.

Other prevention approaches address motor vehicle–related TBIs through legislative actions such as motorcycle helmet laws (now active in 19 states for all riders and in 28 states for riders younger than ages 17–20 years). The National Highway Traffic Safety Administration (NHTSA; Goodwin et al., 2013) has rated motorcycle helmet laws as the most effective countermeasure to reduce crash-related brain injuries by 41% to 69% (Liu et al., 2008). Technological advances in the design of motor vehicles, such as passive-restraint seat belts and airbags, have decreased the incidence of TBI, with the greatest protection offered by the combined use of seat belts and airbags (Huber, Lee, Yang, & King, 2005; Stewart, Girotti, Nikore, & Williamson, 2003; Williams & Croce, 2009; Williams et al., 2008). The first generation of airbags from the late 1990s underwent redesign to modify the speed at which they deploy to reduce airbag-related injuries. Airbags, however, appear to have decreased ability to protect drivers of shorter stature who sit closer to the steering wheel, thus limiting the space in which the airbag can deploy (Cunningham, Brown, Gradwell, & Nee, 2000). As public health professionals continue to design and implement evidence-based intervention programs aimed at reducing preventable TBIs, the burden of caring for people with TBI in the United States should lessen (Coronado, Thurman, Greenspan, & Weissman, 2009).

Causes of and Risk Factors for Traumatic Brain Injury

The lack of a unified surveillance system for TBI in the United States creates a challenge in identifying the incidence and causes of TBI in the population (Coronado et al., 2011; see Figure 1.1). Older adults and children ages 15 to 19 years account for the highest incidence of hospitalization for TBI resulting from falls and motor vehicle crashes, respectively (Coronado et al., 2012). The leading cause of TBI-related deaths is violence involving firearms, whether the injury is attributable to homicide, suicide, or unintentional injury. Between 1997 and 2007, TBI resulting from firearm violence decreased by 1% (from 7.2% to 6.2%; Coronado et al., 2012). People at risk for intentional TBI from gunshot wounds and blunt trauma from assault are typically male, minority (i.e., Black, Hispanic, other non-White ethnicity), young (i.e., ages 15–24 years), and low income (Hanks et al., 2003). The penetrating brain injuries associated with intentional TBI have higher rates of death and severe injury (Kazim, Shamim, Tahir, Enam, & Waheed, 2011).

Over the past 2 decades, a combination of prevention awareness and technological changes, such as increased seat belt and child safety seat use, increased number of vehicles equipped with airbags, and decreased incidence of driving while intoxicated, has led to a steady decrease in TBI-associated deaths resulting from vehicle crashes (Coronado et al., 2011). Yet motor vehicle–related TBIs remain the second leading cause of TBI-related deaths. The popularity of certain passenger vehicles appears to have caused a shift in the type and severity of injuries observed in motor vehicle crashes (Braitman, Ferguson, & Elharam, 2007; Trowbridge, McKay, & Maio, 2007). A retrospective

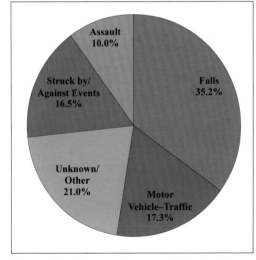

Figure 1.1. Causes of traumatic brain injury.

Source. From *Traumatic Brain Injury in the United States: Emergency Department Visits, Hospitalizations, and Deaths 2002–2006* (p. 18), by M. Faul, L. Xu, M. M. Wald, & V. G. Coronado, 2010, Atlanta: Centers for Disease Control and Prevention, National Center for Injury Prevention and Control. In the public domain.

study of more than 400 people admitted to the medical center of the University of Medicine and Dentistry of New Jersey (Siegel et al., 2001) showed that for both front- and side-impact crashes between sedans and sport utility vehicles, vans, or light trucks, the pattern of injury changed: Thorax and intrathoracic organ injuries increased, and TBI increased in severity. Despite airbag deployment and seat belt use, incidence of severe TBI rose, as did the incidence of facial lacerations. These injuries appeared to be a result of the greater mass, hood height, and width of sport utility vehicles, vans, and light trucks compared with sedans.

Overall, TBI-related deaths have continued to decrease except for deaths resulting from falls, which are predicted to continue to increase because of the demographic age-related shift in the U.S. population (Coronado et al., 2012). Falls are the leading cause of ED visits and TBI-associated death and disability in older adults (Coronado et al., 2012). Physiological changes associated with aging, use of certain medications, and impaired balance and lower-extremity function lead to a greater risk of TBI in people older than age 65 (Faul, Xu, Wald, & Coronado, 2010).

Sports- and recreation-related TBIs have been estimated at 1.6 million to 3.8 million per year in the United States, with the highest incidence in children and young adults ages 10 to 19. TBI-related visits to EDs were highest among teens engaged in sports such as football, basketball, soccer, and baseball or softball. Bicycling-related TBIs were highest in all age groups (Coronado et al., 2012). Among professional athletes who participate in contact sports, repetitive concussions can result in **chronic traumatic encephalopathy** (CTE; see Box 1.1) with symptoms

---

Box 1.1. Chronic Traumatic Encephalopathy

Chronic traumatic encephalopathy (CTE; previously termed *punch-drunk syndrome* and *dementia pugilistica*) can be definitively diagnosed only postmortem (Martland, 1928; Millspaugh, 1937). CTE has been reported to affect some people exposed to repeated mild traumatic brain injury (mTBI), *concussion* (defined as a traumatically induced transient disturbance of brain function), or even repetitive subconcussive blows to the head, especially in the context of competitive sports (e.g., football, wrestling, soccer, boxing, basketball, hockey) and military combat (Baugh, Robbins, Stern, & McKee, 2014; Baugh et al., 2012; Goldstein et al., 2012; Lehman, Hein, Baron, & Gersic, 2012; McCrory et al., 2009; McCrory, Zazryn, & Cameron, 2007). For example, Lehman et al. (2012) examined mortality and morbidity data for 3,439 retired National Football League players who had played for five pension-credited seasons between 1959 and 1988. Their neurodegenerative mortality rate was 3 times higher than that of the general U.S. population, and when Alzheimer's disease and amyotrophic lateral sclerosis were considered, the rate was 4 times higher.

Neuropathologically, CTE is characterized by accumulation of hyperphosphorylated τ and transactive response DNA-binding protein 43; enlargement of the **lateral** and **third ventricles;** and neuronal loss, anterior cavum septi pellucidi and posterior fenestrations, and damage to other parts of the brain, including the hippocampus and the medial temporal cortex (Baugh et al., 2012). CTE is distinct from postconcussive symptoms, and symptom onset is typically years or decades after the repetitive trauma believed to cause CTE (Baugh et al., 2014). Clinically, CTE is characterized by disturbances in **mood,** including irritability, **anxiety,** depression, and hopelessness and suicidality; disturbances in behavior, including impulsivity, poor impulse control, disinhibition, and aggression; altered cognitive processing severe enough in some cases to warrant a diagnosis of major neurocognitive disorder; and motor dysfunction, including Parkinsonism, **ataxia** and **dysarthria,** and balance and gait disturbances. Although repetitive blows to the head are recognized as being necessary for CTE, not all people exposed to repetitive head injury develop CTE, which suggests that other factors play a role. Apolipoprotein e4 has been associated with severity of cognitive impairment in professional boxers (Jordan et al., 1997) and with worse outcome after moderate to severe TBI (Chiang, Chang, & Hu, 2003; Zhou et al., 2008), but evidence for an association of apolipoprotein e4 with CTE is currently inconclusive (Baugh et al., 2012; Gavett, Stern, & McKee, 2011). Most studies of CTE are limited to case reports, and much more research is needed to fully understand the nature of CTE (Gavett et al., 2011; Stern et al., 2013).

of **major neurocognitive disorder** (i.e., dementia) and increased risk of depression and suicide (Saulle & Greenwald, 2012).

Risk factors for TBI are complex and interdependent. Age-related physiological changes and comorbidities place older adults at greater risk for TBI, specifically fall-related TBI (Coronado, Thomas, Sattin, & Johnson, 2005). Men consistently sustain more TBIs than women do and are more likely than women to die from a TBI. This higher incidence has been attributed to risk-taking behavior, participation in more contact sports, and overall higher rates of general injury (Coronado et al., 2012). Race and ethnicity affect clinical outcomes, with Black and Hispanic males having a higher death rate and decreased likelihood of discharge to a rehabilitation facility (Bowman, Martin, Sharar, & Zimmerman, 2007). Approximately 44% of TBI events involve alcohol use by either the person causing the injury or the person sustaining the injury (Traumatic Brain Injury Model Systems National Data and Statistical Center, 2010).

Nonintentional TBIs can occur as a result of a variety of normal daily activities. Although TBI can occur in almost any work setting, some work environments pose a greater risk (e.g., construction, transportation, and agriculture industries; Tiesman, Konda, & Bell, 2011). Although data connecting the increased use of mobile communication devices while driving to incidence of TBI have not been studied to date, the overall rise of distracted driving is of public concern. Seventy-one percent of teens and young adults admit to composing and sending texts while driving, and 78% report having read text messages while driving (NHTSA, 2014). In motor vehicle crashes, 18% of fatalities are related to distracted driving (NHTSA, 2014). The benefits are still to be determined of public awareness campaigns and legislation related to distracted driving for the reduction of TBI injuries and fatalities resulting from motor vehicle crashes.

> Age-related physiological changes and comorbidities place older adults at greater risk for TBI, specifically fall-related TBI.

Classification of Injuries

TBI is typically classified as either closed or open penetrating. *Closed TBIs* are caused by the rapid oscillating movement of the brain within the skull during falls or motor vehicle accidents; the movement results in bruised and torn brain tissue and blood vessels. *Open penetrating TBIs* are caused by bullets or other objects piercing the brain or by compound or depressed skull fractures in which the dura mater is torn and the brain substance is exposed (Yokobori & Bullock, 2012). Penetrating injuries are associated with high rates of certain medical complications, especially in the pulmonary and central nervous systems (Long, 2012).

A brain injury may be temporally classified as primary or secondary. *Primary brain injury* occurs at the time of injury and may present as a **focal injury** or as a **coup–contrecoup injury;** it involves visible bruising of the brain tissue, typically at the **frontal** and **temporal lobes** because of the irregular interior skull features in these areas (Frosch, Anthony, & DeGirolami, 2005; Yokobori & Bullock, 2012). For example, acceleration injuries common in motor vehicle accidents can result in bruising as the brain moves violently back and forth across the irregular surfaces within the skull. Contrecoup bruising can occur in an opposite pole (e.g., **occipital lobe**), but these bruises are less severe because of the smoother surface of the skull in these areas. ***Diffuse axonal injuries*** are caused by straining and shearing of **axons** throughout the **white matter** of the brain and are accompanied by **petechial hemorrhages** (Johnson, Stewart, & Smith, 2012; Yokobori & Bullock, 2012). *Secondary brain injuries* (e.g., brain herniation, **anoxia,** local infarcts) occur after the initial injury and result from the cascading series of events that occur when the brain responds to the initial injury. Secondary injuries can lead to even greater insult to the brain and brain function (Kochanek, Clark, & Jenkins, 2012).

Classification of TBI severity as *mild, moderate,* or *severe* requires the combination of several factors and is not an exact science. Table 1.1 provides an overview of the guidelines used to classify injury severity. Classifications of injury severity can have significant variability in the clinical presentation within these categories because the actual brain injury may be combined with secondary brain injury and other bodily injuries (Sherer, Struchen, Yablon, Wang, & Nick, 2008). The initial **Glasgow Coma Scale** (GCS; Teasdale & Jennett, 1976) score (which consists of initiation of eye opening, best verbal response, and best motor response), the duration of **coma,** the length of *posttraumatic amnesia* (PTA; the period from the commencement of coma until reliable, consistent, and accurate ongoing **memory** returns), and the presence of abnormal findings on neuroimaging are used to classify injuries as *mild, moderate,* or *severe.*

There is lack of consistency in which GCS score is used to rate severity of injury. Commonly used scores are GCS on admission to the ED, lowest GCS in the first 24 hours, and highest GCS in the first 24 hours (Sherer et al., 2008), all of which have been found to be equally as accurate in predicting mortality (Settervall, de Sousa, & Fürbringer e Silva, 2011). Some authors have suggested that only a GCS score of 15 should be considered mild, and scores of 13 and 14 should be considered moderate (Culotta, Sementilli, Gerold, & Watts, 1996; Gómez, Lobato, Ortega, & De La Cruz, 1996). Guidelines for classification of TBI as *mild, moderate,* or *severe* also vary on the basis of the length of time the person is unconscious (American Psychiatric Association [APA], 2013; Andriessen et al., 2011; Malec et al., 2007; Posner, Saper, Schiff, & Plum, 2007), as well as on the length of coma or time to follow commands. GCS and PTA are now the predominant indicators of severity. Similarly, current definitions of mTBI have replaced the idea of duration of loss of **consciousness** as the sole criterion with a range of symptoms (including loss of consciousness) that may indicate mTBI. Most clients with TBI seen by occupational therapists in rehabilitation settings are in the severe category, and the fatality rate for clients with this level of injury severity is approximately 46% (Andriessen et al., 2011).

Table 1.1. Classification of Traumatic Brain Injury Severity

| Level of Severity | Initial Glasgow Coma Scale Score | Loss of Consciousness | Posttraumatic Amnesia | | Neuroimaging Studies |
			Russell Criteria (Russell & Smith, 1961)	Mississippi Criteria (Nakase-Richardson et al., 2011)	
Mild[a]	13–15	<30 min or <1 hr (Posner et al., 2007)	<5 min (very mild; Vollmer & Dacey, 1991), 0–1 hr	0–24 hr	Normal
Moderate	9–12	>30 min to <24 hr or 1–6 hr (Posner et al., 2007)	1–24 hr	12–28 days	Normal or abnormal
Severe	3–8	>24 hr or >6 hr (Posner et al., 2007)	>1 day and <7 days	29–70 days	Focal abnormalities
Very severe			>7 days	>70 days	

[a]Initial Glasgow Coma Scale score of 13–15, loss of consciousness, or posttraumatic amnesia is indicative of mild severity. For moderate, severe, and very severe injuries, all criteria must be met.

Occupational therapists on neurological rehabilitation units may also encounter clients with nontraumatic brain injuries. Clients who have sustained **hypoxic brain damage** and cerebral anoxia (e.g., from partial drowning, smoke asphyxiation, or cardiac arrest) are surviving as a result of improved emergency medicine (Wilson, Harpur, Watson, & Morrow, 2003). In addition, clients with aneurysms and arterial–venous malformations, tumors, exposure to toxic substances (e.g., carbon monoxide poisoning, drug overdose), or brain infections (e.g., meningitis, encephalitis) may be placed on a TBI treatment unit because their clinical symptoms and behaviors may resemble those of people who have sustained a TBI.

Underlying Brain Pathology

No direct relationship exists between the presence or absence of linear skull fractures and severity of brain injury. Linear skull fractures may occur without any concomitant brain injury; however, skull fractures can be found in as many as 70% of people with **contusions** or intracranial **hematomas** (Macpherson, Macpherson, & Jennett, 1990). Depressed skull fractures and basilar skull fractures carry an increased risk of infection because of the exposure of the brain tissue to external material and pathogens (Frosch et al., 2005). The use of prophylactic antibiotics in patients with linear types of skull fractures is controversial (Yokobori & Bullock, 2012). A recent meta-analysis found a lack of evidence supporting the use of prophylactic antibiotics in patients with and without **cerebrospinal fluid** (CSF) leaks (Ratilal, Costa, Sampaio, & Pappamikail, 2011).

Cerebral edema—swelling of the brain tissues secondary to abnormal fluid accumulation—may be cytotoxic, vasogenic, or osmotic. *Cytotoxic cerebral edema* is secondary to neuronal damage such as diffuse axonal injury; *vasogenic cerebral edema* results from a disruption of the **blood–brain barrier;** and *osmotic cerebral edema* results from leakage of CSF into the periventricular white matter or obstruction of normal CSF pathways (Kochanek et al., 2012). Treatment of cerebral edema is necessary when it begins to elevate intracranial pressure (ICP).

Elevated ICP can result from the development of any lesion or event that causes an increase in the volume of the skull contents. During the acute medical management of the patient in the ED or in the intensive care unit (ICU), ICP may be monitored by placing a pressure gauge in the lateral ventricles, subarachnoid space, or epidural space. Normal ICP is 5 to 15 millimeters of mercury (mm Hg) when measured in the lateral ventricles. Treatment to lower ICP is typically initiated when pressure readings are above the threshold of 20 mm Hg (Brain Trauma Foundation, 2007). Cerebral perfusion pressure (CPP) may be calculated by subtracting the ICP from the mean arterial blood pressure. CPP readings greater than or equal to 50 mm Hg suggest adequate cerebral blood flow autoregulation.

Elevated ICP or decreased CPP is treated with a combination of client positioning, hyperventilation, ventricular drainage through shunts, and medications such as barbiturates or osmotic diuretics (e.g., mannitol; Brain Trauma Foundation, 2007; Sanchez, Kahn, & Bullock, 2012; Yokobori & Bullock, 2012). Current evidence (Brain Trauma Foundation, 2007) has indicated that steroids do not improve outcome or lower ICP in patients with severe brain injuries. Osmotic diuretics, such as mannitol, may be beneficial preoperatively in patients with hematomas, but continuous infusion in patients who do not have an operable intracranial hematoma can raise

ICP and cause renal failure when used in higher doses (Tsai & Shu, 2010; Wakai, McCabe, Roberts, & Schierhout, 2003). Individualized management of elevated ICP is based on analysis of serial neurological and imaging exams to monitor ICP measurements and cerebral blood flow to maintain the patient's ICP at a threshold to support the physical changes in the brain (Chesnut, 2014; Lazaridis et al., 2014). Uncontrolled elevated ICP accounts for most TBI-related deaths because it can cause cardiovascular insufficiency, brain herniation, or both (Yokobori & Bullock, 2012).

Occupational therapists working with clients in the ICU need to monitor the effects that interventions such as **range of motion** (ROM) exercises and serial casting have on the client's ICP. Therapists must also observe for potential elevation of ICP in various phases of the client's recovery. Clients with shunts may have a shunt malfunction during later rehabilitation and display symptoms of elevated ICP: headache, stiff neck, vomiting, decrease in vital signs and consciousness, and increased motor or sensory loss or a sudden halting of steady progress in the recovery of motor function. Reporting such symptoms to the physician can contribute valuable information to the medical management of the client.

Elevated ICP may cause secondary anoxic brain injuries that affect the *watershed areas* of the brain—those that are rich in capillary supply (e.g., the hippocampus, basal **ganglia, cerebellum;** Long, 2012; Wilson et al., 2003). The brain's volume may increase in response to cerebral edema associated with bruising and contusions or the presence of space-occupying lesions such as hematomas. The increasing pressure of the brain contents within the closed environment of the skull results in displacement of brain tissue or brain herniation.

In their classic work on the diagnosis of stupor and coma, Plum and Posner (1982; Posner et al., 2007) described the major patterns of **supratentorial herniation:** *falcine,* in which the cingulate herniates across the falx cerebri; *uncal,* in which the medial aspect of the temporal lobe herniates medially and downward across the tentorium cerebelli; and *transtentorial* or *central displacement,* in which the **diencephalon** is pushed downward with or without lateral displacement. Each type of herniation shows a corresponding pattern of clinical symptoms that may include *papilledema,* a fixed dilation of the pupil resulting from pressure on the third cranial nerve; posturing of the limbs (i.e., **decorticate** or **decerebrate**); and respiratory and cardiac changes resulting from the increasing pressure on the **brainstem.** Brain herniation may also cause compression of the **posterior cerebral artery,** thereby resulting in a focal infarct that presents with **homonymous hemianopsia** and hippocampal damage resulting from posterior cerebral artery blood distribution (Yuh & Gean, 2012).

Clients who show evidence of enlarged ventricles and posttraumatic **hydrocephalus** on computed tomography (CT) scans will typically have a shunt placed to assist with CSF drainage. Obstructive hydrocephalus is common in patients who have sustained **subarachnoid hemorrhages** because the cells in the accumulating blood block CSF reabsorption in the subarachnoid space (Levine & Flanagan, 2012; Yokobori & Bullock, 2012). Clinically, these patients may present with a stiff neck, headache, restlessness, and blood in the CSF on lumbar puncture. Posttraumatic hydrocephalus affects about 50% of people with severe TBI; however, only 11% of those with severe hydrocephalus require surgery and shunt placement (Mazzini et al., 2003). Posttraumatic hydrocephalus influences the functional outcome from TBI and is a prognostic factor for posttraumatic epilepsy (Mazzini et al., 2003).

Hematomas form when blood from injured vessels collects and occupies the limited space within the closed skull. These space-occupying lesions are named by the location in which they form and can be life threatening because they may obstruct CSF circulation and distort brain tissue, causing herniation (Frosch et al., 2005; Yokobori & Bullock, 2012; Yuh & Gean, 2012).

Subdural hematomas collect between the dura mater and the brain's surface. Subdural hematomas are further classified by the rate at which they develop (i.e., acute, subacute, or chronic). Chronic subdural hematomas are more common in clients who are older than age 65 or in clients with alcoholism as a result of alcohol-associated brain atrophy and stretching of the dural veins (Frosch et al., 2005; Yokobori & Bullock, 2012; Yuh & Gean, 2012). Even apparently minor injuries, such as a shower curtain rod falling on someone's head, can result in trauma to the brain and dural veins.

Epidural hematomas form in the space between the dura mater and the skull. Epidural hematomas are usually the result of lacerations of the middle meningeal artery and are more common in young clients. The clinical manifestations (e.g., alterations in wakefulness) are varied and can be confusing, and a severe injury can be missed in its early stages (Frosch et al., 2005). Subdural and epidural hematomas are usually surgically evacuated through burr holes (i.e., holes drilled into the skull) or craniotomies in which a larger section of the skull is opened.

Intracerebral hematomas form deep in the white matter of the brain. They present as deep contusions in the brain, and their clinical signs depend on their location and size. Needle aspiration through burr holes may be considered if the site can be accessed without additional damage to the brain. Unlike epidural and subdural hematomas, in which the primary damage is caused by bleeding, surgery for intracerebral hematomas is less likely to restore function (Bullock et al., 2006).

Neurodiagnostic Testing

Occupational therapists reviewing the medical chart of a patient with TBI may see the results of a range of neurodiagnostic tests used to assist in the management of the client's neurological recovery. Electroencephalograms (EEGs) and evoked potentials may be conducted to look at the responsiveness of the **neurons** (Vernet, Bashir, Enam, Kumru, & Pascual-Leone, 2012). CT scans, magnetic resonance imaging (MRI), and X rays may be completed to review the brain and skull for lesions (Yuh & Gean, 2012). The neurosurgical staff may perform angiograms to identify damage to the brain's circulatory system and positron emission transaxial tomography to explore the brain's metabolism (Ricker, Arenth, & Wagner, 2012).

Postinjury Recovery and Complications

Because of the often violent nature of the incident causing the TBI, clients may experience traumatic injuries to multiple body systems and structures. It is not uncommon to see people with TBI and coexisting spinal cord injuries, amputations, or peripheral nerve injuries and fractures. Differences in the size and weight of vehicles involved in a crash may result in injuries to the thorax and intrathoracic organs of the occupants of the smaller and lighter vehicle. The invasive nature of some medical management procedures can result in potential infections. Immobility during the lengthy recovery can cause **deep vein thrombosis.** Additionally, clients with TBI may experience **heterotopic ossification** or seizures.

Early recognition of the risk for HO is essential to medically manage the condition and prevent future functional limitations.

Heterotopic ossification (HO) is the ectopic formation of new bone in soft-tissue structures surrounding the joints (Vanden Bossche & Vanderstraeten, 2005). Early recognition of the risk for HO is essential to medically manage the condition and prevent future functional limitations. The medical literature has indicated that 11% to 73% of people who sustain a TBI will develop HO, with a larger percentage of HO occurring in women (as a result of hormonal influence) and in clients with severe brain injuries or long-bone fractures (Simonsen, Sonne-Holm, Krasheninnikoff, & Engberg, 2007). Monitoring of clients' alkaline phosphatase blood levels, bone scans, and clinical examination for signs of inflammation (e.g., increased joint stiffness, limited ROM, warmth, swelling, erythema) will aid in the diagnosis of HO.

HO may initially be managed by administering anti-inflammatory drugs, functional positioning, and mobilization. Surgical excision of the HO is typically performed 12 to 18 months after onset when the bone shows evidence of maturation (Vanden Bossche & Vanderstraeten, 2005). Clients with a **central nervous system** (CNS) injury who develop HO show gains in motion postsurgery equal to those of clients whose HO resulted from localized bony trauma. However, clients with CNS injuries such as TBI who develop HO have a higher occurrence of bone regrowth (Baldwin et al., 2011).

Posttraumatic seizures are classified as *early* when they occur within 7 days of the TBI or *late* when they occur after 7 days post-TBI (Brain Trauma Foundation, 2007). Continuous EEG monitoring may be performed for patients suspected of having subclinical seizure activity. Prophylactic medication to prevent seizures has been a standard protocol in clients with TBI, but physicians must balance the risk of seizure with the neurobehavioral side effects of seizure medications. Seizures are more common in clients who have sustained penetrating TBIs, with approximately 50% experiencing a seizure. Other factors such as presence of a hematoma, depressed skull fracture, or cortical contusion appear to increase the risk of developing posttraumatic seizures. A recent meta-analysis of medical management of seizures recommended routine seizure prophylaxis for only the first week after TBI (Brain Trauma Foundation, 2007) unless the patient shows clinical or electrographic evidence of seizure activity (Sanchez et al., 2012).

Incidence and Definition of *Mild Traumatic Brain Injury*

Although there is no universally accepted definition of *mTBI,* the most commonly used definition comes from the American Congress of Rehabilitation Medicine (1993, p. 86), which has defined *mTBI* as a traumatically induced physiological disruption of brain function, as manifested by at least one of the following:

- Any period of loss of consciousness;
- Any loss of memory for events immediately before or after the accident;
- Any alteration in mental state at the time of the accident (e.g., feeling dazed, disoriented, or confused); and
- Focal neurological deficit(s) that may or may not be transient;

but where the severity of the injury does not exceed the following:

- Loss of consciousness of approximately 30 minutes or less;
- After 30 minutes, an initial GCS of 13–15; and
- PTA lasting not longer than 24 hours.

Approximately 25% of people who are injured in a motor vehicle crash sustain an mTBI (Cassidy, Boyle, & Carroll, 2014). Although 15% of people with a diagnosis of mTBI have an acute intracranial lesion identified through head CT, fewer than 1% of these people require neurosurgical intervention (Bruns & Jagoda, 2009). Of the 1.4 million people released from EDs with mTBI, approximately 420,000 (30%) show ongoing postconcussive symptoms (PCS) at 1 week postinjury (Ponsford, Cameron, Fitzgerald, Grant, & Mikocka-Walus, 2011). PCS symptoms may not be recognized by ED personnel (Powell, Ferraro, Dikmen, Temkin, & Bell, 2008), resulting in a lack of referral for follow-up assessment of rehabilitation needs. Because patients in this category of severity typically do not have observable abnormalities on neuroimaging and may score in the normal range on the GCS, ED physicians may need to conduct a more extensive review of possible symptoms before discharge so appropriate follow-up care can be recommended.

Current evidence-based guidelines for ED physicians strongly recommend educating people regarding PCS (see Box 1.2); the potential influence of PCS on work, school, or sports; and when to seek additional medical intervention (Jagoda, 2010; Jagoda et al., 2009). Monitoring of clients discharged from EDs with scales such as the Rivermead Post-Concussion Symptoms Questionnaire (Eyres, Carey, Gilworth, Neumann, & Tennant, 2005) may prevent symptoms from becoming chronic and may minimize the functional effects of the injury (Prigatano & Gale, 2011; Willer & Leddy, 2006). The Abbreviated Westmead Post-Traumatic Amnesia Scale (Meares, Shores, Taylor, Lammél, & Batchelor, 2011), another scale used with patients with suspected mTBI, extends the content of the verbal section of the GCS to include items testing the client's **orientation** and adds a short-term visual memory task (i.e., recall of three objects). The testing is done hourly during the period of time in which the client is being observed in the ED to provide a prospective rather than a retrospective measure of PTA and a more accurate diagnosis of mTBI.

The diagnostic criteria for mTBI differ substantially between the *International Statistical Classification of Diseases and Related Health Problems* (10th rvsn.; World Health Organization [WHO], 2004) definition of **postconcussion syndrome** and the *Diagnostic and Statistical Manual of Mental Disorders* (5th ed.; APA, 2013)

Box 1.2. Common Symptoms of Mild Traumatic Brain Injury

Physical Symptoms
- Headache
- Nausea
- Vomiting
- Blurred or double vision
- Seeing stars or lights
- Balance problems
- Dizziness
- Sensitivity to light or noise
- Tinnitus

Behavioral and Emotional Symptoms
- Drowsiness
- **Fatigue** or lethargy
- Irritability
- Depression
- Anxiety
- Sleeping more than usual
- Difficulty falling asleep

Cognitive Symptoms
- Feeling slowed down
- Feeling in a fog or dazed
- Difficulty concentrating
- Difficulty remembering

Source. From "Management of Concussion and Post-Concussion Syndrome," by B. Willer & J. J. Leddy, 2006, *Current Treatment Options in Neurology, 8*, p. 418. Copyright © 2006 by Springer Science and Bus Media B V. Adapted with permission.

definition of **mild neurocognitive disorder** resulting from TBI (previously called *postconcussional disorder*) in relation to the cutoff time between acute and persistent symptoms; the reliance on neuropsychological testing versus patient complaints for diagnosis; and the physical, cognitive, and emotional symptoms (Ruff, 2011). Guidelines on the diagnosis and assessment of mTBI include strong recommendations for the early diagnosis of mTBI through a combined assessment of clinical factors and symptoms using standardized tools and the monitoring of persistent somatic, cognitive, and emotional or behavioral symptoms (Marshall, Bayley, McCullagh, Velikonja, & Berrigan, 2012). Early diagnosis and management are vital to successful recovery from mTBI. Consistent evidence has supported the beneficial effects of client education interventions that focus on the common symptoms and course of recovery along with advice on **coping** with the symptoms and reintegrating into daily life activities (Marshall et al., 2012; mTBI Guidelines Development Team, 2010).

A growing awareness of sports-related concussions and their potential effects on functioning and fulfillment of role responsibilities led the American Academy of Neurology (2010) to develop guidelines for managing athletes with sports-related concussion. These guidelines recognize the potential for symptoms from a single event as well as the potential for multiple events to result in cumulative symptoms (Iverson, Echemendia, Lamarre, Brooks, & Gaetz, 2012).

After their injury, people with mTBI may experience difficulties with cognitive tasks that involve **attention,** fluency, and speed of processing (Marshall et al., 2012; Ponsford et al., 2011; Ruff, 2011; Williams, Potter, & Ryland, 2010). There is a lack of consensus on the persisting nature of functional limitations from mTBI. Some studies have reported that people who sustained mTBI have continuing PCS 3 to 12 months postinjury that result in difficulties performing daily activities that require memory and **concentration** (Lundin, de Boussard, Edman, & Borg, 2006; Ponsford et al., 2011). Several meta-analyses have offered strong support for the argument that the vast majority of people who sustain mTBI return to normal cognitive functioning by 3 months. These studies have suggested that remaining symptoms can be attributed to non–brain-based etiologies such as secondary gain, psychological problems, or physical problems. However, incomplete recovery from mTBI may exist and may not have been captured in these meta-analyses because of methodological issues (e.g., definition of mTBI, complexity of cognitive testing) and attrition rates (Ruff, 2011).

Although more than 80% of people discharged from EDs after mTBI return to work within 1 year (Iverson, Silverberg, Lange, & Zasler, 2012), the long-term consequences for people with continuing PCS may result in an altered life. The structured nature of office-based cognitive testing may not tap into the more complex cognitive skills needed to perform **instrumental activities of daily living** (IADLs) such as grocery shopping, financial management, work tasks, or driving a vehicle in often busy and crowded real-world environments with multiple distractions (Toglia & Golisz, 2012). Development of **posttraumatic stress disorder** after mTBI has been observed both in the military population (Vanderploeg, Belanger, & Curtiss, 2009) and in 17% of the civilian population (Hoffman, Dikmen, Temkin, & Bell, 2012), resulting in lower levels of **life satisfaction** even 3 years postinjury (Benedictus, Spikman, & van der Naalt, 2010).

Other persistent problems reported in people after mTBI include balance disorders, sleep disturbances, headaches, vision disorders, and fatigue (Cassidy et al., 2014; Lundin et al., 2006; mTBI Guidelines Development Team, 2010). These symptoms, combined with persisting cognitive issues, can limit full resumption of life roles and tasks on return to work or school environments after the injury. The lack of any visible impairment and the classification of the injury as mild may diminish the perception that any actual brain injury occurred. The person may doubt the cause of functional changes and experience **stress.** Gradual resumption of previous occupations and life roles after mTBI, combined with psychological support and intervention addressing specific impairments, is recommended. It is estimated that fewer than 10% of people who sustain mTBI experience persisting difficulties that affect their role performance, and the neuropathological versus psychosocial contributions to the persisting symptoms remain an issue of debate (Ruff, 2011).

Measuring Recovery

TBI is often referred to as the *silent epidemic* because the associated impairments and limitations are not readily apparent to the casual observer. Physical evidence or signs of the injury may be lacking. Cognitive, emotional, sensory, and motor impairments, however, may permanently change a person's ability to live independently, work competitively, and engage in stable, meaningful social and family relationships (CDC, 2012). People with TBI often report that transportation, government policies, attitudes, and the natural environment are barriers to their **community integration** and participation in society (Rapport, Hanks, & Bryer, 2006; Whiteneck, Gerhart, & Cusick, 2004).

The specific mechanisms that mediate TBI recovery are not completely understood (Stein, 2000). Theories related to ***diaschisis*** (i.e., a temporary disruption to function immediately after the injury), compensation, and adaptive **plasticity** of remaining and intact brain structures have been proposed to explain functional recovery after TBI (Nudo & Dancause, 2012). A single tool may not be capable of measuring the quantitative and qualitative physical, cognitive, and functional changes throughout each phase of recovery. In addition, because outcome can be measured from both an objective or clinician-rated and a subjective or client-rated perspective, the members of the health care team, client, and family may describe a good outcome differently (Koskinen et al., 2011). A good medical recovery as defined by the health care team may not be perceived as such by the client if he or she is unable to resume previously valued roles and meaningful activities. During initial medical treatment in the ICU, survival is the desired outcome. Although this goal may satisfy the health care team at this phase of recovery, the family usually wants to know the long-term outcome: "Will my family member ever be the same as before the injury?" Clients and family members are concerned about the ultimate outcome, which may not be known for years.

Several factors may influence the final clinical and functional outcomes after TBI. Clients who are relatively young at the time of TBI have been shown to have a more positive outcome and require less inpatient rehabilitation (Kothari & DiTommaso, 2012). Older adults who sustain a TBI may have more chronic health conditions and age-related physiological changes that result in additional complexity and challenges during rehabilitation. They typically make slower recoveries and have shorter lengths of stay in inpatient rehabilitation and lower discharge **FIM**™ (Uniform Data System for Medical Rehabilitation, 1997) motor and cognitive ratings (Graham et al., 2010). Older adults are more likely to be discharged to a postacute medical facility (Cuthbert et al., 2011) and are less likely (<10% chance) to achieve a good recovery on the Glasgow Outcome Scale (GOS; Brown, Elovic, Kothari, Flanagan, & Kwasnica, 2008). The 2002 enactment of the Medicare inpatient prospective payment system has had an influence on TBI rehabilitation length of stay and may account for the changes in the length of stay noted in more recent studies (Hoffman et al., 2003).

Gender differences have been found in both recovery and discharge disposition after TBI. Women younger than age 50 tend to present more frequently with brain swelling and elevated ICP than do men of the same age with injuries of similar severity; this pattern suggests that younger women may benefit from aggressive monitoring and treatment of elevated ICP (Farin, Deutsch, Biegon, & Marshall, 2003). Women of all ages are more likely to be discharged to long-term care facilities (Brown, Colantonio, & Kim, 2012).

At different points in recovery, various assessments may be helpful in evaluating the client's severity of injury and predicting potential outcomes (see Table 1.2). Valid and reliable assessments can help quantify clients' **functional impairments,** the burden of care experienced by caregivers, and appropriate rehabilitation supports to meet client and family needs (Nichol et al., 2011). Methods used to measure initial TBI severity may not predict the long-term outcome and final classification of injury severity. Great variety exists in the clinical presentation and functional outcomes of the group of clients classified as having severe injuries (Sherer et al., 2008).

The GCS is a standard assessment used in the acute phases of TBI recovery to rate the neurological status of the **cerebral cortex** (the verbal response component; *V*), upper brainstem (the motor response component; *M*), and reticular activating system (the eye-opening component; *E*). The GCS requires training for high interrater reliability, appropriate scoring at defined intervals using a consistent EVM or EMV sequence, and consideration of confounding scoring variables such as endotracheal intubation, sedation, neuromuscular blocking agents, or spinal or eye trauma (Zuercher, Ummenhofer, Baltussen, & Walder, 2009). Without training and appropriate scoring, clients may receive artificially lowered initial GCS scores that underestimate their level of consciousness or overestimate the severity of the injury. Emerging assessments of neurological recovery such as the Neurological Outcome Scale for Traumatic Brain Injury, an adaptation of the National Institutes of Health Stroke Scale, and the Full Outline of UnResponsiveness scale may help provide information to the team and family (Fischer et al., 2010; Jalali & Rezaei, 2014; Wilde, McCauley, et al., 2010).

The Rancho Los Amigos Levels of Cognitive Functioning Scale is often used in rehabilitation programs to describe recovery of cognitive and behavioral functioning.

The Rancho Los Amigos Levels of Cognitive Functioning Scale (LCFS; Hagen, Malkmus, & Durham, 1972) is often used in rehabilitation programs to describe recovery of cognitive and behavioral functioning. The original scale, developed in 1972, consists of 8 levels that describe clients ranging from those with an absence of purposeful responses to those with community levels of recovery and the ability to display purposeful and appropriate behaviors. The LCFS is typically used in acute medical and inpatient rehabilitation settings, as described in Chapters 5 and 6 of this text. Both interrater and test–retest reliability of the 8-level LCFS were found to be acceptable in a study of 40 patients with TBI admitted to an acute

Table 1.2. Commonly Used Traumatic Brain Injury Outcome Assessments

Outcome Assessment	Clinical Notes
Brain Injury Community Rehabilitation Outcome–39 (BICRO–39; Powell et al., 1998)	The BICRO–39 contains 39 items structured into 8 domains (personal care, mobility, self-organization, partner–child contact, parent–sibling contact, socializing, productive employment, psychological well-being). All items are rated on a 6-point scale, with some domains rating frequency and other domains rating degree of assistance. Total scores range from 0 to 195, with lower scores representing better outcome.
Craig Handicap Assessment and Reporting Technique–Short Form (CHART–SF; Whiteneck et al., 1992)	The CHART–SF focuses on occupation, physical independence, mobility, social integration, and economic self-sufficiency after brain injury. Uses the *ICF* framework to measure the degree to which impairments and disabilities restrict participation.
Disability Rating Scale (Rappaport et al., 1982)	This 30-point scale quantifies the progress of clients with TBI from coma to community in 4 categories: consciousness, cognitive ability, dependence on others, and employability.
FIM™ (Uniform Data System for Medical Rehabilitation, 1997) and Functional Assessment Measure (FAM; Hall, 1997)	The FAM is a 12-item addition to the FIM that relates to community functioning (e.g., car transfers, employability, adjustment to limitations, swallowing function). The advantage of this assessment is that it makes the FIM more sensitive to the problems of clients with TBI.
Glasgow Outcome Scale (GOS; Teasdale & Jennett, 1976) and Glasgow Outcome Scale–Extended (GOS–E; Wilson et al., 1998)	The original GOS classified patient outcomes into 5 categories (dead, **vegetative,** severely disabled, moderately disabled, good recovery). The extended version of the scale separates the last 3 categories into lower and upper categories, resulting in a total of 8 categories. The GOS–E provides a structured interview to determine the final rating.
Mayo–Portland Adaptability Inventory–4 (Malec & Lezak, 2003)	This observational assessment is designed for interdisciplinary assessment at the community level of recovery. It measures physical function (including pain and mobility), cognitive capacity, emotional status, social behavior, self-care, work, and driving status. The patient's status on 30 functional items is rated, based on team consensus, on a 4-category scale: no impairment, impairment on clinical examination but does not interfere with everyday function, impairment does interfere with everyday function, and complete or nearly complete loss of function.
Participation Assessment With Recombined Tools–Objective (PART–O; Whiteneck et al., 2011)	The PART–O is a 24-item assessment based on 3 legacy instruments of participation: Community Integration Questionnaire–II, POPS, and the CHART–SF. Objective data measure frequency of engagement in activities related to 6 of the 9 areas of the *ICF* (domestic life, interpersonal interactions and relationships, major life areas, and community, social, and civic life).
Participation Objective, Participation Subjective (POPS; Brown et al., 2004)	The 26 items of the POPS are sorted into 5 categories: domestic life; major life activities; transportation; interpersonal interactions and relationships; and community, recreational, and civic life. The client rates frequency and satisfaction with participation.
Participation Profile (PAR-PRO; Ostir et al., 2006)	The PAR-PRO measures frequency of participation in 20 items selected from the *ICF* domains of participation (e.g., domestic life, interpersonal interactions and relationships, major life areas such as work or education) using a 5-point scale. Data are collected at 3 points in time (admission, discharge, and follow-up). Preinjury data are used as a benchmark for follow-up.
Quality of Life After Brain Injury (QOLIBRI; von Steinbuechel et al., 2005)	The QOLIBRI is a 37-item scale divided into 4 satisfaction subscales that assess thinking, **feelings** and **emotions,** autonomy in daily life, and social aspects, and 2 "bothered" subscales that assess negative feelings and restrictions.
Rehabilitation Institute of Chicago–Functional Assessment Scale (RIC–FAS; Cichowski, 1998)	The RIC–FAS consists of 89 items organized into the domains of medical management, health maintenance, self-care, mobility, communication, cognitive, psychosocial, community integration, and vocational. Items are scored by the health care team using a 7-point ordinal scale similar to the FIM.
Reintegration to Normal Living Index (RNLI; Wood-Dauphinee et al., 1988)	The RNLI contains 11 items presented in a visual analog scale to assess people's reintegration into social activities after trauma or illness. Eight items look at daily functioning in 7 domains (e.g., self-care, family roles, personal relationships), and 3 items look at perception of self.
Satisfaction With Life Scale (Diener et al., 1985)	The client scores level of agreement with 5 statements about life satisfaction on a 7-point Likert scale. Statements address satisfaction with the past (1 item), present (3 items), and future (1 item).
Short Form–36 Health Survey (SF–36; Ware et al., 1994)	The SF–36 is a short generic health survey of 36 items related to functional health and well-being. It has been researched extensively.

Note. ICF = International Classification of Functioning, Disability and Health (World Health Organization, 2001); TBI = traumatic brain injury.

rehabilitation facility (Gouvier, Blanton, LaPorte, & Nepomuceno, 1987). A 10-level LCFS (Table 1.3), introduced by Hagen in 1998, expanded the higher levels of the scale to refine and expand the descriptions of clients' behaviors relevant to out-patient and community settings (discussed in Chapter 7). This 10-level version of the scale has not been validated, and the staff at Rancho Los Amigos continue to

Table 1.3. Rancho Los Amigos Levels of Cognitive Functioning (1998 Revised Scale)

Rancho Cognitive Level	Cognitive, Behavioral, Psychosocial, and Functional Characteristics
Level I: No response; total assistance	• Complete absence of observable change in behavior when presented with visual, auditory, tactile, **proprioceptive, vestibular,** or painful stimuli
Level II: Generalized response; total assistance	• Demonstrates generalized reflex response to painful stimuli • Responds to repeated auditory stimuli with increased or decreased activity • Responds to external stimuli with generalized physiological changes, gross body movement, or not-purposeful vocalization • These responses may be the same regardless of type and location of stimulation • Responses may be significantly delayed
Level III: Localized response; total assistance	• Demonstrates withdrawal or vocalization to painful stimuli • Turns toward or away from auditory stimuli • Blinks when strong light crosses **visual field** • Follows moving object passed within visual field • Responds to discomfort by pulling at tubes or restraints • Responds inconsistently to simple commands • Responses are directly related to type of stimulus • May respond to some people (especially family and friends) but not to others
Level IV: Confused, agitated; maximal assistance	• Alert and in heightened state of activity • Purposeful attempts to remove restraints or tubes or crawl out of bed • May perform motor activities such as sitting, reaching, and walking but without any apparent purpose or on another's request • Very brief and usually nonpurposeful moments of sustained alternatives and divided attention • Absent **short-term memory** • May cry out or scream out of proportion to stimulus even after its removal • May exhibit aggressive or flight behavior • Mood may swing from euphoric to hostile with no apparent relationship to environmental events • Unable to cooperate with treatment efforts • Verbalizations are frequently incoherent or inappropriate to activity or environment
Level V: Confused, inappropriate, nonagitated; maximal assistance	• Alert, not agitated, but may wander randomly or with a vague intention of going home • May become agitated in response to external stimulation, lack of environmental structure, or both • Not oriented to person, place, or time • Frequent brief periods of nonpurposeful, sustained attention • Severely impaired recent memory, with confusion of past and present in reaction to ongoing activity • Absent goal-directed problem solving, self-monitoring behavior • Often demonstrates inappropriate use of objects without external direction • May be able to perform previously learned tasks when they are structured and cues are provided • Unable to learn new information • Able to respond appropriately to simple commands fairly consistently with external structures and cues • Responses to simple commands without external structure are random and nonpurposeful in relation to command • Able to converse on a social, automatic level for brief periods of time when provided external structure and cues • Verbalizations about present events become inappropriate and confabulatory when external structure and cues are not provided
Level VI: Confused, appropriate; moderate assistance	• Inconsistently oriented to person, time, and place • Able to attend to highly familiar tasks in nondistracting environment for 30 min with moderate redirection • Remote memory has more depth and detail than recent memory • Vague recognition of some staff • Able to use assistive memory aid with maximal assistance • Emerging awareness of appropriate response to self, family, and basic needs • Moderate assist to problem-solve barriers to task completion • Supervised for old learning (e.g., self-care) • Shows carryover for relearned familiar tasks (e.g., self-care) • Maximal assistance for new learning with little or no carryover • Unaware of impairments, disabilities, and safety risks • Consistently follows simple directions • Verbal expressions are appropriate in highly familiar and structured situations
Level VII: Automatic–appropriate; minimal assistance for routine daily living skills	• Consistently oriented to person and place in highly familiar environments; moderate assistance for orientation to time • Able to attend to highly familiar tasks in a nondistracting environment for at least 30 min with minimal assistance to complete tasks • Able to use assistive memory devices with minimal assistance • Minimal supervision for new learning; demonstrates carryover of new learning

(Continued)

Table 1.3. Rancho Los Amigos Levels of Cognitive Functioning (1998 Revised Scale) *(cont.)*

Rancho Cognitive Level	Cognitive, Behavioral, Psychosocial, and Functional Characteristics
	• Initiates and carries out steps to complete familiar personal and household routines but has shallow recall of what he or she has been doing • Able to monitor accuracy and completeness of each step in routine personal and household **activities of daily living** and modify plan with minimal assistance • Superficial awareness of his or her condition but unaware of specific impairments and disabilities and the limits they place on his or her ability to safely, accurately, and completely carry out household, community, work, and **leisure** tasks • Unrealistic planning; unable to think about consequences of a decision or action • Overestimates abilities • Unaware of others' needs and feelings; unable to recognize inappropriate social interaction behavior • Oppositional or uncooperative
Level VIII: Purposeful and appropriate; standby assistance for routine daily living skills	• Consistently oriented to person, place, and time • Independently attends to and completes familiar tasks for 1 hr in a distracting environment • Able to recall and integrate past and recent events • Uses assistive memory devices to recall daily schedule, create to-do lists, and record critical information for later use with standby assistance • Initiates and carries out steps to complete familiar personal, household, community, work, and leisure routines with standby assistance; can modify the plan when needed with minimal assistance • Requires no assistance once new tasks or activities are learned • Aware of and acknowledges impairments and disabilities when they interfere with task completion but requires standby assistance to take appropriate corrective action • Thinks about consequences of a decision or action with minimal assistance • Overestimates or underestimates abilities • Acknowledges others' needs and feelings and responds appropriately with minimal assistance • Depressed, irritable; low tolerance for frustration; easily angered and argumentative • Self-centered • Uncharacteristically dependent or independent • Able to recognize and acknowledge inappropriate social interaction behavior while it is occurring; takes corrective action with minimal assistance
Level IX: Purposeful and appropriate; standby assistance on request for daily living skills	• Independently shifts back and forth between tasks and completes them accurately for at least 2 consecutive hr • Uses assistive memory devices to recall daily schedule, create to-do lists, and record critical information for later use with assistance when requested • Initiates and carries out steps to complete familiar personal, household, work, and leisure tasks independently; completes unfamiliar personal, household, work, and leisure tasks with assistance when requested by others • Aware of and acknowledges impairments and disabilities when they interfere with task completion and takes appropriate corrective action; requires standby assistance to anticipate a problem before it occurs and to take action to avoid it • Able to think about consequences of decisions or actions with assistance when requested by others • Accurately estimates abilities but requires standby assistance to adjust to task demands • Acknowledges others' needs and feelings and responds appropriately with standby assistance • May continue to be depressed • May be easily irritable • May have low tolerance for frustration • Able to self-monitor appropriateness of social interaction with standby assistance
Level X: Purposeful and appropriate; modified independent	• Able to handle multiple tasks simultaneously in all environments but may require periodic breaks • Able to independently procure, create, and maintain own assistive memory devices • Independently initiates and carries out steps to complete familiar and unfamiliar personal, household, community, work, and leisure tasks; may require more than the usual amount of time, compensatory strategies, or both to complete them • Anticipates impact of impairments and disabilities on ability to complete activities of daily living and takes action to avoid problems before they occur; may require more than the usual amount of time, compensatory strategies, or both • Able to independently think about consequences of decisions or actions but may require more than the usual amount of time, compensatory strategies, or both to select the appropriate decision or action • Accurately estimates abilities and independently adjusts to task demands • Able to recognize the needs and feelings of others and automatically respond in an appropriate manner • Periodic periods of depression may occur • Irritability and low tolerance for frustration when sick, fatigued, or under emotional stress • Social interaction behavior is consistently appropriate

Source. From *The Rancho Los Amigos Levels of Cognitive Functioning: The Revised Levels* (3rd ed.), by C. Hagen, 1998, Downey, CA: Los Amigos Research and Education Institute. Copyright © 1998 by Los Amigos Research and Education Institute.
Note. hr = hour/hours; min = minutes.

use the original 8-level scale because they believe it better fits the acute rehabilitation patient (http://dhs.lacounty.gov/wps/portal/dhs/rancho). The Rancho levels are applicable in the first weeks or months after the injury, although the rate of progression and the level of plateau cannot be predicted. Clients typically exhibit characteristics of several adjoining levels at a time and may skip some levels or appear stuck at others for a period.

The FIM is used to track admission and discharge change in the inpatient rehabilitation setting. The FIM, however, is not sensitive to the gradual and subtle changes expected after discharge from acute inpatient rehabilitation. The Functional Assessment Measure (FAM; Hall, 1997; Hall et al., 1996) was developed as an adjunct to the FIM to specifically address the major functional areas that are relatively less emphasized in the FIM (i.e., cognitive, communication, psychosocial adjustment, community functioning). The Rehabilitation Institute of Chicago–Functional Assessment Scale (RIC–FAS; Cichowski, 1998) is often used in combination with the FIM and FAM to provide a comprehensive measurement of outcome (Groswasser, Schwab, & Salazar, 1997). The RIC–FAS measures awareness of disability, behavioral control, pragmatics, written expression, reading comprehension, money management, and community recreation reintegration.

Almost 4 decades since it was first described, the GOS (Teasdale & Jennett, 1976) remains the most widely used method of measuring outcome in people who have sustained severe brain injuries. Wilson, Pettigrew, and Teasdale (1998) described an improved and extended 8-point scale, the GOS–E. This scale uses a structured, question-based interview to assign an outcome category based on WHO (2001) categories of impairment, activity limitation, and participation restriction. Other common outcome assessments include the Mayo–Portland Adaptability Inventory (Malec & Lezak, 2003) and the Disability Rating Scale (Rappaport, Hall, Hopkins, Belleza, & Cope, 1982).

More recently, the *International Classification of Functioning, Disability and Health (ICF;* WHO, 2001) concept of *participation* has received greater attention as clinicians and researchers have struggled with the challenges of measuring this concept (Eyssen, Steultjens, Dekker, & Terwee, 2011; Magasi & Post, 2010; Whiteneck, 2010). Occupational therapists, with their broad perspective on the influence of the interaction among person, task, and environment on one's ability to engage in meaningful occupations, have a vital role in defining and measuring participation. Mallinson and Hammel (2010, p. S29) described participation as occurring "at the intersection of what the person can do, wants to do, has the opportunity to do, and is not prevented from doing." Community integration and participation scales typically measure engagement in social activity, independent living, and employment.

Simply measuring the frequency of a person's performance of a select group of activities in his or her community does not constitute meaningful participation. People's choice of activities, the meaningfulness of the activities to their roles, and the desired occupational pattern of performance all contribute to people's level of satisfaction with their level of participation. Objective measures need to be combined with subjective perspectives to capture a comprehensive understanding of participation. Clients with TBI frequently identify a difference between desired and actual occupational participation with their transition from the hospital to their home and community (Turner, Ownsworth, Cornwell, & Fleming, 2009). This insider–outsider perspective on recovery is important to consider in ensuring that the client's decisional autonomy, values, and goals are considered in the rehabilitation plan (Brown, 2010).

Commonly used community participation scales, such as the Community Integration Questionnaire–II (CIQ–II; Willer, Rosenthal, Kreutzer, Gordon, & Rempel, 1993) and the Craig Handicap Assessment and Reporting Technique–Short Form (CHART–SF; Whiteneck, Charlifue, Gerhart, Overholser, & Richardson, 1992), attempt to objectively measure the clinician's or outsider's perspective on the client's level of participation by scoring the frequency of participation with a "more is better" concept. Newer assessments such as the 20-item Participation Profile (Ostir et al., 2006) use the principles, definitions, and domains of the *ICF* to measure home and community participation and address Commission on Accreditation of Rehabilitation Facilities standards for inpatient rehabilitation. Other participation assessments such as the Participation Objective, Participation Subjective (POPS; Brown et al., 2004) provide both a comparison of the frequency of the person's participation with normative data and the client's satisfaction with his or her level of engagement in personally meaningful activities. A working group of the TBI Model Systems program is currently developing a new instrument, the Participation Assessment with Recombined Tools–Objective, that pools items from the CHART–SF, CIQ–II, POPS, and Mayo–Portland Participation Index (Malec, 2004) to capture the objective and subjective aspects of participation (Whiteneck et al., 2011).

As time progresses from the initial injury and the client's recovery becomes more stable, measurement of long-term outcomes becomes more reliable. Perceived health-related quality-of-life measures such as the Satisfaction With Life Scale (Diener, Emmons, Larsen, & Griffin, 1985) or the Quality of Life After Brain Injury (von Steinbuechel, Petersen, & Bullinger, 2005) have been recommended for use with people with TBI by the TBI Outcomes Workgroup (Wilde, Whiteneck, et al., 2010). These measures may assist clinicians in identifying areas in which the person with TBI may require intervention to achieve greater satisfaction; however, impairments in self-awareness have been linked to higher estimates of health-related **quality of life** (Sasse et al., 2012). It is important to recognize that recovery of functional status after TBI correlates with depressive symptoms (Hudak, Hynan, Harper, & Diaz-Arrastia, 2012), but there appears to be a lack of association between the frequency of and satisfaction with participation in specific activity and overall perceived quality of life after TBI (Johnston, Goverover, & Dijkers, 2005). Clients with mTBI experience psychosocial issues and lower life satisfaction even 3 years after their injury (Stålnacke, 2007). Clients with TBI and depression may need psychological counseling and medication, but they may also benefit from occupational therapy intervention focused on function and psychosocial needs.

In 2010, the TBI Outcomes Workgroup, which is composed of scientific experts from a variety of federal agencies, developed recommendations for a set of common data elements, including outcome measures, so data are consistently collected across TBI studies. The goals of using a set of common data elements are to

1. Document the natural course of recovery after TBI,
2. Enhance the prediction of later outcome,
3. Measure the effects of treatment, and
4. Facilitate comparisons across studies (Wilde, Whiteneck, et al., 2010, p. 1651).

> Other participation assessments such as the Participation Objective, Participation Subjective provide both a comparison of the frequency of the person's participation with normative data and the client's satisfaction with his or her level of engagement in personally meaningful activities.

This initial set of common data elements continues to be expanded and updated on the Federal Interagency Traumatic Brain Injury Research Informatics System website (http://fitbir.nih.gov/). The set of common data elements attempt to capture information on the *ICF* classifications of impairments, activity limitations, and participation restrictions and identify measures as core, supplemental, or emerging.

The Center for Outcome Measurement in Brain Injury, a collaborative project of the partners of the TBI Model Systems, maintains an online resource of outcome measures for brain injury rehabilitation (http://www.tbims.org/combi). The Rehabilitation Measures Database (http://www.rehabmeasures.org), developed through collaboration between the Center for Rehabilitation Outcomes Research at the Rehabilitation Institute of Chicago and the Department of Medical Social Sciences Informatics group at Northwestern University's Feinberg School of Medicine, provides a comprehensive list of outcome measures. This database can assist clinicians and researchers in identifying reliable and valid evidence-based instruments to assess client outcomes during all phases of rehabilitation.

Family and Cultural Issues

TBI can change the entire family system and create lifelong challenges and caregiver burden. Instruments such as the Family Needs Questionnaire–Revised (Kreutzer & Marwitz, 2008) assist the health care team in identifying the family's need for informational, emotional, or instrumental support. Patterns of coping with the brain injury of a family member vary greatly. Families with preinjury dysfunctional patterns of interaction or coping may struggle to manage the increased demands on their time and responsibilities. Better preinjury family functioning and reliance on positive coping skills are associated with greater independence in IADLs, improved community and social integration, and reduced caregiver stress in clients with mild to moderate injuries (Sady et al., 2010; Sander, Maestas, Sherer, Malec, & Nakase-Richardson, 2012).

Identifying at-risk families during rehabilitation and providing early and ongoing team-based family support and education may improve the client's community integration. Short-term (i.e., 12 sessions) cognitive–behavioral group-based intervention focusing on **psychoeducation,** support, and coping skills can increase family members' perceived **self-efficacy** and emotional adjustment (Backhaus, Ibarra, Klyce, Trexler, & Malec, 2010). Couple or marital relationships may be strained after one partner experiences a TBI. The stressors caused by the TBI need to be acknowledged. The relationship is more likely to remain intact when the couple is older and has been together longer and the injured partner has sustained a less severe and nonviolent injury. Intervention programs, led by marriage and family therapists, psychologists, or social workers, that provide education and support are important in maintaining the ongoing relationship and minimizing the risk of separation or divorce (Kreutzer, Marwitz, Hsu, Williams, & Riddick, 2007).

The health care team must consider cultural patterns of dealing with illness and injury to understand families' responses to the injury and resulting disability. Enlisting the family as a partner in the provision of care, with cultural sensitivity, can support the client with TBI throughout the recovery. Expectations for family, home, and community participation after TBI may vary in different cultures, and current measures of TBI outcome may have racial and ethnic biases (Arango-Lasprilla & Kreutzer, 2010; Sander, Clark, & Pappadis, 2010). For health care providers to be culturally competent in their care, they must consider the client's and family's cultural values, beliefs, and practices because these factors influence the family's ways of communicating, behaving, interpreting, seeking help, and problem solving (Arango-Lasprilla & Kreutzer, 2010). Disparities in access to health care may result from socioeconomic status, language barriers, immigration status, or cultural beliefs about medicine and rehabilitation that place ethnic minorities at greater risk for poor outcomes (Gary, Arango-Lasprilla, & Stevens, 2009).

Occupational Therapy and the Client With Traumatic Brain Injury

Occupational therapists may work in all kinds of settings, ranging from acute care hospitals to community-based practices, with clients who have sustained TBI. Although often considered a specialty area of occupational therapy practice, working with clients who have TBI can require therapists to tap into every intervention approach and strategy learned in their educational preparation—biomechanical, neurological, and psychosocial—because of the wide variety of potential impairments. Recent emphasis in the medical and rehabilitation community on evidence-based practice (Badjatia et al., 2008; Brasure et al., 2012; Bullock et al., 2006; Cicerone et al., 2011; Cifu, Kreutzer, Kolakowsky-Hayner, Marwitz, & Englander, 2003; Scottish Intercollegiate Guidelines Network, 2009; Thompson & Mauk, 2011; U.S. Department of Veterans Affairs, 2009) should improve the quality of care and lead to increasingly effective interventions and, thus, improved outcomes.

Rehabilitation professionals recognize the need for evidence-based guidelines to be structured yet flexible enough to accommodate variability in locale, epidemiology of injury, intervention, and prehospital care system. The *Occupational Therapy Practice Guidelines for Adults With Traumatic Brain Injury* (Golisz, 2009) provide occupational therapy practitioners and external audiences access to the best available evidence and recommendations for occupational therapy intervention with this population. Therapists practicing with this population must continually monitor the literature for new or updated evidence both within and external to the profession to ensure that their intervention with clients with TBI is evidence based.

Occupational therapists specializing in TBI rehabilitation may choose to pursue national certification as a brain injury specialist from the Academy of Certified Brain Injury Specialists. To obtain this certification, therapists must provide evidence that they have met the required work experience and training and must pass an examination.

Occupational therapists must constantly consider the life context of the individual client with TBI. What influence might the client's cultural, social, physical, and spiritual contexts have on his or her current and future performance (American Occupational Therapy Association, 2014)? Who exactly is the client? The therapist may at times need to take a broad perspective of the client that includes the family, friends, and colleagues. Coma and impaired awareness of the physical and cognitive changes resulting from the injury may require the therapist to gather information from others about the occupations in which the client engaged before the injury and his or her typical patterns of performance.

TBI rehabilitation requires teamwork to address the overlapping functional implications of physical and cognitive impairments. Occupational therapists, as vital members of the health and rehabilitation team, offer a holistic perspective on the client with TBI. By honoring clients' previous roles and meaningful occupations and acknowledging clients' current limitations and goals, occupational therapists partner with clients, families, and colleagues to help the client with TBI achieve meaningful participation in life.

References

American Academy of Neurology. (2010). *Position statement on sports concussion.* Retrieved from http://www.aan.com/globals/axon/assets/7913.pdf

American Congress of Rehabilitation Medicine. (1993). Definition of mild traumatic brain injury. *Journal of Head Trauma Rehabilitation, 8,* 86–87. http://dx.doi.org/10.1097/00001199-199309000-00010

American Occupational Therapy Association. (2014). Occupational therapy practice framework: Domain and process (3rd ed.). *American Journal of Occupational Therapy, 68*(Suppl. 1), S1–S48. http://dx.doi.org/10.5014.ajot.2014.682006

American Psychiatric Association. (2013). *Diagnostic and statistical manual of mental disorders* (5th ed.). Arlington, VA: Author.

Andriessen, T. M., Horn, J., Franschman, G., van der Naalt, J., Haitsma, I., Jacobs, B., . . . Vos, P. E. (2011). Epidemiology, severity classification, and outcome of moderate and severe traumatic brain injury: A prospective multicenter study. *Journal of Neurotrauma, 28,* 2019–2031. http://dx.doi.org/10.1089/neu.2011.2034

Arango-Lasprilla, J. C., & Kreutzer, J. S. (2010). Racial and ethnic disparities in functional, psychosocial, and neurobehavioral outcomes after brain injury. *Journal of Head Trauma Rehabilitation, 25,* 128–136. http://dx.doi.org/10.1097/HTR.0b013e3181d36ca3

Backhaus, S. L., Ibarra, S. L., Klyce, D., Trexler, L. E., & Malec, J. F. (2010). Brain injury coping skills group: A preventative intervention for patients with brain injury and their caregivers. *Archives of Physical Medicine and Rehabilitation, 91,* 840–848. http://dx.doi.org/10.1016/j.apmr.2010.03.015

Badjatia, N., Carney, N., Crocco, T. J., Fallat, M. E., Hennes, H. M., Jagoda, A. S., . . . Wright, D. W. (2008). Guidelines for prehospital management of traumatic brain injury, 2nd edition. *Prehospital Emergency Care, 12,* S1–S52. http://dx.doi.org/10.1080/10903120701732052

Baldwin, K., Hosalkar, H. S., Donegan, D. J., Rendon, N., Ramsey, M., & Keenan, M. A. (2011). Surgical resection of heterotopic bone about the elbow: An institutional experience with traumatic and neurologic etiologies. *Journal of Hand Surgery, 36,* 798–803. http://dx.doi.org/10.1016/j.jhsa.2011.01.015

Baugh, C. M., Robbins, C. A., Stern, R. A., & McKee, A. C. (2014). Current understanding of chronic traumatic encephalopathy. *Current Treatment Options in Neurology, 16,* 30. http://dx.doi.org/10.1007/s11940-014-0306-5

Baugh, C. M., Stamm, J. M., Riley, D. O., Gavett, B. E., Shenton, M. E., Lin, A., . . . Stern, R. A. (2012). Chronic traumatic encephalopathy: Neurodegeneration following repetitive concussive and subconcussive brain trauma. *Brain Imaging and Behavior, 6,* 244–254. http://dx.doi.org/10.1007/s11682-012-9164-5

Benedictus, M. R., Spikman, J. M., & van der Naalt, J. (2010). Cognitive and behavioral impairment in traumatic brain injury related to outcome and return to work. *Archives of Physical Medicine and Rehabilitation, 91,* 1436–1441. http://dx.doi.org/10.1016/j.apmr.2010.06.019

Bowman, S. M., Martin, D. P., Sharar, S. R., & Zimmerman, F. J. (2007). Racial disparities in outcomes of persons with moderate to severe traumatic brain injury. *Medical Care, 45,* 686–690. http://dx.doi.org/10.1097/MLR.0b013e31803dcdf3

Brain Injury Association of America. (n.d.). *Brain injury definitions.* Retrieved from http://biausa.fyrian.com/about-brain-injury.htm#definitions

Brain Trauma Foundation, American Association of Neurological Surgeons, & Congress of Neurological Surgeons. (2007). Guidelines for the management of severe traumatic brain injury, 3rd edition. *Journal of Neurotrauma, 24*(Suppl. 1), S1–S106. http://dx.doi.org/10.1089/neu.2007.9999

Braitman, K. A., Ferguson, S. A., & Elharam, K. (2007). Changes in driver fatality rates and vehicle incompatibility concurrent with changes in the passenger vehicle fleet. *Public Health Reports, 122,* 319–328. Retrieved from http://www.ncbi.nlm.nih.gov/pmc/articles/PMC1847494/pdf/phr122000319.pdf

Brasure, M., Lamberty, G. J., Sayer, N. A., Nelson, N. W., MacDonald, R., Ouellette, J., & Wilt, T. J. (2012). *Multidisciplinary postacute rehabilitation for moderate to severe traumatic brain injury in adults* (AHRQ Pub. No. 12-EHC101-EF). Rockville, MD: Agency for Healthcare Research and Quality. Retrieved from http://www.effectivehealthcare.ahrq.gov/reports/final.cfm

Brown, A. W., Elovic, E. P., Kothari, S., Flanagan, S. R., & Kwasnica, C. (2008). Congenital and acquired brain injury: 1. Epidemiology, pathophysiology, prognostication, innovative treatments, and prevention. *Archives of Physical Medicine and Rehabilitation, 89*(Suppl. 1), S3–S8. http://dx.doi.org/10.1016/j.apmr.2007.12.001

Brown, M. (2010). Participation: The insider's perspective. *Archives of Physical Medicine and Rehabilitation, 91*(Suppl.), S34–S37. http://dx.doi.org/10.1016/j.apmr.2009.11.030

Brown, M., Dijkers, M. P., Gordon, W. A., Ashman, T., Charatz, H., & Cheng, Z. (2004). Participation Objective, Participation Subjective: A measure of participation combining outsider and insider perspectives. *Journal of Head Trauma Rehabilitation, 19,* 459–481. http://dx.doi.org/10.1097/00001199-200411000-00004

Brown, S. B., Colantonio, A., & Kim, H. (2012). Gender differences in discharge destination among older adults following traumatic brain injury. *Health Care for Women International, 33,* 896–904. http://dx.doi.org/10.1080/07399332.2012.673654

Bruns, J. J., Jr., & Jagoda, A. S. (2009). Mild traumatic brain injury. *Mount Sinai Journal of Medicine, 76,* 129–137. http://dx.doi.org/10.1002/msj.20101

Bullock, M. R., Chesnut, R., Ghajar, J., Gordon, D., Hartl, R., Newell, D. W., . . . Wilberger, J.; Surgical Management of Traumatic Brain Injury Author Group. (2006). Surgical management of traumatic parenchymal lesions. *Neurosurgery, 58*(Suppl.), S25–S46, discussion Si–iv. http://dx.doi.org/10.1227/01.NEU.0000210365.36914.E3

Cassidy, J. D., Boyle, E., & Carroll, L. J. (2014). Population-based, inception cohort study of the incidence, course, and prognosis of mild traumatic brain injury after motor vehicle collisions. *Archives of Physical Medicine and Rehabilitation, 95*(Suppl.), S278–S285. http://dx.doi.org/10.1016/j.apmr.2013.08.295

Centers for Disease Control and Prevention. (2007). *Heads Up: Facts for physicians about mild traumatic brain injury (mTBI).* Atlanta: Author. Retrieved from http://www.cdc.gov/concussion/headsup/pdf/Facts_for_Physicians_booklet-a.pdf

Centers for Disease Control and Prevention. (2012). *Traumatic brain injury.* Retrieved November 11, 2012, from http://www.cdc.gov/TraumaticBrainInjury/index.html

Chesnut, R. M. (2014). A conceptual approach to managing severe traumatic brain injury in a time of uncertainty. *Annals of the New York Academy of Sciences, 1345,* 99–107. http://dx.doi.org/10.1111/nyas.12483

Chiang, M. F., Chang, J. G., & Hu, C. J. (2003). Association between apolipoprotein E genotype and outcome of traumatic brain injury. *Acta Neurochirurgica, 145,* 649–653, discussion 653–654. http://dx.doi.org/10.1007/s00701-003-0069-3

Cicerone, K. D., Langenbahn, D. M., Braden, C., Malec, J. F., Kalmar, K., Fraas, M., . . . Ashman, T. (2011). Evidence-based cognitive rehabilitation: Updated review of the literature from 2003 through 2008. *Archives of Physical Medicine and Rehabilitation, 92,* 519–530. http://dx.doi.org/10.1016/j.apmr.2010.11.015

Cichowski, K. (1998). *Rehabilitation Institute of Chicago–Functional Assessment Scale, Version V (RIC–FAS V).* Chicago: Rehabilitation Institute of Chicago.

Cifu, D. X., Kreutzer, J. S., Kolakowsky-Hayner, S. A., Marwitz, J. H., & Englander, J. (2003). The relationship between therapy intensity and rehabilitative outcomes after traumatic brain injury: A multicenter analysis. *Archives of Physical Medicine and Rehabilitation, 84,* 1441–1448. http://dx.doi.org/10.1016/S0003-9993(03)00272-7

Coronado, V. G., McGuire, L. C., Faul, M., Sugerman, D. E., & Pearson, W. S. (2012). Traumatic brain injury epidemiology and public health issues. In N. D. Zasler, D. I. Katz, & R. D. Zafonte (Eds.), *Brain injury medicine* (2nd ed., pp. 84–100). New York: Demos.

Coronado, V. G., Thomas, K. E., Sattin, R. W., & Johnson, R. L. (2005). The CDC Traumatic Brain Injury Surveillance System: Characteristics of persons aged 65 years and older hospitalized with a TBI. *Journal of Head Trauma Rehabilitation, 20,* 215–228. http://dx.doi.org/10.1097/00001199-200505000-00005

Coronado, V. G., Thurman, D. J., Greenspan, A. I., & Weissman, B. M. (2009). Epidemiology. In J. Jallo & C. M. Loftus (Eds.), *Neurotrauma and critical care of the brain* (pp. 3–19). New York: Thieme.

Coronado, V. G., Xu, L., Basavaraju, S. V., McGuire, L. C., Wald, M. M., Faul, M. D., . . . Hemphill, J. D.; Centers for Disease Control and Prevention. (2011). Surveillance for traumatic brain injury–related deaths—United States, 1997–2007. *Morbidity and Mortality Weekly Report (MMWR) Surveillance Summaries, 60,* 1–32.

Culotta, V. P., Sementilli, M. E., Gerold, K., & Watts, C. C. (1996). Clinicopathological hetero-geneity in the classification of mild head injury. *Neurosurgery, 38,* 245–250. http://dx.doi.org/10.1097/00006123-199602000-00002

Cunningham, K., Brown, T. D., Gradwell, E., & Nee, P. A. (2000). Airbag-associated fatal head injury: Case report and review of the literature on airbag injuries. *Journal of Accident and Emergency Medicine, 17,* 139–142. http://dx.doi.org/10.1136/emj.17.2.139

Cuthbert, J. P., Corrigan, J. D., Harrison-Felix, C., Coronado, V., Dijkers, M. P., Heinemann, A. W., & Whiteneck, G. G. (2011). Factors that predict acute hospitalization discharge disposition for adults with moderate to severe traumatic brain injury. *Archives of Physical Medicine and Rehabilitation, 92,* 721–730, e3. http://dx.doi.org/10.1016/j.apmr.2010.12.023

Defense and Veterans Brain Injury Center. (2012). *DoD worldwide numbers for TBI.* Retrieved from http://www.dvbic.org/dod-worldwide-numbers-tbi

Diener, E., Emmons, R. A., Larsen, R. J., & Griffin, S. (1985). The Satisfaction With Life Scale. *Journal of Personality Assessment, 49,* 71–75. http://dx.doi.org/10.1207/s15327752jpa4901_13

Eyres, S., Carey, A., Gilworth, G., Neumann, V., & Tennant, A. (2005). Construct validity and reliability of the Rivermead Post-Concussion Symptoms Questionnaire. *Clinical Rehabili-tation, 19,* 878–887. http://dx.doi.org/10.1191/0269215505cr905oa

Eyssen, I. C., Steultjens, M. P., Dekker, J., & Terwee, C. B. (2011). A systematic review of instru-ments assessing participation: Challenges in defining participation. *Archives of Physical Medicine and Rehabilitation, 92,* 983–997. http://dx.doi.org/10.1016/j.apmr.2011.01.006

Farin, A., Deutsch, R., Biegon, A., & Marshall, L. F. (2003). Sex-related differences in patients with severe head injury: Greater susceptibility to brain swelling in female patients 50 years of age and younger. *Journal of Neurosurgery, 98,* 32–36. http://dx.doi.org/10.3171/jns.2003.98.1.0032

Faul, M., Xu, L., Wald, M. M., & Coronado, V. G. (2010). *Traumatic brain injury in the United States: Emergency department visits, hospitalizations, and deaths 2002–2006.* Atlanta: Centers for Disease Control and Prevention, National Center for Injury Prevention and Control. Retrieved from http://www.cdc.gov/traumaticbraininjury/pdf/blue_book.pdf

Fischer, M., Rüegg, S., Czaplinski, A., Strohmeier, M., Lehmann, A., Tschan, F., . . . Marsch, S. C. (2010). Inter-rater reliability of the Full Outline of UnResponsiveness score and the Glasgow Coma Scale in critically ill patients: A prospective observational study. *Critical Care, 14,* R64. http://dx.doi.org/10.1186/cc8963

Frosch, M. P., Anthony, D. C., & DeGirolami, U. (2005). The central nervous system. In V. Jumar, A. K. Abbas, & N. Fausto (Eds.), *Robbins and Cotran pathologic basis of disease* (pp. 1347–1419). Philadelphia: Elsevier.

Gary, K. W., Arango-Lasprilla, J. C., & Stevens, L. F. (2009). Do racial/ethnic differences exist in post-injury outcomes after TBI? A comprehensive review of the literature. *Brain Injury, 23,* 775–789. http://dx.doi.org/10.1080/02699050903200563

Gavett, B. E., Stern, R. A., & McKee, A. C. (2011). Chronic traumatic encephalopathy: A potential late effect of sport-related concussive and subconcussive head trauma. *Clinics in Sports Medicine, 30,* 179–188, xi. http://dx.doi.org/10.1016/j.csm.2010.09.007

Goldstein, L. E., Fisher, A. M., Tagge, C. A., Zhang, X.-L., Velisek, L., Sullivan, J. A., . . . McKee, A. C. (2012). Chronic traumatic encephalopathy in blast-exposed military veterans and a blast neurotrauma mouse model. *Science Translational Medicine, 4,* 134ra160. http://dx.doi.org/10.1126/scitranslmed.3003716

Golisz, K. M. (2009). *Occupational therapy practice guidelines for adults with traumatic brain injury.* Bethesda, MD: AOTA Press.

Gómez, P. A., Lobato, R. D., Ortega, J. M., & De La Cruz, J. (1996). Mild head injury: Differ-ences in prognosis among patients with a Glasgow Coma Scale score of 13 to 15 and analysis of factors associated with abnormal CT findings. *British Journal of Neurosurgery, 10,* 453–460. http://dx.doi.org/10.1080/02688699647078

Goodwin, A., Kirley, B., Sandt, L., Hall, W., Thomas, L., O'Brien, N., & Summerlin, D. (2013, April). *Countermeasures that work: A highway safety countermeasures guide for State Highway Safety Offices,* 7th edition (Report No. DOT HS 811 727). Washington, DC: National Highway Traffic Safety Administration. Retrieved from http://www.nhtsa.gov/staticfiles/nti/pdf/811727.pdf

Gouvier, W. D., Blanton, P. D., LaPorte, K. K., & Nepomuceno, C. (1987). Reliability and validity of the Disability Rating Scale and the Levels of Cognitive Functioning Scale in monitoring recovery from severe head injury. *Archives of Physical Medicine and Rehabilitation, 68,* 94–97.

Graham, J. E., Radice-Neumann, D. M., Reistetter, T. A., Hammond, F. M., Dijkers, M., & Granger, C. V. (2010). Influence of sex and age on inpatient rehabilitation outcomes among older adults with traumatic brain injury. *Archives of Physical Medicine and Rehabilitation, 91,* 43–50. http://dx.doi.org/10.1016/j.apmr.2009.09.017

Groswasser, Z., Schwab, K., & Salazar, A. M. (1997). Assessment of outcome following traumatic brain injury in adults. In R. M. Herndon (Ed.), *Handbook of neurologic rating scales* (pp. 187–208). New York: Demos Vermande.

Hagen, C. (1998). *The Rancho Los Amigos Levels of Cognitive Functioning: The revised levels* (3rd ed.). Downey, CA: Los Amigos Research and Educational Institute.

Hagen, C., Malkmus, D., & Durham, P. (1972). *Levels of Cognitive Functioning.* Downey, CA: Rancho Los Amigos Hospital.

Hall, K. M. (1997). The Functional Assessment Measure (FAM). *Journal of Rehabilitation Outcomes, 1,* 63–65.

Hall, K. M., Mann, N., High, W. M., Wright, J. M., Kreutzer, J. S., & Wood, D. (1996). Functional measures after traumatic brain injury: Ceiling effects of FIM, FIM+FAM, DRS, and CIQ. *Journal of Head Trauma Rehabilitation, 11,* 27–39. http://dx.doi.org/10.1097/00001199-199610000-00004

Hanks, R. A., Wood, D. L., Millis, S., Harrison-Felix, C., Pierce, C. A., Rosenthal, M., . . . Kreutzer, J. (2003). Violent traumatic brain injury: Occurrence, patient characteristics, and risk factors from the Traumatic Brain Injury Model Systems project. *Archives of Physical Medicine and Rehabilitation, 84,* 249–254. http://dx.doi.org/10.1053/apmr.2003.50096

Herring, S. A., Cantu, R. C., Guskiewicz, K. M., Putukian, M., Kibler, W. B., Bergfeld, J. A., . . . Indelicato, P. A.; American College of Sports Medicine. (2011). Concussion (mild traumatic brain injury) and the team physician: A consensus statement—2011 update. *Medicine and Science in Sports and Exercise, 43,* 2412–2422. http://dx.doi.org/10.1249/MSS.0b013e3182342e64

Hoffman, J. M., Dikmen, S., Temkin, N., & Bell, K. R. (2012). Development of posttraumatic stress disorder after mild traumatic brain injury. *Archives of Physical Medicine and Rehabilitation, 93,* 287–292. http://dx.doi.org/10.1016/j.apmr.2011.08.041

Hoffman, J. M., Doctor, J. N., Chan, L., Whyte, J., Jha, A., & Dikmen, S. (2003). Potential impact of the new Medicare prospective payment system on reimbursement for traumatic brain injury inpatient rehabilitation. *Archives of Physical Medicine and Rehabilitation, 84,* 1165–1172. http://dx.doi.org/10.1016/S0003-9993(03)00232-6

Huber, C. D., Lee, J. B., Yang, K. H., & King, A. I. (2005). Head injuries in airbag-equipped motor vehicles with special emphasis on AIS 1 and 2 facial and loss of consciousness injuries. *Traffic Injury Prevention, 6,* 170–174. http://dx.doi.org/10.1080/15389580590931644

Hudak, A. M., Hynan, L. S., Harper, C. R., & Diaz-Arrastia, R. (2012). Association of depressive symptoms with functional outcome after traumatic brain injury. *Journal of Head Trauma Rehabilitation, 27,* 87–98. http://dx.doi.org/10.1097/HTR.0b013e3182114efd

Hukkelhoven, C. W., Steyerberg, E. W., Rampen, A. J., Farace, E., Habbema, J. D., Marshall, L. F., . . . Maas, A. I. (2003). Patient age and outcome following severe traumatic brain injury: An analysis of 5,600 patients. *Journal of Neurosurgery, 99,* 666–673. http://dx.doi.org/10.3171/jns.2003.99.4.0666

Iverson, G. L., Echemendia, R. J., Lamarre, A. K., Brooks, B. L., & Gaetz, M. B. (2012). Possible lingering effects of multiple past concussions. *Rehabilitation Research and Practice, 2012,* 316575. http://dx.doi.org/10.1155/2012/316575

Iverson, G. L., Silverberg, N., Lange, R. T., & Zasler, N. D. (2012). Mild traumatic brain injury. In N. D. Zasler, D. I. Katz, & R. D. Zafonte (Eds.), *Brain injury medicine* (2nd ed., pp. 434–469). New York: Demos.

Jagoda, A. S. (2010). Mild traumatic brain injury: Key decisions in acute management. *Psychiatric Clinics of North America, 33,* 797–806. http://dx.doi.org/10.1016/j.psc.2010.09.004

Jagoda, A. S., Bazarian, J. J., Bruns, J. J., Jr., Cantrill, S. V., Gean, A. D., Howard, P. K., . . . Whitson, R. R. (2009). Clinical policy: Neuroimaging and decisionmaking in adult mild traumatic brain injury in the acute setting. *Journal of Emergency Nursing, 35,* e5–e40. http://dx.doi.org/10.1016/j.jen.2008.12.010

Jalali, R., & Rezaei, M. (2014). A comparison of the Glasgow Coma Scale score with Full Outline of UnResponsiveness scale to predict patients' traumatic brain injury outcomes in intensive care units. *Critical Care Research and Practice, 2014,* 289803. http://dx.doi.org/10.1155/2014/289803

Johnson, V. E., Stewart, W., & Smith, D. H. (2012). Axonal pathology in traumatic brain injury. *Experimental Neurology, 246,* 35–43. http://dx.doi.org/10.1016/j.expneurol.2012.01.013

Johnston, M. V., Goverover, Y., & Dijkers, M. (2005). Community activities and individuals' satisfaction with them: Quality of life in the first year after traumatic brain injury. *Archives of Physical Medicine and Rehabilitation, 86,* 735–745. http://dx.doi.org/10.1016/j.apmr.2004.10.031

Jordan, B. D., Relkin, N. R., Ravdin, L. D., Jacobs, A. R., Bennett, A., & Gandy, S. (1997). Apolipoprotein E epsilon4 associated with chronic traumatic brain injury in boxing. *JAMA, 278,* 136–140. http://dx.doi.org/10.1001/jama.1997.03550020068040

Kazim, S. F., Shamim, M. S., Tahir, M. Z., Enam, S. A., & Waheed, S. (2011). Management of penetrating brain injury. *Journal of Emergencies, Trauma, and Shock, 4,* 395–402. http://dx.doi.org/10.4103/0974-2700.83871

Kochanek, P. M., Clark, R. S. B., & Jenkins, L. W. (2012). Pathobiology of secondary brain injury. In N. D. Zasler, D. I. Katz, & R. D. Zafonte (Eds.), *Brain injury medicine* (2nd ed., pp. 148–161). New York: Demos.

Koskinen, S., Hokkinen, E. M., Wilson, L., Sarajuuri, J., Von Steinbüchel, N., & Truelle, J. L. (2011). Comparison of subjective and objective assessments of outcome after traumatic brain injury using the *International Classification of Functioning, Disability and Health (ICF). Disability and Rehabilitation, 33,* 2464–2478. http://dx.doi.org/10.3109/09638288.2011.574776

Kothari, S., & DiTommaso, C. (2012). Prognosis: A practical, evidence-based approach. In N. D. Zasler, D. I. Katz, & R. D. Zafonte (Eds.), *Brain injury medicine* (2nd ed., pp. 248–278). New York: Demos.

Kreutzer, J. S., & Marwitz, J. H. (2008). *The Family Needs Questionnaire–Revised.* Richmond, VA: National Resource Center for Traumatic Brain Injury.

Kreutzer, J. S., Marwitz, J. H., Hsu, N., Williams, K., & Riddick, A. (2007). Marital stability after brain injury: An investigation and analysis. *NeuroRehabilitation, 22,* 53–59.

Lazaridis, C., DeSantis, S. M., Smielewski, P., Menon, D. K., Hutchinson, P., Pickard, J. D., & Czosnyka, M. (2014). Patient-specific thresholds of intracranial pressure in severe traumatic brain injury. *Journal of Neurosurgery, 120,* 893–900. http://dx.doi.org/10.3171/2014.1.JNS131292

Lehman, E. J., Hein, M. J., Baron, S. L., & Gersic, C. M. (2012). Neurodegenerative causes of death among retired National Football League players. *Neurology, 79,* 1970–1974. http://dx.doi.org/10.1212/WNL.0b013e31826daf50

Levine, J., & Flanagan, S. R. (2012). Traumatic brain injury in the elderly. In N. D. Zasler, D. I. Katz, & R. D. Zafonte (Eds.), *Brain injury medicine* (2nd ed., pp. 420–433). New York: Demos.

Liu, B. C., Ivers, R., Norton, R., Boufous, S., Blows, S., & Lo, S. K. (2008). Helmets for preventing injury in motorcycle riders. *Cochrane Database of Systematic Reviews, 2008,* CD004333. http://dx.doi.org/10.1002/14651858.CD004333.pub3

Long, D. F. (2012). Diagnosis and management of late intracranial complications of traumatic brain injury. In N. D. Zasler, D. I. Katz, & R. D. Zafonte (Eds.), *Brain injury medicine* (2nd ed., pp. 726–747). New York: Demos.

Lundin, A., de Boussard, C., Edman, G., & Borg, J. (2006). Symptoms and disability until 3 months after mild TBI. *Brain Injury, 20,* 799–806. http://dx.doi.org/10.1080/02699050600744327

Macpherson, B. C., Macpherson, P., & Jennett, B. (1990). CT evidence of intracranial contusion and haematoma in relation to the presence, site and type of skull fracture. *Clinical Radiology, 42,* 321–326. http://dx.doi.org/10.1016/S0009-9260(05)82145-2

Magasi, S., & Post, M. W. (2010). A comparative review of contemporary participation measures' psychometric properties and content coverage. *Archives of Physical Medicine and Rehabilitation, 91*(Suppl.), S17–S28. http://dx.doi.org/10.1016/j.apmr.2010.07.011

Malec, J. F. (2004). The Mayo–Portland Participation Index: A brief and psychometrically sound measure of brain injury outcome. *Archives of Physical Medicine and Rehabilitation, 85,* 1989–1996. http://dx.doi.org/10.1016/j.apmr.2004.01.032

Malec, J. F., Brown, A. W., Leibson, C. L., Flaada, J. T., Mandrekar, J. N., Diehl, N. N., & Perkins, P. K. (2007). The Mayo Classification System for Traumatic Brain Injury Severity. *Journal of Neurotrauma, 24,* 1417–1424. http://dx.doi.org/10.1089/neu.2006.0245

Malec, J. F., & Lezak, M. D. (2003). *Manual for the Mayo–Portland Adaptability Inventory (MPAI–4).* Retrieved November 25, 2012, from http://tbims.org/combi/mpai/manual.pdf

Mallinson, T., & Hammel, J. (2010). Measurement of participation: Intersecting person, task, and environment. *Archives of Physical Medicine and Rehabilitation, 91*(Suppl.), S29–S33. http://dx.doi.org/10.1016/j.apmr.2010.04.027

Marshall, S., Bayley, M., McCullagh, S., Velikonja, D., & Berrigan, L. (2012). Clinical practice guidelines for mild traumatic brain injury and persistent symptoms. *Canadian Family Physician/Medecin de Famille Canadien, 58,* 257–267, e128–e140.

Martland, H. S. (1928). Punch drunk. *JAMA, 91,* 1103–1107. http://dx.doi.org/10.1001/jama.1928.02700150029009

Mazzini, L., Campini, R., Angelino, E., Rognone, F., Pastore, I., & Oliveri, G. (2003). Posttraumatic hydrocephalus: A clinical, neuroradiologic, and neuropsychologic assessment of long-term outcome. *Archives of Physical Medicine and Rehabilitation, 84,* 1637–1641. http://dx.doi.org/10.1053/S0003-9993(03)00314-9

McCrory, P., Davis, G., & Makdissi, M. (2012). Second impact syndrome or cerebral swelling after sporting head injury. *Current Sports Medicine Reports, 11,* 21–23. http://dx.doi.org/10.1249/JSR.0b013e3182423bfd

McCrory, P., Meeuwisse, W., Johnston, K., Dvorak, J., Aubry, M., Molloy, M., & Cantu, R. (2009). Consensus statement on concussion in sport: The 3rd International Conference on Concussion in Sport held in Zurich, November 2008. *Journal of Athletic Training, 44,* 434–448. http://dx.doi.org/10.4085/1062-6050-44.4.434

McCrory, P., Zazryn, T., & Cameron, P. (2007). The evidence for chronic traumatic encephalopathy in boxing. *Sports Medicine, 37,* 467–476. http://dx.doi.org/10.2165/00007256-200737060-00001

Meares, S., Shores, E. A., Taylor, A. J., Lammél, A., & Batchelor, J. (2011). Validation of the Abbreviated Westmead Post-Traumatic Amnesia Scale: A brief measure to identify acute cognitive impairment in mild traumatic brain injury. *Brain Injury, 25,* 1198–1205. http://dx.doi.org/10.3109/02699052.2011.608213

Menon, D. K., Schwab, K., Wright, D. W., & Maas, A. I.; Demographics and Clinical Assessment Working Group of the International and Interagency Initiative Toward Common Data Elements for Research on Traumatic Brain Injury and Psychological Health. (2010). Position statement: Definition of traumatic brain injury. *Archives of Physical Medicine and Rehabilitation, 91,* 1637–1640. http://dx.doi.org/10.1016/j.apmr.2010.05.017

Millspaugh, J. A. (1937). Dementia pugilistica. *United States Naval Medical Bulletin, 35,* 297–303.

mTBI Guidelines Development Team. (2010). *Guidelines for mild traumatic brain injury and persistent symptoms.* Toronto, ON: Ontario Neurotrauma Foundation. Retrieved from http://onf.org/system/attachments/60/original/Guidelines_for_Mild_Traumatic_Brain_Injury_and_Persistent_Symptoms.pdf

Nakase-Richardson, R., Sherer, M., Seel, R. T., Hart, T., Hanks, R., Arango-Lasprilla, J. C., . . . Hammond, F. (2011). Utility of post-traumatic amnesia in predicting 1-year productivity following traumatic brain injury: Comparison of the Russell and Mississippi PTA classification intervals. *Journal of Neurology, Neurosurgery, and Psychiatry, 82,* 494–499. http://dx.doi.org/10.1136/jnnp.2010.222489

National Center for Injury Prevention and Control. (2008). *CDC compendium of effective fall interventions: What works for community-dwelling older adults* (2nd ed.). Atlanta: Centers for Disease Control and Prevention. Retrieved from http://www.cdc.gov/HomeandRecreationalSafety/pdf/CDC_Falls_Compendium_lowres.pdf

National Conference of State Legislatures. (2014). *Traumatic brain injury legislation.* Retrieved August 17, 2014, from http://www.ncsl.org/research/health/traumatic-brain-injury-legislation.aspx

National Highway Traffic Safety Administration. (2014). *Distraction.gov: Get the facts.* Retrieved from http://www.distraction.gov/

Nichol, A. D., Higgins, A. M., Gabbe, B. J., Murray, L. J., Cooper, D. J., & Cameron, P. A. (2011). Measuring functional and quality of life outcomes following major head injury: Common scales and checklists. *Injury, 42,* 281–287. http://dx.doi.org/10.1016/j.injury.2010.11.047

Nudo, R. J., & Dancause, N. (2012). Neuroscientific basis for occupational and physical therapy interventions. In N. D. Zasler, D. I. Katz, & R. D. Zafonte (Eds.), *Brain injury medicine* (2nd ed., pp. 1133–1148). New York: Demos.

Ostir, G. V., Granger, C. V., Black, T., Roberts, P., Burgos, L., Martinkewiz, P., & Ottenbacher, K. J. (2006). Preliminary results for the PAR-PRO: A measure of home and community participation. *Archives of Physical Medicine and Rehabilitation, 87,* 1043–1051. http://dx.doi.org/10.1016/j.apmr.2006.04.024

Plum, F., & Posner, J. B. (1982). *The diagnosis of stupor and coma.* Philadelphia: F. A. Davis.

Ponsford, J., Cameron, P., Fitzgerald, M., Grant, M., & Mikocka-Walus, A. (2011). Long-term outcomes after uncomplicated mild traumatic brain injury: A comparison with trauma controls. *Journal of Neurotrauma, 28,* 937–946. http://dx.doi.org/10.1089/neu.2010.1516

Posner, J. B., Saper, C. B., Schiff, N. D., & Plum, F. (2007). *Plum and Posner's diagnosis of stupor and coma* (4th ed.). Oxford, England: Oxford University Press.

Powell, J. H., Beckers, K., & Greenwood, R. J. (1998). Measuring progress and outcome in community rehabilitation after brain injury with a new assessment instrument—The BICRO–39 scales. Brain Injury Community Rehabilitation Outcome. *Archives of Physical Medicine and Rehabilitation, 79,* 1213–1225. http://dx.doi.org/10.1016/S0003-9993(98)90265-9

Powell, J. M., Ferraro, J. V., Dikmen, S. S., Temkin, N. R., & Bell, K. R. (2008). Accuracy of mild traumatic brain injury diagnosis. *Archives of Physical Medicine and Rehabilitation, 89,* 1550–1555. http://dx.doi.org/10.1016/j.apmr.2007.12.035

Prigatano, G. P., & Gale, S. D. (2011). The current status of postconcussion syndrome. *Current Opinion in Psychiatry, 24,* 243–250. http://dx.doi.org/10.1097/YCO.0b013e328344698b

Rappaport, M., Hall, K. M., Hopkins, K., Belleza, T., & Cope, D. N. (1982). Disability Rating Scale for severe head trauma: Coma to community. *Archives of Physical Medicine and Rehabilitation, 63,* 118–123.

Rapport, L. J., Hanks, R. A., & Bryer, R. C. (2006). Barriers to driving and community integration after traumatic brain injury. *Journal of Head Trauma Rehabilitation, 21,* 34–44. http://dx.doi.org/10.1097/00001199-200601000-00004

Ratilal, B. O., Costa, J., Sampaio, C., & Pappamikail, L. (2011). Antibiotic prophylaxis for preventing meningitis in patients with basilar skull fractures. *Cochrane Database of Systematic Reviews, 2011,* CD004884. http://dx.doi.org/10.1002/14651858.CD004884.pub3

Ricker, J. H., Arenth, P. M., & Wagner, A. K. (2012). Functional neuroimaging. In N. D. Zasler, D. I. Katz, & R. D. Zafonte (Eds.), *Brain injury medicine* (2nd ed., pp. 218–229). New York: Demos.

Ruff, R. M. (2011). Mild traumatic brain injury and neural recovery: Rethinking the debate. *NeuroRehabilitation, 28,* 167–180. http://dx.doi.org/10.3233/NRE-2011-0646

Russell, W. R., & Smith, A. (1961). Post-traumatic amnesia in closed head injury. *Archives of Neurology, 5,* 4–17. http://dx.doi.org/10.1001/archneur.1961.00450130006002

Sady, M. D., Sander, A. M., Clark, A. N., Sherer, M., Nakase-Richardson, R., & Malec, J. F. (2010). Relationship of preinjury caregiver and family functioning to community integration in adults with traumatic brain injury. *Archives of Physical Medicine and Rehabilitation, 91,* 1542–1550. http://dx.doi.org/10.1016/j.apmr.2010.07.012

Sanchez, J. J., Kahn, D. E., & Bullock, M. R. (2012). Development of acute care guidelines and effect on outcome. In N. D. Zasler, D. I. Katz, & R. D. Zafonte (Eds.), *Brain injury medicine* (2nd ed., pp. 367–384). New York: Demos.

Sander, A. M., Clark, A., & Pappadis, M. R. (2010). What is community integration anyway? Defining meaning following traumatic brain injury. *Journal of Head Trauma Rehabilitation, 25,* 121–127. http://dx.doi.org/10.1097/HTR.0b013e3181cd1635

Sander, A. M., Maestas, K. L., Sherer, M., Malec, J. F., & Nakase-Richardson, R. (2012). Relationship of caregiver and family functioning to participation outcomes after postacute rehabilitation for traumatic brain injury: A multicenter investigation. *Archives of Physical Medicine and Rehabilitation, 93,* 842–848. http://dx.doi.org/10.1016/j.apmr.2011.11.031

Sasse, N., Gibbons, H., Wilson, L., Martinez-Olivera, R., Schmidt, H., Hasselhorn, M., . . . von Steinbüchel, N. (2012). Self-awareness and health-related quality of life after traumatic brain injury. *Journal of Head Trauma Rehabilitation, 28,* 464–472. http://dx.doi.org/10.1097/HTR.0b013e318263977d

Saulle, M., & Greenwald, B. D. (2012). Chronic traumatic encephalopathy: A review. *Rehabilitation Research and Practice, 2012,* 816069. http://dx.doi.org/10.1155/2012/816069

Scottish Intercollegiate Guidelines Network. (2009). *Early management of patients with a head injury*. Retrieved November 25, 2012, from http://www.sign.ac.uk/pdf/sign110.pdf

Selassie, A. W., Zaloshnja, E., Langlois, J. A., Miller, T., Jones, P., & Steiner, C. (2008). Incidence of long-term disability following traumatic brain injury hospitalization, United States, 2003. *Journal of Head Trauma Rehabilitation, 23,* 123–131. http://dx.doi.org/10.1097/01.HTR.0000314531.30401.39

Settervall, C. H., de Sousa, R. M., & Fürbringer e Silva, S. C. (2011). In-hospital mortality and the Glasgow Coma Scale in the first 72 hours after traumatic brain injury. *Revista Latino-Americana de Enfermagem, 19,* 1337–1343.

Sherer, M., Struchen, M. A., Yablon, S. A., Wang, Y., & Nick, T. G. (2008). Comparison of indices of traumatic brain injury severity: Glasgow Coma Scale, length of coma and post-traumatic amnesia. *Journal of Neurology, Neurosurgery, and Psychiatry, 79,* 678–685. http://dx.doi.org/10.1136/jnnp.2006.111187

Siegel, J. H., Loo, G., Dischinger, P. C., Burgess, A. R., Wang, S. C., Schneider, L. W., . . . Tenenbaum, N. (2001). Factors influencing the patterns of injuries and outcomes in car versus car crashes compared to sport utility, van, or pick-up truck versus car crashes: Crash Injury Research Engineering Network Study. *Journal of Trauma, 51,* 975–990. http://dx.doi.org/10.1097/00005373-200111000-00024

Simonsen, L. L., Sonne-Holm, S., Krasheninnikoff, M., & Engberg, A. W. (2007). Symptomatic heterotopic ossification after very severe traumatic brain injury in 114 patients: Incidence and risk factors. *Injury, 38,* 1146–1150. http://dx.doi.org/10.1016/j.injury.2007.03.019

Stålnacke, B. M. (2007). Community integration, social support and life satisfaction in relation to symptoms 3 years after mild traumatic brain injury. *Brain Injury, 21,* 933–942. http://dx.doi.org/10.1080/02699050701553189

Stein, D. G. (2000). Brain injury and theories of recovery. In A. L. Christensen & B. P. Uzzell (Eds.), *International handbook of neuropsychological rehabilitation* (pp. 9–32). New York: Kluwer Academic.

Stern, R. A., Daneshvar, D. H., Baugh, C. M., Seichepine, D. R., Montenigro, P. H., Riley, D. O., . . . McKee, A. C. (2013). Clinical presentation of chronic traumatic encephalopathy. *Neurology, 81,* 1122–1129. http://dx.doi.org/10.1212/WNL.0b013e3182a55f7f

Stewart, T. C., Girotti, M. J., Nikore, V., & Williamson, J. (2003). Effect of airbag deployment on head injuries in severe passenger motor vehicle crashes in Ontario, Canada. *Journal of Trauma, 54,* 266–272. http://dx.doi.org/10.1097/01.TA.0000038699.47295.2D

Teasdale, G., & Jennett, B. (1976). Assessment and prognosis of coma after head injury. *Acta Neurochirurgica, 34,* 45–55. http://dx.doi.org/10.1007/BF01405862

Thompson, H. J., & Mauk, K. (2011). *Care of the patient with mild traumatic brain injury*. Glenview, IL: American Association of Neuroscience Nurses & Association of Rehabilitation Nurses. Retrieved from http://www.rehabnurse.org/uploads/files/cpgmtbi.pdf

Tiesman, H. M., Konda, S., & Bell, J. L. (2011). The epidemiology of fatal occupational traumatic brain injury in the U.S. *American Journal of Preventive Medicine, 41,* 61–67. http://dx.doi.org/10.1016/j.amepre.2011.03.007

Toglia, J. P., & Golisz, K. M. (2012). Therapy for activities of daily living: Theoretical and practical perspectives. In N. D. Zasler, D. I. Katz, & R. D. Zafonte (Eds.), *Brain injury medicine* (2nd ed., pp. 1162–1177). New York: Demos.

Traumatic Brain Injury Model Systems National Data and Statistical Center. (2010). *Model systems brochure*. Retrieved from https://www.tbindsc.org/

Trowbridge, M. J., McKay, M. P., & Maio, R. F. (2007). Comparison of teen driver fatality rates by vehicle type in the United States. *Academic Emergency Medicine, 14,* 850–855. http://dx.doi.org/10.1111/j.1553-2712.2007.tb02317.x

Tsai, S. F., & Shu, K. H. (2010). Mannitol-induced acute renal failure. *Clinical Nephrology, 74,* 70–73. http://dx.doi.org/10.5414/CNP74070

Turner, B., Ownsworth, T., Cornwell, P., & Fleming, J. (2009). Reengagement in meaningful occupations during the transition from hospital to home for people with acquired brain injury and their family caregivers. *American Journal of Occupational Therapy, 63,* 609–620. http://dx.doi.org/10.5014/ajot.63.5.609

Uniform Data System for Medical Rehabilitation. (1997). *Guide for the Uniform Data Set for Medical Rehabilitation (including the FIM™ instrument), version 5.1*. Buffalo, NY: Author.

U.S. Department of Veterans Affairs. (2009). *VA/DoD clinical practice guidelines for management of concussion/mild traumatic brain injury (mTBI)*. Washington, DC: Author.

Vanden Bossche, L., & Vanderstraeten, G. (2005). Heterotopic ossification: A review. *Journal of Rehabilitation Medicine, 37,* 129–136. http://dx.doi.org/10.1080/16501970510027628

Vanderploeg, R. D., Belanger, H. G., & Curtiss, G. (2009). Mild traumatic brain injury and posttraumatic stress disorder and their associations with health symptoms. *Archives of Physical Medicine and Rehabilitation, 90,* 1084–1093. http://dx.doi.org/10.1016/j.apmr.2009.01.023

Vernet, M., Bashir, S., Enam, S. F., Kumru, H., & Pascual-Leone, A. (2012). Electrophysiologic techniques. In N. D. Zasler, D. I. Katz, & R. D. Zafonte (Eds.), *Brain injury medicine* (2nd ed., pp. 230–246). New York: Demos.

Vollmer, D. G., & Dacey, R. G., Jr. (1991). The management of mild and moderate head injuries. *Neurosurgery Clinics of North America, 2,* 437–455.

von Steinbuechel, N., Petersen, C., & Bullinger, M.; QOLIBRI Group. (2005). Assessment of health-related quality of life in persons after traumatic brain injury—Development of the QOLIBRI, a specific measure. *Acta Neurochirurgica, 93*(Suppl.), 43–49. http://dx.doi.org/10.1007/3-211-27577-0_6

Wakai, A., McCabe, A., Roberts, I., & Schierhout, G. (2003). Mannitol for acute traumatic brain injury. *Cochrane Database of Systematic Reviews, 2003,* CD001049. http://dx.doi.org/10.1002/14651858.CD001049.pub5

Ware, J. E., Kosinski, M., & Keller, S. K. (1994). *SF–36® Physical and Mental Health Summary Scales: A user's manual.* Boston: Health Institute.

Whiteneck, G. G. (2010). Issues affecting the selection of participation measurement in outcomes research and clinical trials. *Archives of Physical Medicine and Rehabilitation, 91*(Suppl.), S54–S59. http://dx.doi.org/10.1016/j.apmr.2009.08.154

Whiteneck, G. G., Charlifue, S. W., Gerhart, K. A., Overholser, J. D., & Richardson, G. N. (1992). Quantifying handicap: A new measure of long-term rehabilitation outcomes. *Archives of Physical Medicine and Rehabilitation, 73,* 519–526.

Whiteneck, G. G., Dijkers, M. P., Heinemann, A. W., Bogner, J. A., Bushnik, T., Cicerone, K. D., . . . Millis, S. R. (2011). Development of the Participation Assessment with Recombined Tools—Objective for use after traumatic brain injury. *Archives of Physical Medicine and Rehabilitation, 92,* 542–551. http://dx.doi.org/10.1016/j.apmr.2010.08.002

Whiteneck, G. G., Gerhart, K. A., & Cusick, C. P. (2004). Identifying environmental factors that influence the outcomes of people with traumatic brain injury. *Journal of Head Trauma Rehabilitation, 19,* 191–204. http://dx.doi.org/10.1097/00001199-200405000-00001

Whitmore, R. G., Thawani, J. P., Grady, M. S., Levine, J. M., Sanborn, M. R., & Stein, S. C. (2012). Is aggressive treatment of traumatic brain injury cost-effective? *Journal of Neurosurgery, 116,* 1106–1113. http://dx.doi.org/10.3171/2012.1.JNS11962

Wilde, E. A., McCauley, S. R., Kelly, T. M., Levin, H. S., Pedroza, C., Clifton, G. L., . . . Moretti, P. (2010). Feasibility of the Neurological Outcome Scale for Traumatic Brain Injury (NOS-TBI) in adults. *Journal of Neurotrauma, 27,* 975–981. http://dx.doi.org/10.1089/neu.2009.1193

Wilde, E. A., Whiteneck, G. G., Bogner, J., Bushnik, T., Cifu, D. X., Dikmen, S., . . . von Steinbuechel, N. (2010). Recommendations for the use of common outcome measures in traumatic brain injury research. *Archives of Physical Medicine and Rehabilitation, 91,* 1650–1660, e17. http://dx.doi.org/10.1016/j.apmr.2010.06.033

Willer, B., & Leddy, J. J. (2006). Management of concussion and post-concussion syndrome. *Current Treatment Options in Neurology, 8,* 415–426. http://dx.doi.org/10.1007/s11940-006-0031-9

Willer, B., Rosenthal, M., Kreutzer, J., Gordon, W. A., & Rempel, R. (1993). Assessment of community integration following rehabilitation for traumatic brain injury. *Journal of Head Trauma Rehabilitation, 8,* 75–87. http://dx.doi.org/10.1097/00001199-199308020-00009

Williams, R. F., & Croce, M. A. (2009). Are airbags effective in decreasing trauma in auto accidents? *Advances in Surgery, 43,* 139–145. http://dx.doi.org/10.1016/j.yasu.2009.03.003

Williams, R. F., Fabian, T. C., Fischer, P. E., Zarzaur, B. L., Magnotti, L. J., & Croce, M. A. (2008). Impact of airbags on a Level I trauma center: Injury patterns, infectious morbidity, and hospital costs. *Journal of the American College of Surgeons, 206,* 962–968, discussion 968–969. http://dx.doi.org/10.1016/j.jamcollsurg.2007.12.016

Williams, W. H., Potter, S., & Ryland, H. (2010). Mild traumatic brain injury and postconcussion syndrome: A neuropsychological perspective. *Journal of Neurology, Neurosurgery, and Psychiatry, 81,* 1116–1122. http://dx.doi.org/10.1136/jnnp.2008.171298

Wilson, F. C., Harpur, J., Watson, T., & Morrow, J. I. (2003). Adult survivors of severe cerebral hypoxia—Case series survey and comparative analysis. *NeuroRehabilitation, 18,* 291–298.

Wilson, J. T. L., Pettigrew, L. E. L., & Teasdale, G. M. (1998). Structured interviews for the Glasgow Outcome Scale and the Extended Glasgow Outcome Scale: Guidelines for their use. *Journal of Neurotrauma, 15,* 573–585. http://dx.doi.org/10.1089/neu.1998.15.573

Wood-Dauphinee, S. L., Opzoomer, M. A., Williams, J. I., Marchand, B., & Spitzer, W. O. (1988). Assessment of global function: The Reintegration to Normal Living Index. *Archives of Physical Medicine and Rehabilitation, 69,* 583–590.

World Health Organization. (2001). *International classification of functioning, disability and health.* Geneva: Author.

World Health Organization. (2004). *International statistical classification of diseases and related health problems* (10th rvsn). Geneva: Author.

Yokobori, S., & Bullock, M. R. (2012). Pathobiology of primary traumatic brain injury. In N. D. Zasler, D. I. Katz, & R. D. Zafonte (Eds.), *Brain injury medicine* (2nd ed., pp. 137–147). New York: Demos.

Yuh, E. L., & Gean, A. D. (2012). Structural neuroimaging. In N. D. Zasler, D. I. Katz, & R. D. Zafonte (Eds.), *Brain injury medicine* (2nd ed., pp. 367–384). New York: Demos.

Zaloshnja, E., Miller, T., Langlois, J. A., & Selassie, A. W. (2008). Prevalence of long-term disability from traumatic brain injury in the civilian population of the United States, 2005. *Journal of Head Trauma Rehabilitation, 23,* 394–400. http://dx.doi.org/10.1097/01.HTR.0000341435.52004.ac

Zhou, W., Xu, D., Peng, X., Zhang, Q., Jia, J., & Crutcher, K. A. (2008). Meta-analysis of APOE4 allele and outcome after traumatic brain injury. *Journal of Neurotrauma, 25,* 279–290. http://dx.doi.org/10.1089/neu.2007.0489

Zuercher, M., Ummenhofer, W., Baltussen, A., & Walder, B. (2009). The use of Glasgow Coma Scale in injury assessment: A critical review. *Brain Injury, 23,* 371–384. http://dx.doi.org/10.1080/02699050902926267

CHAPTER 2

Neuroanatomy of Traumatic Brain Injury

Fred Feuchter, PhD; Gordon Muir Giles, PhD, OTR/L, FAOTA; and Christina C. Lewis, PhD

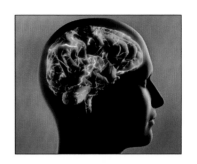

Learning Objectives

After completion of this chapter, readers will be able to

- Identify the basic structure of the cerebrum;
- Identify the basic subcomponents and organization of a neuron;
- Identify the layered structure of typical isocortex;
- Differentiate primary, unimodal, and heteromodal cortex;
- Identify the components and brain structures involved in vision, language, attention, and memory;
- Identify the cortical and subcortical circuits that are important for executive functions and behavioral control;
- Recognize the causes of primary and secondary damage to the brain associated **traumatic brain injury** (TBI);
- Recognize the damage to cranial nerves associated with TBI and their associated features; and
- Identify the pathophysiological processes associated with primary and secondary brain injury.

Key Words

- **association cortex**
- **axon**
- **basal nuclei**
- **central nervous system**
- **cerebral cortex**
- **cerebrum**
- **cranial nerves**
- **dendrites**
- **glia**
- **gray matter**
- **isocortex**
- **neural networks**
- **nucleus**
- **white matter**

Introduction

This chapter provides a review of the organization of the human **central nervous system** (CNS) and focuses specifically on the cerebral networks that, when damaged by traumatic brain injury (TBI), result in functional and behavioral changes that are the focus of occupational therapy intervention. The chapter describes a way of understanding how gene expression affects behavior and how behavior, in turn, affects gene expression. Although the chapter describes brain regions, it focuses on the interrelated systems underlying the processes that may be affected after TBI. This and the other chapters in this publication and Self-Paced Clinical Course together form a basis for understanding the ways in which performance can break down after TBI and for interventions that may help clients redevelop or compensate for neurological deficits.

Overview of the Central Nervous System

The CNS consists of the brain and the spinal cord. The brain has several anatomical subdivisions including the **cerebrum, diencephalon, brainstem,** and **cerebellum** (Figure 2.1). Each division exhibits a unique morphology and is associated with specific neural activities that are not replicated elsewhere in the CNS. For instance, the primary region that receives input from the retina about what a person sees is located in the far posterior of the cerebrum, and the area that directs automatic aversive movements when the eyes detect an object moving rapidly toward the head is located in the upper regions of the midbrain. Similarly, the area that receives pain information from the right big toe is on the inner surface of the left **cerebral hemisphere,** but the area responsible for creating new memories (say, from stubbing that toe) is buried deep within that hemisphere in the medial temporal lobe.

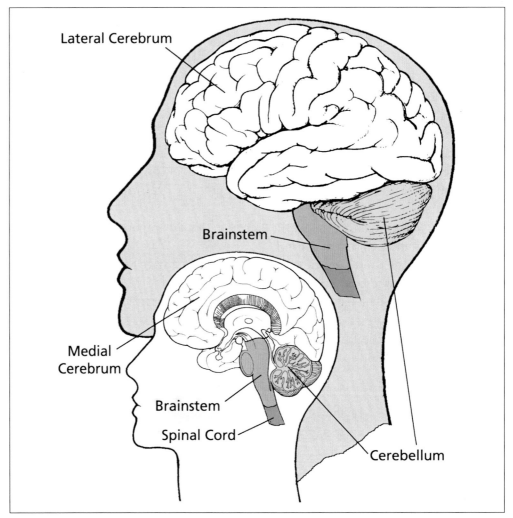

Figure 2.1. Anatomical subdivisions of the brain, including the lateral and medial cerebrum, brainstem, and cerebellum.

Source. F. Feuchter.

It is perfectly reasonable to expect that damage to a specific region of the CNS will result in loss of the neurological functions associated with the damaged region. Complex neurological tasks, however, such as the execution of purposeful movements, analysis of competing sensory inputs, and performance of cognitive processes, involve both simultaneous and sequential processing within multiple areas of the CNS. Although specific functions can be localized to specific regions of the CNS, most neurological processing takes place across **neural networks** of interconnected sites in the CNS, each of which processes specific information related to the specific neurological task. Each region may play a role in multiple functions and participate in many separate and distinct networks. Therefore, specific types of neurological dysfunction may be related either to damage to specific CNS sites or to disruptions of the interconnections among those sites. Diffuse damage to **neurons** in the **corpus callosum** is common after even mild TBI, and damage to the hemispheric **white matter,** brainstem, and cerebellum is more common after severe TBI (Blumbergs et al., 1995).

Although specific functions can be localized to specific regions of the CNS, most neurological processing takes place across neural networks of interconnected sites in the CNS.

Neurons

Nervous tissue consists of neurons and their supporting cells, **glia** (also called *neuroglia*). The primary form of neuron-to-neuron communication is through slender cytoplasmic extensions, known as ***axons,*** that form **synapses** for the release of **neurotransmitters** (Figure 2.2). The function of the axons is to transmit neural signals away from the cell body, and the function of the **dendrites,** which are typically on the opposite pole of the neuron, is to receive signals. Each neuron communicates with an average of 10^4 to 10^5 other neurons, and many axons are quite long, especially those communicating between the brain and spinal cord. Therefore, much of the volume of the brain and CNS consists of the axons and dendrites interconnecting the neurons. Chemical neurotransmitters released from the **presynaptic** neuron bind to dendrites of the **postsynaptic** neuron in the area of the synapse, changing the resting membrane potential of the cell body (-70 mV). If the membrane potential changes enough to reach the threshold value (usually -59 mV), an electrical impulse or action potential is initiated, with calcium ions flowing into the neuron and resulting in neurotransmitter release.

The neuronal cell bodies are grouped into layers or clusters at specific sites within the CNS. For instance, in the cerebrum, the neuronal cell bodies are confined to six layers from the external surface, known as the ***cerebral cortex,*** and to globular clusters deep within the center of the cerebrum, known as ***basal nuclei*** (historically referred to as *basal ganglia*). The rest of the cerebrum consists of billions of axons interconnecting neurons that are nearby, in the opposite hemisphere, or elsewhere in the CNS (see the "Cytoarchitecture of the Cerebral Cortex" section later in this chapter). Areas of the CNS that consist predominantly of axons and dendrites are known as *white matter* because the abundance of the fatty insulating **myelin** makes it appear light in color. Areas that contain nonmyelinated or thinly myelinated neuronal cell bodies are known as ***gray matter.*** Collections of neuronal cell bodies in the CNS are referred to as ***nuclei,*** and those in the **peripheral nervous system** are referred to as ***ganglia*** (Purves & Augustine, 2004).

It is generally accepted that the action of one neuron on another is most often unidirectional, propagating a neural signal from the presynaptic axon terminal of

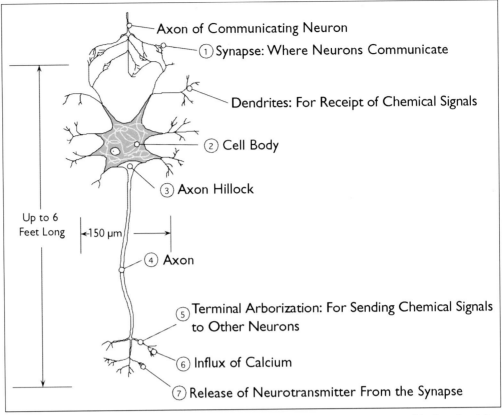

Figure 2.2. The neuron. (1) Chemical neurotransmitters released from neurons bind to dendrites in the area of the synapse. (2) Binding changes the resting potential of the membrane in the cell body (−70 mV). If the potential changes enough to reach the threshold value (usually −59 mV), an action potential is initiated from the axon hillock (3), which travels down the axon (4) to the terminus (5), resulting in calcium ions flowing into the neuron (6). The influx of calcium causes release of the neurotransmitter in the direction of the next neuron's dendrites (7). The activity of neurons can be blocked by blocking the energy supply necessary to maintain membrane potential, blocking the binding of the neurotransmitter to dendrites, or blocking release of the neurotransmitter into the synaptic cleft.

Source. F. Feuchter.

the first (presynaptic) neuron to different sites on the second (postsynaptic) neuron. The postsynaptic neuron can also send information upstream to the presynaptic neuron (retrograde transmission). Examples of substances that can exert their effects via retrograde neurotransmission are endocannabinoids, nitrous oxide, and neurotrophic factors, which can stimulate the **genome** of the presynaptic neuron.

Although the synapse has traditionally dominated the conceptual model of neurotransmission, other mechanisms, such as **neuromodulation** and **nonsynaptic diffusion neurotransmission** (NDN), have also been considered to support and complement synaptic transmission. In neuromodulation, several classes of neurotransmitters regulate diverse populations of CNS neurons (Stahl, 2008). In contrast to direct synaptic transmission, neuromodulators secreted by a small group of neurons diffuse throughout large areas of the nervous system, thereby exerting their effect on numerous neurons. Examples of neuromodulators include dopamine, serotonin, **acetylcholine,** and histamine. NDN involves the diffusion of neurotransmitters through the **extracellular fluid** and other neuroactive substances released at sites that may be remote from the target cells, with the resulting activation of extrasynaptic receptors (Stahl, 2008). An example of NDN is dopamine in the **prefrontal cortex.** Some substances, such as nitric oxide, diffuse both through the extracellular fluid and across the cellular membranes to act within the cell. NDN is postulated to play a role in expansive and sustained functions such as **mood** and sleep. Because receptor up-regulation and down-regulation in response to brain damage may be among the methods of compensating for the damage, NDN may play a role in brain **plasticity** (Bach-y-Rita, 1995).

The timing and the pattern of neurotransmission, as well as the type of transmission and the specific neurotransmitter, are all important in brain functioning. Some neurotransmitter signals exhibit a fast onset, starting within milliseconds of the receptors being occupied by the neurotransmitter. Two of the best examples of fast-onset signals are those elicited by the neurotransmitters glutamate and γ-aminobutyric acid (GABA). Glutamate almost uniformly stimulates the neuron it contacts, and GABA almost uniformly inhibits the neuron it contacts. Both glutamate and GABA can cause fast-onset chemical signaling by rapidly altering the excitability of the neurons. Signals from other neurotransmitters (e.g., dopamine, serotonin) can take longer to develop, ranging from many milliseconds to several seconds. Sometimes neurotransmitters with slow onset are also called *neuromodulators* because their actions may last long enough to carry over and modulate a subsequent neurotransmission by another neurotransmitter (Stahl, 2008).

All of this chemical back-and-forth may provoke structural changes at the synapses that increase the ease of neurotransmission and create a mini-network. The nature of the effects of a neurotransmitter on the target cell is dependent on its chemical composition. Neurotransmitters arriving at the cell membrane will either trigger the actions of second messengers within the cell (i.e., protein-based neurotransmitters) or diffuse across the membrane, eventually reaching the cell nucleus and ultimately resulting in either the initiation or the inhibition of gene expression (i.e., steroid-based neurotransmitters). In the case of protein-based neurotransmitters, the second messengers are signal transducers that pass along the neural signal from the cell membrane to the intracellular environment, which ultimately change the physiology via myriad mechanisms. In the case of steroid-based neurotransmitters, the behavior of the cell is altered once a change in gene expression has been triggered, and a second biochemical cascade is initiated. Collectively, through these processes, irrespective of the composition of the neurotransmitters, patterns of neuronal firing related to a person's experiences or activities can lead to modification of neuronal connections and the development of networks. Thus, the function of chemical neurotransmission is not so much to have a presynaptic neurotransmitter communicate with its postsynaptic receptors as it is to have a presynaptic genome converse with a postsynaptic genome (Stahl, 2008). In this way, chemical neurotransmission may lead to alterations in behavior patterns—that is, people's experiences and what they do can lead to structural brain changes and ultimately to enduring changes in patterns of thought, **emotion,** and behavior (Stahl, 2008).

Glial Cells

Neurons perform the essential communication functions of the brain, but the glial cells (neuroglia) outnumber them as much as tenfold. Unlike neurons, glial cells are not electrically excitable and do not propagate action potentials.

Rather, they maintain the appropriate microenvironment essential for neuronal functions and provide neurons with physical and mechanical support (*glia* means "glue"). Although glial cells do not participate directly in synaptic interactions, their supportive functions help organize synaptic contacts and maintain the signaling abilities of neurons (Sharma & Vijayaraghavan, 2001; Ullian, Sapperstein, Christopherson, & Barres, 2001). The three main varieties of glial cells are (1) **astrocytes,** (2) **oligodendrocytes,** and (3) **microglia.**

Overview of the Cerebrum

The cerebrum is associated with **consciousness** and controls the most complex and highest order functions of the brain, such as language, perception, voluntary movement, understanding of spatial relationships, decision making, **memory,** and emotions. The cerebrum is more developed in humans than in other animals and is the newest and most highly evolved portion of the brain. It consists of the cerebral cortex, which forms the visible surface of the brain, and the subcortical basal nuclei, which are buried deep within the cerebrum and are not visible except by slicing the brain in horizontal or coronal planes.

Cerebral Hemispheres

The cerebrum is divided into left and right hemispheres, which are separated by the deep **longitudinal fissure.** The surface of each hemisphere consists of numerous folds, known as *gyri* (singular *gyrus*), and intervening grooves, known as *sulci* (singular *sulcus*). Although certain gyri and sulci are present in almost every human brain, no two brains have exactly the same folding patterns. The outer surface of the cerebrum, the *cerebral cortex,* is composed of gray matter that is organized into six layers of neurons. The highly folded nature of the cortical surface allows for the presence of many more neurons than could be accommodated if the brain surface were not folded. The **lateral ventricles,** which lie deep below the cortical surface, may become enlarged because of the loss of **subcortical** gray and white matter (loss of cells in the basal nuclei and loss of axons or myelin in the white matter) that occurs in **diffuse axonal injury** after TBI.

It is noteworthy that the folding of the cerebrum increases in tandem with progression up the phylogenetic tree (i.e., the more complex the animal, the more folded its cerebrum). Brain size generally varies with the size of an animal (i.e., larger animals have larger brains); however, relative to their size, humans have the largest frontal lobe of any animal.

Each cerebral hemisphere can be divided into six lobes: (1) **frontal,** (2) **parietal,** (3) **temporal,** (4) **occipital,** (5) **insular,** and (6) **limbic** (Figure 2.3, top). The lateral surface of each hemisphere is split by a deep groove known as the ***lateral sulcus*** (or ***Sylvian fissure***), which gives the hemisphere the shape of a boxing glove. The cortex lying inferior to this groove (i.e., the thumb of the glove) is called the *temporal lobe* because it is situated beneath the temporal bone (and temple region) of the skull. About midway between the anterior and posterior aspects of the cerebrum, another groove, the ***central sulcus (of Rolando),*** runs vertically from the lateral sulcus to the vertex. The cerebrum anterior to the central sulcus is the *frontal lobe* and that immediately posterior to the central sulcus is the *parietal lobe.* The most posterior region of the cerebrum is the *occipital lobe,* which is not very well delineated from the parietal lobe and continues on the lateral and medial surfaces of

Brain size generally varies with the size of an animal (i.e., larger animals have larger brains); however, relative to their size, humans have the largest frontal lobe of any animal.

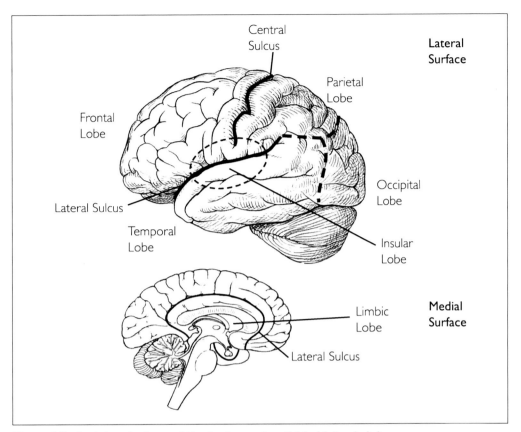

Figure 2.3. Each hemisphere of the brain can be divided into six lobes.
Source. F. Feuchter.

the posterior aspect of the hemisphere. The remaining two of the six lobes cannot be seen on the surface. However, if the borders of the lateral sulcus are spread apart, additional cortex is revealed: the *insular lobe* (see Figure 2.3, top). The sixth region, the *limbic lobe,* cannot be viewed clearly unless the brain is cut in the midsagittal plane (see Figure 2.3, bottom). The limbic lobe consists of the gyrus immediately surrounding the corpus callosum (the **cingulate gyrus,** described in the "Networks of Attention" section) and the medial surface of the temporal lobe.

Cytoarchitecture of the Cerebral Cortex

Within the cerebral cortex, two basic types of neurons can be found: (1) neurons with large, pyramidal (pyramid-shaped) cell bodies and (2) smaller, nonpyramidal neurons with multiple morphologies, often referred to collectively as *granular neurons.* The pyramidal cells represent about 75% of the population of neurons. They have long axons that may leave the cortex and communicate with other brain regions or extend to distant cortical sites. In contrast, many of the granular neurons have shorter axons that do not leave the cerebral cortex and compose the intracortical circuitry.

Most of the cerebral cortex (about 95%) exhibits a well-defined *lamellar* (i.e., layerlike) organization, with the cells arranged in six layers, numbered I through VI from the surface inward (Figure 2.4). This organization is unique to the evolution of the human brain and is therefore referred to as the *neocortex,* or "new cortex." The multiple layering of neurons is related to the organization of the inputs and outputs. For instance, synapses for receiving nonspecific thalamic input are in Layers I and II,

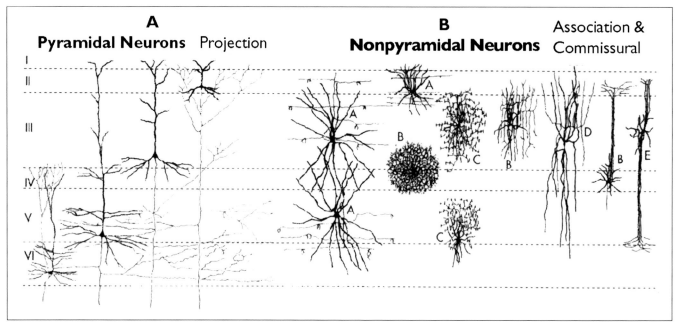

Figure 2.4. The cerebral cortex has a well-defined *lamellar* (i.e., layerlike) appearance with neurons arranged in six layers, numbered I through VI from the surface inward. **(A)** Pyramidal neurons in different layers have characteristically different soma sizes and patterns of distribution of axon collaterals. **(B)** Nonpyramidal neurons come in a variety of sizes and shapes; many have names attributable to their shape. Basket cells (A) are usually large and make basket-shaped endings that partially surround the cell bodies of pyramidal cells. Other kinds of smaller multipolar cells (B) may have elaborate dendritic and axonal arborizations. Chandelier cells (C) have vertically oriented synaptic "candles" that end on the initial segments of pyramidal cell axons. Bipolar cells (D) have dendrites that both ascend and descend, and double bouquet cells (E) have axons that both ascend and descend.

Source. From *The Human Brain* (5th ed., p. 528), by J. Nolte, 2002, St. Louis: Mosby. Copyright © 2002 by Elsevier. Used with permission.

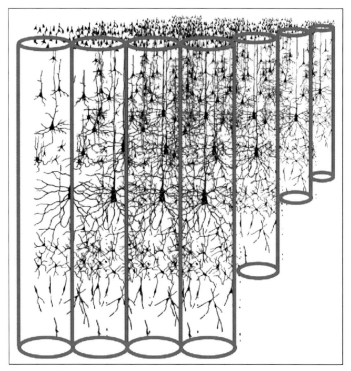

Figure 2.5. Cortical columns. All the neurons within a column are concerned with a single, specific aspect of a neurological task.

Source. F. Feuchter.

whereas synapses for receiving input from specific thalamic nuclei are in Layer IV. Layer III contains neurons that send information to and receive information from nearby cortical areas and the other cerebral hemisphere. Layer V is the location of large pyramidal cells that send output to distant sites such as the brainstem, spinal cord, and basal nuclei. Cells in Layer VI are the source of **corticothalamic fibers.**

The functional unit of the cerebral cortex at the microscopic level is the ***cortical column*** (Figure 2.5; Mountcastle, 1998). All the neurons within a column share in common a specific aspect of a neurological task. For example, a column in the visual cortex may be responsible for detecting an edge at a certain angle at a small spot of the retina. Cortical columns are about 50 to 500 μm in diameter and extend vertically through all six layers of the cortex. Each column contains neurons that receive inputs from extracortical sites (specific and nonspecific) and other areas within the cortex, and each additionally has neurons responsible for sending signals out to other cortical areas. When large numbers of columns in a given region of the cerebral cortex are involved in the specific functions characteristic of that region and span all six well-defined cell layers (i.e., of the neocortex), they are referred to as ***isocortex*** ("same cortex"). Other areas with fewer than six layers are referred to as ***allocortex*** ("other cortex"), whereas those with between three and six layers are referred to as ***mesocortex*** ("middle cortex"). Allocortex and mesocortex represent evolutionarily older cortex and are found mostly in the medial portions of the temporal lobe, the insula, and the limbic lobe.

The cell layers are not uniform across the neocortex. Rather, different regions vary in thickness of the layers and relative proportions of pyramidal and granular neurons. Most areas of isocortex are ***homotypic isocortex;*** that is, they display the prototypical six layers of varying thickness and differing proportions of neurons (Figure 2.6). Certain areas, however, show extreme variations of the homotypic pattern and are referred to as ***heterotypic isocortex.*** Heterotypic cortex of the granular variety contains almost entirely granular neurons and no pyramidal cells, whereas agranular heterotypic cortex consists almost entirely or entirely of pyramidal neurons. Differences in layering can be related to functions within a region. For instance, motor and premotor regions consist almost exclusively of agranular cortex, as one might expect, because the agranular pyramidal cells have long projection axons for carrying motor commands to distant sites where they are needed. The primary motor and sensory cortices are illustrated in Figure 2.7. The primary receptive regions for

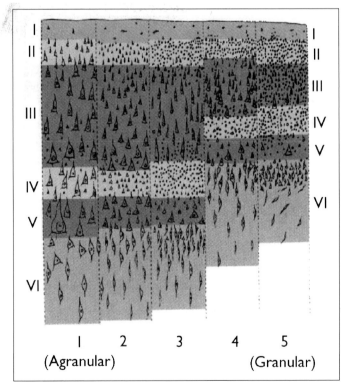

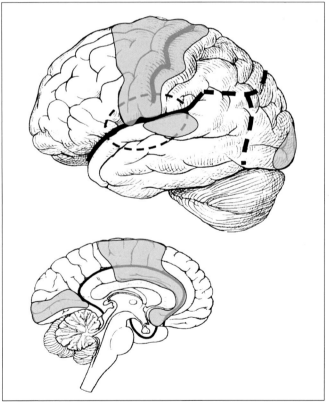

Figure 2.6. Neocortex regions vary in thickness of the layers and relative proportions of agranular (pyramidal) and granular neurons. Most areas of the isocortex are *homotypic isocortex;* that is, they display the prototypical six layers of varying thickness and differing proportions of neurons.

Source. From *The Human Brain* (5th ed., p. 530), by J. Nolte, 2002, St. Louis: Mosby. Copyright © 2002 by Elsevier. Used with permission.

Figure 2.7. The primary motor and sensory cortices. The primary receptive regions for hearing, vision, and somatosensory functions (shaded) consist of granular cortex. The unshaded portion is association cortex, which shows homotypic structure.

Source. F. Feuchter.

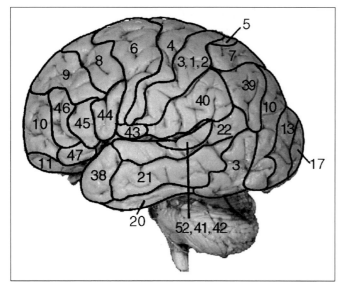

Figure 2.8. Each numbered Brodmann's area denotes a region of the cortex that has a microscopic appearance, cell composition, and thickness of layers that differentiate it from other areas. Many of the Brodmann's areas are used today as a way of describing particular areas of the cortex, but only some of those areas can be associated with single functions.

Source. F. Feuchter.

hearing, vision, and somatosensory functions consist of granular cortex; granular cells typically process information locally and interconnect regional cortical sites.

Most of the remaining cortex is **association cortex,** which shows homotypic structure (see the unshaded portion of Figure 2.7). The association cortex can be further divided into ***unimodal association cortices,*** which process a single kind of sensory modality (e.g., visual, auditory, or somatosensory association areas), and *unimodal motor association cortex,* which deals exclusively with programming movements. Lesions in unimodal association areas lead to complex deficits in sensory perception, but the elemental sensations remain intact. *Heteromodal association cortex* receives input from multiple unimodal areas. Neurons in heteromodal association cortex are responsible for the integration of sensory or sensorimotor material or, in some cases, fire in response to stimuli having some motivational significance. This pattern makes sense when one considers awareness of objects or events in the real world: A person is aware of objects and events not along a single perceptual plane but rather across modes of perception. For example, bacon has a certain odor; tastes salty; and has attributes of shape, color, and texture that are quite specific. **Heteromodal association areas** can be found in prefrontal regions and the posterior parietal and temporal lobes. Lesions in heteromodal areas result in complex deficits involving both cognitive and affective functions.

The concept that the variation in the appearance of the cortex might be related to function has led to use of a map to delineate areas of the cortex that are identical in their microscopic appearance. The map divides the brain into areas on the basis of their cytoarchitecture known as ***Brodmann's areas*** (Figure 2.8), named after the German scientist Korbinian Brodmann (1868–1918) who developed it. Although many of the Brodmann's areas are used today as a way of describing particular areas of the cortex, only some of those areas can be associated with a single function, with many apparently serving multiple functions. For instance, the primary motor area is Brodmann's area 4; the primary somatosensory areas are Brodmann's areas 1, 2, and 3; and the **primary visual area** is Brodmann's area 17. The complex tasks of the cerebrum, such as those embodied in higher-level cognitive functions, can be localized to larger regions of cortex that overlap many of the Brodmann's areas.

Functional Areas of Cerebral Cortex

The current understanding of the cerebral cortex is that local networks of neurons in specific anatomical areas are activated during the performance of mental tasks. Each local network is composed of multiple interconnected cortical columns and performs a particular operation during a mental task. Most mental activity involves sequential processing of information by multiple networks. For example, information from the retina is sent first to the primary visual cortex, but this information is

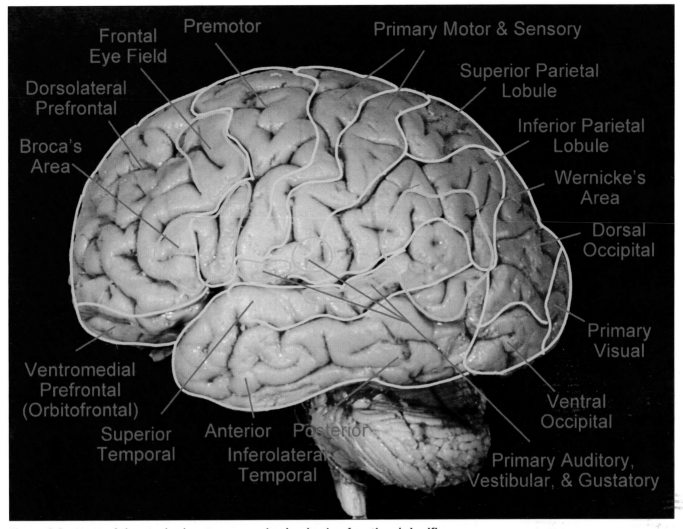

Figure 2.9. Areas of the cerebral cortex recognized as having functional significance.
Source. F. Feuchter.

coded as edges on certain locations on the retina. The input about edges is passed to other nearby areas of the occipital lobe to generate a representation of the visible object and then to the parietal lobe before an understanding of what is being seen is generated. If the task is to name the visible object, additional networks for the retrieval of the name from memory and for verbalization are involved.

Many areas of the cerebral cortex recognized as having a particular functional significance are shown in Figure 2.9, and recognized function–location associations are summarized in Table 2.1.

Lateralization

The issues of lateralization and localization of function in the human brain are complex. Many basic perceptual and motor functions are *lateralized* (i.e., one hemisphere governs the **contralateral** half of the body). Higher order attentional, representational, and processing capacities tend to exhibit *hemispheric specialization*, which is the tendency for one hemisphere to carry out more than 50% of a particular function. Many conditions that were initially thought to be basic

Table 2.1. Summary of Functions of Brain Regions

Region	Function
Frontal Lobe	
Primary motor cortex	Major source of cells (upper motor neurons) for the descending motor pathways that are essential for the voluntary control of movement and that are part of the reflex circuits of brainstem and spinal cord
	Located in the precentral gyrus (Brodmann's area 4)
Premotor cortex	Planning and initiation of voluntary movement, guidance of limb trajectory based on cerebellar input
	Located anterior to the primary motor cortex within the lateral surface of the frontal lobe (part of Brodmann's area 6)
Supplementary motor cortex	Planning of complex movements with motor sequences derived from basal nuclei input, bilateral movements
	Located within the medial surface of the frontal lobe, in the superior frontal gyrus anterior to the primary motor cortex (part of Brodmann's area 6)
Frontal eye field	Direction of eye movement into the contralateral visual hemisphere, volitional saccadic eye movements
	Located in the rostral portion of the premotor cortex and in the posterior portion of the middle frontal gyrus (Brodmann's area 8)
Broca's area	Production of language, both written and spoken
	Located in the inferior frontal gyrus of the dominant hemisphere, usually left (Brodmann's areas 44 and 45)
Area for **prosody**	Musical aspects of speech, production and recognition of the rhythmic and tonal aspects (*prosody*) of speech that convey much of its emotional meaning, equivalent of Broca's or Wernicke's areas or both
	Located in the inferior frontal gyrus of the nondominant hemisphere, usually right
Prefrontal cortex	**Executive functions** of the brain; receipt of inputs from sensory, motor association, and limbic areas; decision making, planning, and selection of appropriate responses in social situations; problem solving
	Located anterior to the premotor and supplementary motor cortical areas
Dorsolateral	Critical role in working memory; **attention** and problem solving; massive connectivity with somatosensory, visual, and auditory association areas of the cortex (Brodmann's areas 8, 9, and 46)
	Left: Verbal intellectual capacities; creative, flexible, verbal thinking; verbal fluency
	Right: Nonverbal intellectual capacities; creative, flexible, nonverbal thinking; design fluency
Ventromedial	Interconnection with limbic structures, emotional aspects of planning and decision making, emotional behaviors and reactions, social conduct, impulse control, judgment, planning, decision making, triggering of bodily states associated with emotions (Brodmann's area 10)
Superomedial	Emotional behavior, emotional aspects of planning and decision making, motivation, basic drive states, maintenance of adaptive state of **arousal** and alertness, personality characteristics (Brodmann's areas 6, 8, 10, and 12)
Occipital Lobe	
Primary visual cortex	Perception of edges
	Located in the banks of the calcarine sulcus (Brodmann's area 17)
Ventral	*Left:* Perception of shapes and contours (features), color perception and naming, reading, face recognition (features); the "what" recognition system
	Right: Perception of shapes and contours (global), color perception, nonverbal pattern recognition, face recognition (holistic); the "what" recognition system
Dorsal	*Left:* Depth and motion perception, **stereopsis,** visual attention, recognition of identity from movement; the "where" recognition system
	Right: Depth and motion perception, stereopsis, visual attention, visually guided reaching, recognition of identity from movement, mental rotation; the "where" recognition system
Parietal Lobe	
Primary **somatosensory cortex**	Primary sensory perception of touch, vibration, temperature, and pain
	Located in the postcentral gyrus (Brodmann's areas 1, 2, and 3)
Superior	Integration of tactile and visual information, sensory and visually guided movements
Inferior	*Left:* Tactile object recognition, verbatim repetition
	Right: Tactile object recognition, self-perception, mapping of physical and emotional states, placement of oneself in space
Wernicke's area	Comprehension of language, both written and spoken
	Located in the posterior part of the superior temporal gyrus of the dominant hemisphere, usually left (Brodmann's area 22)

(Continued)

Table 2.1. Summary of Functions of Brain Regions *(cont.)*

Region	Function
Temporal Lobe	
Primary auditory cortex	Primary auditory sensation
	Located in the transverse temporal gyri (Brodmann's areas 41 and 42)
Superior	*Left:* Speech perception and comprehension, processing of temporal aspects of auditory signals
	Right: Processing and comprehension of nonverbal sounds, music, timbre, prosody, perception of spectral aspects of aural signals
Inferolateral	*Posterior:* Visual object recognition, face recognition
	Anterior left: Common and proper noun retrieval, retrieval of verbal information from memory
	Anterior right: Comprehension of emotional meanings of nonverbal stimuli, retrieval of nonverbal information from memory
Medial	*Left:* Anterograde verbal memory, acquisition of new verbal information
	Right: Anterograde nonverbal memory, acquisition of new nonverbal information

perceptual problems are really disorders of higher order processing and integration. Examples of higher order processing disorders that interfere with basic functions include neglect syndromes and **prosopagnosia.**

Other Hemispheric Specialization

Table 2.1 provides an overview of lateralization. Lateralized functions include language functions and the hemispheric association of holistic versus analytic modes of **information processing.** The right side is responsible for the analysis of the gestalt of a figure, outside contour, and holistic elements, and the left side is responsible for a local detail-by-detail analysis (Kaplan, 1988). In addition, a lack of awareness is associated with right-sided brain damage, whereas depression and catastrophic reactions are associated with left-sided brain damage.

White Matter of the Cerebrum

The bulk of the cerebrum consists of white matter, composed of the axons that interconnect different areas of the cortex with each other and with distant sites. Normal functioning of the cerebral cortex requires intact connections among its component parts and with other parts of the CNS. The fibrous nature of the brain is not apparent on sliced sections but can be seen clearly in specimens that have been pulled apart (Figures 2.10 and 2.11). Three kinds of axons are present in the white matter and are defined by where they travel: (1) projection axons, (2) long axons, and (3) short axons. Projection axons carry, or project, impulses to and from sites outside the cerebrum. **Projection fibers** originate either in the cerebrum and synapse in the brainstem or originate in the **thalamus** and synapse in the cerebrum. The bundle of fibers carrying projection axons is called the *internal capsule;* the internal capsule lies deep within the cerebrum, where it is tightly compacted (see Figure 2.10). In locations near the cerebral cortex, the bundle of projection fibers is referred to as the ***corona radiata*** because it is expanded and resembles a fan (*corona* means "crown"; *radiata* means "to spread out from a center or be arranged in a radial pattern").

Long and short association fibers interconnect various sites within the same cerebral hemisphere (see Figure 2.11). The major long-fiber bundles are known as the *occipitofrontal fasciculus* and the *arcuate fasciculus,* but many other bundles also exist.

Three kinds of axons are present in the white matter and are defined by where they travel: (1) projection axons, (2) long axons, and (3) short axons.

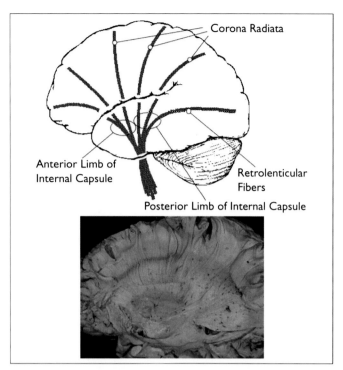

Figure 2.10. Projection axons leave the cerebrum and enter the brainstem or enter the cerebrum from the thalamus. They carry impulses to and from sites outside the cerebrum.

Source. F. Feuchter.

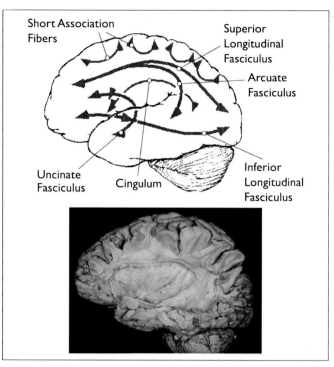

Figure 2.11. Long and short association fibers interconnect various sites within the same cerebral hemisphere. The fibrous nature of the brain is not apparent on sliced sections but can be seen clearly on specimens that have been pulled apart.

Source. F. Feuchter.

The fibers connecting one gyrus to another are simply called *short association fibers.* Finally, bundles of fibers interconnect mirror-image sites in the opposite hemisphere; these site-to-site connections across the hemispheres are known as ***commissural fibers,*** the most prominent collection of which is the corpus callosum (Figure 2.12), which, as mentioned earlier, is highly susceptible to damage in TBI.

Cerebral Networks

Our current understanding of information processing in the cerebral cortex is based on the concept of multiple networks. The local networks of cortical columns, which perform a particular operation of a mental task, are interconnected with other sites in the brain that perform other aspects of the task. Thus, multiple brain areas form large networks that are involved in higher cognitive functions. This view expands on the earlier view that the cerebrum operates on the basis of serial, unidirectional processing from primary sensory to association to motor areas in the manner of an elaborate reflex arc. Discoveries about the cortical connections of primates have led to the idea that information processing occurs in simultaneous parallel processes in large-scale networks. This model of cortical functioning takes into account that heteromodal association areas interconnect reciprocally not only with unimodal areas and with each other but also with paralimbic and limbic areas necessary for motivation, learning, and memory. Essentially, simultaneous activation of the various functional areas in a cortical network occurs during task performance. Many of the functional networks also involve subcortical structures.

Most of the cerebral surface is classified as association cortex and is responsible for the complex processing that follows the arrival of input from primary sensory cortices and that leads to the generation of behavior via connections to the primary motor cortex. Higher order cerebral functions depend on both local cortical functions and distributed network functions; for example, reading depends on vision and language. Numerous subcortical structures participate in such integrative functions. For example, complex behavioral functions (*executive functions*) are managed via a range of frontal subcortical circuits. Thus, specific neurobehavioral deficits can be caused not only by focal cortical lesions but also by lesions that involve only subcortical structures or by lesions that disrupt cortical–cortical or cortical–subcortical network connections.

Knowledge about the functions of cortical regions comes primarily from observations of patients with damage to one or another of these areas. Noninvasive neuroimaging of neurologically healthy people, functional mapping during neurosurgery, and electrophysiological analysis of comparable brain regions in nonhuman primates have generally confirmed the clinical deductions (Squire & Wixted, 2011). Together, the studies indicate that the parietal association cortex has particular responsibility for attending to stimuli in the external and internal environments, the temporal association cortex is important in identifying the nature of such stimuli, and the frontal association cortex is especially important in planning and controlling appropriate behavioral responses.

That TBI from a major impact or blow may damage localized regions of neurons and cortical columns is intuitive. TBI caused by excessive rotation of the brain, as in severe whiplash or **coup–contrecoup injury,** may result in widespread damage to white matter tracts that interconnect various regions and form the intrinsic cerebral networks. Several critical brain networks are described next.

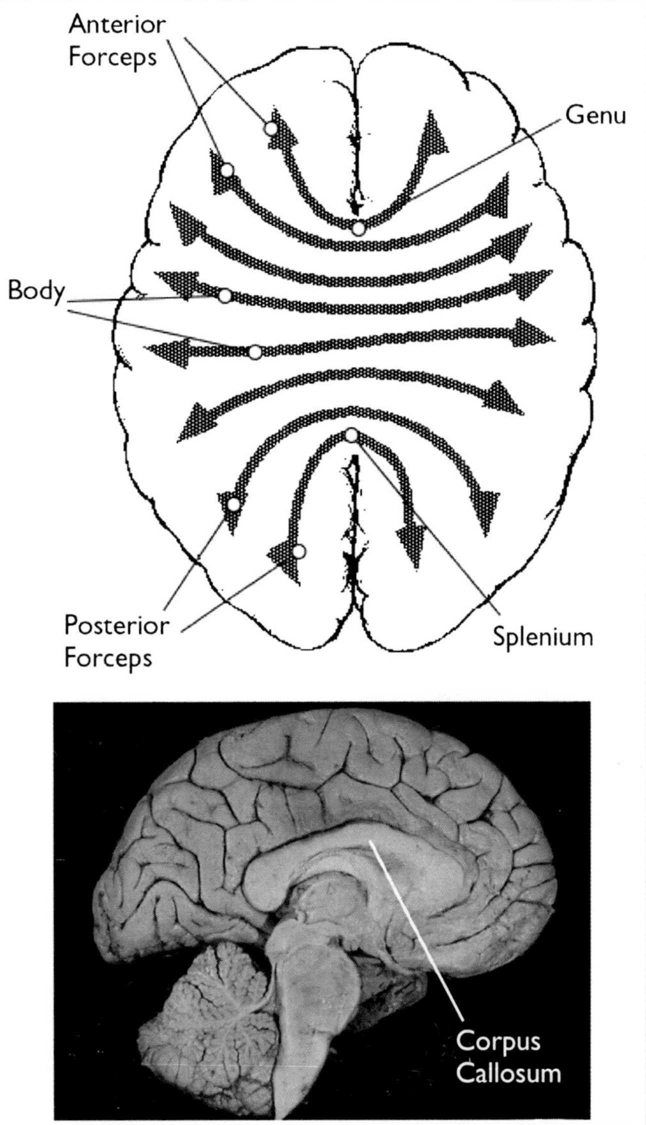

Figure 2.12. Bundles of fibers interconnect identical sites between the two hemispheres. These fibers are known as *commissural fibers,* the most prominent of which is the corpus callosum.

Source. F. Feuchter.

> Specific neurobehavioral deficits can be caused not only by focal cortical lesions but also by lesions that involve only subcortical structures or by lesions that disrupt cortical–cortical or cortical–subcortical network connections.

Visual Networks

Among the earliest investigated and best understood of the cerebral networks is the system for processing visual stimuli. The general organizational features of the visual system have been well established in all primates, including human beings, from decades of detailed study of patients with permanently impaired vision and from laboratory experiments with nonhuman primates. Input from the visual system is the trigger for many forms of higher mental activity, such as pattern recognition, the construction of mental images in the absence of outside stimuli, and the interpretation of symbols involved in reading.

When examining the specifics of vision, it is useful to divide the **visual fields** into right and left halves because the parts of the retina of each eye that receive light from the left half of the visual field send the information to the right half of the visual cortex through their connections. Similarly, the parts of the retina of each eye that receive light from the right half of the visual field send the information to the left half of the visual cortex (Figure 2.13). Thus, the information from the right visual world is received and analyzed on the left side of the cerebrum, whereas the information from the left visual world is received and analyzed on the right side of the cerebrum. Each cell in the visual cortex receives its input only from a particular part of the retina and, hence, from a particular part of the visual field, which is

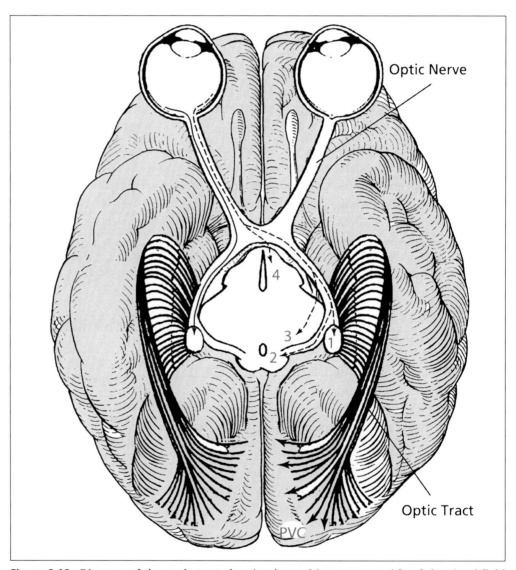

Figure 2.13. Diagram of the optic tract showing how objects on one side of the visual field send information to the contralateral visual cortex. (1) Lateral geniculate nucleus, (2) superior colliculus, (3) pretectal region, (4) hypothalamus.

Source. F. Feuchter.

Note. PVC = primary visual cortex.

called the *receptive field of the cell.* Therefore, the cells of the retina and the corresponding cells of the visual cortex to which they report have a precise topographic relationship, called *retinotopic* because it defines a particular place on the retina. In this organizational scheme, adjacent regions of the retina (and thus visual field) are connected to cells in the primary visual cortex that are also located adjacent to each other. Additionally, the cells in the corresponding location on the other retina are also connected to cells in primary visual cortex in areas adjacent to those from the other eye.

The axons in the optic nerve synapse in the **lateral geniculate nucleus** (LGN) of the *thalamus* (the sensory relay center for all sensory inputs except **olfaction**). From the thalamus, the optic tract fibers radiate to the primary visual cortex. Additionally, the optic nerve fibers communicate with three other important areas of the brain: (1) The **superior colliculus** of the brainstem receives input from the optic nerve to coordinate reflexive eye and head movement, (2) the pretectal region of the midbrain receives input from the optic nerve to control the pupillary light reflex, and (3) the **suprachiasmatic nucleus** of the hypothalamus receives input from the optic nerve to regulate **diurnal rhythms** and hormonal levels.

Information flow from the retina through the optic nerves and tracts appears to follow one of three main data streams on the basis of shape, movement, and color. This organization is preserved in the LGN and passed on to the primary visual area V1 (Brodmann's area 17). However, the color, shape, and movement information from the thalamus is sent to different and specific neurons within V1 for processing and then subsequently sent on to different areas of the occipital lobe known as *extrastriate visual cortex* (described later in this section). Within V1, a population of cells known as *blob cells* process information about color, including the perception and discrimination of color and the learning and memory of the color of objects. Also within V1 are the *interblob cells,* which exhibit orientation and location specificity; are not motion sensitive; and are used in object perception, discrimination, learning, and memory or in **spatial orientation.** These interblob cells are the shape- and form-processing cells and the location-processing cells of V1. A second subset of interblob cells respond preferentially to moving stimuli without a preference for the direction of movement. A third subset respond preferentially to movement in a particular direction. The motion-sensitive V1 interblob cells detect object movement, direction, and velocity and guide eye movements. Motion-sensitive interblob cells are the motion-detecting cells of V1.

The medioposterior surfaces of the occipital lobe are devoted to primary vision (Brodmann's area 17; Figure 2.14). Bundles of nerve fibers innervating the primary visual cortex form a clear stripe visible to the naked eye termed the *striate cortex* (*striate* means "striped"). The striate cortex is split by a prominent sulcus known as the *calcarine fissure,* which marks the division between the inputs received from the upper versus lower halves of the visual field. The input is inverted, with the striate cortex inferior to the calcarine fissure receiving input from the upper half of the visual field and the striate cortex superior to the calcarine fissure receiving input from the lower half of the visual field. Moreover, the volume of striate cortex receiving input from specific areas of the retina varies depending on the location within the retina. Significantly more striate cortex is devoted to analyzing input from central parts of the retina, especially the **macula lutea.** Peripheral parts of

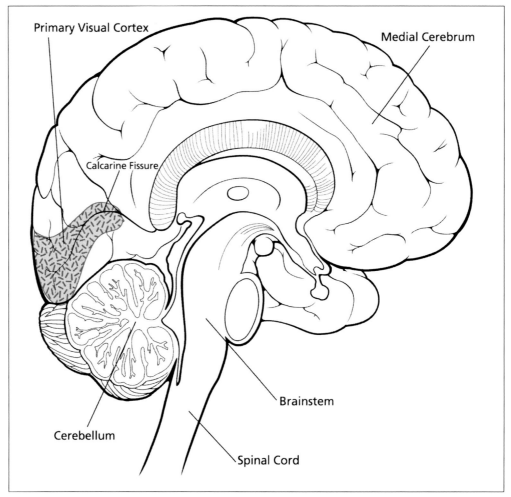

Figure 2.14. The primary visual region is located predominantly on the medioposterior surfaces of the occipital lobe.

Source. F. Feuchter.

the retina send information about the periphery of the visual field, such as moving objects, but visual objects that receive attentional focus are visualized with the macula lutea. The macula lutea occupies about 1% of the entire surface area of the retina, but information from the macula lutea is reported by approximately 50% of the fibers within the optic nerve to cells occupying about 50% of the striate cortex (Figure 2.15).

The most acute vision (i.e., that which occurs at the macula lutea), is analyzed in the visual cortex at the most posterior pole of the occipital lobe, with the ***fovea,*** the central region of the macula lutea region of the retina, represented on the external surface at the posterior tip of the lobe. Retinal cells located more laterally in the retina report to cortical cells located more anteriorly on the medial surface of the occipital lobe. The most peripheral retinal cells send input to the most anterior portions of the striate cortex.

Recordings from individual cells have shown that the visual system is organized into maps, each of which represents the "picture" viewed by the retina. The maps are organized in a hierarchical manner, each corresponding to a distinct area of the brain responsible for carrying out a particular type of analysis of the

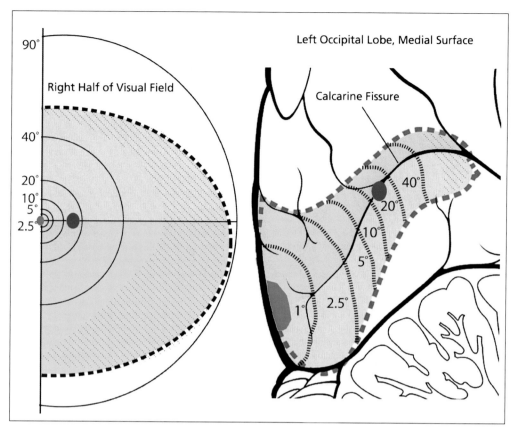

Figure 2.15. Diagram illustrating the volume of visual cortex devoted to either central or peripheral parts of the retina. On the left side of the diagram, the right half of the visual field is shown, with the superior part in light blue and the inferior part in yellow. The red dot indicates the macula lutea, which focuses on objects on which attention is fixed, and the blue dot is the blind spot. The concentric semicircles indicate distance from the macula on the retina in degrees, and the region with the hatch lines is the part seen with only one eye. On the right side of the diagram, the corresponding representation of the visual field on the primary visual cortex is shown. The part of the visual field within 40° of the macula is represented on most of the primary visual cortex, with peripheral regions less well represented. The field is inverted, and the area of most acute vision is located on the most posterior part of the lobe.

Source. F. Feuchter.

visual information sent to the brain. The primary visual cortical cells respond most strongly to form, movement, or color. However, complete analysis of the information coming from the visual fields, and therefore pattern recognition, involves sequential processing through several areas that go from the primary visual area in the back of the brain into adjacent areas of the occipital, temporal, and parietal lobes. These areas of visual processing have been referred to as *extrastriate cortex* and *visual association cortex* (Figure 2.16). Researchers have determined that the monkey may have as many as 34 separate extrastriate visual association regions, each analyzing a different attribute of the visual field.

In humans, the extrastriate cortex includes all of the occipital lobe areas surrounding the primary visual cortex (Brodmann's areas 18 and 19). The extrastriate cortex has been subdivided into as many as three functional visual areas (V2, V3, and V4). Each visual area contains neurons, the receptive fields of which together represent the entire visual field. Visual information enters through the primary visual cortex and travels through the rest of the areas in sequence.

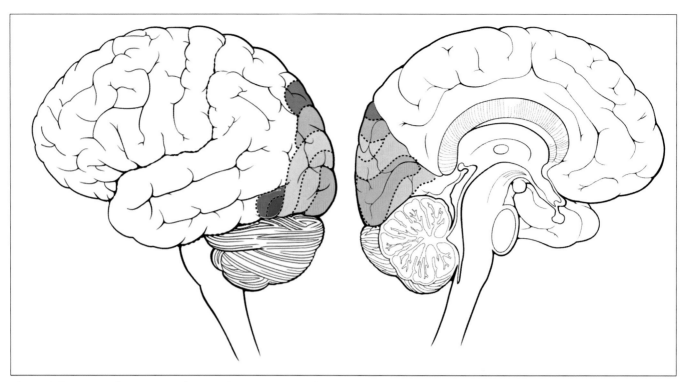

Figure 2.16. Several regions in the visual association and extrastriate cortices, each specialized for carrying out a particular type of analysis of the visual information sent to the brain.

Source. F. Feuchter.

The visual association cortex extends anteriorly from the extrastriate cortex to encompass adjacent areas of the posterior parietal lobe and much of the posterior temporal lobe (Brodmann's areas 7, 20, 37, and 39). These areas receive visual input from the extrastriate cortex, which sends color, shape and form, location, and motion information to different areas of the visual association cortex. Several areas of the visual association cortex have been described in humans, including V5, medial temporal superior, and superior temporal sulcus, all of which analyze various aspects of motion. Other areas analyze faces and specific body parts, and still others analyze various aspects of location and space.

The network of visual analysis in the extrastriate occipital cortex sends out two main streams of information, the *dorsal/where* stream and the *ventral/what* stream. Data regarding attributes of the stimulus, such as position of an object in space and its movement, are sent anteriorly toward the parietal lobe in the data stream constituting the dorsal/where system (Figure 2.17). Also known as the *dorsal visual pathway,* the dorsal/where stream stretches from the primary visual cortex in the occipital lobe forward into the parietal lobe. The dorsal/where stream is believed to be involved in the guidance of actions and the recognition of where objects are in space. The dorsal/where stream commences with purely visual functions in the occipital lobe before gradually transferring to spatial awareness at its termination in the parietal lobe. The posterior parietal cortex is essential for the perception and interpretation of spatial relationships, accurate body image, and the learning of tasks involving coordination of the body in space.

The dorsal/where stream is interconnected with the parallel ventral/what stream, which runs anteriorly from V1 into the temporal lobe. The ventral/what

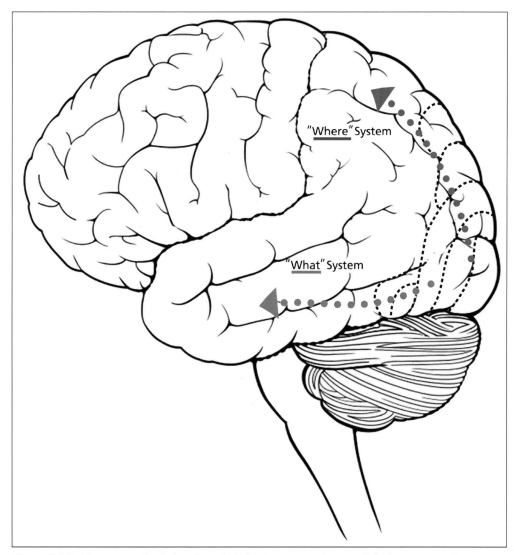

Figure 2.17. The network of visual analysis in the extrastriate occipital cortex sends out two main streams of information, the *dorsal/where* stream and the *ventral/what* stream. Data regarding attributes of the stimulus, such as position of an object in space and its movement, are sent anteriorly toward the parietal lobe in the data stream constituting the dorsal/where stream. The ventral/what stream is associated with object recognition and form representation and has strong connections to the medial temporal lobe (involved in the encoding of explicit memories).

Source. F. Feuchter.

stream is associated with object recognition and form representation and has strong connections to the medial temporal lobe (involved in the encoding of explicit memories), the limbic system (involved in emotions), and the dorsal/where stream (which deals with object locations and motion). All the areas in the ventral/what stream are influenced by extraretinal factors in addition to the nature of the stimulus in the receptive field. These factors include attention, working memory, and stimulus salience. Thus, the ventral/what stream does not merely provide a description of the elements in the visual world; it also plays a crucial role in judging the significance of these elements.

Researchers in neurophysiology have emphasized the importance of bidirectional signaling within these systems, with multiple reciprocal connections, and it is postulated that when a visual image of an object is created in the absence of visual stimuli (i.e., in imagination), the extrastriate areas of the brain that are activated are the same as those involved in actively viewing the same object when it is physically present. Positron emission tomography studies have provided abundant evidence that multiple visual areas of the human brain contribute to the formation of visual imagery. It is clear that the elements of the ventral/what and dorsal/where pathways within the visual system can be engaged in forming visual imagery.

Additional brain areas outside the visual area can also be activated when forming mental imagery, including the basal nuclei and **anterior cingulate gyrus,** which are elements of the attentional networks of the brain (see the "Networks of Attention" section). Attentional networks are central to the types of top-down processing that occur in many of the brain networks.

Language Networks

Symbolic language, as far as is known, is a uniquely human ability. Much of a person's conscious life consists of concepts represented by words. Therefore, by examining what occurs in the brain as a person understands and expresses words, researchers can examine much of the process of conscious thought.

Figure 2.18 illustrates a model proposed by Norman Geschwind (1926–1984), an important U.S. behavioral neurologist, who described the successive participation of several brain areas as research participants read and spoke a written word (Geschwind, 1979). Although the model is consistent with observed deficits after human brain damage, it does not account for people's flexibility in language-processing strategies during different kinds of language-related tasks. For instance, when research participants were presented with a noun and asked to generate an appropriate verb, different areas of the brain were activated in addition to those activated during the reading task (Figure 2.19). The activated areas included the anterior cingulate region, the left prefrontal and left posterior temporal cortices, and the right half of the cerebellum.

The additional demands of verb generation thus appear to be supported by a network of widely separated brain areas not involved in the basic functions of reading. Moreover, the change in brain activity after practice and associated improved performance on the verb-generating task suggest that as the task is learned, the brain regions involved in the task change. The pathway used might depend on the degree to which a task has become automatic because participation of frontal areas typically associated with the management of novel experience diminishes as a task becomes automatized.

Networks of Attention

The ability to attend to and identify internal and external stimuli with relevance to the self is a fundamental component of cognitive functioning. Several different but interlinked attentional systems have been examined. The **covert visual orienting network** is active in shifting attention from one focus to another in the

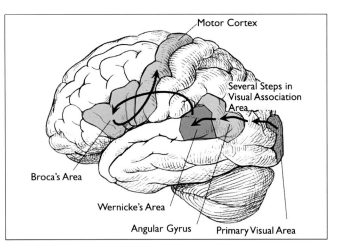

Figure 2.18. The model proposed by Geschwind (1979) is consistent with observed deficits after human brain injury, but it does not account for flexibility in language-processing strategies during different kinds of language-related tasks.

Source. From *Images of Mind* (p. 108), by Michael I. Posner and Marcus E. Raichle. Copyright © 1994, 1997 by Scientific American Library. Reprinted by permission of Henry Holt and Company, LLC.

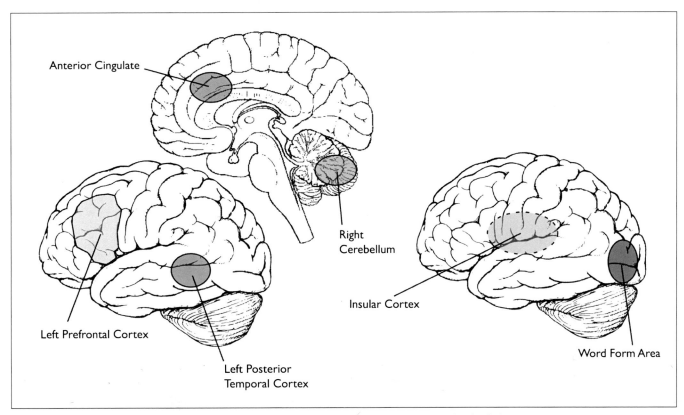

Figure 2.19. Geschwind (1979) presented research participants with a noun and asked them to generate an appropriate verb; different areas of the brain were activated in addition to those activated on the reading task. The activated areas included the anterior cingulate region, the left prefrontal and left posterior temporal cortices, and the right half of the cerebellum. *Left diagrams:* The generation task requires the combined activation of four brain areas, which may constitute at least part of an executive attention network. *Right diagram:* When practice has made responses automatic, an entirely different set of areas is activated, including areas in the insular cortex of both hemispheres.

Source. From *Images of Mind* (p. 124), by Michael I. Posner and Marcus E. Raichle. Copyright © 1994, 1997 by Scientific American Library. Reprinted by permission of Henry Holt and Company, LLC.

external environment. When one attends to an object in the environment, one usually looks at that object (i.e., moves the eyes to place the image on the *retinal fovea,* the central region of the macula lutea) (Posner & Petersen, 1990). One can also visually focus attention on objects in the environment without moving the eyes. The circuitry proposed by Posner and Petersen (1990) is shown in Figure 2.20. The right parietal lobe, known for many years to play a significant role in selective attention, initiates movement of the focus of attention to a new location. It seems likely that the superior colliculus in the midbrain plays a role in moving visual covert attention from one location to another, much as it does for eye movements.

The role of the *pulvinar region* of the thalamus (a region known to be involved in visual and attentional processing) is suspected to be that of enhancing input from the new location while filtering out much of the unattended information before passing the information forward to the frontal lobe. Once attention has shifted to a new location and the new content is transmitted forward in the brain, the **executive attention network** is engaged (Figure 2.21). The task of the executive attention network is ***detection***—conscious recognition that an object is present, along with recognition of the object's identity and its significance. Detection plays a special role in selecting a target from many alternatives, a process known as *target detection.*

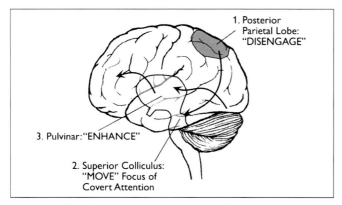

Figure 2.20. **The proposed circuitry of the covert visual orienting network, which is active in shifting attention from one focus to another in the external environment.** The three areas of the orienting network perform three functions required to orient attention: (1) The focus of attention is first disengaged from a cue; (2) then moved to the expected target location; and, (3) finally, there is enhanced focus on the new target location.

Source. From *Images of Mind* (p. 168), by Michael I. Posner and Marcus E. Raichle. Copyright © 1994, 1997 by Scientific American Library. Reprinted by permission of Henry Holt and Company, LLC.

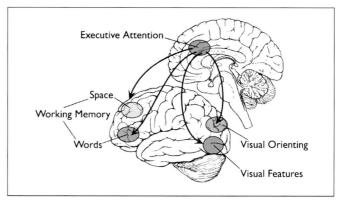

Figure 2.21. **Once attention has shifted to a new location and the new content is transmitted forward in the brain, the executive attention network is engaged in the task of** *detection*—**conscious recognition that an object is present, along with recognition of the object's identity and its significance.**

Source. From *Images of Mind* (p. 173), by Michael I. Posner and Marcus E. Raichle. Copyright © 1994, 1997 by Scientific American Library. Reprinted by permission of Henry Holt and Company, LLC.

Target detection absorbs attention in a way that resists interference by other signals and thus represents a different kind of attention than merely orienting to a cue. The anterior cingulate gyrus appears to have executive control over information processing and is linked to frontal lobe regions involved in working memory (see the "Networks of Memory" section, which follows) and to posterior regions for visual orienting and feature identification. Damage to medial prefrontal structures (anterior cingulate gyrus) diminishes both the speed and the amount of human activity. The medial sagittal structures are part of a system that includes brainstem structures that are responsible for tonic arousal. Tonic arousal appears to be subserved by pathways originating in the **locus coeruleus** and terminating in frontal areas with the function lateralized to the right (Posner & Petersen, 1990).

Another brain network, the **vigilance network** (Figure 2.22), appears to maintain a sustained state of alertness. Sometimes a person must minimally attend to environmental stimuli to be vigilant about a future event (i.e., maintain a state of expectancy). In this state, physical changes in the brain and body occur that have a quieting effect; heart rate slows, and electrical activity in the brain is reduced. Subjectively, the person feels calm as he or she tries to avoid any stray thoughts. Although total brain activity decreases, activity in the right frontal and right parietal areas increases; these areas may be part of a network responsible for maintaining the alert state. As activation in the right prefrontal and right parietal regions increases, the anterior cingulate region for target detection quiets. In tasks in which a person needs to suspend activity while waiting for infrequent signals, it is important not to carry out any mental activity that might interfere with detecting an external event. The vigilance network affects activity in both the executive attention network and the covert visual orienting network. During the vigilant state, the orienting system is tuned so that it acts faster. Thus, in highly alert states, response time is reduced.

It is useful to view attention as a set of networks carrying out particular functions. The interactions among the networks, however, suggest that these networks make up a single attentional system that underlies the unity of people's subjective experience of the world.

Networks of Memory

Although memory is often thought of as a single phenomenon, remembering in daily life involves multiple memory systems, each of which is dependent on different sets of neural structures and pathways. Memory involves the acquisition, storage, and retrieval of knowledge, and the capabilities of human memory systems for retention are highly varied, ranging from milliseconds to many decades. Additionally, the learning can be intentional or unintentional, and retrieval of information may occur in the presence or absence of awareness that something is being remembered. Thus, memory can be categorized qualitatively, on the basis of whether it is available to introspection, or temporally, depending on the time over which the retention may occur. In this section, memory systems are grouped temporally into **immediate, short-term,** and **working memory** types and qualitatively into explicit (declarative) and implicit (nondeclarative) memory types. Table 2.2 summarizes the memory functions and their neuroanatomical correlates.

Immediate, Short-Term, and Working Memory

Immediate memory (also called *sensory memory*) involves the automatic holding of ongoing sensory experiences in mind for very short periods of time (i.e., seconds or even fractions of seconds), maintaining very briefly how a stimulus looked (*iconic* or *visual sensory memory*), sounded (*echoic* or *auditory sensory information*), or felt (*tactile* or *haptic memory*). The capacity of each sensory memory system is large because each sensory memory system is subserved by its own cortical area (i.e., visual, auditory, sensory, and motor cortices). *Short-term memory* (*active* or *primary memory*) allows the processing and temporary storage of information needed to carry out activities as diverse as understanding, learning, and reasoning for a limited amount of material to be readily accessible for a brief period of time (i.e., several seconds). Simple short-term memory does not require the rehearsal of information but can be extended with rehearsal. *Chunking* temporally consolidates information to create spatial or nonspatial contexts that reduce information decay and facilitate encoding. These processes associated with short-term memory occur in the prefrontal cortex.

Working memory (which conceptually overlaps with short-term memory) involves holding knowledge briefly in awareness (seconds to minutes) while it is being used to perform a specific mental operation (e.g., planning, organizing, problem solving, paying attention). Working memory is limited in both duration and

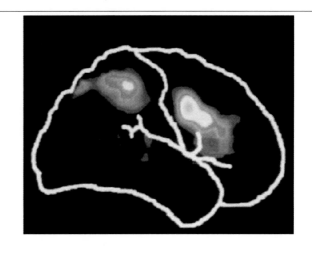

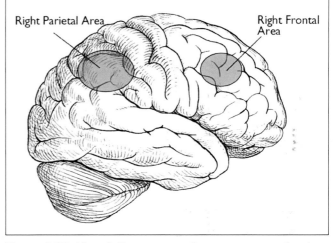

Figure 2.22. The vigilance network appears to maintain a sustained state of alertness. This positron emission tomography scan (top) shows activity increasing in the right frontal and right parietal lobes, the proposed sites of the vigilance network, when the person was required to maintain a state of alertness. Areas of the right parietal and right frontal lobes (bottom) may constitute a vigilance network that maintains the alert state.

Source. From Images of Mind (p. 176), by Michael I. Posner and Marcus E. Raichle. Copyright © 1994, 1997 by Scientific American Library. Reprinted by permission of Henry Holt and Company, LLC.

Table 2.2. Summary of Memory Systems

		Immediate, Short-Term, and Working Memory		
Memory Type	**Duration Before Decay**	**Function**	**Neuroanatomical Components**	**Description**
Immediate (sensory memory)	Iconic (<1 s)	Visual sensory memory	Photoreceptors of retina and visual cortex (occipital lobe)	Is not under conscious control Awareness is present but cannot be suppressed Fast-decaying stores of information Allows retention of information after original stimulus is removed
	Echoic (<4 s)	Auditory sensory memory	Hair cells in inner ear and auditory cortex (superior temporal lobe)	
	Haptic and tactile (<2 s)	**Proprioceptive** and tactile sensory memory with subcomponents (see final section of the table)	Sensory receptors located throughout body (cutaneous and kinesthetic), primary somatosensory cortex (Harris et al., 2002; Zhou & Fuster, 1996), and several distinct areas of parietal lobe (Gallace & Spence, 2009) (see final section of the table)	
Short-term	8–10 s, or minutes if rehearsal is used	Simple serial recall (stores 7 ± 2 items; error-free limit 3 items); exhibits temporal decay, but duration may be extended by rehearsal; chunk capacity limits (Camos & Tillmann, 2008)	Prefrontal cortex	Does not correlate with measures of intelligence or aptitude (Cowan, 2008)
Working	8–10 s, or minutes if rehearsal is used (same as short-term)	Active maintenance and manipulation of limited amounts of information; function is influenced by passage of time, load, rehearsability, distraction; important to attention, language, reasoning, and problem solving	Prefrontal cortex and posterior regions of association cortex; supported by sustained activity in the brain areas that process the specific perceptual information to be retained (modality-specific cortex; e.g., recall of faces, posterior fusiform gyrus; Ranganath, 2004)	Does correlate with measures of intelligence or aptitude (Cowan, 2008) Not completely distinct from short-term memory Used to describe both storage and processing components (Smith & Jonides, 1997)
		Phonological loop: Formation and maintenance of memories associated with verbal information (Cowan, 2008)	Frontal cortex, mostly left	
		Visuospatial sketchpad: Formation and maintenance of memories associated with visual and spatial information (Cowan, 2008)	Frontal cortex, mostly right	

(Continued)

Immediate, Short-Term, and Working Memory

Table 2.2. Summary of Memory Systems (*cont.*)

	Memory Type	Function	Neuroanatomical Components	Description
Explicit (Long-Term) Memory	Episodic Medium range (0–3 yr)	Memory for events with perceptual and temporal correlates attached	MTL structures, diencephalic (anterior and medial thalamus, mammillary bodies); may be associated with time-dependent dendritic spine formation (Ranganath, 2004; Restivo et al., 2009; Squire & Wixted, 2011)	Initially responsible for all supraspan recall of ongoing events (Squire & Wixted, 2011)
	Episodic Remote (>3 yr)		MTL structures and cortical areas associated with specific modalities (e.g., visual memory and calcarine cortex). Remote episodic memory may be completely dependent on cortex (the standard model) or contextually rich memories may always involve hippocampus and cortex (multiple trace theory; Nadel & Moscovitch, 1997). Consistent with the standard model, both views suggest prefrontal cortex may be important in integrating multiple cortical regions.	Very remote episodic memories may be more factlike or semantic in quality without spatial or perceptual attributes (Squire & Wixted, 2011)
	Semantic	Knowledge of the world (e.g., facts, dates); general knowledge without acquisition context	MTL structures and the same neocortical areas that performed the perceptual processing and analysis at the time of learning; impaired with extensive temporal lobe damage bilaterally	Impairment in initial processing may not be separable from recall; therefore, anterior and retrograde deficits co-occur Organized by semantic category (e.g., asymmetric ability to recognize animate vs. inanimate objects in category-specific amnesia)

(Continued)

Table 2.2. Summary of Memory Systems (cont.)

	Memory Type	Function	Neuroanatomical Components	Description
Implicit Memory	Perceptual priming	Object identification	Modality-specific cortex	Allows for efficient processing, decreased recognition latency, and improved accuracy when encountering a pre-experienced object or concept
	Conceptual priming	Activation of knowledge structures	Modality-specific cortex	
	Motor skills learning	Motor skills acquisition	Basal nuclei, cerebellum, frontal participation during learning and execution	Acquisition of skills through experience
	Operant conditioning	S–R (stimulus–response)	Putamen; DF cortex (pre- and postcentral); DL striatum (putamen), motor cortex	Allows the automatic initiation of behavioral sequences in the context of a sensory stimulus (Yin & Knowlton, 2006)
		A–O (action–outcome)	VL prefrontal cortex, caudate; DM striatum	Allows for the control of actions according to their anticipated outcomes / Knowledge of the causal relationship between action and outcome, goal expectancy (Yin & Knowlton, 2006)
	Associative conditioning (**habit** learning)	Mapping of relationships established through repetitive pairings	Basal nuclei, dorsal striatum, cerebellum	Actions controlled by goals
	Habituation	Reduction in response to repetitive stimuli (Yin & Knowlton, 2006)	Basal nuclei, cerebellum	Actions controlled by stimuli (Yin & Knowlton, 2006)
	Sensitization	Increased response to repetitive stimuli (Yin & Knowlton, 2006)	Limbic cortex, basal nuclei, cerebellum	
Haptic and Tactile Memory	Haptic and tactile	Roughness, texture, spatial discrimination of stimuli	Cutaneous mechanoreceptors, parietal operculum (Gallace & Spence, 2009)	Long-term structure is poorly understood; it is believed that memory for tactile and haptic information is located in the same areas in which initial processing takes place. Haptic memory has implicit and short-term explicit components (Gallace & Spence, 2009; Zhou & Fuster, 1996).
		Size and shape of stimuli	Cutaneous mechanoreceptors, anterior parietal lobe (Zhou & Fuster, 1996)	
		Location of stimuli	Superior parietal lobe, temporoparietal junction (Gallace & Spence, 2009)	

Note. DF = dorsofrontal; DL = dorsolateral; DM = dorsomedial; MTL = medial temporal lobe (includes the hippocampus and adjacent entorhinal, perirhinal, and parahippocampal cortices); s = second/seconds; VL = ventrolateral; yr = years.

capacity, and therefore the relevant information must be maintained via rehearsal. The *phonological loop* is the brain's "inner ear" and "inner voice," which allow the rehearsal of verbal information to prevent its decay, such as when repeating a phone number until the number is dialed. The *visuospatial sketchpad* is the "mind's eye," which allows the brain to visualize something and to place it into context. Working memory engages the frontal cortex, and its ability correlates with intelligence or aptitude, in contrast to short-term memory, which does not.

Explicit and Implicit Memory

Long-term memory entails the retention of information in more permanent forms of storage (i.e., days, weeks, or even a lifetime). Material in working memory can enter into long-term memory in various ways, including by conscious rehearsal or practice. Medium-term (i.e., minutes to hours to years) and long-term (i.e., decades) recall of material is subserved by two fundamental types of memory systems, **explicit memory** and **implicit memory.** These memory systems differ fundamentally in their retrieval processes and accordingly engage distinct neuroanatomical structures and pathways across different time scales (explicit) or under different conditions (implicit; Eustache & Desgranges, 2008).

Explicit memories may be retrieved automatically or through introspective processing because people "know that they know" the information that is being retrieved. In contrast, implicit memories may or may not be associated with introspective processing, and people may or may not be aware that they know the information retrieved. Explicit memory encompasses the retrieval of *episodic memories* (i.e., personally experienced events, specific history of what happened where and when in an autobiographical context; Tulving, 2001, 2002) and *semantic memories* (i.e., words, concepts, general facts and information about the world, independent of temporal and sensory personal experience and without autobiographical context; Eustache & Desgranges, 2008). *Implicit* (or *procedural*) memory is the memory of actions. It includes **priming,** motor-skill learning, cognitive skills, operant conditioning, associative conditioning, habituation, and sensitization.

The two main regions of the brain that appear to be critical to explicit memory formation are (1) the medial temporal lobe (MTL), including the hippocampus and adjacent entorhinal, perirhinal, and parahippocampal cortical areas, and (2) the medial diencephalic areas, including the thalamic **mediodorsal nucleus, anterior nucleus of the thalamus, mammillary bodies,** and other diencephalic nuclei lining the **third ventricle** (Squire & Wixted, 2011). The medial temporal and medial diencephalic memory areas are interconnected both with each other and with widespread regions of cortex by a variety of pathways, crucial for memory consolidation and retrieval (Eichenbaum, 2001; Frankland & Bontempi, 2005; Polyn, Natu, Cohen, & Norman, 2005).

The MTL seems to have a time-limited role in the storage and retrieval of explicit memories. Over time, memories gradually reorganize and become permanently stored outside the MTL. Engagement of hippocampal–cortical networks leads to gradual strengthening of cortical–cortical connections, which eventually allows memories to become independent of the hippocampus and to be gradually integrated with preexisting cortical memories (i.e., the hippocampus is a fast learner and the cortex a slow one; Frankland & Bontempi, 2005). Thus, hippocampal damage preferentially affects recent but not remote memories (Frankland & Bontempi, 2005).

The medial temporal lobe (MTL) seems to have a time-limited role in the storage and retrieval of explicit memories. Over time, memories gradually reorganize and become permanently stored outside the MTL.

Most authorities view the role of the hippocampus as limited to explicit memory. However, some theorists have suggested that the hippocampus may be involved in all forms of complex, integrative memory functioning and not restricted to memories available to conscious introspection (Henke, 2010). Episodic memory is probably the most functionally important form of memory and also that which is most susceptible to **impairment** after TBI. Semantic memories are encoded with the participation of the MTL structure, are believed to be widely distributed throughout the neocortex, and are organized categorically (Polyn et al., 2005).

Implicit memory likely involves the construction of motor patterning that makes an action, behavior, or skill become increasingly automatic. Components of the basal nuclei support learning of the causal relationship between action and outcome and between stimulus and response across trials (i.e., instrumental behaviors or operant conditioning; Klimkowicz-Mrowiec, Slowik, Krzywoszanski, Herzog-Krzywoszanska, & Szczudlik, 2008; Knowlton, Mangels, & Squire, 1996; Simons, Schölvinck, Gilbert, Frith, & Burgess, 2006). Priming depends on several cortical areas. Simple associative learning (i.e., classical conditioning) and nonassociative learning (i.e., habituation and sensitization) appear to involve a variety of structures, including the cerebellum (in classical conditioning), **amygdala** (in conditioned fear), cerebral cortex, brainstem nuclei, and even the spinal cord.

Typically, a key distinction between explicit and implicit memory is the number of trials needed for memory formation. For example, the learning of procedures, skills, and habits (implicit memory) typically requires a large number of trials, whereas explicit memory formation requires only one. An additional distinction between explicit and implicit memory is the complexity of the memory itself. For example, episodic memories are complex, involving multiple sensory systems, and therefore elements of the memory can be recalled separately. In contrast, implicit memories, although they may be complex, are typically recalled as a single unit (Henke, 2010).

Frontal Subcortical Networks

The *basal nuclei* are a collection of five subcortical masses of neuronal cell bodies located deep within the white matter of the cerebrum that modulate the output of the frontal cortex through multiple parallel circuits (Figure 2.23). They influence the activity of the cerebral cortex through their extensive connections and thus a range of functionally diverse activities, including motor control and movement, **cognition,** emotion, and motivation. The components of the basal nuclei (see Table 2.3) are (1) the *corpus striatum* ("striped body"), consisting of the **caudate nucleus** and **putamen;** (2) the *globus pallidus* (GP; "pale globe"), consisting of external and internal segments; (3) the *substantia nigra* (SN), consisting of

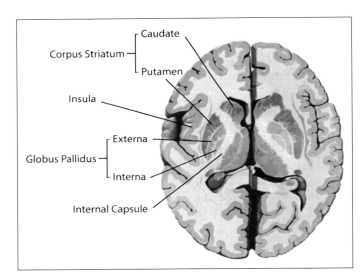

Figure 2.23. Masses of neurons known as *basal nuclei* **are located deep in the cerebrum.** Horizontal (transverse) sections reveal the components of the basal nuclei, surrounded by the white matter and including the internal capsule. The image demonstrates the geographical relationship of the basal nuclei to the cerebral cortex and thalamus. The components are the corpus striatum, consisting of the caudate nucleus and putamen; the globus pallidus, consisting of external and internal segments; the substantia nigra, consisting of the pars reticulata and pars compacta (not shown); and the subthalamic nucleus (not shown).

Source. From *Atlas of Human Anatomy* (5th ed., Plate 109), by F. Netter, 2011, Saunders/Elsevier. Netter illustration from http://www.netterimages.com. Copyright © Elsevier Inc. All rights reserved.

Table 2.3. Functions of the Basal Nuclei

Component Nuclei	Summary of Functions
Corpus striatum	The major input zone of the basal nuclei; it receives excitatory (glutamate) inputs from large areas of the cerebral cortex, substantia nigra, and thalamus.
Caudate	The medial part of the striatum, connected with prefrontal and other association areas of cortex. Involved primarily in cognitive functions and less directly in movement.
Putamen	The lateral part of the striatum, involved most prominently in the motor functions of the basal nuclei. Receives input from the primary somatosensory and somatomotor areas of the cortex and from the substantia nigra. The putamen projects output to the globus pallidus, which in turn projects to the premotor and supplementary motor areas via the thalamus.
Globus pallidus	Main output from the basal nuclei; relays information from the striatum to the thalamus.
Externa	Receives inputs from the striatum and sends output to the subthalamic nucleus.
Interna	Receives inputs from the striatum and subthalamic nucleus and sends inhibitory (GABA) projections to the thalamus.
Substantia nigra	Main output from the basal nuclei that sends inhibitory (GABA) projections to the thalamus.
Pars reticulata	Contains loosely arranged neurons that receive input from the striatum and subthalamic nucleus and send output to the thalamus.
Pars compacta	Contains closely packed, pigmented dopaminergic neurons that send their output to the striatum.
Subthalamic nucleus	Located ventral and inferior to the thalamus. Receives input from the striatum as part of the indirect pathway and participates in modulation of motor behavior by sending excitatory (glutamate) inputs to the global pallidus interna or substantia nigra pars reticulata and ultimately the thalamus.

Note. GABA = γ-aminobutyric acid.

the pars reticulata (SNpr) and pars compacta (SNpc); and (4) the **subthalamic nucleus** (STN). Collectively, these components of the basal nuclei are part of a complex network of multiple information loops that extend from the cerebral cortex through the basal nuclei and on to the thalamus, from where they subsequently loop back to the cortex. This basal nuclei circuitry modulates cortical output (see Box 2.1).

The location of the cortical starting and ending points of each loop determines their function, and the interconnections within the basal nuclei determine whether the activity is released or inhibited. The body of the caudate is separated from the putamen by the *internal capsule,* which is a collection of white matter fibers projecting to and from the cerebral cortex, but remains connected to the putamen via cellular bridges. The GP lies just medial to the putamen and has external (GPe) and internal (GPi) segments. The SN lies inferior to the internal capsule and has both ventral components (SNpr) and dorsal components (SNpc). The STN is located ventral and inferior to the thalamus but just above the most rostral aspect of the SN. **Afferents** reach the basal nuclei from the cortex via the **striatum** and STN, and **efferents** leave the basal nuclei via the GP and the SN.

The *prefrontal cortex* is the anterior portion of the frontal lobe, lying just in front of the motor and premotor cortical areas. The functions of the prefrontal cortex are thought to be accomplished by a division of labor among five distinct and reciprocal subcortical networks that are involved in modulation of motor and cognitive functions in the cerebrum and share the following features: (1) They begin

Box 2.1. Pathways of the Frontal Subcortical Circuits

Inputs to the basal nuclei arrive via the striatum or the subthalamic nucleus, and outputs leave via the internal segment of the globus pallidus (GPi), the closely related substantia nigra pars reticulata (SNpr), or both. Within the basal nuclei are a variety of complex excitatory and inhibitory connections that enable the organism to fine-tune behavior control and mediate learning. Also within the basal nuclei are several parallel pathways for different functions, including general motor control, eye movements, and cognitive and emotional functions. Inputs from major cortical regions are received by the striatum and subsequently directed to the basal nuclei via one of four distinct pathways: (1) *direct,* (2) *indirect,* (3) *subthalamic,* or (4) *striosomal.* These distinct pathways enable the organism to tailor activity to environmental circumstances and to base behavior on assessment of outcome and reward.

Cortical projections into the striatum are topographically oriented, but multiple cortical neurons terminate on a far more limited number of striatal neurons (i.e., the input compression ratio is high), leading to a considerable reduction in specificity. Certain regions of cerebral cortex may project to more than one region of the striatum, supporting functional integration. Both the regional integration and the reduction from many to few neurons support response pattern formation. Similarities between different patterns of inputs allow for importantly similar events and circumstances to be responded to in the same way. In this way, the same adaptive behavior can occur in the context of different but similar stimulus situations.

Outputs from the basal nuclei arise from the GPi and from the SNpr. Neurons in the GPi have a very high spontaneous firing rate, such that this region is tonically active. The tonic activity in the GPi inhibits activity in the thalamus, preventing the thalamus from activating the downstream cortical neurons to which it connects. Therefore, the basal nuclei can be viewed as inhibiting cortical responsiveness in their normal state. By activating the striatum, cortical activity inhibits the activity in the GPi (which otherwise acts to inhibit thalamic activity), allowing the thalamus to release behavior mediated by the cortex.

Both the direct and the indirect pathways are excitatory in their connections from the cortex to the striatum but ultimately differ in their effects on the GPi or SNpr, the main outputs from the basal nuclei. Thus, these pathways ultimately differ in their ability to activate or inhibit basal nuclei–mediated cortical motor areas. The direct pathway travels from the striatum directly to the GPi or SNpr. The indirect pathway takes a detour from the striatum first to the external segment of the globus pallidus (GPe) and then to the subthalamic nucleus (STN) before finally reaching the GPi or the SNpr, from which all outputs exit the basal nuclei. The net effect of excitatory input from the cortex via the direct pathway will be excitation of the thalamus, which will in turn facilitate behavior through its cortical connections. In contrast, the net effect of excitation of the indirect pathway will be inhibition of the thalamus, resulting in inhibition of behavior through its connections with the cortex. The two pathways are believed to operate in opposite directions but in balance. Activation of the direct pathway causes the GPi to release inhibition on the thalamus and thus to ultimately enable release behavior of wanted actions. In contrast, activation of the indirect pathway causes the STN to activate the GPi, which suppresses thalamic activity, preventing release behavior, and thus ultimately inhibits closely related but unwanted actions.

The subthalamic pathway connects cortical regions directly to the STN. The striosomal pathway connects certain regions of the cortex to "islands" of neurons or *striosomes* (hence *striosomal*) to the substantia nigra via the putamen. These pathways operate at a much faster rate because they have fewer synapses. When the subthalamic, or "hyperdirect," pathway is active, it suppresses all behavior and thus enables the organism to not respond. When the striosomal pathway is active, it allows information about rewards and behavioral states to be integrated with information about behavioral control. The interaction between cortical and subcortical structures in some ways mirrors the integration of automatic with higher-order control. Because most behaviors involve some level of automatic responsiveness but may from time to time require adaptation or change because of different circumstances, it is possible to see how cortically mediated adaptation and subcortically mediated automatic behaviors can interact to facilitate the accomplishment of adaptive behaviors in a person.

Of the four pathways within each subcortical circuit, the predominant two (direct and indirect) go through the basal nuclei. The direct (cortical activation) pathway travels from the striatum to the GPi or the SNpr, with the net effect being excitation of the thalamus, which in turn facilitates action through its connections with the motor and premotor cortex. The indirect (cortical inactivation) pathway takes a detour from the striatum first to the GPe and then to the STN before reaching the GPi or the SNpr. The net effect of excitation of the indirect pathway is inhibition of the thalamus, resulting in inhibition of actions through connections back to the cortex.

in the anterior frontal gray matter; (2) they have reciprocal connections primarily through the basal nuclei and thalamus; (3) each has its own direct and indirect pathways, which are not exclusive of one another; and (4) they end in the prefrontal cortex, where they began. One circuit is primarily associated with motor control and arises in the supplementary motor area. A second circuit relates primarily to oculomotor control and arises in the frontal eye fields. The remaining three circuits relate to executive control, behavioral inhibition, and skill development (Bonelli & Cummings, 2008; Cummings, 1993; see Tables 2.4 and 2.5). Damage to these

Table 2.4. Frontal Subcortical Circuits Involved With Behavior Control

	Frontal Subcortical Circuit				
	Dorsolateral Prefrontal System		**Orbitofrontal System**		**Anterior Cingulate System**
Neuronal groups	1. Brodmann's areas 9, 10 (DL) 2. DL caudate 3. DM globus pallidus; substantia nigra 4. VA & DM thalamic nuclei		1. Brodmann's areas 10 (IM), 11 2. VM caudate 3. DM globus pallidus; substantia nigra 4. VA & DM thalamic nuclei		1. Brodmann's area 24 2. V striatum (VM caudate, V putamen, nucleus accumbens, olfactory tubercle) 3. RM & V globus pallidus 4. DM thalamic nuclei
Circuit-specific behaviors	Organization, executive planning, attention		Inhibition, reward; mediates socially appropriate behavior & empathy		Motivated behavior, error correction, wakefulness, arousal
Cognitive & behavioral abnormalities associated with pathology	Executive dysfunction; poor planning; inability to generate hypotheses; inability to change tasks, filter environmental distractions, or organize or plan		Disinhibition, impulsivity, tactlessness, inability to shift responses		Impaired motivation (*abulia*), **apathy,** reduced creative thought, poor response inhibition, impaired emotional display
Vascular supply (rostral to caudal)	DL caudate	MCA (lenticulostriate aa.)	VM caudate	ACA (Heubner's a.)	Caudate nucleus: accumbens V striatum	ACA (Heubner's a. & penetrating aa.)
	Internal capsule (IM head of caudate)	ACA (Heubner's a.)	Internal capsule (IM head of caudate)	ACA (Heubner's a.)	Internal capsule (IM head of caudate)	ACA (Heubner's a.)
	Internal capsule: inferior genu	ACA (Heubner's a.)	Caudate: entire head	ACA & MCA (penetrating aa.)	Caudate: entire head	ACA & MCA (penetrating aa.)
	Caudate: entire head	ACA & MCA (penetrating aa.)	V & VA thalamus	Posterior communicating (tuberothalamic a.)		
	Globus pallidus	MCA (lenticulostriate aa.) ACA (ant. choroidal a.)	DM thalamus	Posterior communicating (paramedian aa.)	Globus pallidus	MCA (lenticulostriate aa.) ACA (ant. choroidal a.)
	V & VA thalamus	Posterior communicating (tuberothalamic a.)			DM thalamus	Posterior communicating (paramedian aa.)
	DM thalamus	Posterior communicating (paramedian aa.)			DM thalamus & mammillothalamic tracts	ICA (paramedian a.)
	DM thalamus & mammillo-thalamic tracts	ICA (paramedian a.)				

Note. a. = arteria (artery); aa. = arteriae (arteries); ACA = **anterior cerebral artery;** ant. = anterior; DL = dorsolateral; DM = dorsomedial; ICA = internal carotid artery; IM = inferomedial; MCA = **middle cerebral artery;** RM = rostromedial; V = ventral; VA = ventral anterior; VM = ventromedial.

Table 2.5. Basal Nuclei Circuitry

	Direct Pathway	Indirect Pathway	Subthalamic	Striosomal
Role	*Cortical input into striatum:* Initiation of action; establishing adaptive patterns; releases behavior or movement	*Cortical input into striatum:* "Braking"; switching from one action to the next; inhibits closely related unwanted behavior or movement	*"Hyperdirect pathway":* Response inhibition; enables nonresponse; suppresses all behavior; stops response faster than indirect pathway owing to fewer synapses	Allows for evaluation of information for reward; influences similar behavior in the future; instrumental learning
Overall circuitry	Cortex → striatum → pallidus → thalamus → cortical motor areas	Cortex → striatum → pallidus → thalamus → cortical motor areas	Cortex → subthalamic nucleus → pallidus or substantia nigra → thalamus → cortical motor areas	Cortex → striatum → pallidus → cortical motor areas
Effects of cortical input to the basal nuclei	Cortex activates striatum	Cortex activates striatum	Cortex activates subthalamic nucleus	Cortex activates putamen
Specific route through the basal nuclei	1. Cortex ↓ 2. striatum ↓ 3. GPi/SNpr ↓ 4. thalamus ↓ 5. cortical motor areas	1. Cortex ↓ 2. striatum ↓ 3. GPe ↓ 4. STN ↓ 5. GPi, SNpr ↓ 6. thalamus ↓ 7. cortical motor areas	1. Cortex ↓ 2. STN ↓ 3. GPi or SNpr ↓ 4. thalamus ↓ 5. cortical motor areas	1. Cortex ↓ 2. putamen ↓ 3. SNpc/SNpr ↓ 4. back through basal nuclei
Effects of basal nuclei (GPi, SNpr) on thalamus	Excitatory	Inhibitory	Inhibitory	No direct involvement with thalamus
Effects of thalamus on cortex	Thalamus activated

Results in release of behavior; releases inhibition of cortex; cortex activated | Thalamus not activated

Results in suppression of behavior; cortex not activated | Thalamus not activated

Results in suppression of behavior; cortex not activated | No direct connection

Evaluation of reward influences future behavior |
| Summary of activity | Active when required, depending on the circumstances or needs of the organism; allows wanted behavior | Active when required, depending on the circumstances or needs of the organism; inhibits unwanted behavior | Allows person to think before responding; therefore, important in impulse control | Assessment of the value of behavior for the organism; allows instrumental learning |

Note. Green type = excitatory, activation via glutamate; red type = inhibitory, inactivation via γ-aminobutyric acid; GPe = globus pallidus externa; GPi = globus pallidus interna; SNpc = substantia nigra pars compacta; SNpr = substantia nigra pars reticulata; STN = subthalamic nuclei.

systems is central to the executive function and behavioral inhibition deficits that are a frequent consequence of TBI.

The dorsolateral prefrontal system is primarily associated with organization, executive planning, and executive attention (Figure 2.24). The orbitofrontal system is primarily associated with response inhibition, reward, and the mediation of empathy and socially appropriate behavior (Figure 2.25). The anterior cingulate system is associated with motivation, error correction, and arousal (Figure 2.26). In general, most cortical areas project afferents to the striatum, which subsequently funnel them down through the GP and SN and on to the thalamus from which they are then redirected in a loop back to the frontal lobe.

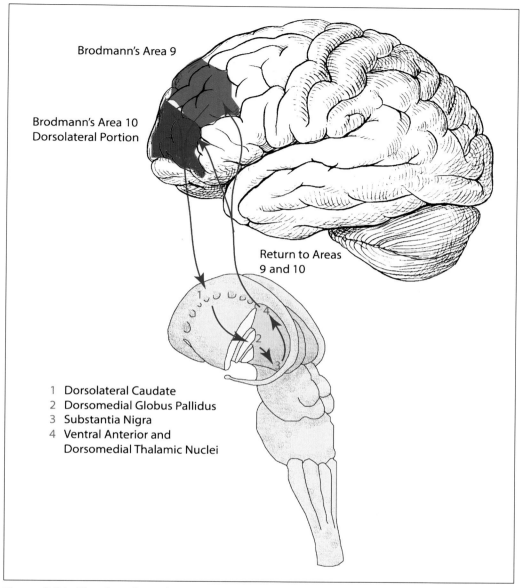

Brodmann's Area 9

Brodmann's Area 10
Dorsolateral Portion

Return to Areas
9 and 10

1 Dorsolateral Caudate
2 Dorsomedial Globus Pallidus
3 Substantia Nigra
4 Ventral Anterior and
   Dorsomedial Thalamic Nuclei

Figure 2.24. The dorsolateral prefrontal system is primarily associated with organization, executive planning, and executive attention.

Source. F. Feuchter.

Brainstem and Cranial Nerves

The brainstem lies at the base of the brain, linking the cerebral hemispheres above with the spinal cord below. It is composed of three segments: (1) the midbrain, (2) the pons, and (3) the **medulla oblongata.** The brainstem regulates the basic processes necessary for life—respiration, heart rate, sleeping, eating, maintenance of a conscious and alert state—and provides innervation to the viscera. The brainstem is also the origin of most *cranial nerves* (CNs; III–XII), which consist of nerve fibers that have at least one or more of the following neural functions:

1. *Somatic sensory* (afferent) fibers transmit general sensory information of
   the body (i.e., touch, pressure, vibration, temperature, pain) from the skin
   and mucous membranes to the CNS;

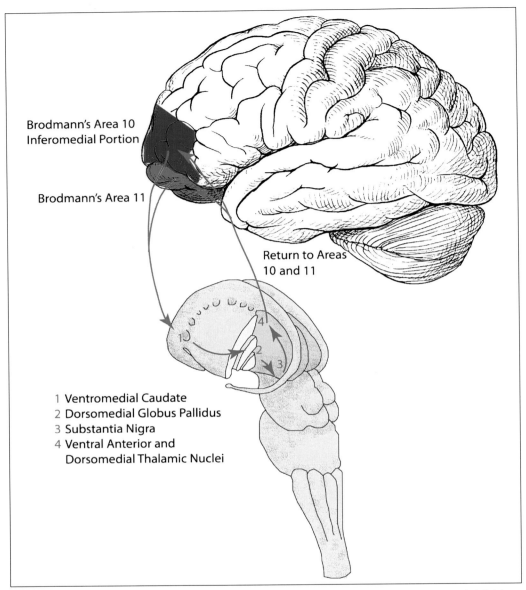

Brodmann's Area 10
Inferomedial Portion

Brodmann's Area 11

Return to Areas
10 and 11

1 Ventromedial Caudate
2 Dorsomedial Globus Pallidus
3 Substantia Nigra
4 Ventral Anterior and
   Dorsomedial Thalamic Nuclei

Figure 2.25. The orbitofrontal system is primarily associated with response inhibition, reward, and the mediation of empathy and socially appropriate behavior.

Source. F. Feuchter.

2. *Visceral sensory* (afferent) fibers transmit sensory information from the viscera (i.e., blood pressure, gut distention, mucosal irritation of throat and airways) to the CNS (e.g., afferent arm of cough reflex);

3. *Special sensory* (afferent) fibers transmit information associated with the special senses (i.e., smell, vision, hearing, balance, taste) to the CNS;

4. *Somatic motor* (efferent) fibers; axons of somatic motor neurons provide neural regulation of muscles under voluntary control (i.e., those that are striated); and

5. *Visceral motor* (efferent) fibers; axons of autonomic (parasympathetic or sympathetic) or visceral motor neurons provide neural regulation to smooth muscle, cardiac muscle, and glandular tissue (under involuntary control).

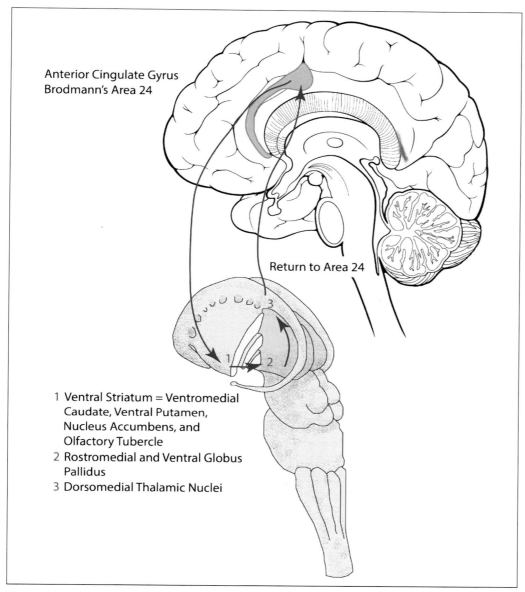

Figure 2.26. The anterior cingulate system is associated with motivation, error correction, and arousal.

Source. F. Feuchter.

Some CNs are purely sensory (CNs I, II, and VIII), some are purely motor (CNs III, IV, VI, XI, and XII), and some have both sensory and motor functions (CNs V, VII, IX, and X; see Tables 2.6, 2.7, and 2.8). CN damage is somewhat rare in mild TBI (**Glasgow Coma Scale** [GCS] 13–15) and almost a certainty in moderate to severe TBI (GCS 3–12). At all levels of severity of TBI, CN I is the most commonly injured (Coello, Canals, Gonzalez, & Martín, 2010; Jin et al., 2010) because of its particularly vulnerable anatomical journey through the ethmoid bone of the skull.

Loss of consciousness in TBI is believed to result from rotational forces that lead to stretching of the brainstem (Ivancevic, 2009); severe damage to the brainstem can result in death. Increased intracranial pressure (ICP) can result in the brainstem

Table 2.6. Origin, Route, and Functions of the Cranial Nerves

Number and Name	Origin and Route	Functions
I: Olfactory	Olfactory receptors originate in mucosa on the roof of the nasal cavity and travel to temporal lobes of the cerebrum via the olfactory bulbs.	*Afferent:* Special sense of smell (olfaction) *Efferent:* None
II: Optic	Ganglion cells transmit visual information from the retina via the optic nerves to the lateral geniculate nucleus of the thalamus and ultimately to the primary visual cortex of the occipital lobe.	*Afferent:* Special sense of vision *Efferent:* None

III: Oculomotor	Originates from the mesencephalon (midbrain) of the brainstem and travels through the orbit to reach muscles of the globe.	*Afferent:* None
		Efferent:
		1. Somatic motor to the following extraocular muscles produces movement of the globe:
		  • Inferior oblique (IO): Elevates globe when globe adducted; *extorts* (laterally rotates) globe when globe abducted
		  • Superior rectus (SR): Elevates globe
		  • Medial rectus (MR): Adducts globe
		  • Inferior rectus (IR): Depresses globe
		  • Levator palpebrae superioris: Raises (opens) eyelid
		  Note: The superior oblique (SO) is innervated by the trochlear nerve (IV), and the lateral rectus (LR) is innervated by the abducens nerve (VI), as discussed in the sections below.
		2. Visceral motor (parasympathetic) to sphincter pupillae (pupil constriction) and to ciliary body (allows lens to become more rounded for near vision via **accommodation** reflex)
		
		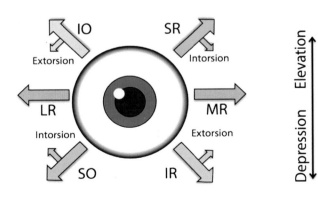

IV: Trochlear	Mesencephalon (midbrain)	*Afferent:* None *Efferent:* Somatic motor to the superior oblique muscle; contraction causes depression of the globe (directs gaze inferolaterally) when the globe is adducted and inward rotation of the globe (*intorsion*) when the globe is abducted. The superior oblique muscle assists in directing gaze inferolaterally from the adducted position and acts as a pulley to redirect the globe's line of action down and out (*trochlea* refers to an anatomical structure that resembles or functions like a pulley).

(Continued)

Table 2.6. Origin, Route, and Functions of the Cranial Nerves *(cont.)*

Number and Name	Origin and Route	Functions
V: Trigeminal	Metencephalon (pons)	*Afferent:*
		Somatic sensory:
		V_1 (opthalmic): Cutaneous sensation from the skin of face overlying maxilla, including upper lip, gums, maxillary teeth, mucosa of the nose, lateral aspect of external nose, as well as the maxillary sinuses and palate
		V_2 (maxillary): Cutaneous sensation from middle one-third of face (upper lip, gums, upper teeth, anterior cheek, lateral external nose) as well as palate
		V_3 (mandibular): Cutaneous sensation from lower one-third of face (lower lip, gums, lower teeth, palate), mucosa of mouth, and anterior two-thirds of tongue

Distribution of Sensory Fibers of Trigeminal Nerve Divisions

Number and Name	Origin and Route	Functions
		Efferent:
		Somatic:
		V_1 (opthalmic): None
		V_2 (maxillary): None
		V_3 (mandibular): Muscles of mastication as well as the following:
		• Tensor tympani: Tenses tympanic membrane to prevent damage to internal ear when exposed to loud sounds
		• Tensor veli palatini: Tenses soft palate during swallowing
		• Mylohyoid: Depresses mandible during swallowing and speaking
		• Anterior belly of digastric: Depresses mandible during swallowing and speaking
VI: Abducens	Metencephalon (pons)	*Afferent:* None
		Efferent: Somatic motor to lateral rectus muscle (allows abduction of globe)
VII: Facial	Taste receptors on tongue and posterior border of metencephalon (pons)	*Afferent:*
		1. Special sense of taste to anterior two-thirds of tongue (sweet, salty) and soft palate
		2. Somatic sensory fibers transmit cutaneous sensation for small region surrounding external auditory meatus
		Efferent:
		1. Somatic motor to the muscles of facial expression and scalp, as well as the stapedius of middle ear, stylohyoid, and posterior belly of digastric muscles
		2. Visceral motor (parasympathetic) or secretomotor to the sublingual and submandibular salivary glands as well as the lacrimal gland

(Continued)

Table 2.6. Origin, Route, and Functions of the Cranial Nerves *(cont.)*

Number and Name	Origin and Route	Functions
VIII: Vestibulocochlear	Receptors of the inner ear and grooves between the pons and medulla	*Afferent:* Special sense of hearing (cochlea) and of equilibrium and motion (vestibular apparatus and semicircular canals) *Efferent:* None
IX: Glossopharyngeal	Receptors of the tongue, carotid artery, and mucosa of pharynx; convey sensory information to the rostral end of the medulla	*Afferent:* 1. Special sense of taste to posterior one-third of tongue (bitter, sour) 2. Somatic sensory from posterior one-third of tongue, soft palate, nasopharynx, mucosa of pharynx, eustachian tube, tympanic membrane and cavity 3. Visceral sensory: Carotid sinus (baroreceptors) and carotid body (O_2– CO_2 chemoreceptors) at bifurcation of carotid artery *Efferent:* 1. Somatic motor to stylopharyngeus muscle 2. Visceral motor (parasympathetic) to pharyngeal plexus and secretomotor to parotid gland
X: Vagus	Rootlets (8–10) from the lateral aspects of the medulla and brainstem to various viscera	*Afferent:* 1. Special sense of taste to epiglottis 2. Somatic sensory from mucosa of pharynx and larynx 3. Visceral sensory from aortic sinus and body in aortic arch and mucosa of pharynx and larynx (reflex afferents for cough) *Efferent:* 1. Somatic motor to the voluntary muscles of larynx and superior esophagus (palatoglossus and levator veli palatini) 2. Visceral motor (parasympathetic) to smooth muscle and glands of the viscera of thorax and abdomen (esophageal, pulmonary, cardiac plexuses)
XI: Spinal accessory	Arise as rootlets from the sides of the spinal cord in the superior 5–6 cervical segments	*Afferent:* None *Efferent:* Somatic motor to sternocleidomastoid and trapezius muscles
XII: Hypoglossal	Rootlets between pyramids and olives of the medulla	*Afferent:* None *Efferent:* Somatic motor to extrinsic and intrinsic muscles of the tongue (except palatoglossus)

Note. V_1 = first branch of the trigeminal nerve (cranial nerve V); also referred to as the *opthalmic division*. V_2 = second branch of the trigeminal nerve (cranial nerve V); also referred to as the *maxillary division*. V_3 = third branch of the trigeminal nerve (cranial nerve V); also referred to as the *mandibular division*.

being forced downward toward the **foramen magnum,** which leads to compression of brainstem structures and may also result in death, which is one reason why ICP is closely monitored in the acute stage of recovery from TBI. Mechanical trauma or stretching of the CNs may occur in TBI and disrupt the functions controlled by these nerves, including the control of eye movement, hearing, and motor and sensory functions of the face and neck.

Cerebellum

The cerebellum ("little brain") accounts for only about 10% of the mass of the brain, but it contains more neurons than all other components of the CNS combined. It is located inferior to the cerebrum and *caudal* (posterior) to the brainstem. The cerebellum is attached to the brainstem via the *cerebellar peduncles*, three pairs of short, thick fiber bundles that contain the afferent and efferent fibers of each half of the cerebellum. The *superior cerebellar peduncle* contains the major output from the cerebellum to the thalamus. The *middle cerebellar peduncle* is the largest and is composed of afferents to the cerebellum arising from the pontine nuclei of the

Table 2.7. Cranial Nerve Injuries: Presentation and Causes

Number and Name	Clinical Testing	Presentation of Neural Lesion	Causes, Frequency, and Characteristics in Moderate and Severe TBI
I: Olfactory	• Assessed by exposure to pure, nonirritating odors. • Serial, quantified testing can be performed, and each nostril should be tested separately.	• *Anosmia* (loss of the sense of smell), *hyposmia* (diminished sense of smell), or *parosmia* (distorted sense of smell whereby an unpleasant odor is perceived in place of the natural one) can result from a lesion anywhere along the olfactory pathway and is often accompanied by a decreased sense of taste. • Patients with unilateral lesions are not usually aware of the deficit because olfaction can be compensated by the contralateral nostril.	• Head injury is the most common cause of the loss of olfaction. • The olfactory nerve is the most commonly damaged CN in head injury. • TBI involving any of the components of the olfactory pathways or any interpreting centers of the brain can disturb olfaction. • Fractures of the cribriform plate of the ethmoid bone can damage the olfactory nerves. • Scarring of tissues of the cribriform plate post-TBI may compress the olfactory nerves. • Shearing forces or abrasive injuries from frontal or occipital blows can shear or stretch olfactory nerve fibers. • Compression of the olfactory bulbs as a result of **hemorrhage,** edema, or **contusion** and abrasion will compromise function of the olfactory nerves. • Coup–contrecoup injuries produce severe acceleration–deceleration forces that avulse the olfactory nerve.
II: Optic	• Swinging flashlight test is used to search for an afferent pupillary defect. • Alterations in visual acuity and fields can be determined by a Snellen chart but should be well documented, and patient should be referred to specialists for close observation for potential deterioration.	• Optic nerve damage may result in partial or total blindness in a single eye (optic nerve) or both eyes (at chiasm) and affect both visual fields (posterior to chiasm along the optic tract). • Blindness can occur in half of the visual field (hemianopsia or hemianopia) or in the whole visual field, but when affecting half often occurs in the same half of the field in each eye (*homonymous hemianopsia*[a]).	• Contusion or rupture of the optic nerves, compression from bone fragments, hemorrhage, or edema from adjacent tissues will affect nerve function. • Immediate loss of vision is due to traumatic injury to the optic nerve (i.e., shearing or contusion resulting from movement of the contents of the orbit and cranium). • Symptomatic **convergence** insufficiency may result from a subdural **hematoma** (Spierer et al., 1995).
III: Oculomotor	• Patient is asked to move the eyes in the directions represented by the muscles supplied by CN III. • In the event of complete disruption of the nerve, all extraocular muscles are paralyzed except the lateral rectus and superior oblique, and the globe would be able to achieve only some abduction, some depression, and intorsion. • Patient may report that ***diplopia*** (double vision—seeing two images instead of one) is worse when looking at near objects and improved when looking at distant objects because convergence is impaired.	• Oculomotor nerve palsy typically presents with vertical and horizontal diplopia that improves when the affected globe is abducted and may occur unilaterally or bilaterally, with the pupil variably involved or spared. • Partial impairment can yield a combination of presentations and in milder form. • Complete disruption of the oculomotor nerve function causes paralysis of all but two of the extraocular muscles (lateral rectus and superior oblique), resulting in ipsilateral *ptosis* (drooping of the eyelid), dilation of the pupil that is unresponsive to light, and the globe directed inferolaterally (i.e., globe is depressed and abducted, appearing down and out).	• Shearing forces associated with TBI or herniation of the brain may damage the oculomotor nerve. • Severe damage to the oculomotor nerve can result in almost total loss of the extraocular muscles supplied by the oculomotor nerve.

(Continued)

Table 2.7. Cranial Nerve Injuries: Presentation and Causes (*cont.*)

Number and Name	Clinical Testing	Presentation of Neural Lesion	Causes, Frequency, and Characteristics in Moderate and Severe TBI
IV: Trochlear	• Recorded diplopia fields are useful for diagnosis and follow-up. • Movement of the superior oblique muscle is tested by prompting the patient to depress the globe while the globe is adducted, to rotate the globe inward (*intorsion*) while the globe is abducted, or both. • Trochlear palsy can be verified by having the patient look up while tucking the chin and tilting the head away from the affected globe. • Vertical diplopia caused by trochlear palsy will be alleviated by the head-tilt and chin-tuck maneuvers, which collectively compensate for the hyperopia and extorsion associated with trochlear nerve palsy.	• Trochlear nerve palsy is the most common cause of vertical strabismus. • Vertical diplopia is worse or present only with near vision and on downward gaze directed to the opposite side of the affected globe (i.e., when looking inferolaterally or down and out). • Typically, patients with trochlear nerve palsy experience difficulty reading and diplopia when going downstairs, with the deficits improving with contralateral head tilt and worsening with ipsilateral head tilt.	• Not commonly affected in isolation. • Trochlear nerve damage is associated with brainstem lesions; lesions in the subarachnoid space; or lesions in the cavernous sinus, superior orbital fissure, orbit, or both.

V: Trigeminal	• Testing involves assessment of all three divisions of the nerve for **somatic sensation.**
	• *Sensory evaluation:* Involves somatic sensation (light touch, pain, vibration, temperatures) tested on face and mucous membranes:
	  • Each trigeminal division is tested and compared with the contralateral side.
	  • Eyelid response to corneal testing with cotton can distinguish CN V from CN VII palsies.
	• *Motor evaluation:* Involves asking the patient to clench jaw, open jaw, and move jaw side to side against resistance.
		• Anesthesia of the face, forehead, scalp, nose, conjunctiva, gingivae, anterior two-thirds of tongue, mucous membrane lining the nasal cavity, hard and soft palates, cheek, and lips may be observed.
		• Muscles of mastication may be paralyzed ipsilaterally (V_3). Corneal drying and decreased salivation may occur.
			• Brainstem lesions and lesions at Meckel's cave and superior orbital fissure may result in extensive loss of trigeminal nerve function because of the proximity of its origin.

VI: Abducens	• Recorded diplopia fields are useful for diagnosis and follow-up. • Movement of the lateral rectus muscle is tested by prompting the patient to laterally rotate (or abduct) the globe. • Minor degrees of lateral rectus limitation are ambiguous after TBI, and testing requires patient cooperation.	• Abducens nerve palsy typically presents as horizontal diplopia that is worse when the affected eye is abducted (i.e., in lateral gaze) or when viewing objects at a distance because the globes must diverge. • With a partial injury, the affected eye is seen at midline at rest, but the patient cannot deviate the eye laterally. • In a complete injury, the patient is unable to abduct the eye, and the affected eye is therefore turned medially. • Combined injuries of CN III, IV, or V can result in the loss of depth perception and problems with reading and visual scanning.	• Abducens nerve injury typically occurs in combination with injuries to the oculomotor, trochlear, or trigeminal nerves.

(Continued)

Table 2.7. Cranial Nerve Injuries: Presentation and Causes *(cont.)*

Number and Name	Clinical Testing	Presentation of Neural Lesion	Causes, Frequency, and Characteristics in Moderate and Severe TBI
VII: Facial	• *Motor evaluation:* The patient is asked to produce facial expressions. • *Special sensory evaluation:* Assesses sweet and salty taste. • The stapedius reflex is evaluated.	• Complete or partial paralysis of facial muscles always occurs with lesions of the facial nerve, although symptoms vary in extent and severity depending on the location of the lesion. • Impaired sense of sweet or salty taste may occur (from the anterior two-thirds of the tongue). • The corneal blink reflex and lacrimal secretions may or may not be affected. • Paralysis of the facial nerve (Bell's palsy) often resolves without surgical intervention. • Loss of the stapedius reflex is manifested by hypersensitivity to loud sounds.	• The facial nerve is highly vulnerable to injury with blunt trauma to the head because of its tortuous course through the temporal bone. • Temporal bone fractures, especially longitudinal and transverse fractures causing cranial trauma, may result in facial nerve damage. • Immediate paralysis may occur as a result of tears of the nerve or bony impingement. • Delayed paralysis (>4–6 days) may occur as a result of the formation of edema or hematoma.
VIII: Vestibulocochlear	• Evaluation of hearing, examination of ocular movements, cerebellar testing, and evaluation of vestibular control of balance and movement are performed. • Tuning forks are used to evaluate hearing via the Weber and Rinne tests. • Positional vertigo usually occurs for ~30 s as a result of sudden changes in position, from lying to sitting or from sitting to standing.	• Posttraumatic positional vertigo (illusory sensation of movement) is the most common manifestation of a CN VIII lesion, with possible ipsilateral tinnitus, hearing loss, and loss of equilibrium. • Patients may experience deficits in perceiving tones or speech (often associated with tinnitus). • **Nystagmus** (oscillating globe movements) and autonomic effects (nausea, vomiting, pallor, sweating, hypotension) may also be observed.	• Blunt trauma to the lateral aspect of the skull or temporal bone fractures may cause vestibulocochlear nerve damage. • Longitudinal fractures of the temporal bone may disrupt the tympanic membrane. • Transverse fractures of the temporal bone are commonly associated with damage to the facial and vestibulocochlear nerves. • Positional vertigo, tinnitus, hearing loss, and deafness may occur after TBI.
IX: Glossopharyngeal	• *Sensory evaluation:* Assesses ipsilateral loss of taste over posterior one-third of tongue and loss of sensation over soft palate and posterior one-third of tongue. • *Motor evaluation:* Usually no obvious deficit results from loss of stylopharyngeus function, but mild **dysphagia** may occur. • *Reflex evaluation:* Gag reflex can be tested with light touch to pharynx, tonsillar area, or base of tongue, which should lead to gagging. • *Autonomic evaluation:* Assess ipsilateral alteration in parotid salivation; carotid sinus nerve dysfunction may lead to tachycardia or bradycardia, hypotension, or all of these.	• Patients may experience loss of somatic sensation in the posterior one-third of the tongue and in the pharynx, with possible mild dysphagia, **dysarthria,** drooling, difficulty initiating swallowing, nasal regurgitation, difficulty managing secretions, choking–coughing episodes while feeding, and food sticking in the throat.	• The glossopharyngeal nerve is only occasionally affected by head trauma. • Lesions or trauma involving the jugular foramen **(basilar skull fracture)** may damage the glossopharyngeal nerve as it exits the skull. • Dysphagia and dysarthria are caused by injury to the glossopharyngeal and vagus nerves.

(Continued)

Table 2.7. Cranial Nerve Injuries: Presentation and Causes *(cont.)*

Number and Name	Clinical Testing	Presentation of Neural Lesion	Causes, Frequency, and Characteristics in Moderate and Severe TBI
X: Vagus	• *Sensory evaluation:* Assessment is difficult because of considerable overlap with CNs VII and IX. • *Motor evaluation:* Soft palate and uvula can be examined at rest and with phonation; laryngeal and pharyngeal function can be evaluated with phonation and swallowing with respirations and coughing via direct laryngoscopy. • *Reflex evaluation:* Gag, cough, and vomiting reflexes can be tested. • *Autonomic evaluation:* Ipsilateral decreased carotid sinus reflex may be observed as a result of reduced vagal outflow. Bilateral vagal dysfunction is associated with tachycardia and other signs of sympathetic overactivity.	• Unilateral paralysis of larynx and palate with hoarseness may result from loss of the recurrent laryngeal nerve. • Aphonia or weak or hoarse voice may result. • Unilateral anesthesia of the larynx will also be present ipsilaterally. • Tachycardia and decreased respiration result if both vagi are cut in the head and neck, and the patient is often unable to breathe or speak as a result of the loss of innervation to both vocal cords. • Locked-in syndrome, which results from damage to the pons, may also be associated with vagal nerve lesions, thereby causing severely decreased bowel sounds and elevated but unchanging pulse.	• The vagus nerve is only occasionally affected by head trauma. • Lesions or trauma involving the jugular foramen (basilar skull fracture) may result in damage to the vagus nerve as it exits the skull. • Dysphagia and dysarthria are caused by injury to the glossopharyngeal and vagus nerves. • Vagus nerve injury results in a hoarse voice.
XI: Spinal accessory	• Motor evaluation of the spinal accessory nerve involves testing the sternocleidomastoid and trapezius muscles against resistance.	• Sternocleidomastoid paresis manifests as weakness in turning head to the opposite side. • Trapezius paresis manifests as shoulder drop, difficulty raising abducted arm above horizontal, and inability to shrug the shoulders. • Lower trapezius function may be spared because of partial innervation of the trapezius from the cervical plexus.	• The spinal accessory nerve is only occasionally affected by head trauma. • Lesions affecting the jugular foramen and the foramen magnum can damage the spinal accessory nerve as it enters or exits the skull.
XII: Hypoglossal	• Observation of the tongue at rest and with protrusion and movement is necessary. Tongue movement to the left and right against resistance may also be examined.	• The affected side of the tongue becomes wrinkled and atrophied. • When the tongue is protruded, the weakness resulting from a nerve lesion causes the tip of the tongue to deviate toward the side of the lesion. • If both nerves are damaged, the tongue cannot protrude. • If one nerve is damaged, the tongue deviates toward the injured side (ipsilateral atrophy). • Dysarthria and dysphagia can occur.	• The hypoglossal nerve is only occasionally affected by head trauma. • Penetrating wounds to the neck may sever the hypoglossal nerve. • Blunt trauma is rarely caused by hyperextension neck injuries.

Note. CN/CNs = cranial nerve/nerves; s = seconds; TBI = traumatic brain injury; V_3 = third branch of the trigeminal nerve.
[a]*Homonymous hemianopsia* is a visual-field defect involving either two right or two left halves of the visual field of both eyes.

Table 2.8. Frequency of Cranial Nerve Injuries by Injury Severity

CN	Mild TBI[a] (Coello et al., 2010), N = 16,440		Moderate to Severe TBI (Jin et al., 2010), N = 3,417		Severe TBI (Keane & Baloh, 2006), N = 291
	% of CN Injuries	% of TBI	% of CN Injuries	% of TBI	% of TBI
I: Olfactory	21.0	0.08	20.5	1.9	14.0
II: Optic	8.1	0.03	22.1	2.0	2.7
III: Oculomotor	11.3	0.04	25.0[a]	2.28[a]	6.6
IV: Trochlear	11.3	0.04			
V: Trigeminal	1.6	0.01			
VI: Abducens	12.9	0.05			2.7
VII: Facial	17.7	0.07	18.3[a]	1.7[a]	3.0
VIII: Vestibulocochlear	11.3	0.04			
IX: Glossopharyngeal	1.6	0.01	7.7[a]	0.7[a]	
X: Vagus	1.6	0.01			
XI: Spinal accessory	1.6	0.01			
XII: Hypoglossal	0	0	1.9[a]	0.2	

Note. CN = cranial nerve; TBI = traumatic brain injury. Mild TBI = Glasgow Coma Scale score of 13–15; moderate to severe TBI = Glasgow Coma Scale score of 3–12. Not all researchers reported data for each CN.
[a]Reported as a group.

contralateral side, which receive input from the cerebral motor cortex. The *inferior cerebellar peduncle* is composed mostly of afferents to the cerebellum arising from the spinal cord and brainstem.

The cerebellum has a layered micro-organization similar to that of the cerebrum, with a more superficial layer of gray matter overlaying a deeper layer of white matter that transmits neural information to and from the cerebellum. Anatomically, the cerebellum is divided into two hemispheres connected in the center by a midline region or zone, the *vermis* ("worm"). Each hemisphere is divided into three lobes: The primary fissure divides the bulk of the cerebellum into (1) *anterior* and (2) *posterior lobes,* and a deeper fissure separates these from the (3) *flocculonodular lobe.* The functional subdivisions of the cerebellum are the (1) *vermis,* which is involved in postural adjustments; (2) *lateral hemisphere,* which is involved in planning movements; (3) *medial hemisphere,* which is involved in adjusting limb movements; and (4) *flocculonodular lobe,* which is involved in balance, eye movement, and spatial orientation (Blumenfeld, 2010; Nolte, 2009).

The main functions of the cerebellum are to (1) coordinate voluntary motor movement through integrated and precise temporal control of muscles to achieve balance, posture, and equilibrium and to (2) provide for the patterning and learning of complex motor routines. These functions are accomplished in the cerebellum through the integration of massive amounts of sensory and other inputs from many regions of the brain and spinal cord and the coordination of ongoing motor movements and planning. Similar to the basal nuclei, the cerebellum has no direct connection to the lower motor neurons but instead influences the lower motor neurons via its interactions with the motor regions of the cortex and brainstem. The cerebellar white matter contains deeply embedded nuclei that receive input from somatosensory and motor cortex and also from association and limbic cortex. In addition to coordinating movement and motor learning, the cerebellum is

The cerebellum has a layered micro-organization similar to that of the cerebrum, with a more superficial layer of gray matter overlaying a deeper layer of white matter.

Table 2.9. Regions of the Cerebellum and Their Specialized Functions

Region	Functions	Typical Presentations of Injury or Lesions
Lateral hemispheres	1. Motor planning for movements of ipsilateral extremities 2. Cognition	• **Ataxia** of the ipsilateral limbs (*appendicular ataxia*) • Hypotonia, hyporeflexia, pendular reflexes • **Dysmetria**, intention tremors, dysdiadochokinesia • Scanning speech
Medial hemispheres	1. Distal limb coordination for ipsilateral extremities; adjusting limb movements 2. Affective and autonomic function	• Ataxia
Vermis	1. Coordination of proximal trunk movements 2. Postural adjustments 3. Some eye movements	• Unsteady drunklike gait (*truncal ataxia*) • Postural instability • Broad-based staggering gait
Flocculonodular lobe	1. Balance and vestibulo–ocular reflex 2. Eye movements 3. Spatial orientation	• Broad-based staggering gait • Side-to-side swaying while standing still • Abnormal eye movements (nystagmus) • Difficulty with **pursuit** eye movements, maintaining eccentric gaze, or making accurate voluntary eye movements • Disturbances in balance, intense vertigo, nausea, and vomiting

involved in nonmotor functions (see Table 2.9). Connections between the lateral hemispheres of the posterior lobe of the cerebellum are thought to be involved in a range of cognitive processes. Numerous clinical reports have indicated that cerebellar damage can be associated with a variety of cognitive and behavioral disturbances (Blumenfeld, 2010).

Although the cerebellum is generally well protected from trauma compared with the frontal and temporal lobes of the cortex, cerebellar damage as a consequence of TBI can occur indirectly, even though the initial mechanical insult is directed to the cerebral cortex (Potts, Adwanikar, & Noble-Haeusslein, 2009). Cerebellar lesions can cause abnormalities of equilibrium, postural control, and coordination of voluntary movement of the body, causing slowness and incoordination that result in a sway and stagger when walking. Additionally, eye movements and balance and **vestibular function** can be disrupted.

Mechanisms of Traumatic Brain Injury

The exact mechanisms by which brain displacement leads to stretch and shear strain on brain tissue and causes brain damage are not fully understood (Feng et al., 2010). TBI occurs when an external mechanical force such as rapid acceleration or deceleration, impact, crush, or penetration by an external object or projectile damages brain tissue, usually by causing rapid deformation to the brain (Figure 2.27). The severe mechanical deformation initiates a chain reaction of pathological events, ultimately leading to neurodegeneration (via excitotoxicity, apoptosis, and necrosis; Ivancevic, 2009). Brain movement occurs relative to the skull even during normal day-to-day activity (Feng et al., 2010), but in the context of rapid acceleration or deceleration, brain function may be temporarily or permanently impaired, and structural damage may occur (Ivancevic, 2009).

Damage from TBI can be focal or diffuse, with the latter being far more frequent (Krave, Al-Olama, & Hansson, 2011). Focal injuries may result from penetration of the skull and dura by an object (i.e., open TBI) or from contact of the brain tissue with the rough inner surface of the skull, such as in the classic coup–contrecoup injury. In coup–contrecoup injury, a contusion develops when the brain strikes

A. Linear Acceleration

Direction of head movement

Direction of force

Results in gliding contusions in parasagittal regions, ischemic lesions in cerebellum, and axonal damage in brainstem

B. Impact Deceleration

Direction of head movement

Resisting force from ground

Results in contrecoup lesions of frontal lobe orbital surfaces and temporal lobe tips

C. Rotational Acceleration

Rotational movement of head

Direction of force against jaw

Results in subdural hematoma and diffuse axonal injury

D. Arterial Injury

Force applied to lateral neck

Results in injury to the carotid artery and compression of the carotid sinus, leading to generalized ischemia

Figure 2.27. Examples of rapid brain movement that can result in traumatic brain injury. (A) Linear acceleration of the head, as in a whiplash injury; **(B)** impact deceleration, as in falling back on the head; **(C)** rotational acceleration, or rapid twisting of the neck; **(D)** arterial injury resulting from a blow to the lateral neck.

Source. F. Feuchter.

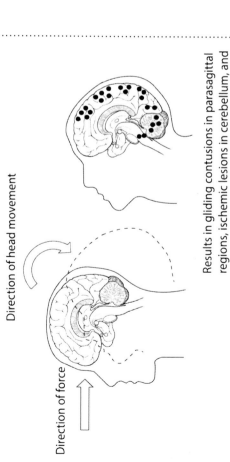
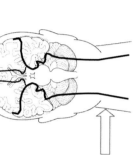
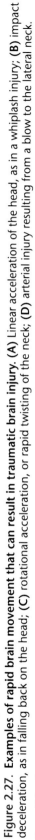

the opposite inner surface of the skull after sudden deceleration. Coup–contrecoup injuries thus commonly occur in the frontal (particularly the orbitofrontal), anterior temporal, and occipital poles of the brain (frontal and temporal contusions are most common in the absence of skull fracture; Ivancevic, 2009).

Certain brain areas are more prone to damage because of the brain's structure and geometry. The anatomical tethering points or attachments of the brain are most robust at the base of the skull, such that deceleration of the skull induces rotation of the brain within the skull on the sagittal axis as well as translational (forward and backward) movement (Feng et al., 2010). Focal injuries may also occur from bleeding in specific locations. *Hematomas* (collections of blood outside of a blood vessel) may occur as a result of TBI and may also cause **focal brain injury.** Hematomas may be epidural, subdural, subarachnoid, or intraventricular (Table 2.10). In an *epidural hematoma,* blood accumulates in the space between the dura mater and the periosteal lining of the inner surface of the skull. In a *subdural hematoma,* blood accumulates between the inner surface of the dura mater and the outer layer of the arachnoid mater. In a *subarachnoid hematoma,* blood accumulates between the arachnoid mater and the pia mater (i.e., in the subarachnoid space). In an *intraventricular hematoma,* blood accumulates in the ventricles. The occurrence of hematomas may result in secondary localized mass effects on the adjacent brain tissue or, if large enough, may cause a midline shift in which the entire brain is forced away by the mass of blood (diffuse injury).

Common causes of diffuse brain injury (DBI) are **cerebral edema** (swelling) and diffuse axonal injury (DAI; sometimes called *traumatic axonal injury*). **Concussion** (mild TBI) results from DAI (Krave et al., 2011). DAI results from mechanical deformation of brain substance (Ivancevic, 2009) and most frequently occurs as a result of impact or dynamic (impulsive) loading, such as in a whiplash injury (Goldsmith, 2001). Brain injury resulting from the application of a static load occurs very infrequently (e.g., when one's head gets caught in a machine press or between elevator doors or when a car comes off a car jack during repairs; Goldsmith, 2001). The severity and distribution of DBI depends to some degree on the type of mechanical force exerted on the brain and its direction (translational force, rotational force in the sagittal plane, flexion vs. extension; Figure 2.27; Krave et al., 2011).

Brain tissue is of heterogeneous consistency (i.e., white matter is stiffer than gray matter, leading to strain where they meet; Bayly et al., 2005) and is *anisotropic* (i.e., the physical and mechanical properties of brain tissue are different when measured in different directions). Consequently, the same amount of force will cause different degrees of damage depending on the direction in which the force is applied (Krave et al., 2011). For example, flexion may cause more severe injury than extension. The presence of DBI may be consistent with little apparent damage in standard neuroimaging studies (magnetic resonance imaging [MRI] or computed tomography). Diffusion tensor imaging provides a way of processing MRI images that more accurately represents damage to white matter tracts from DAI.

Hematomas or brain edema may result in increased ICP. Because the skull is rigid, ICP may force the brainstem down into the foramen magnum (herniation), which, if left untreated, may result in disruption of respiratory function and death. Other consequences of abnormally elevated ICP include restriction in cerebral **perfusion** (cerebral hypoxia, cerebral **ischemia**) and **hydrocephalus.** ICP is measured in millimeters of mercury (mm Hg) and is normally <15 mm Hg for a supine adult. If ICP rises to more than 40 mm Hg, the prognosis is poor. Children appear

The anatomical tethering points or attachments of the brain are most robust at the base of the skull, such that deceleration of the skull induces rotation of the brain within the skull on the sagittal axis as well as translational (forward and backward) movement.

Table 2.10. Characteristics of Epidural, Subdural, and Subarachnoid Hemorrhages

Characteristic	Epidural	Subdural	Subarachnoid
Primary etiology	TBI	TBI	Hemodynamic origin
Location of hemorrhage	• Blood accumulates in the potential space between the dura mater and the periosteal lining of the inner surface of the skull. • Most common site is the lateral temporal area as a result of laceration of the middle meningeal artery.	• Blood accumulates between the inner surface of the dura mater and the outer layer of arachnoid mater (i.e., between the brain and dura).	• Blood accumulates between the arachnoid mater and pia mater (i.e., in the subarachnoid space, where CSF circulates).
Pathogenesis	Caused by blood under arterial pressure. Hematoma displaces the dura, which in turn compresses the brain. Slower onset because of initial protection from the dura mater lying between the blood and brain. 1. Arterial blood (85%) • Dural arteries • Fast bleeding • High pressure • Could become critical within a few hours 2. Venous blood (15%) • Dural sinuses • Develops slowly • Self-limiting	Neurological signs resulting from increased pressure exerted on the adjacent brain and displacement of brain tissue (herniation syndrome). As blood accumulates, pressure on the surface of the brain increases. 1. Venous blood (90%) • Bridging veins draining cerebral hemispheres traveling through the subdural space to empty into the superior sagittal sinus are particularly prone to tearing • May be acute or chronic • Subdural space accommodates slower, chronic hematomas • Slow bleeding • Low pressure	Blood under arterial pressure accumulates in the subarachnoid space, causing increased pressure on the brain, which can be life threatening. 1. Arterial blood • **Circle of Willis**
Typical MOI	MOI may include MVA or sports accidents. • Usually associated with skull fracture (85%–95%)	MOI is commonly related to MVA but may result from other blunt trauma. • 50% occur with skull fracture • Most commonly occurs over the lateral aspects of the cerebral hemispheres	MOI typically results from the rupture of a saccular (berry) aneurysm of the Circle of Willis or less commonly from rupture of an arteriovenous malformation. • May be caused by injury in older adults who have fallen and hit their head • May develop from hemodynamic stress or **hypertension** • Most develop at junctions of communicating branches with the large main cerebral arteries • Increased frequency with age
Onset and course	• May not be recognized • Immediate postinjury unconsciousness followed by a lucid interval (hours or days) and then a relapse into **coma** or death ("talk and die")	• Often manifests within 48 hours of injury • Chronic subdural hematomas (weeks to months) usually occur in older patients with brain atrophy because bridging veins are stretched and have increased vulnerability to tearing after even relatively minor brain trauma or as a result of chronic alcohol abuse	• Sudden, excruciating headache ("worst headache of my life") • Rapid loss of consciousness (hours to days) • Impairment of consciousness may vary from mild dullness to confusion to stupor or coma • If patient survives hemorrhage (50% chance), there is an increased risk of ischemic injury from vasospasm affecting vessels submerged in extravasated blood as well as inflammatory response with cytokine expression that may diffusely impair brain metabolism and cause brain edema

(Continued)

Table 2.10. Characteristics of Epidural, Subdural, and Subarachnoid Hemorrhages *(cont.)*

Characteristic	Epidural	Subdural	Subarachnoid
Signs	• Headache, nausea, vomiting, drowsiness, confusion • Focal neurological deficits • Seizures • Ecchymosis of the skin behind the ear or around the eyes • Uncal herniation with gradual impairment of consciousness	• Focal signs may be present, but clinical manifestations are often not localized and include headache and confusion • Headache, drowsiness, restlessness or agitation, changes in behavior, slowed cognition, confusion, fluctuating levels or loss of consciousness, respiratory changes, homonymous hemianopsia, disconjugate gaze • Seizures	• Severe occipital headache • Nuchal rigidity
Symptoms	• Headache, drowsiness, confusion, alterations in consciousness	• Headache, drowsiness, confusion, alterations in consciousness	• Headache, confusion, alterations in consciousness

Sources. Evans (2006); Ham and Sharp (2012); Kumar, Abbas, Fausto, and Aster (2010); Plum and Posner (1972); Posner, Saper, Schiff, and Plum (2007); Sharp (2014); Sharp et al. (2011); Sharp, Scott, and Leech (2014).

Note. Traumatic aneurysms are somewhat rare, accounting for fewer than 1% of intracranial aneurysms. CSF = **cerebrospinal fluid**; MOI = mechanism of injury; MVA = motor vehicle accident; TBI = traumatic brain injury.

able to tolerate elevated ICP to a greater extent than adults. Because of the potential consequences of elevated ICP, aggressive somatic, pharmacological, and surgical interventions are used to manage it, and monitoring of ICP after TBI is routine.

In addition to the primary injury, the complex response of brain tissue to trauma may result in secondary injury. These secondary injury mechanisms are still being elucidated but involve the activation of endogenous peptides and amino acid mediators that, over the course of hours or days, may cause cellular swelling and death. As these processes become further understood, pharmacological interventions may allow for the interruption of some of these processes and the rescue of neurons that would otherwise be destroyed by these processes.

Several possible mechanisms of neuronal injury from TBI have been described, most of which substantially disrupt various cerebral networks, depending on the type of injury. For instance, the executive attention network is dependent on the tightly coupled activity of two subnetworks, the salience network and the default mode network. DAI caused by TBI damages the structural integrity of these networks and produces abnormalities in network function and cognitive control (Sharp, Scott, & Leech, 2014). Even patients with mild TBI who are mostly free of macroscopic cerebral injury demonstrate abnormal functional connectivity in every brain network identified by independent component analysis of functional MRI data. These networks include visual processing, motor, and limbic as well as numerous circuits believed to underlie executive cognition. Abnormalities include not only function connection deficits but also enhancements that might reflect compensatory neural processes (Stevens et al., 2012).

Pathophysiology of Traumatic Brain Injury

Knowledge of the pathogenesis underlying TBI is necessary for the administration and management of the appropriate therapeutic strategies (see Table 2.11). The cascade of pathophysiological events that follow TBI can be temporally characterized as

Table 2.11. Pathogenesis of Traumatic Brain Injury

Pathophysiological Event	Descriptions and Features	Potential Downstream Effects
		Early or Immediate (Seconds to Days)
Primary injury	• Mechanical damage to cells that occurs at the moment of trauma • Immediate cell death related to physical disruption of membranes • Cells torn, stretched, or compressed • Diffuse axonal injury • Blood vessels damaged	• Diffuse axonal injury • Disruption of axonal membranes • Stretching and activation of ion channels • Cellular dysfunction • Release of neurotransmitters • Activation of multiple and diverse apoptosis pathways • Necrosis • Altered functional connectivity of neural networks as compensation • Disruption of white matter tracts • Brain herniation
Changes in blood flow	• Hypo- or hyperperfusion • Hematoma formation • Cerebral vasospasm • Altered cerebrovascular autoregulation and CO_2 reactivity	• Ischemia and inadequate cerebral oxygenation • Oxidative stress, especially to mitochondria and endoplasmic reticulum • Mitochondrial damage • Cerebral blood flow–glucose metabolism uncoupling • Altered glucose metabolism • Lactic acid accumulation • Failure of ion pumps • Altered neurotransmission • Impaired connectivity
Ionic changes	• Failure of ion pumps • Ionic shifts and imbalances (Ca^{2+}, Na^+, K^+, Mg^+) • Increased influx of Ca^{2+} and Na^+ and efflux of K^+ • Reduced intracellular Mg^+ • Changes in pH • Altered properties of cell membrane and increased membrane permeability	• Alterations in cellular physiology • Nonspecific depolarization and initiation of action potentials • Surge of glutamate release • Excessive excitation leading to neuronal suppression • Enhanced Ca^{2+} availability and toxicity • Neurofilament and microtubule instability • Alterations in neurotransmission • Interruptions in neuronal connectivity • Neurological deficits (e.g., learning, memory, cognition) • Loss of inhibitory neurotransmission • Seizures • Increased compensatory activity of Na^+/K^+ ATPase and glucose utilization • Increased mitochondrial uptake of Ca^{2+} • Altered glucose metabolism • Cellular energy crisis • Increased vulnerability of brain • Activation of multiple and diverse cell death pathways

(Continued)

Table 2.11. Pathogenesis of Traumatic Brain Injury (cont.)

Pathophysiological Event	Descriptions and Features	Potential Downstream Effects
Molecular changes	• Changes in gene expression and stimulation of mRNA	• Altered gene expression and protein production
Edema	• Extracellular and intracellular fluid accumulation • Modified aquaporin expression • Increased brain volume and subsequent pressure	• Neuronal injury, dysfunction, and death • Changes in IQ • Changes in neuronal functioning
Inflammation	• Proinflammatory mediator release • Neurotrophic factor release	• Additional tissue damage and death
Metabolic changes	• Altered glucose utilization • Metabolic derangements • Degenerative and reparative	• Lactic acid accumulation, anaerobic glycolysis • Excitotoxicity • Sudden alterations in excitation or inhibition • Excitotoxic cell death from rapid cytoplasmic changes, including marked cell swelling • Temporary shocklike loss of neural tissue function (*diaschisis*) • Apoptosis • Loss of synapses in widespread regions of injured hemisphere
Metabolic derangements	• Tau protein localized in axonal compartment of neurons • Myelin-associated proteins • Amyloid beta deposits • Neurofibrillary tangles	• Encephalopathy • Altered functional connectivity of neural networks as compensation • Disruption of white matter tracts
Late or Chronic (Weeks to Months)		
Secondary injury	• Delayed cell death in surrounding or distant regions, resulting from both physiological and biochemical changes induced by the insult • Nonmechanical • Possibility of quite extensive damage, perhaps even greater than that resulting directly from injury itself	• Damage to **blood–brain barrier** • Prolonged inflammation • Oxidative stress resulting from free-radical overload and mitochondrial dysfunction • Prolonged and excessive release of glutamate, resulting in excitotoxicity • Calcium and sodium influx • Long-term neuropsychological dysfunction • Prolonged microglial activation and phagocytic clearance of cellular debris • Synaptic reorganization • Degeneration • Alterations in blood flow leading to ischemia and hypoxia • Elevation of intracranial pressure • Cerebral edema

either (1) *early or immediate-phase events* (within seconds to days), which occur as an immediate consequence of the mechanical trauma and physical disruption of brain tissue, or (2) *late- or chronic-phase events* (within months to years; see Table 2.11), which are related to the processes that occur after the trauma itself.

In the early phase, alterations in blood flow (e.g., ischemia, hemorrhage) and DAI are common and can result in dysfunctional cerebrovascular regulation and disrupted neural connectivity. The physical disruption of the cells initiates ionic disturbances, nonspecific depolarization events, and inappropriate initiation of action potentials. Excess excitatory neurotransmitters are then released (especially glutamate), exacerbating extensive neuronal activation and ionic disturbances (Evans, 2006; Giza & Hovda, 2001; Posner, Saper, Schiff, & Plum, 2007). These events culminate in disturbances in cellular physiology, with the activation of multiple apoptotic pathways that lead to widespread cell death and increasing neuronal loss. Additionally, altered blood flow disrupts normal glucose utilization, causing a myriad of metabolic disturbances, including increased glycolysis and lactic acid accumulation, which disrupt cellular and tissue pH and alter membrane permeability. Consequently, cellular transport mechanisms are disrupted and fluid regulation is disturbed, causing edema and additional neuronal dysfunction, injury, or death. Neural connectivity deteriorates as a consequence of these processes (Ham & Sharp, 2012; Sharp et al., 2011), leading to a variety of neurological deficits, loss of inhibitory neurotransmission, and even seizures.

In the late phase of TBI, the chronic pathological processes associated with the secondary injury can be quite extensive and are often even more debilitating than those of the primary injury. These processes include prolonged excessive glutamate release and excitotoxicity, chronic alterations in neurotransmission, axonal disconnection and degeneration, and synaptic reorganization. Impairments in coordination, **attention,** memory, and other cognitive functions are manifestations of the collective underlying neuronal dysfunction (Evans, 2006; Ham & Sharp, 2012; Sharp et al., 2014). In addition to the secondary injury, the late phase may also involve some signs of recovery from TBI, including the recovery of glucose metabolism and improved cerebral blood flow.

> **In the late phase of TBI, the chronic pathological processes associated with the secondary injury can be quite extensive and are often even more debilitating than those of the primary injury.**

Repeated concussion or mild TBI while the brain is still recovering from a previous injury recently has been identified as a significant risk in sports, particularly in youth sports. The risk of this type of injury leading to **chronic traumatic encephalopathy** (previously called *dementia pugilistica*) has also been identified in the context of many professional sports that may include repetitive blows to the head (see Chapter 1 for a discussion of chronic traumatic encephalopathy).

Conclusion

In TBI, acceleration–deceleration or the traumatic impact of the brain against the skull or other object can cause mechanical deformation of the brain and result in structural damage to neurons. Additional sequelae of TBI, such as edema and the release of endogenous cellular substances that result in further injury to the cells, ultimately lead to neurodegeneration. The damage may be *focal,* occurring only in specific regions, or it may be *diffuse,* involving large areas of the brain. Moreover, both focal and diffuse lesions may occur in the same patient. Focal lesions are far less common than diffuse lesions and can result from penetration or acceleration- or deceleration-type injuries. These lesions often occur in areas of the brain that have direct impact with the inner surface of the skull during coup–contrecoup situations and deeper in the brain at anatomical tethering points where movement is restricted. DAI occurs when rotation of the brain causes stretching of axons, especially in areas in which gray and white matter are adjacent and the amount of damage is dependent on the amount and direction of force to which it is exposed (*anisotropy*). All types of axonal damage may be accompanied by edema and hematoma, which may exert localized mass effects, causing midline shift, and increased intracerebral pressure. Whatever the mechanism of trauma or trauma severity, TBI causes neurological impairment by disconnecting intrinsic cerebral networks.

References

Bach-y-Rita, P. (1995). *Nonsynaptic diffusion neurotransmission and late brain reorganization.* New York: Demos Medical.

Bayly, P. V., Cohen, T. S., Leister, E. P., Ajo, D., Leuthardt, E. C., & Genin, G. M. (2005). Deformation of the human brain induced by mild acceleration. *Journal of Neurotrauma, 22,* 845–856. http://dx.doi.org/10.1089/neu.2005.22.845

Blumbergs, P. C., Scott, G., Manavis, J., Wainwright, H., Simpson, D. A., & McLean, A. J. (1995). Topography of axonal injury as defined by amyloid precursor protein and the sector scoring method in mild and severe closed head injury. *Journal of Neurotrauma, 12,* 565–572.

Blumenfeld, H. (2010). *Neuroanatomy through clinical cases* (2nd ed.). Sunderland, MA: Sinauer Associates.

Bonelli, R. M., & Cummings, J. L. (2008). Frontal–subcortical dementias. *Neurologist, 14,* 100–107. http://dx.doi.org/10.1097/NRL.0b013e31815b0de2

Camos, V., & Tillmann, B. (2008). Discontinuity in the enumeration of sequentially presented auditory and visual stimuli. *Cognition, 107,* 1135–1143. http://dx.doi.org/10.1016/j.cognition.2007.11.002

Coello, A. F., Canals, A. G., Gonzalez, J. M., & Martín, J. J. (2010). Cranial nerve injury after minor head trauma. *Journal of Neurosurgery, 113,* 547–555. http://dx.doi.org/10.3171/2010.6.JNS091620

Cowan, N. (2008). What are the differences between long-term, short-term, and working memory? *Progress in Brain Research, 169,* 323–338. http://dx.doi.org/10.1016/S0079-6123(07)00020-9

Cummings, J. L. (1993). Frontal–subcortical circuits and human behavior. *Archives of Neurology, 50,* 873–880. http://dx.doi.org/10.1001/archneur.1993.00540080076020

Eichenbaum, H. (2001). The hippocampus and declarative memory: Cognitive mechanisms and neural codes. *Behavioural Brain Research, 127,* 199–207. http://dx.doi.org/10.1016/S0166-4328(01)00365-5

Eustache, F., & Desgranges, B. (2008). MNESIS: Towards the integration of current multisystem models of memory. *Neuropsychology Review, 18,* 53–69. http://dx.doi.org/10.1007/s11065-008-9052-3

Evans, R. W. (Ed.). (2006). *Neurology and trauma* (2nd ed.). Oxford, England: Oxford University Press.

Feng, Y., Abney, T. M., Okamoto, R. J., Pless, R. B., Genin, G. M., & Bayly, P. V. (2010). Relative brain displacement and deformation during constrained mild frontal head impact. *Journal of the Royal Society, Interface, 7,* 1677–1688. http://dx.doi.org/10.1098/rsif.2010.0210

Frankland, P. W., & Bontempi, B. (2005). The organization of recent and remote memories. *Nature Reviews Neuroscience, 6,* 119–130. http://dx.doi.org/10.1038/nrn1607

Gallace, A., & Spence, C. (2009). The cognitive and neural correlates of tactile memory. *Psychological Bulletin, 135,* 380–406. http://dx.doi.org/10.1037/a0015325

Geschwind, N. (1979). Specializations of the human brain. *Scientific American, 241,* 180–199. http://dx.doi.org/10.1038/scientificamerican0979-180

Giza, C. C., & Hovda, D. A. (2001). The neurometabolic cascade of concussion. *Journal of Athletic Training, 36,* 228–235.

Goldsmith, W. (2001). The state of head injury biomechanics: Past, present, and future: Part 1. *Critical Reviews in Biomedical Engineering, 29,* 441–600. http://dx.doi.org/10.1615/CritRevBiomedEng.v29.i56.10

Ham, T. E., & Sharp, D. J. (2012). How can investigation of network function inform rehabilitation after traumatic brain injury? *Current Opinion in Neurology, 25,* 662–669. http://dx.doi.org/10.1097/WCO.0b013e328359488f

Harris, J. A., Miniussi, C., Harris, I. M., & Diamond, M. E. (2002). Transient storage of a tactile memory trace in primary somatosensory cortex. *Journal of Neuroscience, 22,* 8720–8725.

Henke, K. (2010). A model for memory systems based on processing modes rather than consciousness. *Nature Reviews Neuroscience, 11,* 523–532. http://dx.doi.org/10.1038/nm2850

Ivancevic, V. G. (2009). New mechanics of traumatic brain injury. *Cognitive Neurodynamics, 3,* 281–293. http://dx.doi.org/10.1007/s11571-008-9070-0

Jin, H., Wang, S., Hou, L., Pan, C., Li, B., Wang, H., . . . Lu, Y. (2010). Clinical treatment of traumatic brain injury complicated by cranial nerve injury. *Injury, 41,* 918–923. http://dx.doi.org/10.1016/j.injury.2010.03.007

Kaplan, E. (1988). A process approach to neuropsychological assessment. In T. Boll & B. K. Bryant (Eds.), *Clinical neuropsychology and brain function: Research, measurement, and practice* (pp. 127–167). Washington, DC: American Psychological Association.

Keane, J. R., & Baloh, R. W. (2006). Posttraumatic cranial neuropathies. In R. W. Evans (Ed.), *Neurology and trauma* (2nd ed., pp. 129–145). Oxford, England: Oxford University Press.

Klimkowicz-Mrowiec, A., Slowik, A., Krzywoszanski, L., Herzog-Krzywoszanska, R., & Szczudlik, A. (2008). Severity of explicit memory impairment due to Alzheimer's disease improves effectiveness of implicit learning. *Journal of Neurology, 255,* 502–509. http://dx.doi.org/10.1007/s00415-008-0717-x

Knowlton, B. J., Mangels, J. A., & Squire, L. R. (1996). A neostriatal habit learning system in humans. *Science, 273,* 1399–1402.

Krave, U., Al-Olama, M., & Hansson, H. A. (2011). Rotational acceleration closed head flexion trauma generates more extensive diffuse brain injury than extension trauma. *Journal of Neurotrauma, 28,* 57–70. http://dx.doi.org/10.1089/neu.2010.1431

Kumar, V., Abbas, A. K., Fausto, N., & Aster, J. C. (2010). *Robbins and Cotran pathologic basis of disease* (8th ed.). Philadelphia: Saunders/Elsevier.

Mountcastle, V. B. (1998). *Perceptual neuroscience: The cerebral cortex.* Cambridge, MA: Harvard University Press.

Nadel, L., & Moscovitch, M. (1997). Memory consolidation, retrograde amnesia, and the hippocampal complex. *Current Opinion in Neurobiology, 7,* 217–227. http://dx.doi.org/10.1016/S0959-4388(97)80010-4

Netter, F. (2011). *Atlas of human anatomy* (5th ed.). Philadelphia: Saunders/Elsevier.

Nolte, J. (2002). *The human brain* (5th ed.). St. Louis: Mosby.

Nolte, J. (2009). *The human brain* (6th ed.). Philadelphia: Elsevier.

Plum, F., & Posner, J. B. (1972). *The diagnosis of stupor and coma* (2nd ed.). Philadelphia: F. A. Davis.

Polyn, S. M., Natu, V. S., Cohen, J. D., & Norman, K. A. (2005). Category-specific cortical activity precedes retrieval during memory search. *Science, 310,* 1963–1966. http://dx.doi.org/10.1126/science.1117645

Posner, J. B., Saper, C. B., Schiff, N. D., & Plum, F. (2007). *Plum and Posner's diagnosis of stupor and coma* (4th ed.). Oxford, England: Oxford University Press.

Posner, M. I., & Petersen, S. E. (1990). The attention system of the human brain. *Annual Review of Neuroscience, 13,* 25–42. http://dx.doi.org/10.1146/annurev.ne.13.030190.000325

Posner, M. I., & Raichle, M. E. (1997). *Images of mind.* New York: Henry Holt.

Potts, M. B., Adwanikar, H., & Noble-Haeusslein, L. J. (2009). Models of traumatic cerebellar injury. *Cerebellum, 8,* 211–221. http://dx.doi.org/10.1007/s12311-009-0114-8

Purves, D., & Augustine, G. J. (2004). *Neuroscience* (3rd ed.). Sunderland, CT: Sinauer Associates.

Ranganath, C. (2004). The 3-D prefrontal cortex: Hemispheric asymmetries in prefrontal activity and their relation to memory retrieval processes. *Journal of Cognitive Neuroscience, 16,* 903–907. http://dx.doi.org/10.1162/0898929041502625

Restivo, L., Vetere, G., Bontempi, B., & Ammassari-Teule, M. (2009). The formation of recent and remote memory is associated with time-dependent formation of dendritic spines in the hippocampus and anterior cingulate cortex. *Journal of Neuroscience, 29,* 8206–8214. http://dx.doi.org/10.1523/JNEUROSCI.0966-09.2009

Sharma, G., & Vijayaraghavan, S. (2001). Nicotinic cholinergic signaling in hippocampal astrocytes involves calcium-induced calcium release from intracellular stores. *Proceedings of the*

National Academy of Sciences of the United States of America, 98, 4148–4153. http://dx.doi. org/10.1073/pnas.071540198

Sharp, D. J. (2014). The association of traumatic brain injury with rate of progression of cognitive and functional impairment in a population-based cohort of Alzheimer's disease: The Cache County dementia progression study by Gilbert et al. Late effects of traumatic brain injury on dementia progression. *International Psychogeriatrics, 26,* 1591–1592. http://dx.doi.org/10.1017/S1041610214001689

Sharp, D. J., Beckmann, C. F., Greenwood, R., Kinnunen, K. M., Bonnelle, V., De Boissezon, X., . . . Leech, R. (2011). Default mode network functional and structural connectivity after traumatic brain injury. *Brain, 134*(Pt. 8), 2233–2247. http://dx.doi.org/10.1093/brain/awr175

Sharp, D. J., Scott, G., & Leech, R. (2014). Network dysfunction after traumatic brain injury. *Neurology, 10,* 156–166. http://dx.doi.org/10.1038/nrneurol.2014.15

Simons, J. S., Schölvinck, M. L., Gilbert, S. J., Frith, C. D., & Burgess, P. W. (2006). Differential components of prospective memory? Evidence from fMRI. *Neuropsychologia, 44,* 1388–1397. http://dx.doi.org/10.1016/j.neuropsychologia.2006.01.005

Smith, E. E., & Jonides, J. (1997). Working memory: A view from neuroimaging. *Cognitive Psychology, 33,* 5–42. http://dx.doi.org/10.1006/cogp.1997.0658

Spierer, A., Huna, R., Rechtman, C., & Lapidot, D. (1995). Convergence insufficiency secondary to subdural hematoma. *American Journal of Ophthalmology, 120,* 258–260. http://dx.doi.org/10.1016/S0002-9394(14)72622-4

Squire, L. R., & Wixted, J. T. (2011). The cognitive neuroscience of human memory since H. M. *Annual Review of Neuroscience, 34,* 259–288. http://dx.doi.org/10.1146/annurev-neuro-061010-113720

Stahl, S. M. (2008). *Stahl's essential psychopharmacology* (3rd ed.). Cambridge, England: Cambridge University Press.

Stevens, M. C., Lovejoy, D., Kim, J., Oakes, H., Kureshi, I., & Witt, S. T. (2012). Multiple resting state network functional connectivity abnormalities in mild traumatic brain injury. *Brain Imaging Behavior, 6,* 293–318. http://dx.doi.org/10.1007/s11682-012-9157-4

Tulving, E. (2001). Episodic memory and common sense: How far apart? *Philosophical Transactions of the Royal Society of London, Series B: Biological Sciences, 356,* 1505–1515. http://dx.doi.org/10.1098/rstb.2001.0937

Tulving, E. (2002). Episodic memory: From mind to brain. *Annual Review of Psychology, 53,* 1–25. http://dx.doi.org/10.1146/annurev.psych.53.100901.135114

Ullian, E. M., Sapperstein, S. K., Christopherson, K. S., & Barres, B. A. (2001). Control of synapse number by glia. *Science, 291,* 657–661. http://dx.doi.org/10.1126/science.291.5504.657

Yin, H. H., & Knowlton, B. J. (2006). The role of the basal ganglia in habit formation. *Nature Reviews Neuroscience, 7,* 464–476. http://dx.doi.org/10.1038/nrn1919

Zhou, Y. D., & Fuster, J. M. (1996). Mnemonic neuronal activity in somatosensory cortex. *Proceedings of the National Academy of Sciences of the United States of America, 93,* 10533–10537. http://dx.doi.org/10.1073/pnas.93.19.10533

CHAPTER 3

Neurocognition and Traumatic Brain Injury

*Gordon Muir Giles, PhD, OTR/L, FAOTA,
and M. Tracy Morrison, OTD, OTR/L*

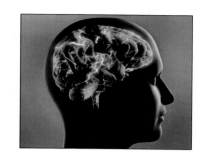

Learning Objectives

After completion of this chapter, readers will be able to

- Identify the epidemiology of cognitive disorders after **traumatic brain injury** (TBI);
- Identify the theoretical foundations and goals of neuropsychological and occupational therapy cognitive evaluation;
- Distinguish top-down and bottom-up approaches to attention, memory, and executive functioning after TBI; and
- Identify the evidence for comprehensive neurological rehabilitation after TBI.

Introduction

Cognitive **impairment** after traumatic brain injury (TBI) can affect occupational performance, independence, and **quality of life** (QoL). Cognitive impairment may also result in reduced engagement in **rehabilitation** and reduced community participation (Cumming, Marshall, & Lazar, 2013). The central focus of occupational therapy is occupational performance (American Occupational Therapy Association [AOTA], 2013, 2014). However, an in-depth understanding of cognitive impairment is central to the work of occupational therapists. Without such an understanding, occupational therapists will have difficulty developing retraining programs that help clients with TBI improve occupational performance. The recent trend has been away from a rigid focus on diagnostic specificity and toward increasing recognition that deficits may be shared across diagnostic categories and that interventions may be implemented across them. This trend has been termed *transdiagnostic* (McEvoy, Nathan, & Norton, 2009). Although the focus of this chapter is TBI-related cognitive dysfunction, much of the content is applicable transdiagnostically to people with **acquired brain injury** (ABI) of various etiologies.

Key Words

- **Cognitive Functional Evaluation**
- **errorless learning**
- **executive functioning**
- **memory**
- **performance-based testing**
- **spaced- and expanding-retrieval techniques**

In this chapter, we describe the frequency and nature of post-TBI cognitive impairment. A short history of cognitive rehabilitation is followed by a discussion of cognitive rehabilitation models. Because understanding **cognition** is important for occupational therapists who are developing occupational performance retraining interventions, we discuss the purpose of neuropsychological testing, focusing on its uses for occupational therapy. We then discuss cognitive and performance-based testing (PBT) from an occupational therapy perspective. The remainder of the chapter includes a brief discussion of cognitive functions of particular importance to occupational therapists working with clients with TBI (**attention, memory, executive function** [EF]) and concludes with a discussion of the principles of holistic neuropsychological rehabilitation (McMillan, 2013).

Epidemiology of Cognitive Impairment After Traumatic Brain Injury

Each year, at least 1.7 million people sustain a TBI, and TBI is a contributing factor in one-third (30.5%) of all injury-related deaths in the United States (Faul, Xu, Wald, & Coronado, 2010). It is common enough that approximately 20% of all people, and as many as 40% of people with a substance use disorder or severe psychiatric illness, have a TBI in their lifetime (Fann et al., 2004; Faul et al., 2010; Kelly, Johnson, Knoller, Drubach, & Winslow, 1997). Most TBIs are mild, but each year 52,000 deaths and 275,000 hospital admissions occur as a result of TBI, and 80,000 to 90,000 people are permanently disabled (Faul et al., 2010). The annual incidence of TBI severe enough to require hospital treatment has been estimated at 200 to 500 per 100,000 population (Ashley, Persel, Clark, & Krych, 1997; Guerrero, Thurman, & Sniezek, 2000; Langlois, Rutland-Brown, & Thomas, 2004; Wade, King, Wenden, Crawford, & Caldwell, 1998).

> The prevalence of TBI-related significant disability in the general population has been estimated at between 100 and 150 per 100,000 population.

The prevalence of TBI-related significant disability in the general population has been estimated at between 100 and 150 per 100,000 population. Currently, up to 5.3 million people in the United States have a TBI-related disability (Faul et al., 2010). TBI occurs most frequently among infants, adolescents ages 15 to 19, and people ages 75 or older. The frequency of occurrence of other conditions that may be treated on a neurological rehabilitation service (e.g., **subarachnoid hemorrhage,** encephalitis, **anoxic** injury of various origins) and that produce lasting disability is unknown but has been estimated at 4 to 16 per 100,000 population (Greenwood & McMillan, 1993; Skandsen et al., 2010).

The severity of the TBI and the severity and duration of the associated cognitive sequelae have a dose–response relationship (Novack, Alderson, Bush, Meythaler, & Canupp, 2000). In cases of a single **concussion,** such as those typical in high school or college sports, the symptoms are most severe immediately after the injury (see Box 3.1), and recovery proceeds over hours and days until, in the vast majority of people, complete resolution of symptoms occurs by Day 7 (McCrea et al., 2009). In injuries that qualify as mild TBI (mTBI) on the basis of standard criteria (see Box 1.2 in Chapter 1), symptoms are typically temporary and self-limiting (Carroll et al., 2004; Dikmen et al., 2009; McCrea et al., 2009).

Historically, debate regarding the sequelae of mTBI has been considerable, but new evidence is leading to an increasing consensus (McCrea et al., 2009). In cases of a single uncomplicated mTBI—that is, one without neuroimaging evidence of injury but with a **Glasgow Coma Scale** (GCS; Teasdale & Jennett, 1974) score of 13 to 15 or time required to follow commands of less than 1 hour—any sequelae are typically resolved within a few weeks, and neuropsychological test scores are indistinguishable

> ## Box 3.1. Concussion
>
> *Concussion* is defined as any physical trauma to the head that results in neurological sequelae and that may or may not meet the minimum criteria for mild traumatic brain injury (De Kruijk, Twijnstra, & Leffers, 2001). Symptoms and signs of concussion may include the following:
>
> - Symptoms
>   - Somatic (e.g., headache)
>   - Cognitive (e.g., feeling like "in a fog")
>   - Emotional (e.g., **emotional lability**)
> - Physical signs (e.g., loss of **consciousness**, amnesia)
> - Behavioral changes (e.g., irritability)
> - Cognitive impairment (e.g., slowed reaction times)
> - Sleep disturbance (e.g., drowsiness).
>
> Evaluation can be accomplished with a variety of sports concussion assessments, such as the Sports Concussion Assessment Tool–2 (SCAT–2; McCrory et al., 2009, p. 435).

from those of neurologically healthy control participants at 1 month (McCrea et al., 2009). McCrea et al. suggested that, contrary to earlier reports, only a very small percentage of civilians with mTBI report symptoms that continue beyond 12 months. In those instances in which a person with an uncomplicated mTBI has enduring sequelae, other factors are implicated, such as preexisting **anxiety** or depression, age-related factors, medical illness, or pain, or there is ongoing litigation (Carroll et al., 2004; Maestas et al., 2014). We should note, however, that these postconcussion or posttrauma symptoms are not unique to people with TBI and may also occur in people with other types of trauma or with chronic pain (Carroll et al., 2004). For these reasons, the remainder of the discussion in this chapter is focused on people with complicated mTBI (see Box 3.2) and moderate to severe TBI.

In people with complicated mTBI (i.e., TBI in which there is evidence of structural damage on neuroimaging, including **contusions** and epidural, subdural, or subarachnoid hemorrhage), impairment may be more severe and long lasting and may more closely approximate the outcomes associated with moderate TBI (De Kruijk, Twijnstra, & Leffers, 2001). Cognitive impairment is a common and often enduring sequela of moderate to severe TBI (Soldatovic-Stajic, Misic-Pavkov, Bozic, Novovic, & Gajic, 2014). Although individual outcomes after moderate to severe TBI vary greatly, when people are grouped by severity of injury on an established severity indicator (e.g., **coma** duration, **posttraumatic amnesia,** GCS score), more severe injuries lead to more severe cognitive impairment (Dikmen, Machamer, Winn, & Temkin, 1995; Soldatovic-Stajic et al., 2014; West, Curtis, Greve, & Bianchini, 2011). For example, Dikmen et al. (1995) found that the longer the coma persisted, the more severe the neuropsychological deficits were, and that the number of symptoms still present at 1 year increased with coma duration.

Dikmen et al. (2009) conducted a systematic review of the occurrence of TBI-related cognitive impairments 6 months or more postinjury and found an association between both penetrating head injury and severe closed-head TBI and long-term cognitive impairments, as well as evidence suggestive of such a relationship with moderate closed-head TBI. The effects of penetrating TBI are moderated by preinjury intelligence, volume of brain tissue lost, and brain region injured, and findings have suggested that penetrating TBI may exacerbate the cognitive effects of normal aging (Dikmen et al., 2009).

Box 3.2. Issues Specific to Mild Traumatic Brain Injury and Cognitive Impairment

Mild traumatic brain injury (mTBI) is a public health concern because in the United States, 100 to 300 people per 100,000 population have an mTBI annually, and many people with mTBI experience emotional, physical, and cognitive dysfunction immediately after injury (Carroll et al., 2004; Maestas et al., 2014). Cognitive problems that may follow mTBI include confusion and impaired attention, recall, and speed of processing. Other symptoms include headache, blurred vision, dizziness, **fatigue**, and sleep disturbance. Most people return to their preinjury level of functioning in 1 month, and continued symptomatology past 3 months is rare. There is evidence that premorbid depression and premorbid **stress** are associated with continuing difficulties after mTBI, and malingering (previously termed *compensation neuroses*) may contribute to symptom maintenance in some instances (Carroll et al., 2004; Maestas et al., 2014). Although actual rates have been difficult to establish, as many as 15% of Iraq and Afghanistan combat veterans may have been exposed to blast-related TBI (Hoge et al., 2008; MacGregor et al., 2010), and research is continuing to establish the effects of blast exposure on the brain, which appear to be different from the effects of noncombat TBI (Elder & Cristian, 2009). The **postconcussion syndrome** that may follow mTBI in some people can be lessened by the provision of limited ongoing education and support.

Wade, King, Wenden, Crawford, and Caldwell (1998) described a prospective randomized controlled trial of psychological and educational support services offered to patients admitted to the hospital for head injury. All adults (*N* = 314) admitted to the hospital in a single British health district after a head injury of any severity were prospectively randomized into a trial group (*n* = 184), who received additional support services provided by a specialist team, or a control group (*n* = 130), who received the standard hospital management and no specialist follow-up services. Most patients were in the mild to moderate TBI severity categories (73%; as defined by posttraumatic amnesia [PTA] estimated retrospectively at 6 months; see Table 1.1 in Chapter 1), and PTA exceeded 7 days in only 10% of cases. Each patient in the trial group was contacted 7 to 10 days after injury and offered assessment, information, support, and advice as needed. Forty-six percent of the trial group also received further outpatient intervention if needed. Patients were assessed for social disability and for postconcussion symptoms at 6 months, and the trial group had significantly less social disability and significantly fewer severe postconcussion symptoms than the control group had. The main benefit of the intervention may have been to minimize the effect of the vicious cycle of anxiety exacerbating postconcussion symptoms and vice versa that is common in patients with TBI. Patients with moderate or severe injuries are not assisted by the limited support that does seem to assist patients with mild injuries and are most likely to have enduring functional deficits. More recent studies and meta-analyses have suggested that people with a history of depression or other psychiatric difficulties that predate the mTBI benefit most from post-mTBI intervention, but there is little evidence that nontargeted interventions for mTBI are effective in improving outcomes (Ghaffar, McCullagh, Ouchterlony, & Feinstein, 2006; Gravel et al., 2013).

This discussion relates to single noncomplex mTBI (without contusions or focal bleeding). However, recognition of the potential consequences of repeated mTBI has been increasing. Particular emphasis is being placed on the risk of mTBI in the context of incomplete recovery from a recent mTBI (Harmon et al., 2013). This new evidence of brain damage that may be a consequence of multiple mTBIs has led to the development of new guidelines and increased supervision of all sports, but especially of professional and school and college sports (Harmon et al., 2013; McCrory et al., 2009). One long-term and temporally distant potential effect of repeated mTBI is **chronic traumatic encephalopathy** (see Box 1.1 in Chapter 1).

The frequency with which cognitive deficits are found after TBI varies not only with the severity of the injury but also with the length of time between injury and follow-up, with cognitive improvement continuing at least within the 6 to 12 months after TBI (Novack, Alderson, et al., 2000). Millis et al. (2001) examined the degree of cognitive recovery between 1 and 5 years after TBI in 182 people with mTBI to severe TBI who received inpatient rehabilitation (i.e., people with mTBI were likely to have had complicated mTBI). They found significant variability in outcome 5 years after TBI, ranging from no measurable impairment to severe impairment on neuropsychological tests. Close to 75% showed performance at or below the 16th percentile on at least one measure, and close to 50% showed performance at or below the 3rd percentile on at least one measure. Change in performance from 1 year to 5 years after injury was also variable, with 22.2% showing improvement, 15.2% declining, and 62.6% remaining unchanged on test measures. Changes between 1 and 5 years after TBI, although statistically significant, were often small and of unclear clinical relevance, such that measurable impairment remained for the majority of people at 5 years after injury.

Skandsen et al. (2010) explored the frequency and severity of cognitive impairment present in 61 patients 3 months after moderate to severe TBI and compared them with a control population. Patients were ages 15 to 65 years with a GCS score of 3 to 13, and their injury was documented by brain imaging. Impaired performance on neuropsychological measures was defined as performance 1.5 standard deviations below that of the control population. According to this criterion, 42% of patients with TBI showed impairment on at least one of the cognitive measures, and deficits were most frequently seen in **information-processing** speed and verbal memory. Deficits at 3 months were associated with functional deficits at 12 months. Sigurdardottir et al. (2014) followed a more severely injured population (GCS score = 3–8) and found that 67% of patients had cognitive impairments at 12 months postinjury, with the most common deficits being in processing speed (58%), memory (57%), and EFs (41%). Taken together, these data demonstrate that although recovery occurs for a considerable period after moderate to severe TBI, significant cognitive impairments are common and enduring sequelae of severe TBI (Millis et al., 2001; Sigurdardottir et al., 2014).

Hawley (2001) studied people with postacute TBI who had been treated on rehabilitation units in the United Kingdom. The participants predominantly had very severe or severe TBI; a smaller proportion had moderate TBI or mTBI. Severity criteria used were similar but not identical to those provided in Table 1.1 in Chapter 1. Most participants reported continuing cognitive impairments. Approximately 63% reported memory problems, approximately 40% had problems with attention, and approximately 30% had impaired safety judgment.

Brief History of Cognitive Rehabilitation

The possibility of reeducating people with impaired brain function has provoked interest since the 1800s (Finger, 1994). This interest intensified after the work of Paul Broca in localizing articulate speech to the frontal brain region, and the earliest efforts to assist recovery from brain damage grew out of aphasiology (Boake, 1991; Finger, 1994). Improvements in neurosurgical procedures at the beginning of the 20th century resulted in more soldiers surviving TBI. Much of the 20th-century progress in rehabilitation came after war as injured service members required reintegration into civilian life. Since World War I, occupational therapists have played a prominent role in this work. After the immediate postwar period, interest in rehabilitation lessened, and the centers of excellence that had developed were disbanded. Advances in the understanding of brain–behavior relationships and the long-term consequences of penetrating brain injury followed World Wars I and II, the Korean and Vietnam Wars, and the Arab–Israeli Six-Day War.

Early pioneers in the 20th century included Shepherd Ivory Franz (1874–1933), Kurt Goldstein (1875–1965), and Alexander R. Luria (1902–1977). Working in the United States, Franz rejected the idea that damage to a specific brain area would necessarily abolish the function of that brain area (i.e., he rejected a strict localizationist position) and argued that specific functional abilities were not localized to any one

Much of the 20th-century progress in rehabilitation came after war as injured service members required reintegration into civilian life.

area of the brain. His work with patients led him to emphasize the critical role of motivation in recovery of function (Finger, 1994). Goldstein made major contributions to assessment and rehabilitation after TBI and described his insights from running a rehabilitation institute in a book published in English as *Aftereffects of Brain Injuries in War: Their Evaluation and Treatment* and subtitled *The Application of Psychologic Methods in the Clinic* (Goldstein, 1942). Goldstein described two types of assessment. One, which he termed *abstract performance testing,* used laboratory psychological tests, and the other, which he termed *concrete labor testing,* used observation of performance in a vocational work site (what we would now call *PBT;* Boake, 1991; Goldstein, 1942).

Luria worked with patients with penetrating TBI and, like Goldstein, emphasized that patients could redevelop abilities after TBI by utilizing alternate strategies that relied on preserved functions. Luria (1966) believed that patients must first consciously adopt a new method of performing a previously automatic skill and then practice it until it approached **automaticity.** He also described the particular problems of people with marked **frontal lobe** impairments and suggested that these patients benefited less from rehabilitation.

The 1970s saw the introduction of the term *cognitive rehabilitation* (Boake, 1991; Gianutsos, 1980). Further advances in acute medical rescue and neurosurgical techniques resulted in many more people surviving with TBI. The 1970s and 1980s also saw increasing recognition of the importance of immersion in a rehabilitative culture for treatment effectiveness and a belief that domain-specific treatment would not resolve the problems of patients with deficits related to frontal lobe impairment, which led rehabilitationists to adopt multidisciplinary milieu approaches (Brasure et al., 2013; McMillan, 2013).

The field of cognitive rehabilitation has evolved considerably since the 1970s. A primary distinction in the field has been that between restitution and substitution approaches, in which *restitution* has focused on the recovery of lost abilities, and *substitution* relates to the development of new ways to circumvent or get around the problem. Another distinction has been between internal and external strategies. Whereas an *internal strategy* relates to a change in the way the person thinks (such as the implementation of formal problem-solving routines), an *external strategy* describes an aid (such as a personal digital assistant [PDA]), an environmental modification, or a reduction in activity demand. Another important distinction has been between **bottom-up approaches** and **top-down approaches**. A *bottom-up approach* is one that focuses on repetitive practice of fundamental cognitive processes such as structured sensory stimulation or repetitive practice in attention skills. A **top-down approach** is one that involves higher processes to regulate lower processes, as in training in self-awareness or **metacognitive** control strategies (Robertson & Murre, 1999).

Cognitive rehabilitation from the 1970s to the present has been continuously evolving but can be divided into three phases: (1) general stimulation and hierarchically based approaches, (2) targeted process-specific approaches, and (3) strategy-driven approaches. Additionally, cognitive rehabilitation has been a major component of milieu-based approaches currently referred to as *holistic neuropsychological rehabilitation* (HNPR). HNPR uses immersion in an interdisciplinary milieu as a therapeutic modality and is intended to promote self-awareness and skill development. Although to some extent all these approaches have existed in parallel, there is currently increased research focus on and a growing evidence base for global strategy–based approaches and for the HNPR approach, which is now seen as the gold standard for cognitive rehabilitation after TBI (Cicerone et al., 2008).

Cognitive Rehabilitation Approaches

General stimulation approaches attempt to place gradually escalating demands on clients' cognitive processing capacity and thereby enhance cognitive functioning (Gianutsos, 1980; Söderback & Normell, 1986a, 1986b). The hope is that cognitive processing responds to cognitive demand in the same way that muscle responds to progressive exercise demand. A key tenet of these approaches is that more fundamental cognitive processes (e.g., naming ability, visual scanning) must be addressed before higher order cognitive processes can be addressed (e.g., reading; Gordon & Hibbard, 1991; Whyte, 1986). Thus, these approaches have been primarily hierarchical, and they have often been directed toward underlying cognitive skills such as attention and memory. Computers have also frequently been used as an adjunct to work with the therapist. Little evidence has supported these approaches, and although they are still used, they cannot in general be considered evidence based.

Process-specific approaches are highly focused and target a specific cognitive process or skill (Gray & Robertson, 1989; Sohlberg & Mateer, 1987a, 1987b). They may also address a cognitive skill and process together, so, for example, a specific attention program may be directed toward the skills required in driving or the scanning attention skill required in reading (Gray & Robertson, 1989; Robertson, Gray, & McKenzie, 1988; Robertson, Gray, Pentland, & Waite, 1990). These approaches may involve behavioral or cognitive compensatory routines, and computers may also be used as part of the retraining program. They may also involve the development of self-awareness and error correction.

A third approach, one that is currently the central focus of work for many occupational therapists working with people with TBI-related cognitive deficits, is the development of programs to improve metacognitive strategies (Polatajko & Mandich, 2004, 2005; Toglia, Johnston, Goverover, & Dain, 2010). These programs involve teaching patients to identify problems, to develop their own methods to overcome these problems, and to implement and evaluate their solutions (Toglia et al., 2010). Strategy training can address global and domain-specific strategies. *Global strategies* are designed to assist clients in developing a general thinking routine, which enables them to develop solutions to a wide range of novel problems that might be encountered in daily life (e.g., Cognitive Orientation to daily Occupational Performance [CO-OP], goal–plan–do–check; Polatajko & Mandich, 2005). Domain-specific cognitive strategies represent mental routines designed to gain mastery of a particular type of problem or situation. Specific strategy training is not aimed at relearning specific tasks but at teaching clients new ways of handling a narrow range of problems in an attempt to compensate for a specific compromised function.

The fourth approach, HNPR, involves individual and group interdisciplinary therapeutic interventions. In the context of a milieu that is intended to provide feedback and support, interdisciplinary interventions include strategy training so that the client develops both new skills to manage the TBI-related impairments and increased self-awareness and a new sense of self. Milieu-based HNPR approaches, which also focus on global strategies, metacognitive control, and emotional self-regulation, are discussed at the end of this chapter.

Table 3.1. Classification of Cognitive Rehabilitation Strategies According to Transfer Distance

Cognitive Rehabilitation Strategy	Definition
1. Global strategy learning	*Global strategy learning* includes approaches such as executive function retraining and interventions intended to increase self-awareness. Instead of attempting to remediate basic cognitive deficits, therapy aims at improving awareness of the impaired cognitive processes. Clients are assisted to develop higher order compensatory strategies using scripts facilitating problem solving, decision making, reasoning, and the like. This type of intervention relies on the skills and experience of the therapist in understanding the whole person and helping clients deconstruct their own performance. These approaches may include formal training aimed at facilitating generalization, but it is assumed that clients will be able to generalize the application of these compensatory strategies to novel situations. Actual task practices are incidental; the central focus of treatment is the strategy (Guidetti & Ytterberg, 2011; Toglia et al., 2010).
2. Domain-specific strategy training	This approach assists clients with managing specific perceptual, cognitive, or functional deficits. The focus is on the strategy rather than on the task itself (e.g., an internal routine to scan the whole environment, manage interpersonal interactions, identify things to be recorded in a personal digital assistant). Training may be provided in such a way as to attempt to maximize the chances for generalization, but generalization is assumed to occur.
3. Function-embedded cognitive retraining	Cognitive retraining is undertaken in a performance context and is specific to the task (e.g., attention retraining during driving reeducation). Although the training is context specific, some authors (e.g., Park, Proulx, & Towers, 1999) have proposed that generalization of skills and improved performance on other tasks will occur, depending on the degree of overlap in processing operations between the training task and the new task, that is, *transfer distance* (the transfer-appropriate processing hypothesis; Park, Moscovitch, & Robertson, 1999).
4. Specific task training	A specific functional behavior is taught, and the therapist attempts to circumvent cognitive deficits that hamper performance by providing a routine (Giles & Clark-Wilson, 1993; Parish & Oddy, 2007). No assumptions are made with respect to generalization across activities. Skills trained may or may not have secondary effects on awareness, mental efficiency, and organization and influence performance in other domains. Improved **self-efficacy** may also positively affect engagement with rehabilitation and therefore other to-be-learned tasks (Parish & Oddy, 2007; Sohlberg & Turkstra, 2011).
5. Environmental modifications and assistive technology	Environmental modifications and simplifications are included in most of the approaches described here. Part of the process of intervention is the simplification of task demands so that skills can be practiced and cueing reduced as the skills are learned. A good match between the client's abilities and environmental demands may be central to success (Evans et al., 2000; Wilson et al., 1994). Several technologically based cognitive prosthetics have been developed to aid task initiation and scheduling and guide tasks in order to bypass memory impairments (Bergman, 2003; Gorman et al., 2003; Wilson, Cockburn, & Baddeley, 2003). This type of cueing system may be used as an ongoing prosthetic or, alternatively, as a way to extend therapy and may become redundant as the client internalizes the routine.

The specific skills-training approach is conceptually distinct from the cognitive rehabilitation approaches just described and has continued to evolve in parallel with them. Rather than target cognitive skills, this approach targets functional and behavioral real-world competencies (occupations). Early cognitive rehabilitationists often derided this approach as superficial because it attempts to remediate not the cognitive dysfunction but rather the performance deficit (Gordon & Hibbard, 1991). Skills-training approaches remain a distinct approach to remediation after cognitive impairment (Giles, 2010), but the importance of developing **habits** and routines relating to needed occupations is gaining greater acceptance across approaches to cognitive rehabilitation (Sohlberg & Mateer, 2011). Because of its special focus on occupation, this approach is of particular interest to occupational therapists in relation to other disciplines involved in cognitive rehabilitation (e.g., speech–language pathologists and neuropsychologists; see Table 3.1).

Cognitive Testing

Neuropsychological testing is the special expertise of neuropsychologists, who have a wide array of tests intended to isolate specific cognitive skills (Evans, 2010; Lezak, Howieson, Bigler, & Tranel, 2012). Testing is office based; testing procedures are intended to allow the test taker to perform the test free of distraction, and the results are intended to describe optimal performance under the best conditions. Test results are related to normative performance (scaled scores) and are meant to be directly related to the client's capacity to use cognitive functions (e.g., **short-term memory** capacity). In this section, we discuss the purposes of neuropsychological testing and the types of information occupational therapists can derive from neuropsychological test reports.

Neuropsychological assessment is concerned with the identification of the *cognitive* (i.e., information-processing) consequences of brain dysfunction and its behavioral manifestations (Evans, 2010; Lowenstein & Acevedo, 2010). Additional goals of such assessment are as follows:

> Neuropsychological assessment is concerned with the identification of the *cognitive* (i.e., information-processing) consequences of brain dysfunction and its behavioral manifestations.

- To determine the presence of organic dysfunction and, more specifically, to aid in diagnosis (Evans, 2010; Lezak et al., 2012). Modern imaging technologies have in many instances replaced this function, but some types of neuropathology cannot be visualized with current imaging techniques (e.g., toxic encephalopathies; Lezak et al., 2012).

- To determine the nature and severity of the cognitive impairment and whether it is a result of TBI (and not preexisting or due to other factors; Evans, 2010). Even when the location of brain damage is known, the specific pattern of cognitive deficits may be quite varied (Lezak et al., 2012).

- To provide realistic information to the client and family members regarding the nature and extent of cognitive impairments (Lezak et al., 2012) and to clarify issues of adjustment to disability versus personality and behavioral changes that may result from the TBI (Lezak et al., 2012). Factual information about cognitive functioning will allow clients with retained self-awareness to understand what has happened to them and to set themselves realistic goals (Lezak et al., 2012).

- To provide information about the implications of the patterns of cognitive functioning (areas of cognitive strength and weakness; Evans, 2010; Lezak et al., 2012). This function of neuropsychological testing may be particularly relevant to occupational therapists because it may influence the parameters of functional retraining programs (Clark-Wilson, Baxter, & Giles, 2014; Giles, 2011) and care planning.

- To determine whether the cognitive impairment has changed over time (Evans, 2010) and to document improvement or deterioration by comparing current test results with those obtained at an earlier time (Lezak et al., 2012). The sensitivity of neuropsychological tests makes them ideally suited for tracking the progress of recovery or deterioration after TBI, which is important in discharge planning, environmental modifications, and caregiver training.

- To use it as part of research into remediation techniques for basic cognitive functions (Evans, 2010).

Although neuropsychologists are increasingly participating in the development and execution of retraining programs, most clients who come in contact with a neuropsychologist after TBI continue to do so for neuropsychological testing. Occupational therapists can use neuropsychological test results in conjunction with their own testing to guide intervention strategies.

Performance-Based and Cognitive Testing in Occupational Therapy

Occupational therapy's focus on occupational performance provides a unique disciplinary perspective to the assessment of cognition (AOTA, 2013). When occupational therapists assess cognition, their assessment is focused on how cognitive deficits contribute to occupational performance dysfunction and more specifically on how to address cognitive deficits so as to address the occupational performance problems identified by the client as of central concern (AOTA, 2013, 2014).

Occupational therapists screen for perceptual and cognitive dysfunction when first evaluating a client and use cognitive testing to understand more about the client's performance deficits, but testing is primarily driven by performance issues (Baum & Katz, 2010; Hartman-Maeir, Katz, & Baum, 2009). Occupational therapists use PBT relevant to the client's level of recovery after TBI, for example, the GCS or the Western Neuro Sensory Stimulation Profile (American Congress of Rehabilitation Medicine, Brain Injury–Interdisciplinary Special Interest Group et al., 2010; Ansell & Keenan, 1989) or the Agitated Behavior Scale (Corrigan, 1989; Corrigan & Bogner, 1994) for clients emerging from coma or the Galveston Orientation and Amnesia Test (Levin, O'Donnell, & Grossman, 1979) or the Orientation Log (O-Log; Jackson, Mysiw, & Corrigan, 1989; Jackson, Novack, & Dowler, 1998; Novack, Dowler, Bush, Glen, & Schneider, 2000) for early rehabilitation patients. Later in recovery, occupational therapists place clients in situations (real or simulated) in which they must use skills, perform real-world tasks, and solve real-world problems that relate to the types of functions that clients must accomplish to successfully fulfill their life roles. This assessment must by necessity also involve the emotional, personality, and behavioral consequences of the neurological dysfunction.

Occupational therapists' PBT may also assess the client for the type of performance errors that occur and the level of assistance or cueing that is required to perform the task successfully (e.g., Executive Function Performance Test [EFPT]; Baum et al., 2008; Morrison et al., 2013). The central advantages of PBT relate to (1) the difficulty of observing natural performance in some contexts (e.g., the acute care hospital; PBT allows the therapist to set up a task of real-world complexity in a context designed to be simple) and (2) the limitation of cognitive testing in the prediction of performance (Manchester, Priestley, & Jackson, 2004; Marcotte, Scott, Kamat, & Heaton, 2010; Priestley, Manchester, & Aram, 2013). Prediction problems associated with cognitive testing are bidirectional. On one hand, people with cognitive impairment may not show deficits in real-world functioning. Varying occupational histories, differences in self-awareness and the capacity for behavioral self-regulation, and life experiences affect the resilience of occupational performance after TBI. This factor could be termed *functional resilience* or *functional reserve*. On the other hand, office-based neuropsychological deficits may suggest an absence of impairment, but the client may nonetheless show marked impairment in real-world functioning (Manchester et al., 2004; Priestley et al., 2013).

PBT may be office based (e.g., the EFPT) or occur in the real world with the unpredictable affordances and interpersonal interactions that are attendant on these settings (e.g., the Multiple Errands Test or Test of Grocery Shopping Skills; Hamera & Brown, 2000; Hamera, Rempfer, & Brown, 2005; Morrison et al., 2013). These performance-based tests may be standardized (e.g., the EFPT) or may have been created

Occupational therapists place clients in situations (real or simulated) in which they must use skills, perform real-world tasks, and solve real-world problems that relate to the types of functions that clients must accomplish to successfully fulfill their life roles.

by the therapist in a way that is specifically tailored to the client's performance requirements, a factor that often provides for high face validity but that without normative standards makes interpretation purely subjective.

Process of Occupational Therapy Evaluation

People with TBI are typically first referred to occupational therapy during coma or during the acute recovery stage, and goals of occupational therapy intervention change rapidly from the prevention of complications and the assessment of emergence from coma to the **activities of daily living** (ADLs) and mobility focus of acute rehabilitation. Occupational therapists are also centrally involved in the ongoing evaluation of cognition and the management of challenging behaviors that may occur during this period. Throughout the recovery process, the occupational therapist assesses for the presence of occupational performance deficits and how cognitive dysfunction may interfere with daily functioning or QoL.

The initial step in the evaluation process is developing the *occupational profile*, which establishes the client's occupational history and experiences; daily habits and routines; and interests, values, and needs (AOTA, 2014). For people with severe TBI in the early stages of recovery, the therapist may need to rely on family or significant-other proxies during the evaluation process, but the client should be engaged in this process as soon as possible. The client's concerns about performing occupations and daily life activities are identified, and his or her priorities are determined (AOTA, 2014). Tools such as the Canadian Occupational Performance Measure (COPM; Law et al., 2014; Phipps & Richardson, 2007) and the Activity Card Sort (ACS; Baum & Edwards, 2008) can help clinicians and clients focus on specific performance-based goals (Wolf, Baum, & Connor, 2009). **Goal Attainment Scaling** may then be used as a client-specific measure of outcome (Hurn, Kneebone, & Cropley, 2006; Kiresuk & Sherman, 1968).

The second step in the evaluation process is the analysis of occupational performance, during which the client's strengths and performance problems are identified (AOTA, 2014). Therapists screen for perceptual and cognitive deficits and to provide a baseline to chart recovery. Evaluation will vary with the severity of the client's injury, stage of recovery, and setting and observed performance problems. Baum and Katz (2010) and Hartman-Maeir et al. (2009) have described the Cognitive Functional Evaluation process to be used by occupational therapists with clients with suspected cognitive disabilities. Hartman-Maier et al. (2009) stated that the interview, cognitive screen, PBT, and environmental assessment should always be performed, and that testing of specific cognitive function and specific measures of cognitive performance should be implemented when other assessments indicate that further information is necessary.

The process is intended to be customized to each person's needs but can include up to six components:

1. The occupational therapist conducts interviews to gather background information from the client or the client's significant others and delineates the client's occupational profile (occupational history, current status, and occupational goals) as well as the client's views regarding the nature of any deficit he or she might have. In addition to interview,

several standardized measures can also be used (e.g., the ACS; Baum &
Edwards, 2008), and use of the COPM is recommended (Law et al., 2014).

2. Cognitive screening tools are used to create a preliminary profile of the
client's cognitive strengths and weaknesses. Appropriate screening methods depend on the client's age, diagnosis, stage of illness, and treatment
setting (e.g., **Mini-Mental State Examination** [Folstein, Folstein,
& McHugh, 1975], Allen Cognitive Level Screen–5 [Riska-Williams et al.,
2007], Loewenstein Occupational Therapy Cognitive Assessment [Katz,
Itzkovich, Averbuch, & Elazar, 1989]).

3. Performance-based measures of functional cognition are intended to cap-
ture occupational performance deficits that would be the target of occu-
pational therapy cognitive intervention (e.g., the Routine Task Inventory
[Katz, 2006], Rabideau Kitchen Task Assessment [Neistadt, 1992],
Assessment of Motor and Process Skills [Fisher & Jones, 2012, 2014],
EFPT).

4. Tests of specific cognitive functions are intended to provide an in-depth
understanding of specific cognitive domains so as to better understand
the client's occupational performance deficits or to aid in the design of
interventions to help the client overcome occupational performance
deficits. Occupational therapists give preference to tests with established
ecological validity (e.g., the Rivermead Behavioural Memory Test [RBMT;
Wilson et al., 1999; Wilson, Cockburn, & Baddeley, 1991, 2003], Test of
Everyday Attention [TEA; Robertson, Ward, Ridgeway, & Nimmo-Smith,
1994], Behavioral Assessment of the Dysexecutive Syndrome [Wilson,
Alderman, Burgess, Emslie, & Evans, 1996]).

5. Specific measures of cognitive performance in occupations determine how
specific cognitive deficits manifest themselves in occupational performance.

6. Environmental assessment is provided by the therapist with information
about the environment and context in which the client needs to function
in his or her daily life. Although we list environmental assessment last,
in reality environmental affordances have a major effect on daily life
activities, and so the environmental assessment is best considered an
ongoing part of the evaluation.

Specific Cognitive Functions

The remainder of this chapter focuses on a limited number of cognitive functions
that are important to the occupational therapist's role of maximizing clients' occupational performance after TBI: attention, memory, insight, and EFs, plus the evidence for postacute holistic neuropsychological rehabilitation. Each section begins
with a discussion of the current understanding of the processes and subsystems
involved in the cognitive function, followed by a discussion of evaluation. Evidence
from systematic reviews is used to summarize the evidence for cognitive rehabilitation in the various domains reviewed (AOTA, 2013). Interventions are categorized
as *bottom-up* or *top-down* and described. Of necessity, discussions are brief, and cita-
tions are included as a point of departure for the reader's future study. Understanding how cognitive functions are disrupted is essential for occupational therapists to
develop individualized intervention programs.

Attention

TBI may cause deficits in many aspects of attention because of its propensity to cause diffuse injury and particularly damage to the frontotemporal juncture and midbrain areas (Ponsford et al., 2014; Schmitter-Edgecombe, 2006; Schmitter-Edgecombe & Nissley, 2000). Attention is not a unitary phenomenon; an understanding of attention as a set of complex interrelated processes clarifies how voluntary control is exerted over relatively automatic processes. Posner and Petersen (1990) described three attentional processes: (1) orienting, (2) target detection, and (3) tonic arousal (see Chapter 2). Other important theoretical models for the role of attention in human functioning have been provided by Norman and Shallice (1986), Schneider and Shiffrin (1977), and Shiffrin and Schneider (1977).

The distinction between conscious and automatic processes may reflect the participation of different neural mechanisms served by different neuroanatomical systems, and it reflects different rehabilitation interventions, one using conscious control (top-down) and the other involving massive practice in responding to attentional demands (bottom-up; Loetscher & Lincoln, 2013; Zoccolotti et al., 2011). Many of the cognitive processes that are disrupted after TBI may be the result of deficits in attention. The following types of attentional processes have been described:

- *Spatial attention:* The ability to detect and allocate attention to different parts of space (see Chapter 2)
- *Selective attention:* The ability to maintain a consistent behavioral set, which requires activation and inhibition of responses that are dependent on the selection of target stimuli from among background stimuli
- *Sustained attention:* The ability to maintain a consistent response set during continuous or repetitive activity and over a long period of time
- *Alternating attention:* The ability to switch response sets as a response to environmental cues so that two activities with distinct response requirements can be performed in sequence
- *Divided attention:* The capacity to divide attention so as to respond to two or more tasks occurring during the same time period (*multitask;* Loetscher & Lincoln, 2013).

Evaluation of Attention

Occupational therapists and others typically assess attention by means of cancellation tasks and sustained vigilance tasks using a computer. Standardized measures of complex attentional processes have been lacking, and the TEA (Robertson et al., 1994) is the first standardized, noncomputerized test of attention for use by occupational therapists. The TEA uses relatively familiar everyday materials and is plausible and acceptable to participants (Robertson et al., 1994). Participants are asked to imagine that they are on vacation in Philadelphia, where they are required to perform several activities. Factor analysis of the standardization sample ($N = 154$) identified four factors: (1) Visual Selective Attention and Speed, (2) Attentional Switching, (3) Sustained Attention, and (4) Auditory–Verbal Working Memory (Robertson, Ward, Ridgeway, & Nimmo-Smith, 1996).

Intervention for Attention Deficits

Meta-analyses and
systematic reviews
have found support for
attention retraining
after TBI.

Meta-analyses and systematic reviews have found support for attention retraining after TBI (Cicerone et al., 2011; Rohling, Faust, Beverly, & Demakis, 2009; Zoccolotti et al., 2011). Zoccolotti et al. (2011) found greater support for strategy application than for repetitive practice (e.g., Attention Process Training [APT–3]) or computer-based practice to improve attention in people with mTBI to severe TBI. In their evidence-based review of cognitive retraining, Cicerone et al. (2011) recommended direct attention training and metacognitive training to promote compensatory strategies and facilitate transfer to real-world tasks (i.e., bottom-up and top-down) for people in the postacute period of TBI recovery, but they found insufficient evidence to recommend its use during the acute recovery period. Ponsford et al. (2014) made similar recommendations that highlighted the use of metacognitive strategy training that focuses on the performance of real-world functional activities. These authors also discussed dual-task training and the use of environmental modifications and cautioned that the evidence to support the remediation of attention through the use of computer-based training is insufficient.

The techniques most frequently used to rehabilitate nonspatial attention are bottom-up, highly structured activities, usually pencil and paper or computer based, that are designed to stress specific attentional systems such as APT–3 (Loetscher & Lincoln, 2013; Park, Proulx, & Towers, 1999; Zoccolotti et al., 2011). In these tasks, clients have to respond selectively to various stimuli with variation in cueing, distraction, stimulus complexity, or other factors. The majority of reports in the literature have used APT–3 (Sohlberg & Mateer, 1987a; Zoccolotti et al., 2011). Occupational therapists may also develop specific functional tasks to stress attentional functions (e.g., graded kitchen activities requiring alternating attention; Zoltan, 2007).

Memory

Although controversy continues about how to divide the different subcomponents of memory (Cowan, 2008; Yin & Knowlton, 2006), there is general agreement that remembering and executing any skilled behavior involve conceptually distinct memory systems and that these memory systems may be differentially impaired by TBI (Baddeley, 2004; Cohen & Conway, 2008).

Structure of Memory

Understanding the effects of TBI on different memory systems offers opportunities to alter the way retraining is provided so as to improve rehabilitation effectiveness (i.e., focusing intervention on relatively spared memory systems). This type of targeted intervention provides an example of how cognitive testing can serve the development of skills retraining programs. A detailed discussion of the various types of memory systems is included in Chapter 2.

Memory Impairment After Traumatic Brain Injury

Memory impairment is common after TBI (Lezak et al., 2012). TBI that is followed by unconsciousness of any duration is typically followed immediately by a period of *posttraumatic amnesia* (PTA; a period of confusion and an inability to form new **episodic memories;** Forrester, Encel, & Geffen, 1994). The presence of PTA limits clients' full participation in rehabilitation and may lead to unpredictable or unsafe behavior. Prospective assessment of PTA duration (which includes the period of coma) is one of the most accurate methods used to infer severity of injury (i.e., loss of both **gray** and **white matter;** Schönberger, Ponsford, Reutens, Beare, & O'Sullivan, 2009) and to predict severity of outcome (Forrester et al., 1994; Perrin et al., 2015).

For example, Nakase-Richardson et al. (2011) found that the odds ratio of return to productive activity at 1 year postinjury decreased by 14% with every additional week of PTA (95% CI [12%, 17%], $p < .0001$). Prospective PTA assessment is more accurate than retrospective assessment because clients may have "islands" of memory function such that questions such as "What is the first thing you can remember?" are unreliable indicators of duration of PTA (Forrester et al., 1994). PTA can be said to be over only once the person is oriented to person, place, and time and is able to recall ongoing events from one day to the next (Forrester et al., 1994). Various methods are used to track PTA's duration prospectively, such as the Galveston Orientation and Amnesia Test (Levin et al., 1979), the O-Log (Jackson et al., 1998; Novack, Dowler, et al., 2000; Penna & Novack, 2007), and the Revised Westmead PTA Scale (Shores et al., 2008).

A new PTA scale developed by Jacobs et al. (2012) for use with people with TBI of all severity levels consists of questions about age, hospital name, day of the week, month, mode of transportation that brought the patient to the hospital, and the recall of three words. The scale is brief and simple to administer but needs further validation before it can be used in routine clinical practice (Jacobs et al., 2012). Typically, at some point PTA resolves, and residual impairment in ongoing memory functioning can be evaluated.

TBI and memory impairment have a dose–response relationship, with more severe injuries resulting in more severe memory impairment (Millis et al., 2001; West et al., 2011). This, however, is only a general rule; other factors such as age contribute to outcome (Millis et al., 2001), and some people with severe injury will have unimpaired memory functions. Memory dysfunction in acute mTBI is characterized by difficulties with attention, verbal memory, and forgetfulness (Lezak et al., 2012). For single mTBI, resolution of memory symptoms can be expected within 3 months (Lezak et al., 2012). After the acute period, various memory subsystems may be impaired, with **working memory** less likely to be impaired (Skandsen et al., 2010) and memory for verbal material most likely to be impaired. Millis et al. (2001) found that 5 years after injury, 71.2% of their sample of patients with complicated mTBI to severe TBI were at least mildly impaired on the Rey Auditory Verbal Learning Test (RAVLT) and that 50.3% were moderately to severely impaired (Lezak et al., 2012; Millis et al., 2001; Rey, 1964). Draper and Ponsford (2009) also found that performance on the RAVLT was significantly more impaired in a sample of people with severe TBI than in age-, gender-, and education-matched controls 10 years after injury.

The functional implications of memory impairment for people with TBI depend on the severity and duration of the various types of memory impairment that may follow from the injury and the array of other factors that affect the person's ability to compensate for the memory dysfunction (e.g., age, previous education, EF impairment; Lezak et al., 2012). In their study of 61 patients 3 months after moderate to severe TBI, Skandsen et al. (2010) found deficits in working memory (7%), visual memory (36%), and verbal memory (29%). In her sample of 50 people (58% post-TBI) with memory impairment 5 to 10 years after rehabilitation, Wilson (1991) found that deterioration was unusual but that 60% of patients had no change in memory functioning over this time period. Himanen et al. (2006), in their 30-year follow-up of people with TBI, found that episodic memory showed continued deterioration. In a Los Angeles head injury survey, Jacobs (1988) studied 142 participants randomly selected from 310 volunteers with predominantly very severe brain injury; 66% were described as oriented, but only 38% were described as remembering recent events, suggesting that for a subset of the population, ongoing memory impairment after severe TBI may be a prominent contribution to functional impairment.

Evaluation of Memory

Screening for acute or severe memory impairment may be accomplished by assessing **orientation.** It should be remembered that impaired orientation, although often a sign of ongoing memory impairment, may occur as an isolated memory impairment or as a part of a delirium. Although some exceptions exist, return of orientation usually occurs in the sequence of person, then place, and then time (Giles & Clark-Wilson, 1999).

To assess orientation to person, the therapist asks the client for his or her name. If the client is unable to speak or write, he or she is provided with a list of names and asked to indicate which one is correct. A client is oriented to place if he or she can state his or her exact location. Clients may also be oriented, however, if they can indicate what town they are in and that they are in a hospital. Many people do not know the names or exact locations of the hospitals in their community. Clients who give a nonspecific response can be told the correct information to determine whether they can retain it. A person is oriented to time if he or she knows the year, month, day of the week, and approximate time of day (many hospitalized people without cerebral pathology miss the day of the month by one or two days; Lezak et al., 2012). A person is at least partially oriented if he or she can state the year, month, whether it is early or late in the month, and the approximate time of day. It is important, however, to assess all aspects of orientation because it is not uncommon for a person to correctly state the day of the week and date but still incorrectly identify the year.

Assessing Other Aspects of Memory

A person can be fully oriented but nonetheless have memory impairment significant enough to interfere with everyday functioning. Numerous tests of memory are available, most of which are in the professional practice area of neuropsychologists (Evans, 2010). Neuropsychologists frequently assess verbal memory (including word-list learning, e.g., the RAVLT, in which the participant is required to learn a list of 15 words over five trials, and the total number of words learned is recorded [Lezak et al., 2012; Rey, 1964]; the California Verbal Learning Test [Delis, Kramer, Kaplan, & Ober, 2000]; and the Logical Memory subtest, which involves recall of a short paragraph-length story [Wechsler, 2009]) and visual memory, which is often tested using complex design reproduction (e.g., the Rey–Osterrieth Complex Figure Test; Corwin & Bylsma, 1993; Shin, Park, Park, Seol, & Kwon, 2006). Less frequently assessed are tactile memory, incidental learning, remote memory, **prospective memory,** and autobiographical memory (Lezak et al., 2012).

Adequate occupational therapy evaluation of memory functioning includes structured interview of the client and the family, standardized testing, and observation of the client in daily life. A combination of methods will allow the therapist to evaluate at what point real-world performance breaks down. Evaluation of memory should include the ability to recall written, visual, and verbal information at 30 seconds and at 30 minutes, and it should include an examination of the client's ability to learn novel behaviors and prospective memory. Behavioral observation of the client performing daily activities will indicate whether his or her memory functioning is adequate for current ADLs or **instrumental activities of daily living** (IADLs).

Prospective memory can be assessed in several ways. The Comprehensive Assessment of Prospective Memory (Chau, Lee, Fleming, Roche, & Shum, 2007; Shum & Fleming, 2008) is a self-report assessment of the client's prospective memory performance in daily life, and a shortened version is available (Man, Fleming, Hohaus, & Shum, 2011). Standardized prospective memory tests are also available (e.g., the Memory for Intentions Screening Test; Woods, Moran, Dawson, Carey, & Grant, 2008). Assigning clients future tasks and seeing whether they remember to perform them or observing prospective memory in complex functional tasks (e.g., planning a menu, shopping, cooking) may also be used.

A standardized test of behavioral memory skills used by occupational therapists, the RBMT (Wilson et al., 2008), is a short (30-minute) assessment that attempts to address prospective memory and has several subtests designed to assess different types of memory disorders; normative data are available for clients up to age 90. Another test to assess memory is the Contextual Memory Test (Toglia, 1993), which has the advantage of allowing clients to predict how well they will perform on the test as a measure of self-awareness of memory functioning.

Intervention for Memory Disorders

In this section, we review the evidence for various interventions for memory disorders that may occur as a result of TBI. We examine the areas in which there is evidence for an approach—internal strategies, external strategies, and specific learning strategies—and we end the discussion of memory with a review of general learning principles.

There has been a recent resurgence in the application of computer-based memory retraining (e.g., APT–3, Lumosity; Lumos Labs, 2010; Sohlberg & Mateer, 2011; Velikonja et al., 2014), but therapy for memory dysfunction directed at correcting the defective process or function (restitution) has been found to be largely ineffective in people with clinically significant impairment, with improvement on the computerized tasks failing to generalize or translate to functional activities (das Nair & Lincoln, 2007; Robertson & Murre, 1999; Rohling et al., 2009; Wilson, Gracey, Malley, Bateman, & Evans, 2009; Zickefoose, Hux, Brown, & Wulf, 2013). A recent review found that the evidence supporting computer-based interventions remains weak (Velikonja et al., 2014).

However, non–computer-based training does have some evidence to support its use (Piras, Borella, Incoccia, & Carlesimo, 2011). In their systematic review, Piras et al. found evidence for the effectiveness of internal strategies (e.g., visual elaboration or visual association of verbal information, verbal elaboration and association) with people with stable brain injury–related memory deficits. However, they found insufficient evidence that such improvement went beyond the tasks that were changed or that there was any improvement in everyday memory functioning. Piras et al. also found evidence for the effectiveness of external strategies and for the use of specific memory retraining strategies to retrain specific skills, along with evidence for **errorless learning.** The vanishing cues and **spaced-retrieval methods** were found to be potentially effective in learning material, but evidence for both procedures was insufficient to support the generalization of this information to daily life activities.

Cicerone et al. (2011) made similar recommendations in their evidence-based review of cognitive retraining and recommended memory strategy training for people with mTBI, use of external strategies directly applicable to function, and errorless learning techniques for specific skills for people with severe memory impairments after TBI. Velikonja et al. (2014) recommended combined internal and external compensatory strategies that consider patient characteristics and functional relevance in the development of retraining methods.

Internal Strategies
The use of internal mnemonic strategies such as visual imagery or verbal elaboration strategies is well recognized to assist in declarative memory in neurologically healthy people (Richardson, 1992, 1995; Richardson, Cermack, Blackford, & O'Connor, 1987), and attempts to apply these techniques to TBI rehabilitation have a long history (Crovitz, 1979; Crovitz, Harvey, & Horn, 1979). Application of many of the more complex visual imagery techniques (e.g., the method of loci) have been criticized on the grounds that they are too effortful (Harris, 1980; Richardson, 1992, 1995), are too dependent on EF and difficult to apply to everyday needs to be applied with people with severe impairments, and do not generalize (Giles & Clark-Wilson, 1999). As a result, they are rarely used (Kaschel et al., 2002). As noted by Kaschel et al., if imagery techniques are to be effective, they need to be used with people with mild post-TBI impairments and tailored to patient needs.

Kaschel et al. (2002) compared the effectiveness of treatment of mild memory problems between 9 patients using visualization as an internal mnemonic strategy and 12 patients receiving various forms of treatment as usual in other treatment settings. Patients in the imagery group received 30 therapy sessions over 10 weeks that focused on the development of visualization skills. Patients went through a multistep process of training in video-assisted visualization, visualizing first objects and then actions until they were proficient at each step. After training in visualization, patients received individualized training with personally relevant memory challenges (e.g., remembering the content of employment-related books and newspaper articles) and prospective memory tasks (e.g., appointments, dates).

Training was then provided with the aim of assisting clients with applying and generalizing the skills that they had learned, including problem identification, the development of an imagery-related strategy for use in the situation, and simulated use of imagery in the situation (within sessions) and transfer of imagery to actual situations (outside sessions). Patients did not show changes in performance on a structured composite neuropsychological test of memory (the Wechsler Memory Scale

[Wechsler, 2009] or the RBMT). However, the results indicated improved memory function for the treatment group relative to the control group on measures of verbal memory (e.g., appointment and story recall) and in family report of functional improvement both immediately and at 3-month follow-up. Kaschel et al.'s findings suggested that highly structured and intensive imagery-based intervention targeted to people with relatively mild memory deficits may be effective in improving day-to-day memory function.

Stringer and Small (2011) described an internal strategy–based training program for people with ABI (including TBI). Patients were evaluated before and after training on simulated functional tasks that tapped declarative and prospective memory. The intervention, ecologically oriented neurorehabilitation of memory, used a manualized treatment approach including a four-step compensatory method: write–organize–picture–rehearse, with patients being taught to apply the method to specific memory content with a minimum of 18 sessions but with the total number of sessions varying depending on the client's progress in acquiring the content of the training. Findings indicated improved performance in everyday memory content across diagnostic groups and severity of impairment.

External Strategies

External aids include passive systems such as checklists, timetables, memory books (Burke, Danick, Bemis, & Durgin, 1994), and daily planners or organizers and active systems such as PDAs (Gentry, Wallace, Kvarfordt, & Lynch, 2008; Kim, Burke, Dowds, Boone, & Park, 2000), mobile phones, and paging systems (Teasdale et al., 2009; Wilson, Scott, Evans, & Emslie, 2003). People who are not neurologically impaired use external (top-down) strategies for remembering more often than they use internal strategies (Harris, 1980). Low-tech memory aids (e.g., day planners) are those most widely used among people with brain injury of various etiologies (Evans, Wilson, Needham, & Brentnall, 2003), but this use may change because both potential users and clinicians are optimistic about the usability of assistive technology (de Joode, van Heugten, Verhey, & van Boxtel, 2010). Various external aids are available, and selection should depend on the client's pattern of impairment, needs, and acceptance of the aid.

Memory aids can be divided into those managed by someone other than the memory-impaired person (typically for people with more severe impairments; e.g., a paging service) and those that are self-managed (Piras et al., 2011). With self-managed aids, a structured approach to training and practice of use are essential because of the client's memory impairment, and several training systems are available in the literature (Burke et al., 1994; Kime, 2006; Sohlberg & Mateer, 1989). Both passive and active memory aids provide scaffolding to assist with EF deficits in that they encourage users to identify what it is they want to remember and to record the pertinent details of the activities and the date and time when they are to be accomplished (McDonald et al., 2011). However, passive external memory aids (e.g., diaries, timetables) require the user to develop a habit of frequent checking, whereas active systems (e.g., mobile phones, paging systems) theoretically reduce the demands on the user for self-initiation (Giles & Shore, 1989) by cueing attention and instructing the user to carry out actions at the intended time (McDonald et al., 2011).

Highly structured and intensive imagery-based intervention targeted to people with relatively mild memory deficits may be effective in improving day-to-day memory function.

McDonald et al. (2011) compared Google Calendar (an active system) and a standard diary (a passive system) as compensatory methods in a group of 12 people with ABI of various etiologies (including 4 people with TBI). Google Calendar was found to be more effective than a standard diary in enhancing prospective memory performance and also proved more popular with participants. Both interventions were least effective with people with the most severe cognitive impairments, but training in the use of the devices was limited. However de Joode, van Heugten, Verhey, and van Boxtel (2013), in a parallel group randomized controlled trial with 34 participants (largest single diagnosis of TBI), compared the use of a customized PDA with the use of paper-and-pencil aids and found no difference. They concluded that the customized PDA was as effective as the standard intervention.

The external cueing system with the most data to support it is NeuroPage, a remote paging service that delivers preprogrammed reminders to people with neurological impairment via pager or smartphone (Wilson, Scott, et al., 2003). This system can be used as a way to learn routines and then discontinued, or it can be used as an ongoing cueing system (Fish, Manly, Emslie, Evans, & Wilson, 2008). In a comparison of use patterns between people with TBI and people with stroke, participants with TBI demonstrated the ability to develop a self-sustaining routine after discontinuing use of the pager, whereas the performance of participants with stroke returned to baseline levels after discontinuing use of the pager. This difference was associated with older age, shorter time since neurological insult, and poorer executive functioning in the poststroke group (Fish et al., 2008).

Specific Learning Strategies
Specific techniques may be used that facilitate the learning of important information.

Overlearning. **Overlearning** (the practice of a skill beyond the point of mastery) has been recognized as effective in increasing retention since the early part of the 20th century (Driskell, Willis, & Copper, 1992; Krueger, 1929; Postman, 1962). Because of the additional time requirements, Healy, Schneider, and Bourne (2012) recommended the use of overlearning only when it is crucial to have the strongest possible representation of the to-be-learned skill. In people with profound memory impairments, specific task routines may be overlearned to the point at which they become automatic and introspective (declarative) remembering becomes unnecessary (Clark-Wilson et al., 2014; Giles, 2010).

Overlearning increases the chances that a skill is consolidated in the person's repertoire of skills and reduces the effort required for performance of the skill (Giles & Clark-Wilson, 1993). There is reason to believe that people with certain types of frontal brain damage may be more susceptible to the effects of overlearning (Brass, Derrfuss, Matthes-von Cramon, & von Cramon, 2003). The efficiency of overlearning when compared with other strategies (e.g., spaced retrieval) is probably influenced by the type and severity of memory impairment, the type of material to be learned (declarative vs. nondeclarative), and retention interval (Rohrer, Taylor, Pashler, Wixted, & Cepeda, 2005). Nonetheless, learning will be more robust if it is continued beyond mastery.

Types of feedback and specific learning schedules. Learning a specific task is likely to be influenced by the type of feedback provided and the type of practice schedule. Feedback may be *intrinsic* (i.e., cutaneous, vestibular, kinesthetic, auditory, and visual information) or *extrinsic* (i.e., information learned from some outside source). Extrinsic feedback augments intrinsic feedback; for example, the therapist lets the client learn something about his or her performance that the client was unaware of from intrinsic feedback. Extrinsic feedback can be further classified as *knowledge of performance* or *knowledge of results*. Although the relative importance of knowledge of performance or knowledge of results may depend on what is being learned, the provision of extrinsic feedback may be necessary after TBI for many people who have significant disruption to their internal sources of feedback.

How practice is structured also appears to contribute significantly to skill learning. *Random practice* versus *blocked practice* refers to the type of variability that is included in a practice session. If, for example, you want the learner to be able to perform three different tasks (Tasks A, B, and C), you could have the learner practice the tasks in blocked (AAABBBCCC) or random (ABCABCABC) format. Giuffrida, Demery, Reyes, Lebowitz, and Hanlon (2009) investigated how different practice schedules affect skill learning in clients with TBI. Participants practiced three tasks (touch typing, use of an adding machine, subway schedule tasks) using a random- ($n = 3$) or a blocked- ($n = 3$) practice schedule. (The blocked-practice group may have been somewhat more impaired.) Practice occurred for 55 minutes per day for 13 days with retention and transfer trials taking place 2 weeks posttraining. Both groups showed a significant increase in performance during skill acquisition and maintained this performance, but acquisition was superior in the blocked-practice condition. However, the random-practice group was able to transfer the learning to another task. These findings are consistent with earlier findings regarding motor-skill learning in that blocked practice facilitates acquisition and random practice appears to facilitate transfer (Shea & Morgan, 1979).

Spaced- and expanding-retrieval techniques. In skill learning, the temporal spacing of practice trials improves retention (Healy, Schneider, & Bourne, 2012). The effect is believed to occur because the act of recall is more powerful in encoding the information than the simple representation of the stimulus association, so the more work that is done in re-creating the memory trace, the deeper the encoding will be. **Spaced-** and **expanding-retrieval techniques** are relatively simple strategies for maximizing the recall of limited amounts of information in people with severe memory disorders. In *spaced retrieval*, recall practice of the to-be-remembered information occurs at identical retention intervals; in *expanding retrieval*, recall practice of the to-be-remembered information occurs at progressively longer retention intervals (Cermak, Verfaellie, Lanzoni, Mather, & Chase, 1996; Schacter, Rich, & Stampp, 1985). The expanding-retrieval technique is essentially a spaced-retrieval technique in which the between-recall interval is gradually increased (e.g., from 2 minutes to 4 minutes to 6 minutes). Failure results in returning to the beginning and representation of the to-be-learned material. The technique is not a way to retrain (i.e., expand) memory capacity; it is a way to memorize information.

In people with cognitive impairments, these techniques have been used primarily with face–name recognition training because this aspect of memory

Spaced- and expanding-retrieval techniques are relatively simple strategies for maximizing the recall of limited amounts of information in people with severe memory disorders.

impairment may be particularly disturbing to people, and improvement can have positive effects on **self-esteem.** The effectiveness of these techniques has been demonstrated in people with various types of brain damage (Clare et al., 2000; Schacter et al., 1985).

Errorless learning. The training method of errorless learning was first proposed by Terrace (1963) and subsequently has been used widely with clinical populations (Giles & Clark-Wilson, 1988; Giles, Ridley, Dill, & Frye, 1997; Hunkin, Squires, Parkin, & Tidy, 1998; Kern, Liberman, Kopelowicz, Mintz, & Green, 2002; Komatsu, Minimua, Kato, & Kashima, 2000; O'Carroll, Russell, Lawrie, & Johnstone, 1999; Parkin, Hunkin, & Squires, 1998). *Trial-and-error learning,* in which the person learns by propagating errors, registering the errors, and correcting the errors on later attempts, may be a superior learning technique for people with relatively mild impairment. However, errorless learning has been shown to be superior in people with TBI with severe memory impairment (Campbell, Wilson, McCann, Kernahan, & Rogers, 2007), and a meta-analysis found large effect sizes for the approach (Kessels & de Haan, 2003). In errorless learning, the therapist provides sufficient support (i.e., cueing, implicit guidance) to prevent the propagation of errors, and support is gradually withdrawn as learning takes place. As a practical matter, it may be very difficult to completely prevent all errors; however, errors can be kept to a minimum (Giles, 2010).

General Learning Principles

Ehlhardt et al. (2008) reviewed transdiagnostic literature from 1986 to 2006 to derive evidence-based practice guidelines for teaching information or activities and procedures to people with memory impairment. They noted that the ways in which the information or task that is being trained, the characteristics of the person, and the training procedures interact are not yet well enough understood to optimize training procedures. Although applications of some of these principles are mutually incompatible (largely depending on whether a declarative information training paradigm or a nondeclarative automatic training paradigm is used), Ehlhardt et al. identified a range of variables as important in training people with memory disorders:

- Selection of appropriate ecologically valid targets
- Task analysis when training multistep tasks
- Use of strategies to promote more effortful processing (e.g., for information, verbal elaboration or imagery; for procedures, self-generation)
- Constraining errors (for errorless learning)
- Reduction of hyperspecificity by introducing stimulus variability with multiple varied exemplars of the to-be-learned material
- Distributed practice
- Adequate practice opportunities.

They also identified sufficient practice as central to learning.

It is clear from studies including neuroimaging that practicing tasks with sufficient frequency leads to cortical restructuring (Draganski et al., 2004; Lövdén, Wenger, Mårtensson, Lindenberger, & Bäckman, 2013; Nudo, Plautz, & Frost, 2001).

However, both therapists and clients may underestimate the amount of practice required for skill development (Ehlhardt et al., 2008; Sohlberg & Turkstra, 2011). Ehlhardt et al. (2008) found that high treatment dosages (a minimum of 6 to 30 or more practice sessions) were associated with successful outcomes when training clients with memory disorders in multistep tasks.

Insight

Various terms have been used to describe the failure of a person with TBI to fully appreciate his or her changed competencies. Terms include **anosognosia** (initially used to describe **denial** of **hemiplegia**), *denial of deficits, impaired self-awareness,* and *lack of insight.* Lack of awareness regarding the injury and the consequences of the injury is characteristic of the delirium and PTA that typically follow moderate to severe TBI and is usually regarded as an orientation deficit rather than a lack of insight. However, once the person is able to retain ongoing events, failure to appreciate the injury and its potential consequences can be regarded as a symptom in its own right. Awareness of deficit often improves with experiences in community life, but lack of insight often continues into the postacute period.

Evidence is contradictory regarding whether lack of insight is associated with severity of injury, as measured by GCS score or duration of PTA (Ergh, Rapport, Coleman, & Hanks, 2002; Prigatano & Altman, 1990), with specific cognitive deficits, or with general intellectual functioning (Bach & David, 2006). Theories have been proposed to explain the observed clinical phenomena, as well as to distinguish organically mediated lack of insight from psychologically motivated lack of insight. None of these attempts have captured the full range of client behaviors, suggesting that they are not completely adequate (Toglia & Kirk, 2000) and that the causes of lack of awareness are multidimensional.

Nonetheless, several useful distinctions have been proposed that have received empirical support (Toglia & Kirk, 2000). After TBI, people are more likely to be able to accurately describe physical (i.e., sensorimotor) deficits than nonphysical deficits, such as deficits in cognitive, emotional, behavioral, or social functioning (Hart, Sherer, Whyte, Polansky, & Novack, 2004; Malouf, Langdon, & Taylor, 2014). The distinctions first suggested by Fleming and Strong (1995) among awareness of the deficits, awareness of the functional consequences of the deficits, and awareness of the realistic goal limitations imposed by the deficits have also received empirical support (Malouf et al., 2014). Crosson et al. (1989) described awareness of deficit as hierarchical, with intellectual awareness at the bottom, emergent awareness at the intermediate level, and anticipatory awareness at the highest level. Toglia and Kirk (2000) built on this framework and emphasized the importance of "online" awareness and awareness that is function or task specific. Attempts to use this model as a framework for the rehabilitation of insight have suggested that people with lack of awareness can learn compensatory skills but that they have no corresponding improvement in general awareness (Toglia et al., 2010).

Lack of insight is frequently reported as a consequence of TBI (Bach & David, 2006) and is frequently assessed using a **discrepancy score,** the difference between the client's rating of an ability or function and a family member's or clinician's rating of that ability or function on a measure such as the Self-Awareness of Deficits Interview (Fleming, Strong, & Ashton, 1996) or the Awareness Questionnaire (Sherer,

Bergloff, Boake, High, & Levin, 1998). Impaired insight makes engaging the client in rehabilitation more difficult (Clark-Wilson et al., 2014) and is associated with behavioral disturbance (Bach & David, 2006), poorer functional recovery (Ropacki, Rickards, Barrera, & Yutsis, 2014), worse rehabilitation outcome (O'Callaghan, McAllister, & Wilson, 2012; Prigatano & Altman, 1990), worse employment outcomes (Sherer, Bergloff, Levin, et al., 1998), and poorer spousal relationships (Burridge, Williams, Yates, Harris, & Ward, 2007).

Lack of insight is one of the central features that occupational therapists must manage in providing rehabilitation to clients after TBI (Clark-Wilson et al., 2014). The impact of lack of self-awareness on rehabilitation and participation is discussed in Chapters 5–7.

Executive Functions

The term *executive functions* describes multiple higher order thinking processes that are needed to manage task complexity and change and to facilitate independent and purposeful participation in home, work, and community life. EFs work to coordinate multiple behaviors—including goal setting, problem solving, inhibition, organization, planning, and multitasking—to support functional task performance (Stuss, 1991). Although EFs are distinct from insight and other metacognitive abilities, they work in concert with self-awareness and personal motivation and are recognized as characteristics of individual personality (Fernandez-Duque, Baird, & Posner, 2000). The frontal lobes, and in particular the **prefrontal cortex,** mediate executive processing through the coordination of cortical and **subcortical** brain regions (Hazy, Frank, & O'Reilly, 2007).

Executive abilities are impaired after **diffuse axonal injury** (i.e., axonal shearing or axonal stretching) to frontal brain regions or subcortical brain regions. TBI may also result in chronic generalized brain swelling and molecular disturbances that delay the recovery process (Walker & Tesco, 2013). After TBI, EF deficits can range in severity but often result in decreased motivation and difficulty initiating, organizing, and planning daily activities (Bottari, Gosselin, Guillemette, Lamoureux, & Ptito, 2011). Many people with TBI experience a decreased tolerance for dynamic and stimulating environments, including **social environments.** These challenges often limit people's participation levels after TBI despite their desire to engage in daily activities. Difficulties with emotional processing coupled with EF deficits may result in heightened frustration and fatigue.

Assessment of Executive Functions

Because EFs coordinate multiple behaviors, they are difficult to identify through traditional measures of cognition (Manchester et al., 2004; Priestley et al., 2013). EFs are best identified through top-down assessments that require the person to establish goals and determine a course of action. Executive abilities are measurable during novel and dynamic test conditions similar to those required to manage the multiple and competing demands of everyday life (Morrison et al., 2013; Shallice & Burgess, 1991). During the clinical assessment of EFs, task complexity can be determined through a person-centered perspective because task complexity and task novelty may increase in the context of cognitive and motor impairments.

The assessment of EFs may include a variety of evaluation methods, including self-report questionnaires, paper-and-pencil tests, or performance-based assessments.

Many self-report measures of EFs ask clients to rate their ability to function in daily life. Questionnaires may also include informant forms for the purpose of response comparison (Odhuba, van den Broek, & Johns, 2005). Self-report and informant-report paper-and-pencil measures are common in the measurement of cognition. However, the ecological validity of self-report measures of EFs is questionable because they may not correspond to clients' real-world functional abilities (Morrison et al., 2013).

Only a few EF measures have psychometric rigor, and these tools require the client to perform single complex tasks or multiple tasks in real-world settings (Baum, Morrison, Hahn, & Edwards, 2003; Morrison et al., 2013). These top-down tests are designed to require the client to self-initiate, problem solve, organize, plan, and manage self-determined functional tasks without prompting from the examiner (Alderman, Burgess, Knight, & Henman, 2003). Many require the examiner to allow time to pass without providing cues, even when the client makes errors or experiences task challenge (Morrison et al., 2013). Performance-based measures of EFs build on the occupational therapy practice of detailed clinical observation of occupational performance (Giles, 2011; Giles & Clark-Wilson, 1993) but use specific methods to support reliable scoring of task performance (Baum et al., 2008; see Poulin, Korner-Bitensky, & Dawson, 2013, for a useful review of stroke-specific EF assessments).

Interventions for Executive Function Deficits

Recent meta-analyses and systematic reviews of intervention for executive dysfunction in TBI have drawn somewhat disparate conclusions (Chung, Pollock, Campbell, Durward, & Hagen, 2013; Cicerone et al., 2011; Poulin, Korner-Bitensky, Dawson, & Bherer, 2012). Cicerone et al. (2011) recommended global (metacognitive) strategy training (self-monitoring and self-regulation) for EF and emotional self-regulation deficits after TBI. They also suggested consideration of group-based interventions for remediation of EF and problem-solving deficits after TBI. However, Chung et al. (2013) concluded that the evidence to support or refute the effectiveness of interventions for executive dysfunction is insufficient.

Although tasks or behaviors that are affected by EF deficits can be practiced and thereby remediated (i.e., a bottom-up intervention), EFs involve solving novel problems, so interventions to remediate EFs cannot be practiced to automaticity. EF remediation involves learning internal thinking routines and is therefore by definition top-down. Therapeutic interventions focused on the rehabilitation of EFs build on clients' self-awareness and personal motivation to improve functional skill performance. Clients with low motivation and decreased self-awareness are unlikely to benefit from interventions targeting EFs (Clark-Wilson et al., 2014). EF training is best achieved through client-centered goals because of the close relationship between motivation and executive processing (Schutz & Wanlass, 2009).

Therapists can support realistic yet client-centered goal development with therapeutic feedback during the occupational interview. The selection of functional tasks for EF training should reflect client-centered goals. After performance-based EF testing, debriefing sessions should focus on the client's ability to develop plans, monitor task performance, detect errors, and generate new strategies to reduce errors. Debriefing sessions encourage problem solving while improving self-efficacy.

Clients with impairments of executive attention are susceptible to daily derailments that challenge their ability to complete personal and work-related goals. Goal derailments may be the result of various influences, including environmental stimuli (e.g., a social context that over- or understimulates the client); behavioral influences (e.g., anxiety or depression); or competing habits, tasks, or activities. *Goal Management Training* (GMT), a clinical intervention based on Duncan's (1986) theory of goal neglect, teaches self-instructional strategies to increase mindfulness and to support the client's functional task performance by increasing self-awareness of attentional drift (Levine et al., 2000, 2011; Schweizer et al., 2008). During GMT, the client is guided to use a predetermined method to review goals, identify constituent subgoals and tasks (e.g., to-do lists), consider task demands, and to stay focused on task completion throughout the task performance:

1. Stop: what I am doing.
2. Define: the main task.
3. List: develop a to-do list.
4. Learn: the steps in the to-do list.
5. Do the task.
6. Check: whether I am doing what I intended to do.

If the client is on track then, he or she proceeds to the next step in the to-do list until the task is completed; if not on track, the client stops, reinitiating Step 1.

According to GMT principles, the client internalizes the behavioral strategy (although it may also have been externally cued) and in so doing compares current behavior and task performance with goal states. Once the GMT process is mastered, the client demonstrates treatment efficacy through self-initiated strategy application that supports task performance. Levine et al. (2000) compared GMT with motor skills training in 30 clients 3 to 4 years after TBI of varying levels of severity. GMT but not motor skills intervention was associated with significantly improved performance on a range of paper-and-pencil tasks designed to mimic real-world tasks considered susceptible to goal neglect. Levine et al. (2011) evaluated GMT among a cohort of clients with chronic stroke. Treatment outcomes were identified through effects on cognitive measures. Despite promising treatment observations, they identified no superiority of GMT over a control condition. A systematic review of 12 studies of GMT found that effective interventions combined GMT with other interventions such as problem-solving training but that the evidence to support the use of GMT alone was insufficient (Krasny-Pacini, Chevignard, & Evans, 2014).

The CO-OP model was developed for children with developmental coordination disorder, but it has been used widely to teach adults with executive dysfunction a strategy to overcome occupational performance deficits. CO-OP teaches a global strategy derived from the work of Meichenbaum (1977; goal–plan–do–check) and uses this global strategy in a process of guided discovery to assist clients in developing their own domain-specific strategies to solve specific performance problems that clients self-identify and choose to address. CO-OP is intended to assist the client in learning a general approach to problem solving that the client is then expected to be able to apply to novel performance problems and use to develop new domain-specific strategies independently (Polatajko & Mandich, 2011). The client is guided in dynamic performance analysis, in which the client identifies performance problems and then identifies and evaluates potential strategies to solve them. The client then implements a strategy and checks to see whether it worked. CO-OP has been used with people with stroke, and some positive results with single cases and small series have been reported (Dawson et al., 2009; McEwen, Polatajko, Huijbregts, & Ryan, 2009).

Finally, EF interventions may take a compensatory approach by providing an external device, for example, a smartphone, to help clients manage their time and monitor their daily accomplishments.

Milieu-Based Comprehensive Holistic Neuropsychological Rehabilitation

Neurobehavioral rehabilitation is an approach to the treatment of postacute cognitive, social, and behavior disorder after TBI that is concerned with reducing disability and increasing community participation. Management of the interpersonal environment is seen as key to the development of prosocial behaviors and the reduction in behavioral problems (McMillan, 2013). *Comprehensive holistic neuropsychological rehabilitation* (a subspecialty of neurobehavioral rehabilitation) is a postacute approach that focuses on the development of awareness, the application of compensatory strategies to reduce the impact of EF and cognitive impairment, and the amelioration of the social and emotional consequences of TBI.

Holistic approaches to rehabilitation after TBI have a long history, with early programs developed by Ben-Yishay et al. (1985), Diller (1976), and Prigatano et al. (1984). Ben-Yishay (1996) and Ben-Yishay et al. (1985) pointed to the importance of holism and described six essential steps in this type of rehabilitation: (1) engagement in the process, (2) awareness of problems, (3) mastery through redevelopment of skills or compensatory routines, (4) *control* (meaning natural execution of needed behaviors), (5) acceptance of the new post-TBI self, and (6) a sense of identity and continuity of the self.

Drawing from the concept of the *therapeutic community*, holistic treatment is transdisciplinary or multidisciplinary and frequently includes occupational therapists. Treatment uses group process and attempts to develop a milieu (including staff and peers) that supports the patient's engagement in the therapeutic process and the development of awareness of impairment and how to use compensatory strategies so as to develop a new awareness of the self as a person with a TBI. The model of treatment is social and educational, although individual treatment of IADLs and social skills typically occurs within this context. Typically, patients with psychiatric illness, **aphasia,** severe functional impairment, or behavior disorder are not accepted into these programs, and patients are required to have some understanding of their problems and agree to participate in the program (McMillan, 2013). Therapy may be inpatient but is typically outpatient and is usually daily for months (McMillan, 2013).

Drawing from the concept of the *therapeutic community,* holistic treatment is transdisciplinary or multidisciplinary and frequently includes occupational therapists.

Evidence Base for a Comprehensive Holistic Neuropsychological Rehabilitation Approach

Despite enthusiasm for the comprehensive holistic neuropsychological rehabilitation approach, recent meta-analyses and systematic reviews of its use in TBI have drawn inconsistent conclusions (Cicerone et al., 2011). Cicerone et al. recommended use of integrated treatment of individualized cognitive and interpersonal therapies in the context of a comprehensive neuropsychological rehabilitation program.

Turner-Stokes (2008) found strong evidence that milieu-based residential multidisciplinary rehabilitation resulted in increased productivity, reduced need for supervision, and increased **social participation** and adjustment and that these benefits were maintained for at least 3 years. Geurtsen, van Heugten, Martina, and Geurts (2010) found that postacute comprehensive rehabilitation programs appeared to be effective in reducing psychosocial problems, providing for a higher level of **community integration** and improved levels of employment, although they stated that clear recommendations could not be made because of poor methodological quality and poor descriptions of the patients treated and the interventions provided.

Brasure et al. (2013) found little evidence for holistic neuropsychological rehabilitation and concluded that current studies provided little information about the overall effectiveness or comparative effectiveness of postacute multidisciplinary rehabilitation for adults with moderate to severe TBI. These authors noted that the absence of evidence is more a reflection of the inadequacy of the available evidence and the need for more rigorously controlled studies in the future.

Interventions That Use the Comprehensive Holistic Neuropsychological Rehabilitation Approach

Cicerone et al. (2008) randomized 68 postacute participants with moderate to severe TBI to receive standard, multidisciplinary rehabilitation or comprehensive holistic neuropsychological rehabilitation. Standard neurorehabilitation consisted primarily of individual, discipline-specific therapies and individual cognitive rehabilitation. The holistic neuropsychological intervention included individual and group treatments for functional deficits, emotional difficulties, and interpersonal behaviors in the context of a therapeutic milieu. Treatment was provided 15 hours per week for 16 weeks. The comprehensive neurological intervention program emphasized feedback on participant performance and participant self-evaluation. Treatment was guided by the assumption that improvements in functioning were the result of the application of retained cognitive abilities and the use of adaptive strategies. Neuropsychological functioning improved in both conditions, but comprehensive holistic neuropsychological rehabilitation was reported to produce greater improvements in community functioning and productivity, self-efficacy, and **life satisfaction.**

A somewhat less intensive version of this type of program was described by Brands, Bouwens, Gregório, Stapert, and van Heugten (2013), who examined the effectiveness of an outpatient neuropsychological rehabilitation program for patients with ABI and their relatives. The participants were 26 patients with ABI (10 with TBI). The intervention consisted of an individually designed process-oriented neuropsychological rehabilitation program that focused on facilitating personal adaptation to cognitive, emotional, and behavioral changes; adapting to these consequences; and rebuilding a new perspective on life. Family and relative involvement was promoted. Treatment was provided in weekly 90-minute sessions provided in modules, and overall intervention duration depended on patient needs and varied greatly (from less than 10 hours to more than 150 hours). Goal Attainment Scaling and measures of QoL and cognitive failures were used as a principal outcome measure. The program had a positive effect on attainment of the patient's individual goals. It was not associated with a higher level of participation or better QoL.

Speicher, Walter, and Chard (2014) described an 8-week interdisciplinary residential treatment program for veterans with **posttraumatic stress disorder** (PTSD) and a history of TBI. Participants were engaged in group and individual therapy, including psychotherapy and **self-management** skills groups (e.g., communication skills, **anger** management, yoga) for more than 20 hours per week. Veterans reported a significant reduction in PTSD symptoms and severity of depression symptoms and improvement in self-identified areas of occupational performance as rated on the COPM.

Conclusion

Progress is continuing in understanding the nature of the cognitive deficits that may follow TBI. Models of brain function are being refined to better account for the problems experienced by people with TBI, especially in the area of EFs. This increased understanding is allowing for improved assessment and the development of theoretically driven intervention methods that have the potential to improve client functioning and QoL. A general difficulty with published reports, however, is that many do not provide sufficient detail about the interventions to replicate them (van Heugten, Gregório, & Wade, 2012).

Two approaches to cognitive rehabilitation are evident in the literature across types of impairment: (1) strategy training (a top-down approach) and (2) direct practice (a bottom-up approach). Bottom-up approaches are of two types and may either address the impaired cognitive processes or attempt to intervene in the affected performance skills. Bottom-up approaches that address the impaired cognitive processes have some limited evidence to support their use in attentional retraining (Cicerone et al., 2011) and, despite the enthusiasm, scant evidence in terms of computer training to enhance memory skills. Specific skills training in the form of errorless skill learning is evidence based for people with severe memory impairments.

References

Alderman, N., Burgess, P. W., Knight, C., & Henman, C. (2003). Ecological validity of a simplified version of the Multiple Errands Shopping Test. *Journal of the International Neuropsychological Society, 9,* 31–44. http://dx.doi.org/10.1017/S1355617703910046

American Congress of Rehabilitation Medicine, Brain Injury–Interdisciplinary Special Interest Group, Disorders of Consciousness Task Force; Seel, R. T., Sherer, M., Whyte, J., Katz, D. I., Giacino, J. T., . . . Zasler, N. (2010). Assessment scales for disorders of consciousness: Evidence-based recommendations for clinical practice and research. *Archives of Physical Medicine and Rehabilitation, 91,* 1795–1813. http://dx.doi.org/10.1016/j.apmr.2010.07.218

American Occupational Therapy Association. (2013). Cognition, cognitive rehabilitation, and occupational performance. *American Journal of Occupational Therapy, 67*(6 Suppl.), S9–S31. http://dx.doi.org/10.5014/ajot.2013.67S9

American Occupational Therapy Association. (2014). Occupational therapy practice framework: Domain and process (3rd ed.). *American Journal of Occupational Therapy, 68*(Suppl. 1), S1–S48. http://dx.doi.org/10.5014/ajot.2014.682006

Ansell, B. J., & Keenan, J. E. (1989). The Western Neuro Sensory Stimulation Profile: A tool for assessing slow-to-recover head-injured patients. *Archives of Physical Medicine and Rehabilitation, 70,* 104–108.

Ashley, M. J., Persel, C. S., Clark, M. C., & Krych, D. K. (1997). Long-term follow-up of post-acute traumatic brain injury rehabilitation: A statistical analysis to test for stability and predictability of outcome. *Brain Injury, 11,* 677–690.

Bach, L. J., & David, A. S. (2006). Self-awareness after acquired and traumatic brain injury. *Neuropsychological Rehabilitation, 16,* 397–414. http://dx.doi.org/10.1080/09602010500412830

Baddeley, A. D. (2004). The psychology of memory. In A. D. Baddeley, M. D. Kopelman, & B. A. Wilson (Eds.), *The essential handbook of memory disorders for clinicians* (pp. 1–13). Chichester, England: Wiley.

Baum, C. M., Connor, L. T., Morrison, T., Hahn, M., Dromerick, A. W., & Edwards, D. F. (2008). Reliability, validity, and clinical utility of the Executive Function Performance Test: A measure of executive function in a sample of people with stroke. *American Journal of Occupational Therapy, 62,* 446–455. http://dx.doi.org/10.5014/ajot.62.4.446

Baum, C. M., & Edwards, D. (2008). *Activity Card Sort* (2nd ed.). Bethesda, MD: AOTA Press.

Baum, C. M., & Katz, N. (2010). Occupational therapy approach to assessing the relationship between cognition and function. In T. D. Marcotte & I. Grant (Eds.), *Neuropsychology of everyday functioning* (pp. 63–90). New York: Guilford.

Baum, C. M., Morrison, T., Hahn, M., & Edwards, D. F. (2003). *Executive Function Performance Test: Test protocol booklet.* St. Louis: Washington University School of Medicine.

Ben-Yishay, Y. (1996). Reflections on the evolution of the therapeutic milieu concept. *Neuropsychological Rehabilitation, 6,* 327–343. http://dx.doi.org/10.1080/713755514

Ben-Yishay, Y., Rattock, J., Lakin, P., Piasetsky, E. B., Ross, B., Silver, S., . . . Ezarachi, O. (1985). Neuropsychologic rehabilitation: Quest for a holistic approach. *Seminars in Neurology, 5,* 252–259. http://dx.doi.org/10.1055/s-2008-1041522

Bergman, M. M. (2003). The essential steps cognitive orthotic. *NeuroRehabilitation, 18,* 31–46.

Boake, C. (1991). History of cognitive rehabilitation following head injury. In J. S. Kreutzer & P. H. Wehman (Eds.), *Cognitive rehabilitation for persons with traumatic brain injury: A functional approach* (pp. 1–12). Baltimore: Paul H. Brookes.

Bottari, C., Gosselin, N., Guillemette, M., Lamoureux, J., & Ptito, A. (2011). Independence in managing one's finances after traumatic brain injury. *Brain Injury, 25,* 1306–1317. http://dx.doi.org/10.3109/02699052.2011.624570

Brands, I. M. H., Bouwens, S. F. M., Gregório, G. W., Stapert, S. Z., & van Heugten, C. M. (2013). Effectiveness of a process-oriented patient-tailored outpatient neuropsychological rehabilitation programme for patients in the chronic phase after ABI. *Neuropsychological Rehabilitation, 23,* 202–215. http://dx.doi.org/10.1080/09602011.2012.734039

Brass, M., Derrfuss, J., Matthes-von Cramon, G., & von Cramon, D. Y. (2003). Imitative response tendencies in patients with frontal brain lesions. *Neuropsychology, 17,* 265–271. http://dx.doi.org/10.1037/0894-4105.17.2.265

Brasure, M., Lamberty, G. J., Sayer, N. A., Nelson, N. W., MacDonald, R., Ouellette, J., & Wilt, T. J. (2013). Participation after multidisciplinary rehabilitation for moderate to severe traumatic brain injury in adults: A systematic review. *Archives of Physical Medicine and Rehabilitation, 94,* 1398–1420. http://dx.doi.org/10.1016/j.apmr.2012.12.019

Burke, J. M., Danick, J. A., Bemis, B., & Durgin, C. J. (1994). A process approach to memory book training for neurological patients. *Brain Injury, 8,* 71–81. http://dx.doi.org/10.3109/02699059409150960

Burridge, A. C., Williams, W. H., Yates, P. J., Harris, A., & Ward, C. (2007). Spousal relationship satisfaction following acquired brain injury: The role of insight and socio-emotional skill. *Neuropsychological Rehabilitation, 17,* 95–105. http://dx.doi.org/10.1080/09602010500505070

Campbell, L., Wilson, F. C., McCann, J., Kernahan, G., & Rogers, R. G. (2007). Single case experimental design study of carer facilitated errorless learning in a patient with severe memory impairment following TBI. *NeuroRehabilitation, 22,* 325–333.

Carroll, L. J., Cassidy, J. D., Peloso, P. M., Borg, J., von Holst, H., Holm, L., . . . Pépin, M.; WHO Collaborating Centre Task Force on Mild Traumatic Brain Injury. (2004). Prognosis for mild traumatic brain injury: Results of the WHO Collaborating Centre Task Force on Mild Traumatic Brain Injury. *Journal of Rehabilitation Medicine, 36,* 84–105. http://dx.doi.org/10.1080/16501960410023859

Cermak, L. S., Verfaellie, M., Lanzoni, S., Mather, M., & Chase, K. A. (1996). Effects of spaced repetitions on amnesia patients' recall and recognition performance. *Neuropsychology, 10,* 219–227. http://dx.doi.org/10.1037/0894-4105.10.2.219

Chau, L. T., Lee, J. B., Fleming, J., Roche, N., & Shum, D. (2007). Reliability and normative data for the Comprehensive Assessment of Prospective Memory (CAPM). *Neuropsychological Rehabilitation, 17,* 707–722. http://dx.doi.org/10.1080/09602010600923926

Chung, C. S., Pollock, A., Campbell, T., Durward, B. R., & Hagen, S. (2013). Cognitive rehabilitation for executive dysfunction in adults with stroke or other adult non-progressive acquired brain damage. *Cochrane Database of Systematic Reviews, 2013*, CD008391. http://dx.doi.org/10.1002/14651858.CD008391.pub2

Cicerone, K. D., Langenbahn, D. M., Braden, C., Malec, J. F., Kalmar, K., Fraas, M., . . . Ashman, T. (2011). Evidence-based cognitive rehabilitation: Updated review of the literature from 2003 through 2008. *Archives of Physical Medicine and Rehabilitation, 92*, 519–530. http://dx.doi.org/10.1016/j.apmr.2010.11.015

Cicerone, K. D., Mott, T., Azulay, J., Sharlow-Galella, M. A., Ellmo, W. J., Paradise, S., & Friel, J. C. (2008). A randomized controlled trial of holistic neuropsychologic rehabilitation after traumatic brain injury. *Archives of Physical Medicine and Rehabilitation, 89*, 2239–2249. http://dx.doi.org/10.1016/j.apmr.2008.06.017

Clare, L., Wilson, B. A., Carter, G., Breen, K., Gosses, A., & Hodges, J. R. (2000). Intervening with everyday memory problems in dementia of Alzheimer type: An errorless learning approach. *Journal of Clinical and Experimental Neuropsychology, 22*, 132–146. http://dx.doi.org/10.1076/1380-3395(200002)22:1;1-8;FT132

Clark-Wilson, J., Baxter, D., & Giles, G. M. (2014). Revisiting the neurofunctional approach: Conceptualising the essential components for the rehabilitation of everyday living skills. *Brain Injury, 28*, 1646–1656. http://dx.doi.org/10.3109/02699052.2014.946449

Cohen, G., & Conway, M. A. (2008). *Memory in the real world* (3rd ed.). Hove, England: Psychology Press.

Corrigan, J. D. (1989). Development of a scale for assessment of agitation following traumatic brain injury. *Journal of Clinical and Experimental Neuropsychology, 11*, 261–277. http://dx.doi.org/10.1080/01688638908400888

Corrigan, J. D., & Bogner, J. A. (1994). Factor structure of the Agitated Behavior Scale. *Journal of Clinical and Experimental Neuropsychology, 16*, 386–392. http://dx.doi.org/10.1080/01688639408402649

Corwin, J., & Bylsma, F. W. (1993). Psychological examination of traumatic encephalopathy. *Clinical Neuropsychologist, 7*, 3–21. http://dx.doi.org/10.1080/13854049308401883

Cowan, N. (2008). What are the differences between long-term, short-term, and working memory? *Progress in Brain Research, 169*, 323–338. http://dx.doi.org/10.1016/S0079-6123(07)00020-9

Crosson, B., Barco, P., Velozo, C., Bolesta, M., Cooper, P., Werts, D., & Brobeck, T. C. (1989). Awareness and compensation in postacute head injury rehabilitation. *Journal of Head Trauma Rehabilitation, 4*, 46–54. http://dx.doi.org/10.1097/00001199-198909000-00008

Crovitz, H. F. (1979). Memory rehabilitation in brain-damaged patients: The airplane list. *Cortex, 15*, 131–134.

Crovitz, H. F., Harvey, M. T., & Horn, R. W. (1979). Problems in the acquisition of imagery mnemonics: Three brain-damaged cases. *Cortex, 15*, 225–234.

Cumming, T. B., Marshall, R. S., & Lazar, R. M. (2013). Stroke, cognitive deficits, and rehabilitation: Still an incomplete picture. *International Journal of Stroke, 8*, 38–45. http://dx.doi.org/10.1111/j.1747-4949.2012.00972.x

das Nair, R., & Lincoln, N. B. (2007). Cognitive rehabilitation for memory deficits following stroke. *Cochrane Database of Systematic Reviews, 2007*, CD002293. http://dx.doi.org/10.1002/14651858.CD002293.pub2

Dawson, D. R., Gaya, A., Hunt, A., Levine, B., Lemsky, C., & Polatajko, H. J. (2009). Using the Cognitive Orientation to Occupational Performance (CO-OP) approach with adults with executive dysfunction following traumatic brain injury. *Canadian Journal of Occupational Therapy, 76*, 115–127. http://dx.doi.org/10.1177/000841740907600209

de Joode, E., van Heugten, C., Verhey, F., & van Boxtel, M. (2010). Efficacy and usability of assistive technology for patients with cognitive deficits: A systematic review. *Clinical Rehabilitation, 24*, 701–714. http://dx.doi.org/10.1177/0269215510367551

de Joode, E. A., van Heugten, C. M., Verhey, F. R. J., & van Boxtel, M. P. J. (2013). Effectiveness of an electronic cognitive aid in patients with acquired brain injury: A multicentre randomised parallel-group study. *Neuropsychological Rehabilitation, 23*, 133–156. http://dx.doi.org/10.1080/09602011.2012.726632

De Kruijk, J. R., Twijnstra, A., & Leffers, P. (2001). Diagnostic criteria and differential diagnosis of mild traumatic brain injury. *Brain Injury, 15*, 99–106. http://dx.doi.org/10.1080/026990501458335

Delis, D. C., Kramer, J. H., Kaplan, E., & Ober, B. A. (2000). *California Verbal Learning Test–Second Edition (CVLT–II)*. San Antonio: Psychological Corporation.

Dikmen, S. S., Corrigan, J. D., Levin, H. S., Machamer, J., Stiers, W., & Weisskopf, M. G. (2009). Cognitive outcome following traumatic brain injury. *Journal of Head Trauma Rehabilitation, 24,* 430–438. http://dx.doi.org/10.1097/HTR.0b013e3181c133e9

Dikmen, S. S., Machamer, J. E., Winn, H. R., & Temkin, N. R. (1995). Neuropsychological outcome at 1-year post head injury. *Neuropsychology, 9,* 80–90. http://dx.doi.org/10.1037/0894-4105.9.1.80

Diller, L. (1976). A model for cognitive retraining in rehabilitation. *Clinical Psychologist, 29,* 13–15.

Draganski, D., Gaser, C., Busch, V., Schuierer, G., Bogdahn, U., & May, A. (2004). Neuroplasticity: Changes in grey matter induced by training. *Nature, 427,* 311–312. http://dx.doi.org/10.1038/427311a

Draper, K., & Ponsford, J. (2009). Long-term outcome following traumatic brain injury: A comparison of subjective reports by those injured and their relatives. *Neuropsychological Rehabilitation, 19,* 645–661. http://dx.doi.org/10.1080/17405620802613935

Driskell, J. E., Willis, R. P., & Copper, C. (1992). Effect of overlearning on retention. *Journal of Applied Psychology, 77,* 615–622. http://dx.doi.org/10.1037/0021-9010.77.5.615

Duncan, J. (1986). Disorganisation of behaviour after frontal lobe damage. *Cognitive Neuropsychology, 3,* 271–290. http://dx.doi.org/10.1080/02643298608253360

Ehlhardt, L. A., Sohlberg, M. M., Kennedy, M., Coelho, C., Ylvisaker, M., Turkstra, L., & Yorkston, K. (2008). Evidence-based practice guidelines for instructing individuals with neurogenic memory impairments: What have we learned in the past 20 years? *Neuropsychological Rehabilitation, 18,* 300–342. http://dx.doi.org/10.1080/09602010701733190

Elder, G. A., & Cristian, A. (2009). Blast-related mild traumatic brain injury: Mechanisms of injury and impact on clinical care. *Mount Sinai Journal of Medicine, 76,* 111–118. http://dx.doi.org/10.1002/msj.20098

Ergh, T. C., Rapport, L. J., Coleman, R. D., & Hanks, R. A. (2002). Predictors of caregiver and family functioning following traumatic brain injury: Social support moderates caregiver distress. *Journal of Head Trauma Rehabilitation, 17,* 155–174. http://dx.doi.org/10.1097/00001199-200204000-00006

Evans, J. J. (2010). Basic concepts and principles of neuropsychological assessment. In J. M. Gurd, U. Kischka, & J. C. Marshall (Eds.), *The handbook of clinical neuropsychology* (2nd ed., pp. 15–27). Oxford, England: Oxford University Press.

Evans, J. J., Wilson, B. A., Needham, P., & Brentnall, S. (2003). Who makes good use of memory aids? Results of a survey of people with acquired brain injury. *Journal of the International Neuropsychological Society, 9,* 925–935. http://dx.doi.org/10.1017OS1355617703960127

Evans, J. J., Wilson, B. A., Schuri, U., Andrade, J., Baddeley, A., Bruna, O., . . . Taussik, I. (2000). A comparison of "errorless" and "trial-and-error" learning methods for teaching individuals with acquired memory deficits. *Neuropsychological Rehabilitation, 10,* 67–101. http://dx.doi.org/10.1080/096020100389309

Fann, J. R., Burington, B., Leonetti, A., Jaffe, K., Katon, W. J., & Thompson, R. S. (2004). Psychiatric illness following traumatic brain injury in an adult health maintenance organization population. *Archives of General Psychiatry, 61,* 53–61. http://dx.doi.org/10.1001/archpsyc.61.1.53

Faul, M., Xu, L., Wald, M. M., & Coronado, V. G. (2010). *Traumatic brain injury in the United States: Emergency department visits, hospitalizations and deaths 2002–2006.* Atlanta: Centers for Disease Control and Prevention, National Center for Injury Prevention and Control. Retrieved from http://www.cdc.gov/traumaticbraininjury/pdf/blue_book.pdf

Fernandez-Duque, D., Baird, J. A., & Posner, M. I. (2000). Awareness and metacognition. *Consciousness and Cognition, 9,* 324–326. http://dx.doi.org/10.1006/ccog.2000.0449

Finger, S. (1994). *Origins of neuroscience: A history of explorations into brain function.* New York: Oxford University Press.

Fish, J., Manly, T., Emslie, H., Evans, J. J., & Wilson, B. A. (2008). Compensatory strategies for acquired disorders of memory and planning: Differential effects of a paging system for patients with brain injury of traumatic versus cerebrovascular aetiology. *Journal of Neurology, Neurosurgery, and Psychiatry, 79,* 930–935. http://dx.doi.org/10.1136/jnnp.2007.125203

Fisher, A. G., & Jones, K. B. (2012). *Assessment of Motor and Process Skills. Vol. 1: Development, standardization, and administration manual* (rev. 7th ed.). Fort Collins, CO: Three Star Press.

Fisher, A. G., & Jones, K. B. (2014). *Assessment of Motor and Process Skills. Vol. 2: User manual* (8th ed.). Fort Collins, CO: Three Star Press.

Fleming, J., & Strong, J. (1995). Self-awareness of deficits following acquired brain injury: Considerations for rehabilitation. *British Journal of Occupational Therapy, 58,* 55–60. http://dx.doi.org/10.1177/030802269505800204

Fleming, J. M., Strong, J., & Ashton, R. (1996). Self-awareness of deficits in adults with traumatic brain injury: How best to measure? *Brain Injury, 10,* 1–15. http://dx.doi.org/10.1080/026990596124674

Folstein, M. F., Folstein, S. E., & McHugh, P. R. (1975). "Mini-Mental State": A practical method for grading the cognitive state of patients for the clinician. *Journal of Psychiatric Research, 12,* 189–198. http://dx.doi.org/10.1016/0022-3956(75)90026-6

Forrester, G., Encel, J., & Geffen, G. (1994). Measuring post-traumatic amnesia (PTA): An historical review. *Brain Injury, 8,* 175–184. http://dx.doi.org/10.3109/02699059409150969

Gentry, T., Wallace, J., Kvarfordt, C., & Lynch, K. B. (2008). Personal digital assistants as cognitive aids for individuals with severe traumatic brain injury: A community-based trial. *Brain Injury, 22,* 19–24. http://dx.doi.org/10.1080/02699050701810688

Geurtsen, G. J., van Heugten, C. M., Martina, J. D., & Geurts, A. C. H. (2010). Comprehensive rehabilitation programmes in the chronic phase after severe brain injury: A systematic review. *Journal of Rehabilitation Medicine, 42,* 97–110. http://dx.doi.org/10.2340/16501977-0508

Ghaffar, O., McCullagh, S., Ouchterlony, D., & Feinstein, A. (2006). Randomized treatment trial in mild traumatic brain injury. *Journal of Psychosomatic Research, 61,* 153–160. http://dx.doi.org/10.1016/j.jpsychores.2005.07.018

Gianutsos, R. (1980). What is cognitive rehabilitation? *Journal of Rehabilitation, 46,* 36–40.

Giles, G. M. (2010). Cognitive versus functional approaches to rehabilitation after traumatic brain injury: Commentary on a randomized controlled trial. *American Journal of Occupational Therapy, 64,* 182–185. http://dx.doi.org/10.5014/ajot.64.1.182

Giles, G. M. (2011). A neurofunctional approach to rehabilitation following brain injury. In N. Katz (Ed.), *Cognition, occupation, and participation across the life span: Neuroscience, neurorehabilitation, and models of intervention in occupational therapy* (3rd ed., pp. 351–381). Bethesda, MD: AOTA Press.

Giles, G. M., & Clark-Wilson, J. (1988). The use of behavioral techniques in functional skills training after severe brain injury. *American Journal of Occupational Therapy, 42,* 658–665. http://dx.doi.org/10.5014/ajot.42.10.658

Giles, G. M., & Clark-Wilson, J. (Eds.). (1993). *Brain injury rehabilitation: A neurofunctional approach.* San Diego: Singular.

Giles, G. M., & Clark-Wilson, J. (Eds.). (1999). *Rehabilitation of the severely brain-injured adult: A practical approach.* Cheltenham, England: Stanley Thornes.

Giles, G. M., Ridley, J. E., Dill, A., & Frye, S. (1997). A consecutive series of adults with brain injury treated with a washing and dressing retraining program. *American Journal of Occupational Therapy, 51,* 256–266. http://dx.doi.org/10.5014/ajot.51.4.256

Giles, G. M., & Shore, M. (1989). The effectiveness of an electronic memory aid for a memory-impaired adult of normal intelligence. *American Journal of Occupational Therapy, 43,* 409–411. http://dx.doi.org/10.5014/ajot.43.6.409

Giuffrida, C. G., Demery, J. A., Reyes, L. R., Lebowitz, B. K., & Hanlon, R. E. (2009). Functional skill learning in men with traumatic brain injury. *American Journal of Occupational Therapy, 63,* 398–407. http://dx.doi.org/10.5014/ajot.63.4.398

Goldstein, K. (1942). *Aftereffects of brain injuries in war: Their evaluation and treatment; the application of psychologic methods in the clinic.* New York: Grune & Stratton.

Gordon, W. A., & Hibbard, M. R. (1991). The theory and practice of cognitive rehabilitation. In J. S. Kreutzer & P. H. Wehman (Eds.), *Cognitive rehabilitation for persons with traumatic brain injury: A functional approach* (pp. 12–22). Baltimore: Paul H. Brookes.

Gorman, P., Dayle, R., Hood, C.-A., & Rumrell, L. (2003). Effectiveness of the ISAAC cognitive prosthetic system for improving rehabilitation outcomes with neurofunctional impairment. *NeuroRehabilitation, 18,* 57–67.

Gravel, J., D'Angelo, A., Carrière, B., Crevier, L., Beauchamp, M. H., Chauny, J. M., . . . Chaillet, N. (2013). Interventions provided in the acute phase for mild traumatic brain injury: A systematic review. *Systematic Reviews, 2,* 63. http://dx.doi.org/10.1186/2046-4053-2-63

Gray, J. M., & Robertson, I. (1989). Remediation of attentional difficulties following brain injury: Three experimental single case studies. *Brain Injury, 3,* 163–170. http://dx.doi.org/10.3109/02699058909004548

Greenwood, R. J., & McMillan, T. M. (1993). Models of rehabilitation programmes for the brain-injured adult: 1. Current service provision. *Clinical Rehabilitation, 7,* 248–255. http://dx.doi.org/10.1177/026921559300700311

Guerrero, J. L., Thurman, D. J., & Sniezek, J. E. (2000). Emergency department visits associated with traumatic brain injury: United States, 1995–1996. *Brain Injury, 14,* 181–186.

Guidetti, S., & Ytterberg, C. (2011). A randomised controlled trial of a client-centered self-care intervention after stroke: A longitudinal pilot study. *Disability and Rehabilitation, 33,* 494–503. http://dx.doi.org/10.3109/09638288.2010.498553

Hamera, E., & Brown, C. E. (2000). Developing a context-based performance measure for persons with schizophrenia: The Test of Grocery Shopping Skills. *American Journal of Occupational Therapy, 54,* 20–25. http://dx.doi.org/10.5014/ajot.54.1.20

Hamera, E., Rempfer, M., & Brown, C. (2005). Performance in the "real world": Update on Test of Grocery Shopping Skills (TOGSS). *Schizophrenia Research, 78,* 111–112, author reply 113–114. http://dx.doi.org/10.1016/j.schres.2005.04.019

Harmon, K. G., Drezner, J. A., Gammons, M., Guskiewicz, K. M., Halstead, M., Herring, S. A., . . . Roberts, W. O. (2013). American Medical Society for Sports Medicine position statement: Concussion in sport. *British Journal of Sports Medicine, 47,* 15–26. http://dx.doi.org/10.1136/bjsports-2012-091941

Harris, J. E. (1980). Memory aids people use: Two interview studies. *Memory and Cognition, 8,* 31–38. http://dx.doi.org/10.3758/BF03197549

Hart, T., Sherer, M., Whyte, J., Polansky, M., & Novack, T. A. (2004). Awareness of behavioral, cognitive, and physical deficits in acute traumatic brain injury. *Archives of Physical Medicine and Rehabilitation, 85,* 1450–1456. http://dx.doi.org/10.1016/j.apmr.2004.01.030

Hartman-Maeir, A., Katz, N., & Baum, C. M. (2009). Cognitive Functional Evaluation (CFE) process for individuals with suspected cognitive disabilities. *Occupational Therapy in Health Care, 23,* 1–23. http://dx.doi.org/10.1080/07380570802455516

Hawley, C. A. (2001). Return to driving after head injury. *Journal of Neurology, Neurosurgery, and Psychiatry, 70,* 761–766.

Hazy, T. E., Frank, M. J., & O'Reilly, R. C. (2007). Towards an executive without a homunculus: Computational models of the prefrontal cortex/basal ganglia system. *Philosophical Transactions of the Royal Society of London, Series B: Biological Sciences, 362,* 1601–1613. http://dx.doi.org/10.1098/rstb.2007.2055

Healy, A. F., Schneider, V. I., & Bourne, L. E. (2012). Empirically valid principles of training. In A. F. Healy & L. E. Bourne (Eds.), *Training cognition: Optimizing efficiency, durability, and generalizability* (pp. 13–39). New York: Psychology Press.

Himanen, L., Portin, R., Isoniemi, H., Helenius, H., Kurki, T., & Tenovuo, O. (2006). Longitudinal cognitive changes in traumatic brain injury: A 30-year follow-up study. *Neurology, 66,* 187–192. http://dx.doi.org/10.1212/01.wnl.0000194264.60150.d3

Hoge, C. W., McGurk, D., Thomas, J. L., Cox, A. L., Engel, C. C., & Castro, C. A. (2008). Mild traumatic brain injury in U.S. soldiers returning from Iraq. *New England Journal of Medicine, 358,* 453–463. http://dx.doi.org/10.1056/NEJMoa072972

Hunkin, N. M., Squires, E. J., Parkin, A. J., & Tidy, J. A. (1998). Are the benefits of errorless learning dependent on implicit memory? *Neuropsychologia, 36,* 25–36. http://dx.doi.org/10.1016/S0028-3932(97)00106-1

Hurn, J., Kneebone, I., & Cropley, M. (2006). Goal setting as an outcome measure: A systematic review. *Clinical Rehabilitation, 20,* 756–772. http://dx.doi.org/10.1177/0269215506070793

Jackson, R. D., Mysiw, W. J., & Corrigan, J. D. (1989). Orientation Group Monitoring System: An indicator for reversible impairments in cognition during posttraumatic amnesia. *Archives of Physical Medicine and Rehabilitation, 70,* 33–36.

Jackson, W. T., Novack, T. A., & Dowler, R. N. (1998). Effective serial measurement of cognitive orientation in rehabilitation: The Orientation Log. *Archives of Physical Medicine and Rehabilitation, 79,* 718–720. http://dx.doi.org/10.1016/S0003-9993(98)90051-X

Jacobs, B., van Ekert, J., Vernooy, L. P., Dieperink, P., Andriessen, T. M., Hendriks, M. P., . . . Vos, P. E. (2012). Development and external validation of a new PTA assessment scale. *BMC Neurology, 12,* 69. http://dx.doi.org/10.1186/1471-2377-12-69

Jacobs, H. E. (1988). The Los Angeles Head Injury Survey: Procedures and initial findings. *Archives of Physical Medicine and Rehabilitation, 69,* 425–431.

Kaschel, R., Della Sala, S., Cantagallo, A., Fahlböck, A., Laaksonen, R., & Kazen, M. (2002). Imagery mnemonics for the rehabilitation of memory: A randomised group controlled trial. *Neuropsychological Rehabilitation, 12,* 127–153. http://dx.doi.org/10.1080/09602010143000211

Katz, N. (2006). *Routine Task Inventory–Expanded manual.* Retrieved from http://www.allen-cognitive-network.org

Katz, N., Itzkovich, M., Averbuch, S., & Elazar, B. (1989). Loewenstein Occupational Therapy Cognitive Assessment (LOTCA) battery for brain-injured patients: Reliability and validity. *American Journal of Occupational Therapy, 43,* 184–192. http://dx.doi.org/10.5014/ajot.43.3.184

Kelly, M. P., Johnson, C. T., Knoller, N., Drubach, D. A., & Winslow, M. M. (1997). Substance abuse, traumatic brain injury and neuropsychological outcome. *Brain Injury, 11,* 391–402. http://dx.doi.org/10.1080/026990597123386

Kern, R. S., Liberman, R. P., Kopelowicz, A., Mintz, J., & Green, M. F. (2002). Applications of errorless learning for improving work performance in persons with schizophrenia. *American Journal of Psychiatry, 159,* 1921–1926. http://dx.doi.org/10.1176/appi.ajp.159.11.1921

Kessels, R. P. C., & de Haan, E. H. F. (2003). Implicit learning in memory rehabilitation: A meta-analysis on errorless learning and vanishing cues methods. *Journal of Clinical and Experimental Neuropsychology, 25,* 805–814. http://dx.doi.org/10.1076/jcen.25.6.805.16474

Kim, H. J., Burke, D. T., Dowds, M. M., Jr., Boone, K. A., & Park, G. J. (2000). Electronic memory aids for outpatient brain injury: Follow-up findings. *Brain Injury, 14,* 187–196. http://dx.doi.org/10.1080/026990500120844

Kime, S. K. (2006). *Compensating for memory deficits using a systematic approach.* Bethesda, MD: AOTA Press.

Kiresuk, T. J., & Sherman, R. E. (1968). Goal Attainment Scaling: A general method for evaluating comprehensive community mental health programs. *Community Mental Health Journal, 4,* 443–453. http://dx.doi.org/10.1007/BF01530764

Komatsu, S., Minimua, M., Kato, M., & Kashima, H. (2000). Errorless and effortful processes involved in the learning of face–name associations by patients with alcoholic Korsakoff's syndrome. *Neuropsychological Rehabilitation, 10,* 113–132. http://dx.doi.org/10.1080/096020100389200

Krasny-Pacini, A., Chevignard, M., & Evans, J. (2014). Goal Management Training for rehabilitation of executive functions: A systematic review of effectiveness in patients with acquired brain injury. *Disability and Rehabilitation, 36,* 105–116. http://dx.doi.org/10.3109/09638288.2013.777807

Krueger, W. C. F. (1929). The effect of overlearning on retention. *Journal of Experimental Psychology, 12,* 71–78. http://dx.doi.org/10.1037/h0072036

Langlois, J. A., Rutland-Brown, W., & Thomas, K. E. (2004). *Traumatic brain injury in the United States: Emergency department visits, hospitalizations, and deaths.* Atlanta: Centers for Disease Control and Prevention, National Center for Injury Prevention and Control.

Law, M., Baptiste, S., Carswell, A., McColl, M. A., Polatajko, H., & Pollock, N. (2014). *The Canadian Occupational Performance Measure* (5th ed.). Ottawa, Ontario: CAOT Publications.

Levin, H. S., O'Donnell, V. M., & Grossman, R. G. (1979). The Galveston Orientation and Amnesia Test: A practical scale to assess cognition after head injury. *Journal of Nervous and Mental Disease, 167,* 675–684. http://dx.doi.org/10.1097/00005053-197911000-00004

Levine, B., Robertson, I. H., Clare, L., Carter, G., Hong, J., Wilson, B. A., . . . Stuss, D. T. (2000). Rehabilitation of executive functioning: An experimental–clinical validation of Goal Management Training. *Journal of the International Neuropsychological Society, 6,* 299–312. http://dx.doi.org/10.1017/S1355617700633052

Levine, B., Schweizer, T. A., O'Connor, C., Turner, G., Gillingham, S., Stuss, D. T., . . . Robertson, I. H. (2011). Rehabilitation of executive functioning in patients with frontal lobe brain damage with Goal Management Training. *Frontiers in Human Neuroscience, 5,* 1–9. http://dx.doi.org/0.3389/fnhum.2011.00009

Lezak, M. D., Howieson, D. B., Bigler, E. D., & Tranel, D. (2012). *Neuropsychological assessment* (5th ed.). New York: Oxford University Press.

Loetscher, T., & Lincoln, N. B. (2013). Cognitive rehabilitation for attention deficits following stroke. *Cochrane Database of Systematic Reviews, 2013,* CD002842. http://dx.doi.org/10.1002/14651858.CD002842.pub2

Lövdén, M., Wenger, E., Mårtensson, J., Lindenberger, U., & Bäckman, L. (2013). Structural brain plasticity in adult learning and development. *Neuroscience and Biobehavioral Reviews, 37,* 2296–2310. http://dx.doi.org/10.1016/j.neubiorev.2013.02.014

Lowenstein, D., & Acevedo, A. (2010). The relationship between activities of daily living and neuropsychological performance. In T. D. Marcotte & I. Grant (Eds.), *Neuropsychology of everyday functioning* (pp. 93–112). New York: Guilford.

Lumos Labs. (2010). *Lumosity: Reclaim your brain.* San Francisco: Dakim.

Luria, A. R. (1966). *Higher cortical functions in man.* New York: Basic Books.

MacGregor, A. J., Shaffer, R. A., Dougherty, A. L., Galarneau, M. R., Raman, R., Baker, D. G., . . . Corson, K. S. (2010). Prevalence and psychological correlates of traumatic brain injury in Operation Iraqi Freedom. *Journal of Head Trauma Rehabilitation, 25,* 1–8. http://dx.doi.org/10.1097/HTR.0b013e3181c2993d

Maestas, K. L., Sander, A. M., Clark, A. N., van Veldhoven, L. M., Struchen, M. A., Sherer, M., & Hannay, H. J. (2014). Preinjury coping, emotional functioning, and quality of life following uncomplicated and complicated mild traumatic brain injury. *Journal of Head Trauma Rehabilitation, 29,* 407–417. http://dx.doi.org/10.1097/HTR.0b013e31828654b4

Malouf, T., Langdon, R., & Taylor, A. (2014). The Insight Interview: A new tool for measuring deficits in awareness after traumatic brain injury. *Brain Injury, 28,* 1523–1541. http://dx.doi.org/10.3109/02699052.2014.922700

Man, D. W., Fleming, J., Hohaus, L., & Shum, D. (2011). Development of the Brief Assessment of Prospective Memory (BAPM) for use with traumatic brain injury populations. *Neuropsychological Rehabilitation, 21,* 884–898. http://dx.doi.org/10.1080/09602011.2011.627270

Manchester, D., Priestley, N., & Jackson, H. (2004). The assessment of executive functions: Coming out of the office. *Brain Injury, 18,* 1067–1081. http://dx.doi.org/10.1080/02699050410001672387

Marcotte, T. D., Scott, J. C., Kamat, R., & Heaton, R. K. (2010). Neuropsychology and the prediction of everyday functioning. In T. D. Marcotte & I. Grant (Eds.), *Neuropsychology of everyday functioning* (pp. 5–38). New York: Guilford.

McCrea, M., Iverson, G. L., McAllister, T. W., Hammeke, T. A., Powell, M. R., Barr, W. B., & Kelly, J. P. (2009). An integrated review of recovery after mild traumatic brain injury (MTBI): Implications for clinical management. *Clinical Neuropsychologist, 23,* 1368–1390. http://dx.doi.org/10.1080/13854040903074652

McCrory, P., Meeuwisse, W., Johnston, K., Dvorak, J., Aubry, M., Molloy, M., & Cantu, R. (2009). Consensus statement on concussion in sport: The 3rd International Conference on Concussion in Sport held in Zurich, November 2008. *Journal of Athletic Training, 44,* 434–448. http://dx.doi.org/10.4085/1062-6050-44.4.434

McDonald, A., Haslam, C., Yates, P., Gurr, B., Leeder, G., & Sayers, A. (2011). Google Calendar: A new memory aid to compensate for prospective memory deficits following acquired brain injury. *Neuropsychological Rehabilitation, 21,* 784–807. http://dx.doi.org/10.1080/09602011.2011.598405

McEvoy, P. M., Nathan, P., & Norton, P. J. (2009). Efficacy of transdiagnostic treatments: A review of published outcome studies and future research directions. *Journal of Cognitive Psychotherapy: An International Quarterly, 23,* 20–33. http://dx.doi.org/10.1891/0889-8391.23.1.20

McEwen, S. E., Polatajko, H. J., Huijbregts, M. P., & Ryan, J. D. (2009). Exploring a cognitive-based treatment approach to improve motor-based skill performance in chronic stroke: Results of three single case experiments. *Brain Injury, 23,* 1041–1053. http://dx.doi.org/10.3109/02699050903421107

McMillan, T. M. (2013). Outcome of rehabilitation for neurobehavioural disorders. *NeuroRehabilitation, 32,* 791–801. http://dx.doi.org/10.3233/NRE-130903

Meichenbaum, D. (1977). *Cognitive–behavior modification: An integrative approach.* New York: Plenum.

Millis, S. R., Rosenthal, M., Novack, T. A., Sherer, M., Nick, T. G., Kreutzer, J. S., . . . Ricker, J. H. (2001). Long-term neuropsychological outcome after traumatic brain injury. *Journal of Head Trauma Rehabilitation, 16,* 343–355. http://dx.doi.org/10.1097/00001199-200108000-00005

Morrison, M. T., Giles, G. M., Ryan, J. D., Baum, C. M., Dromerick, A. W., Polatajko, H. J., & Edwards, D. F. (2013). Multiple Errands Test–Revised (MET–R): A performance-based measure of executive function in people with mild cerebrovascular accident. *American Journal of Occupational Therapy, 67,* 460–468. http://dx.doi.org/10.5014/ajot.2013.007880

Nakase-Richardson, R., Sherer, M., Seel, R. T., Hart, T., Hanks, R., Arango-Lasprilla, J. C., . . . Hammond, F. (2011). Utility of post-traumatic amnesia in predicting 1-year productivity following traumatic brain injury: Comparison of the Russell and Mississippi PTA classification intervals. *Journal of Neurology, Neurosurgery, and Psychiatry, 82,* 494–499. http://dx.doi.org/10.1136/jnnp.2010.222489

Neistadt, M. E. (1992). The Rabideau Kitchen Evaluation–Revised: An assessment of meal preparation skill. *OTJR: Occupation, Participation and Health, 12,* 242–253. http://dx.doi.org/10.1177/153944929201200404

Norman, D. A., & Shallice, T. (1986). Attention to action: Willed and automatic control of behavior. In R. J. Davidson, G. E. Schwartz, & D. Shapiro (Eds.), *Advances in research and theory: Vol. 4. Consciousness and self-regulation* (pp. 1–18). New York: Plenum.

Novack, T. A., Alderson, A. L., Bush, B. A., Meythaler, J. M., & Canupp, K. (2000). Cognitive and functional recovery at 6 and 12 months post-TBI. *Brain Injury, 14,* 987–996. http://dx.doi.org/10.1080/02699050050191922

Novack, T. A., Dowler, R. N., Bush, B. A., Glen, T., & Schneider, J. J. (2000). Validity of the Orientation Log, relative to the Galveston Orientation and Amnesia Test. *Journal of Head Trauma Rehabilitation, 15,* 957–961. http://dx.doi.org/10.1097/00001199-200006000-00008

Nudo, R. J., Plautz, E. J., & Frost, S. B. (2001). Role of adaptive plasticity in recovery of function after damage to motor cortex. *Muscle and Nerve, 24,* 1000–1019. http://dx.doi.org/10.1002/mus.1104

O'Callaghan, A., McAllister, L., & Wilson, L. (2012). Insight vs readiness: Factors affecting engagement in therapy from the perspectives of adults with TBI and their significant others. *Brain Injury, 26,* 1599–1610. http://dx.doi.org/10.3109/02699052.2012.698788

O'Carroll, R. E., Russell, H. H., Lawrie, S. M., & Johnstone, E. C. (1999). Errorless learning and the cognitive rehabilitation of memory-impaired schizophrenic patients. *Psychological Medicine, 29,* 105–112. http://dx.doi.org/10.1017/S0033291798007673

Odhuba, R. A., van den Broek, M. D., & Johns, L. C. (2005). Ecological validity of measures of executive functioning. *British Journal of Clinical Psychology, 44,* 269–278. http://dx.doi.org/10.1348/014466505X29431

Parish, L., & Oddy, M. (2007). Efficacy of rehabilitation for functional skills more than 10 years after extremely severe brain injury. *Neuropsychological Rehabilitation, 17,* 230–243. http://dx.doi.org/10.1080/09602010600750675

Park, N. W., Moscovitch, M., & Robertson, I. H. (1999). Divided attention impairments after traumatic brain injury. *Neuropsychologia, 37,* 1119–1133. http://dx.doi.org/10.1016/S0028-3932(99)00034-2

Park, N. W., Proulx, G., & Towers, W. M. (1999). Evaluation of the Attention Process Training programme. *Neuropsychological Rehabilitation, 9,* 135–154. http://dx.doi.org/10.1080/713755595

Parkin, A. J., Hunkin, N. M., & Squires, E. J. (1998). Unlearning John Major: The use of errorless learning in the reacquisition of proper names following herpes simplex encephalitis. *Cognitive Neuropsychology, 15,* 361–375. http://dx.doi.org/10.1080/026432998381131

Penna, S., & Novack, T. A. (2007). Further validation of the Orientation and Cognitive Logs: Their relationship to the Mini-Mental State Examination. *Archives of Physical Medicine and Rehabilitation, 88,* 1360–1361. http://dx.doi.org/10.1016/j.apmr.2007.07.005

Perrin, P. B., Niemeier, J. P., Mougeot, J.-L., Vannoy, C. H., Hirsch, M. A., Watts, J. A., . . . Whitney, M. P. (2015). Measures of injury severity and prediction of acute traumatic brain injury outcomes. *Journal of Head Trauma Rehabilitation, 30,* 136–142. http://dx.doi.org/10.1097/HTR.0000000000000026

Phipps, S., & Richardson, P. (2007). Occupational therapy outcomes for clients with traumatic brain injury and stroke using the Canadian Occupational Performance Measure. *American Journal of Occupational Therapy, 61,* 328–334. http://dx.doi.org/10.5014/ajot.61.3.328

Piras, F., Borella, E., Incoccia, C., & Carlesimo, G. A. (2011). Evidence-based practice recommendations for memory rehabilitation. *European Journal of Physical and Rehabilitation Medicine, 47,* 149–175.

Polatajko, H. J., & Mandich, A. (2004). *Enabling occupation in children: The Cognitive Orientation to daily Occupational Performance.* Ottawa, Ontario: CAOT Publications.

Polatajko, H. J., & Mandich, A. (2005). Cognitive Orientation to daily Occupational Performance. In N. Katz (Ed.), *Cognition and occupation across the life span* (pp. 237–259). Bethesda, MD: AOTA Press.

Polatajko, H. J., & Mandich, A. (2011). Cognitive Orientation to daily Occupational Performance (CO-OP): A cognitive-based intervention for children and adults. In N. Katz (Ed.), *Cognition, occupation, and participation across the life span: Neuroscience, neurorehabilitation, and models of intervention in occupational therapy* (3rd ed., pp. 299–321). Bethesda, MD: AOTA Press.

Ponsford, J., Bayley, M., Wiseman-Hakes, C., Togher, L., Velikonja, D., & McIntyre, A.; INCOG Expert Panel. (2014). INCOG recommendations for management of cognition following traumatic brain injury, Part II: Attention and information processing speed. *Journal of Head Trauma Rehabilitation, 29,* 321–337. http://dx.doi.org/10.1097/HTR.0000000000000072

Posner, M. I., & Petersen, S. E. (1990). The attention system of the human brain. *Annual Review of Neuroscience, 13,* 25–42. http://dx.doi.org/10.1146/annurev.ne.13.030190.000325

Postman, L. (1962). Retention as a function of degree of overlearning. *Science, 135,* 666–667. http://dx.doi.org/10.1126/science.135.3504.666

Poulin, V., Korner-Bitensky, N., & Dawson, D. R. (2013). Stroke-specific executive function assessment: A literature review of performance-based tools. *Australian Occupational Therapy Journal, 60,* 3–19. http://dx.doi.org/10.1111/1440-1630.12024

Poulin, V., Korner-Bitensky, N., Dawson, D. R., & Bherer, L. (2012). Efficacy of executive function interventions after stroke: A systematic review. *Topics in Stroke Rehabilitation, 19,* 158–171. http://dx.doi.org/10.1310/tsr1902-158

Priestley, N., Manchester, D., & Aram, R. (2013). Presenting evidence of executive functions deficit in court: Issues for the expert neuropsychologist. *Journal of Personal Injury Law, 4,* 240–247.

Prigatano, G. P., & Altman, I. M. (1990). Impaired awareness of behavioral limitations after traumatic brain injury. *Archives of Physical Medicine and Rehabilitation, 71,* 1058–1064.

Prigatano, G. P., Fordyce, D. J., Zeiner, H. K., Roueche, J. R., Pepping, M., & Wood, B. C. (1984). Neuropsychological rehabilitation after closed head injury in young adults. *Journal of Neurology, Neurosurgery, and Psychiatry, 47,* 505–513. http://dx.doi.org/10.1136/jnnp.47.5.505

Rey, A. (1964). *L'examen clinique en psychologie* [The clinical examination in psychology]. Paris: Presses Universitaires de France.

Richardson, J. T. E. (1992). Imagery mnemonics and memory remediation. *Neurology, 42,* 283–286. http://dx.doi.org/10.1212/WNL.42.2.283

Richardson, J. T. E. (1995). The efficacy of imagery mnemonics in memory remediation. *Neuropsychologia, 33,* 1345–1357. http://dx.doi.org/10.1016/0028-3932(95)00068-E

Richardson, J. T. E., Cermack, L. S., Blackford, S. P., & O'Connor, M. (1987). The efficacy of imagery mnemonics following brain damage. In M. A. McDaniel & M. Pressley (Eds.), *Imagery and related mnemonic processes* (pp. 303–328). New York: Springer.

Riska-Williams, L., Allen, C. A., Austin, S., David, S., Earhart, C., & McCraith, D. B. (2007). *Manual for the ACLS–5 and LACLS–5.* Camarillo, CA: ACLS and LACLS Committee.

Robertson, I., Gray, J., & McKenzie, S. (1988). Microcomputer-based cognitive rehabilitation of visual neglect: Three multiple-baseline single-case studies. *Brain Injury, 2,* 151–163. http://dx.doi.org/10.3109/02699058809150939

Robertson, I. H., Gray, J. M., Pentland, B., & Waite, L. J. (1990). Microcomputer-based rehabilitation for unilateral left visual neglect: A randomized controlled trial. *Archives of Physical Medicine and Rehabilitation, 71,* 663–668.

Robertson, I. H., & Murre, J. M. J. (1999). Rehabilitation of brain damage: Brain plasticity and principles of guided recovery. *Psychological Bulletin, 125,* 544–575. http://dx.doi.org/10.1037/0033-2909.125.5.544

Robertson, I. H., Ward, T., Ridgeway, V., & Nimmo-Smith, I. (1994). *The Test of Everyday Attention.* Bury St. Edmunds, England: Thames Valley Test Company.

Robertson, I. H., Ward, T., Ridgeway, V., & Nimmo-Smith, I. (1996). The structure of normal human attention: The Test of Everyday Attention. *Journal of the International Neuropsychological Society, 2,* 525–534. http://dx.doi.org/10.1017/S1355617700001697

Rohling, M. L., Faust, M. E., Beverly, B., & Demakis, G. (2009). Effectiveness of cognitive rehabilitation following acquired brain injury: A meta-analytic re-examination of Cicerone et al.'s (2000, 2005) systematic reviews. *Neuropsychology, 23,* 20–39. http://dx.doi.org/10.1037/a0013659

Rohrer, D., Taylor, K., Pashler, H., Wixted, J. T., & Cepeda, N. J. (2005). The effect of overlearning on long-term retention. *Applied Cognitive Psychology, 19,* 361–374. http://dx.doi.org/10.1002/acp.1083

Ropacki, S., Rickards, T., Barrera, K., & Yutsis, M. (2014). C-69: The relationship between self-awareness and functional outcomes in brain injury rehabilitation. *Archives of Clinical Neuropsychology, 29,* 599. http://dx.doi.org/10.1093/arclin/acu038.250

Schacter, D. L., Rich, S. A., & Stampp, M. S. (1985). Remediation of memory disorders: Experimental evaluation of the spaced-retrieval technique. *Journal of Clinical and Experimental Neuropsychology, 7,* 79–96. http://dx.doi.org/10.1080/01688638508401243

Schmitter-Edgecombe, M. (2006). Implications of basic science research for brain injury rehabilitation: A focus on intact learning mechanisms. *Journal of Head Trauma Rehabilitation, 21,* 131–141. http://dx.doi.org/10.1097/00001199-200603000-00006

Schmitter-Edgecombe, M., & Nissley, H. M. (2000). Effects of divided attention on automatic and controlled components of memory after severe closed-head injury. *Neuropsychology, 14,* 559–569. http://dx.doi.org/10.1037/0894-4105.14.4.559

Schneider, W., & Shiffrin, R. M. (1977). Controlled and automatic human information processing: I. Detection, search, and attention. *Psychological Review, 84,* 1–66. http://dx.doi.org/10.1037/0033-295X.84.1.1

Schönberger, M., Ponsford, J., Reutens, D., Beare, R., & O'Sullivan, R. (2009). The relationship between age, injury severity, and MRI findings after traumatic brain injury. *Journal of Neurotrauma, 26,* 2157–2167. http://dx.doi.org/10.1089/neu.2009.0939

Schutz, L. E., & Wanlass, R. L. (2009). Interdisciplinary assessment strategies for capturing the elusive executive. *American Journal of Physical Medicine and Rehabilitation, 88,* 419–422. http://dx.doi.org/10.1097/PHM.0b013e3181a0e2d3

Schweizer, T. A., Levine, B., Rewilak, D., O'Connor, C., Turner, G., Alexander, M. P., . . . Stuss, D. T. (2008). Rehabilitation of executive functioning after focal damage to the cerebellum. *Neurorehabilitation and Neural Repair, 22,* 72–77. http://dx.doi.org/10.1177/1545968307305303

Shallice, T., & Burgess, P. W. (1991). Deficits in strategy application following frontal lobe damage in man. *Brain, 114,* 727–741. http://dx.doi.org/10.1093/brain/114.2.727

Shea, J. B., & Morgan, R. L. (1979). Contextual interference effects on the acquisition, retention, and transfer of a motor skill. *Journal of Experimental Psychology: Human Learning and Memory, 5,* 179.

Sherer, M., Bergloff, P., Boake, C., High, W., Jr., & Levin, E. (1998). The Awareness Questionnaire: Factor structure and internal consistency. *Brain Injury, 12,* 63–68. http://dx.doi.org/10.1080/026990598122863

Sherer, M., Bergloff, P., Levin, E., High, W. M., Jr., Oden, K. E., & Nick, T. G. (1998). Impaired awareness and employment outcome after traumatic brain injury. *Journal of Head Trauma Rehabilitation, 13,* 52–61. http://dx.doi.org/10.1097/00001199-199810000-00007

Shiffrin, R. M., & Schneider, W. (1977). Controlled and automatic information processing: II. Perceptual learning, automatic attending, and a general theory. *Psychological Review, 84,* 127–190. http://dx.doi.org/10.1037/0033-295X.84.2.127

Shin, M. S., Park, S. Y., Park, S. R., Seol, S. H., & Kwon, J. S. (2006). Clinical and empirical applications of the Rey–Osterrieth Complex Figure Test. *Nature Protocols, 1,* 892–899. http://dx.doi.org/10.1038/nprot.2006.115

Shores, E. A., Lammél, A., Hullick, C., Sheedy, J., Flynn, M., Levick, W., & Batchelor, J. (2008). The diagnostic accuracy of the Revised Westmead PTA Scale as an adjunct to the Glasgow Coma Scale in the early identification of cognitive impairment in patients with mild traumatic brain injury. *Journal of Neurology, Neurosurgery, and Psychiatry, 79,* 1100–1106. http://dx.doi.org/10.1136/jnnp.2007.132571

Shum, D., & Fleming, J. (2008). *Comprehensive Assessment of Prospective Memory: Manual.* Brisbane, Queensland, Australia: Griffith University and University of Queensland.

Sigurdardottir, S., Andelic, N., Wehling, E., Roe, C., Anke, A., Skandsen, T., . . . Schanke, A. K. (2014). Neuropsychological functioning in a national cohort of severe traumatic brain injury: Demographic and acute injury–related predictors. *Journal of Head Trauma Rehabilitation, 30,* E1–E12. http://dx.doi.org/10.1097/HTR.0000000000000039

Skandsen, T., Finnanger, T. G., Andersson, S., Lydersen, S., Brunner, J. F., & Vik, A. (2010). Cognitive impairment 3 months after moderate and severe traumatic brain injury: A prospective follow-up study. *Archives of Physical Medicine and Rehabilitation, 91,* 1904–1913. http://dx.doi.org/10.1016/j.apmr.2010.08.021

Söderback, I., & Normell, L. A. (1986a). Intellectual function training in adults with acquired brain damage: An occupational therapy method. *Scandinavian Journal of Rehabilitation Medicine, 18,* 139–146.

Söderback, I., & Normell, L. A. (1986b). Intellectual function training in adults with acquired brain damage: Evaluation. *Scandinavian Journal of Rehabilitation Medicine, 18,* 147–153.

Sohlberg, M. M., & Mateer, C. A. (1987a). *APT: Attention Process Training manual.* Puyallup, WA: Association for Neuropsychological Research and Development.

Sohlberg, M. M., & Mateer, C. A. (1987b). Effectiveness of an attention-training program. *Journal of Clinical and Experimental Neuropsychology, 9,* 117–130. http://dx.doi.org/10.1080/01688638708405352

Sohlberg, M. M., & Mateer, C. A. (1989). Training use of compensatory memory books: A three-stage behavioral approach. *Journal of Clinical and Experimental Neuropsychology, 11,* 871–891. http://dx.doi.org/10.1080/01688638908400941

Sohlberg, M. M., & Mateer, C. A. (2011). *Attention Process Training APT–3: A direct attention training program for persons with acquired brain injury.* Youngsville, NC: Lash & Associates/ Training Inc.

Sohlberg, M. M., & Turkstra, L. (2011). *Optimizing cognitive rehabilitation: Effective instructional methods.* New York: Guilford.

Soldatovic-Stajic, B., Misic-Pavkov, G., Bozic, K., Novovic, Z., & Gajic, Z. (2014). Neuropsychological and neurophysiological evaluation of cognitive deficits related to the severity of traumatic brain injury. *European Review for Medical and Pharmacological Sciences, 18,* 1632–1637.

Speicher, S. M., Walter, K. H., & Chard, K. M. (2014). Interdisciplinary residential treatment of posttraumatic stress disorder and traumatic brain injury: Effects on symptom severity and occupational performance and satisfaction. *American Journal of Occupational Therapy, 68,* 412–421. http://dx.doi.org/10.5014/ajot.2014.011304

Stringer, A. Y., & Small, S. K. (2011). Ecologically-oriented neurorehabilitation of memory: Robustness of outcome across diagnosis and severity. *Brain Injury, 25,* 169–178. http://dx.doi.org/10.3109/02699052.2010.541894

Stuss, D. T. (1991). Self-awareness and the frontal lobes: A neuropsychological perspective. In J. Strauss & G. R. Goethals (Eds.), *The self: Interdisciplinary approaches* (pp. 255–278). New York: Springer-Verlag.

Teasdale, G., & Jennett, B. (1974). Assessment of coma and impaired consciousness: A practical scale. *Lancet, 2,* 81–84. http://dx.doi.org/10.1016/S0140-6736(74)91639-0

Teasdale, T. W., Emslie, H., Quirk, K., Evans, J., Fish, J., & Wilson, B. A. (2009). Alleviation of carer strain during the use of the NeuroPage device by people with acquired brain injury. *Journal of Neurology, Neurosurgery, and Psychiatry, 80,* 781–783. http://dx.doi.org/10.1136/jnnp.2008.162966

Terrace, H. S. (1963). Discrimination learning with and without "errors." *Journal of the Experimental Analysis of Behavior, 6,* 1–27. http://dx.doi.org/10.1901/jeab.1963.6-1

Toglia, J. P. (1993). *The Contextual Memory Test.* Tucson, AZ: Therapy Skill Builders.

Toglia, J., Johnston, M. V., Goverover, Y., & Dain, B. (2010). A multicontext approach to promoting transfer of strategy use and self regulation after brain injury: An exploratory study. *Brain Injury, 24,* 664–677. http://dx.doi.org/10.3109/02699051003610474

Toglia, J., & Kirk, U. (2000). Understanding awareness deficits following brain injury. *NeuroRehabilitation, 15,* 57–70.

Turner-Stokes, L. (2008). Evidence for the effectiveness of multi-disciplinary rehabilitation following acquired brain injury: A synthesis of two systematic approaches. *Journal of Rehabilitation Medicine, 40,* 691–701. http://dx.doi.org/10.2340/16501977-0265

van Heugten, C., Gregório, G. W., & Wade, D. (2012). Evidence-based cognitive rehabilitation after acquired brain injury: A systematic review of content of treatment. *Neuropsychological Rehabilitation, 22,* 653–673. http://dx.doi.org/10.1080/09602011.2012.680891

Velikonja, D., Tate, R., Ponsford, J., McIntyre, A., Janzen, S., & Bayley, M.; INCOG Expert Panel. (2014). INCOG recommendations for management of cognition following traumatic brain injury, Part V: Memory. *Journal of Head Trauma Rehabilitation, 29,* 369–386. http://dx.doi.org/10.1097/HTR.0000000000000069

Wade, D. T., King, N. S., Wenden, F. J., Crawford, S., & Caldwell, F. E. (1998). Routine follow up after head injury: A second randomized controlled trial. *Journal of Neurology, Neurosurgery, and Psychiatry, 65,* 177–183.

Walker, K. R., & Tesco, G. (2013). Molecular mechanisms of cognitive dysfunction following traumatic brain injury. *Frontiers in Aging Neuroscience, 5,* 29. http://dx.doi.org/10.3389/fnagi.2013.00029

Wechsler, D. (2009). *Wechsler Memory Scale–Fourth Edition (WMS–IV): Technical and interpretive manual.* San Antonio: Pearson.

West, L. K., Curtis, K. L., Greve, K. W., & Bianchini, K. J. (2011). Memory in traumatic brain injury: The effects of injury severity and effort on the Wechsler Memory Scale–III. *Journal of Neuropsychology, 5,* 114–125. http://dx.doi.org/10.1348/174866410X521434

Whyte, J. (1986). Outcome evaluation in the remediation of attention and memory deficits. *Journal of Head Trauma Rehabilitation, 1,* 64–71. http://dx.doi.org/10.1097/00001199-198609000-00010

Wilson, B. A. (1991). Long-term prognosis of patients with severe memory disorders. *Neuropsychological Rehabilitation, 1,* 117–134. http://dx.doi.org/10.1080/09602019108401386

Wilson, B. A., Alderman, N., Burgess, A. W., Emslie, H., & Evans, J. J. (1996). *Behavioral Assessment of the Dysexecutive Syndrome.* Bury St. Edmunds, England: Thames Valley Test Company.

Wilson, B. A., Baddeley, A., Evans, J. J., & Shiel, A. (1994). Errorless learning in the rehabilitation of memory-impaired people. *Neuropsychological Rehabilitation, 4,* 307–326. http://dx.doi.org/10.1080/09602019408401463

Wilson, B. A., Clare, E., Baddeley, A. D., Cockburn, J., Watson, P., & Tate, R. (1999). *The Rivermead Behavioural Memory Test–Extended version.* London: Pearson Assessment.

Wilson, B. A., Cockburn, J., & Baddeley, A. D. (1991). *The Rivermead Behavioural Memory Test.* Bury St. Edmunds, England: Thames Valley Test Company.

Wilson, B. A., Cockburn, J., & Baddeley, A. D. (2003). *The Rivermead Behavioural Memory Test* (2nd ed.). London: Pearson Assessment.

Wilson, B. A., Gracey, F., Malley, D., Bateman, A., & Evans, J. J. (2009). The Oliver Zangwill Centre approach to neuropsychological rehabilitation. In B. A. Wilson, F. Gracey, J. J. Evans, & A. Bateman (Eds.), *Neuropsychological rehabilitation: Theory, models, therapy, and outcome* (pp. 47–67). Cambridge, England: Cambridge University Press.

Wilson, B. A., Greenfield, E., Clare, E., Baddeley, A. D., Cockburn, J., Watson, P., & Crawford, J. (2008). *The Rivermead Behavioural Memory Test* (3rd ed.). London: Pearson.

Wilson, B. A., Scott, H., Evans, J., & Emslie, H. (2003). Preliminary report of a NeuroPage service within a health care system. *NeuroRehabilitation, 18,* 3–8.

Wolf, T. J., Baum, C., & Connor, L. T. (2009). Changing face of stroke: Implications for occupational therapy practice. *American Journal of Occupational Therapy, 63,* 621–625. http://dx.doi.org/10.5014/ajot.63.5.621

Woods, S. P., Moran, L. M., Dawson, M. S., Carey, C. L., & Grant, I.; HIV Neurobehavioral Research Center Group. (2008). Psychometric characteristics of the Memory for Intentions Screening Test. *Clinical Neuropsychology, 22,* 864–878. http://dx.doi.org/10.1080/13854040701595999

Yin, H. H., & Knowlton, B. J. (2006). The role of the basal ganglia in habit formation. *Nature, 7,* 464–476. http://dx.doi.org/10.1038/nm1919

Zickefoose, S., Hux, K., Brown, J., & Wulf, K. (2013). Let the games begin: A preliminary study using Attention Process Training–3 and Lumosity™ brain games to remediate attention deficits following traumatic brain injury. *Brain Injury, 27,* 707–716. http://dx.doi.org/10.3109/02699052.2013.775484

Zoccolotti, P., Cantagallo, A., De Luca, M., Guariglia, C., Serino, A., & Trojano, L. (2011). Selective and integrated rehabilitation programs for disturbances of visual/spatial attention and executive function after brain damage: A neuropsychological evidence-based review. *European Journal of Physical and Rehabilitation Medicine, 47,* 123–147.

Zoltan, B. (2007). *Vision, perception, and cognition: A manual for the evaluation and treatment of the adult with acquired brain injury* (4th ed.). Thorofare, NJ: Slack.

Section II: Traumatic Brain Injury Rehabilitation Across the Continuum of Recovery and Community Reintegration

CHAPTER 4

The Case of Diane Archer

Kathleen M. Golisz, OTD, OTR/L

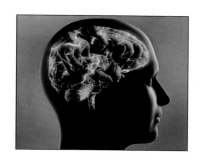

Learning Objectives

After completion of this chapter, readers will be able to

- Identify key elements of a client's occupational profile that may influence occupational therapy intervention;
- Identify physiological signs of brain injury and the methods used to measure their severity; and
- Identify the typical medical-based interventions provided to an individual with **traumatic brain injury** (TBI) in the emergency department.

Introduction

This chapter introduces the case of Diane Archer, a young woman who sustained a traumatic brain injury (TBI). By revisiting her through the four phases of recovery—(1) preinjury, (2) medical treatment, (3) **rehabilitation,** and (4) survivorship (Chesnut et al., 1999)—the case highlights the role of the occupational therapist in the neuro-rehabilitation of an adult with a TBI. As you revisit the case at each phase of recovery in the chapters ahead, consider the evidence supporting the occupational therapist's intervention and additional approaches that might support Diane's recovery.

Diane Archer might be viewed as leading the perfect life. Diane, who is 28 years old, grew up in a middle-class family in a suburban environment near a major metropolitan city. She is the only daughter and the youngest child in a family of German descent. Her two older brothers were always protective of Diane and challenged her to succeed in meeting her goals. She grew up as somewhat of a tomboy, always attempting to participate in her brothers' activities. Her parents instilled a strong work ethic in their children, and each child participated in assigned weekly household and yard chores. Although Diane did not have a large extended family, the neighborhood in which she grew up was close, and the families frequently socialized.

During her high school years, Diane excelled both academically and athletically. She was involved in several school sports and was popular with her peers. Diane did have her appendix removed at age 16 but otherwise had no medical issues requiring medications or hospitalization except for the birth of her daughter at age 25.

Diane graduated from college with a bachelor's degree in accounting and immediately began to work as an accountant with a small publishing firm in the nearby city. During the year that Diane worked for this company, she lived in an apartment in the city and enjoyed the rich cultural and social life that the city offered. Occasional weekend trips to her parents' house and weekly calls kept her connected with her old neighborhood. At age 23, she met her future husband, Tom, who worked as a draftsman in an architectural firm. He lived and worked about 30 minutes from her parents' home.

Diane and Tom were married in her hometown when she was 24. They decided to purchase an old house in a town that was within an hour's drive of her parents and brothers because both Diane and Tom wanted their children to experience childhood in a supportive community environment, like they had. Diane found a job with a large, competitive publishing company approximately 20 minutes from home. Tom's job also was within commuting distance from their new home. The two were constantly busy fixing up the interior and landscape of their new house and enjoying dinners and other activities (e.g., hiking, skiing, tennis, game nights) with a group of close friends. Diane also enjoyed reading and cooking for their dinner parties.

Tom and Diane's daughter, Kate, was born when Diane was 25, as has been mentioned. Diane's pregnancy was uneventful, and Kate's delivery was normal. Diane enjoyed an extended 4-month maternity leave before returning to her job at the publishing company. Kate is enrolled in a day care center that is on the way to Diane's job. Tom and Diane hope to have another child before Kate is 5.

Those who know Diane describe her as energetic, efficient, detail oriented, competitive, quick to laugh, and great at multitasking. If one were to ask Diane what her primary life roles were, she would list them as mother, wife, accountant, daughter, sister, aunt, and friend. She would be quick to say that the first two roles are tied in importance.

The Accident

Diane was late picking up Kate from day care. She was driving fast down a suburban two-lane road when a deer jumped out in front of her car. She swerved to miss the deer, and her car went off the road, head-on into a tree. Diane was wearing her seat belt, and even though her front airbag deployed when her car hit the tree, her head hit the side window and the door frame as her car did not have side airbags. A passing motorist called 911.

Diane was unconscious when the police and emergency medical service (EMS) arrived on the scene approximately 10 minutes after the accident. She had a large cut on her forehead and left temple area and an apparent fracture of her left lower leg. Diane's breathing was shallow and rapid. Her left pupil showed a sluggish reaction to light. She had an abnormal flexor response in her right upper extremity to pain stimulus, and she did not open her eyes or speak. Because the physical evidence suggested a TBI, the EMS crew began transport to the regional trauma center. During transport, Diane's vital signs showed a heart rate of 100, a respiratory rate of 16, and blood pressure of 90/60. Her oxygen saturation rate was dropping, but the cardiac monitor showed a normal sinus rhythm. The EMS crew reported her preadmission **Glasgow Coma Scale** score as 5 (eye opening = 1, motor score = 3, verbal score = 1). A cervical collar was placed, an intravenous drip was started, and Diane was intubated at the scene prior to transport to the trauma center.

Emergency Department of the Trauma Center

In the emergency department (ED) of the trauma center, a team of emergency medical personnel awaited Diane's arrival. Because of the information radioed in from the EMS team, a neurosurgeon was called to the ED. In an orchestrated but rapid pace, the team assessed Diane's condition from the moment the ambulance reached the ED bay. X rays of Diane's head and neck cleared her of any neck injuries but showed a linear fracture of the left temporal skull. A computed tomography (CT) scan showed a left epidural **hematoma** with herniation of the left **temporal lobe** into the tentorial notch. Diane was administered a bolus of mannitol in the CT room and rushed to surgery for a craniotomy to repair a tear in her middle meningeal artery, evacuate the hematoma, and place a ventriculo–peritoneal pressure gauge to monitor and treat her elevating intracranial pressure.

Trauma Center Intensive Care Unit

In the intensive care unit, Diane was noted to posture in **decorticate** position on her right upper extremity. The endotracheal and **nasogastric tubes** inserted in the ED remained in place to ensure adequate ventilation and nutrition, respectively. Orders were written for the rehabilitation team to evaluate and treat Diane.

The case continues at the end of the chapter on **coma** recovery (Chapter 5).

Reference

Chesnut, R. M., Carney, N., Maynard, H., Mann, N. C., Patterson, P., & Helfand, M. (1999). Summary report: Evidence for the effectiveness of rehabilitation for persons with traumatic brain injury. *Journal of Head Trauma Rehabilitation, 14,* 176–188. http://dx.doi. org/10.1097/00001199-199904000-00007

CHAPTER 5

Rehabilitation of the Patient With a Disorder of Consciousness

Robin McNeny, OTR/L

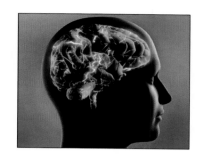

Learning Objectives

After completion of this chapter, readers will be able to

- Identify the primary client factors that may be impaired in patients with **traumatic brain injury** (TBI) at Rancho Los Amigos Levels of Cognitive Functioning I, II, or III (Hagen, Malkmus, & Durham, 1972);
- Select the most appropriate measures and tools to evaluate the patient at the coma level of recovery;
- Identify contextual supports and barriers to responses from the comatose patient; and
- Identify methods for engaging in client- and family-centered care with patients who have impaired interaction or awareness skills.

Key Words

- arousal
- assessment
- coma
- family
- positioning
- sensory stimulation

Introduction

The patient with a disorder of **consciousness** is a very special patient for the occupational therapist. Unlike many patients with whom the occupational therapist interacts in a professional relationship, the patient who has a disorder of consciousness is unable to actively participate in a therapeutic relationship. Therefore, the therapist bears an uncommon responsibility in the therapeutic process to gather information that enables him or her to infer the patient's preinjury personality and possible **rehabilitation** goals. This chapter focuses on the occupational therapist's role with patients with disorders of consciousness resulting from traumatic brain injury (TBI). It emphasizes the importance of expanding the definition of *patient* to include family and friends and the need for continued evaluation of the patient, primarily through structured observation.

Understanding Disorders of Consciousness

Coma has long been used as an all-encompassing term to describe a state of unarousability after significant injury or illness. The application of the global term *coma* to describe all people experiencing unconsciousness has come under scrutiny over the past decade. To improve accuracy in diagnosis, nomenclature based on behavioral response was developed that distinguishes coma from other states of altered consciousness, such as the **vegetative state** or the **minimally conscious state** (MCS). This nomenclature has gained wide acceptance and has been commonly used in clinical practice since it was first published (American Congress of Rehabilitation Medicine [ACRM], 1995; see Table 5.1 for differences in the observed behaviors of patients in coma, vegetative state, and MCS). The chief feature of coma after severe TBI is a total loss of awareness and the inability to attain **arousal,** whether spontaneously or via a stimulus (ACRM, 2010; Posner, Saper, Schiff, & Plum, 2007).

Arousal is critical to consciousness and is the state of being awake and responsive. Arousal is the basis for the attention and purposeful responses critical to daily function. The absence of arousal, characteristic of coma after TBI, arises from injury to the ascending reticular activating system or **brainstem** or from diffuse cortical or **subcortical** brain injury (ACRM, 1995; Davis & Gimenez, 2003; Edlow et al., 2012; Silva et al., 2010).

The **Glasgow Coma Scale** (GCS; Teasdale & Jennett, 1974), one of the most common scales used to rate disorders of consciousness, characterizes the patient's best visual, verbal, and motor responses at a point in time. Overall GCS scores range between 3 and 15, and patients with scores of 8 or less are diagnosed as being in coma (Teasdale & Jennett, 1974). These patients typically show no spontaneous eye opening, no purposeful movement, and no vocalization. They are not aware of, nor do they interact with, their environment. The patient in coma makes no observable response when presented with stimulation, and the sleep–wake cycle is absent (Katz, Zasler, & Zafonte, 2012). Clinical observations of a patient in coma correspond to Level I on the Rancho Los Amigos Levels of Cognitive Functioning (RLA LCF; see Table 1.3 in Chapter 1).

Most people in coma resulting from a severe TBI emerge from coma within 3 to 4 weeks postinjury (Katz, Polyak, Coughlan, Nichols, & Roche, 2009; Schnakers, Giacino, & Laureys, 2010), and cases of more prolonged coma are rare (ACRM, 1995). In fact, coma nearly always evolves into a vegetative state, which then progresses into an MCS (ACRM, 1995; Katz et al., 2012; Schnakers et al., 2010).

Table 5.1. Comparison of Coma, Vegetative State, and Minimally Conscious State

Observed Behaviors	Coma (RLA LCF I)	Vegetative State (RLA LCF II)	Minimally Conscious State (RLA LCF III)
Eye opening	No	Yes	Yes
Sleep–wake cycle	No	Yes	Yes
Visual tracking	No	No	Often
Object recognition	No	No	Inconsistent
Command following	No	No	Inconsistent
Communication	No	No	Inconsistent
Stimulus-contingent behavior or **emotion**	No	No	Inconsistent

Source. From "Facts About the Vegetative and Minimally Conscious States After Severe Brain Injury," by M. Sherer, M. Vaccaro, J. Whyte, J. T. Giacino, and the Consciousness Consortium, in *Resources Offered by the MSKTC to Support Individuals Living With Traumatic Brain Injury* (p. 76), by Model Systems Knowledge Translation Center, 2013, Washington, DC: Author. Copyright © 2013 by the Model Systems Knowledge Translation Center. Adapted with permission.
Note. RLA LCF = Rancho Los Amigos Levels of Cognitive Functioning.

The *vegetative state,* which corresponds to RLA LCF II, is characterized by continued unconsciousness even though the patient's vegetative functions, such as respiration, digestion, and sleep–wake cycle, return. Artificial support of autonomic functions may no longer be required. Patients in the vegetative state open their eyes, but they remain unable to interact with the environment. They do not follow commands and are unable to visually track (ACRM, 1995; Gosseries et al., 2011; Katz & Black, 1999; Silva et al., 2010). The patient in a vegetative state at RLA LCF II can make some generalized responses, such as grossly moving when presented with a painful stimulus. The patient's response may be the same regardless of the nature of the stimulation. When patients at RLA LCF II demonstrate random and nonpurposeful responses to stimuli or alterations in the environment, the responses are quite often delayed and lack consistency over time. The patient at RLA LCF II remains dependent in all activities.

Disagreement exists about when the term **persistent vegetative state** should be applied to an unconscious person. The Quality Standards Subcommittee of the American Academy of Neurology (1995) recommended use of the term *persistent* at 1 month postinjury, with the term *permanent* applied 12 months after a traumatic injury. Although neuroimaging and electrophysiological procedures are evolving, no current evidence exists that injury characteristics or the appearance of lesions on neuroimaging can significantly predict recovery from a vegetative state as measured by the Disability Rating Scale (Whyte et al., 2005). Although the prognosis for meaningful recovery from a vegetative state that lasts longer than 3 months is poor, applying the term *persistent* to the vegetative state just 1 month after injury may have implications for the patient's access to rehabilitation services (ACRM, 1995).

Recent consideration of the term *vegetative state* by a group of clinicians in Europe has led to the development of a new term: *unresponsive wakefulness syndrome.* The term removes the negative connotation of the word *vegetative,* which is often distressing to the families of people with TBI. In addition, *unresponsive wakefulness* seems a more apt description of the patient's level of function at this stage of early recovery—unresponsive although wakeful (Gosseries et al., 2011; Laureys et al., 2010). This term has not yet gained widespread use in the United States.

Patients who have progressed beyond the coma and the vegetative state are described as being in the MCS. The term *minimally conscious* was coined by the Aspen Neurobehavioral Conference Work Group to denote a state of severely altered consciousness characterized by limited environmental or self-awareness. The MCS corresponds to a GCS score of 12 and RLA LCF III (Katz et al., 2012).

The patient at RLA LCF III makes more localized, inconsistent, but reproducible and appropriate responses to stimulation. Patients at RLA LCF III might withdraw purposefully when given an injection; moan when turned; blink when a bright overhead light is turned on; or pull at intravenous lines, **gastrostomy tubes,** and catheters. The patient might respond more consistently to a particular person, such as a spouse or parent. Careful, skilled assessment of responses at this stage of early recovery is required to determine whether the responses are purposeful or reflexive (Cruse & Chennu, 2012; Giacino et al., 1997, 2002). Understanding the nature of the patient's level of responsiveness is important in setting goals, offering a prognosis to the family, and planning treatment. The patient at RLA LCF III continues to be fully dependent in **activities of daily living** (ADLs), communication, and mobility.

Global Ratings of Disorders of Consciousness

The RLA LCF is the classic tool used by TBI rehabilitation professionals, including occupational therapists, to categorize the patient's functional response to and interaction with the environment. First developed as an 8-level scale in the early 1970s by Chris Hagen and his colleagues at Rancho Los Amigos Rehabilitation Hospital, the Rancho Levels of Cognitive Functioning was later revised to include 10 levels (see Table 1.3 in Chapter 1). Professionals in the field of TBI rehabilitation use the RLA LCF widely to describe patients' performance and progress (Hagen et al., 1972; Katz et al., 2012). The GCS, developed in 1974, continues to be used today by first responders and emergency personnel to classify the state of unconsciousness of a person with a TBI from the point of initial emergency treatment and beyond (Teasdale & Jennett, 1974). Professionals working in the field of TBI rehabilitation recognized that the GCS alone was not sufficient to assess people with TBI.

Behavioral assessment methods remain the gold standard for assessment of patients with disorders of consciousness, yet these types of assessments are subject to diagnostic errors related to the examiner (e.g., inexperience, brief or infrequent exams), the patient (e.g., underlying sensory or motor impairments, **fatigue,** medical sedation), or the environment (e.g., noise, temperature, lighting, positioning) (ACRM, 2010; Giacino & Smart, 2007). One of the dilemmas in assessing patients with disorders of consciousness is the high degree of interrater variability in tool use. Some studies have shown that misdiagnosis of disorders of consciousness is more common than originally thought (Giacino et al., 2002). Inconsistency in patient responsiveness is one barrier to accuracy in assessment. Clinically, a lack of clarity about a patient's actual level of responsiveness affects the quality of decision making regarding therapeutic intervention as well as the use of medications. Also, accuracy in diagnosis is vital to team and family long-term planning discussions. Families want the team to predict their loved one's ultimate level of function. The treatment team's clear understanding of the patient's level of unconsciousness should be the basis for giving family members information concerning prognosis and the patient's level of function (ACRM, 2010).

A variety of additional assessment tools have been developed over the past 3 decades to precisely rate the patient's responsiveness to stimuli in a meaningful way. While providing an accurate clinical picture of the patient's responsiveness, these measures also facilitate decision making and planning within the rehabilitation team (Giacino & Smart, 2007). The selection by clinicians of a good assessment tool to measure responsiveness is essential, and numerous tools are available from which to choose. The Disorders of Consciousness Task Force of the ACRM, which consisted of brain injury specialists, analyzed 13 assessment tools developed to measure levels of unconsciousness. The task force's analysis of the tools included specification of the evidence of standardization, content validity, reliability, and criterion and construct validity for each tool. The task force also made recommendations about each tool's clinical usefulness. Table 5.2 summarizes the task force's general recommendations.

No assessment tool was fully endorsed by the task force (ACRM, 2010), but of the assessments it analyzed, the Coma Recovery Scale–Revised (CRS–R) was the single scale supported with only minor reservations (Giacino, Kalmar, & Whyte, 2004). The CRS–R has excellent content validity and acceptable standardized administration and

> One of the dilemmas in assessing patients with disorders of consciousness is the high degree of interrater variability in tool use.

Table 5.2. Assessment Scales for Disorders of Consciousness: Recommendations Based on the ACRM Special Task Force Analysis

Recommendation	Assessment Scale
Recommended with minor reservations	• Coma Recovery Scale–Revised (Giacino et al., 2004)
Recommended with moderate reservations	• Disorders of Consciousness Scale (Pape et al., 2005) • Sensory Modality Assessment and Rehabilitation Technique (Gill-Thwaites & Munday, 1999) • Sensory Stimulation Assessment Measure (Rader & Ellis, 1994) • Wessex Head Injury Matrix (Shiel et al., 2000) • Western Neuro Sensory Stimulation Profile (Ansell & Keenan, 1989)
Recommended with major reservations	• Coma/Near Coma Scale (Rappaport et al., 1992)
Not recommended for bedside assessment at this time	• Comprehensive Level of Consciousness Scale (Stanczak et al., 1984) • Full Outline of UnResponsiveness Score (Wijdicks, 2006) • Glasgow-Liège Scale (Born, 1988) • Innsbruck Coma Scale (Benzer et al., 1991) • Loewenstein Communication Scale (Borer-Alafi et al., 2002) • Swedish Reaction Level Scale–1985 (Stålhammar & Starmark, 1986)

Source. American Congress of Rehabilitation Medicine (2010).

scoring procedures, but its criterion validity is unproven (ACRM, 2010), and raters' level of experience influences the reliability of CRS–R scores (Løvstad et al., 2010). The CRS–R assesses the patient's auditory, visual, motor, oromotor–verbal, and communication functions and scores the patient's level of arousal. Key elements of the CRS–R denote emergence from the MCS, and other elements signal that the patient has transitioned into the MCS. The CRS–R has been found to be a well-studied interdisciplinary tool for discriminating between the vegetative state and the MCS (ACRM, 2010).

Tools used by professionals in the field of TBI rehabilitation vary from facility to facility. The RLA LCF and the GCS are commonly used in TBI rehabilitation programs; therefore, occupational therapists working in the field of TBI rehabilitation should be skilled in the use of both. Given the variety of assessment tools available, including some home-grown, facility-specific tools, the occupational therapist working in a program for people with TBI must become competent with whatever tools and scales a particular program uses. Ongoing reviews of evidence supporting the design and validity of assessments for disorders of consciousness will help refine the selection of best practice tools to inform the health care team.

Identifying the Patient

The occupational therapist usually encounters the patient with a disorder of consciousness in the intensive care unit (ICU) of a hospital. In some cases, physicians induce coma in a patient with a brain injury to control brain swelling and the brain's metabolic function. Medically induced comas are a form of treatment after brain injury, not the direct result of trauma to the brain, and are therefore not addressed in this chapter.

As a result of current trends in health care driven by insurance coverage, payer constraints, availability of services, and cost containment, patients with disorders of consciousness are being placed in a variety of settings. In addition to being treated in acute care hospitals, patients with TBI may be placed in skilled nursing facilities, subacute rehabilitation facilities, special coma care programs, acute rehabilitation programs, or at home with personalized care from family and health care professionals. The occupational therapist may encounter patients with disorders of consciousness in any of these treatment venues (Katz et al., 2012).

Patients with a disorder of consciousness present to the occupational therapist with a range of clinical problems, among which is the inability to establish a therapeutic relationship with the therapist. For this reason, occupational therapists working with patients with disorders of consciousness must expand their perception of the client to include families and significant others who serve as surrogates in the clinician–client relationship.

The occurrence of a TBI resulting in severe disability evokes a variety of reactions and disrupts family units and the social networks of the injured person. Common family reactions to severe TBI include depression, **anger,** guilt, prolonged emotional distress, and **anxiety** (Godwin, Schaat, & Kreutzer, 2012; Verhaeghe, van Zuuren, Defloor, Duijnstee, & Grypdonck, 2007). Traumatic brain injuries, as the name implies, occur suddenly, shocking families and significant others and causing confusion and disequilibrium (Engli & Kirsivali-Farmer, 1993). Hope for recovery appears to sustain family members as they transition through what has been described as three phases of protection: (1) protecting life, (2) protecting from suffering, and (3) protecting what remains to rebuild life (Verhaeghe, van Zuuren, Grypdonck, Duijnstee, & Defloor, 2010a, 2010b).

Understanding the family's process of protecting enables the occupational therapist to provide support to the family and significant others at this difficult time. The long-term nature of recovery from TBI requires health care professionals to recognize and bolster the precious resources and critical supporting role family and friends provide in the patient's care program over the course of recovery. The long-term outcome of the patient with TBI may depend on the psychosocial health of the family unit (Kreutzer, Marwitz, Godwin, & Arango-Lasprilla, 2010; Vangel, Rapport, & Hanks, 2011).

Frequently, families and the treatment teams partner well to help the patient in the early stages of recovery. However, initial strong emotional responses among family members can make it very difficult, if not impossible, for the team, including the occupational therapist, to establish a therapeutic relationship with the family. The family's primary focus may be on whether the patient with TBI is going to survive, so interventions from the occupational therapist may seem irrelevant and intrusive. However, the persistent kindness and patience of the clinician can often ease the family's anxiety. The therapist's expression of concern can forge a working partnership between the family and the clinicians as a trusting relationship develops.

Identifying the client when the patient has a disorder of consciousness requires thinking beyond traditional boundaries. Appropriate expansion of the concept of *client* to include others close to the person with the TBI can contribute to a more comprehensive occupational therapy evaluation and program of intervention.

Compiling the Patient's Occupational Profile

Gathering the occupational profile for a patient with a disorder of consciousness is a time-intensive but highly valuable process. Given the pressure occupational therapists feel to be productive in the clinical setting, there is a temptation to bypass the compilation of a thorough occupational profile. However, a complete occupational profile is crucial to comprehensive client-centered intervention planning and implementation (McNeny, 2007).

Because the patient is unable to participate in the development of the occupational profile, the therapist uses all reliable sources available to compile the patient's occupational history. He or she uses information about the patient's life experiences, daily living patterns, and perhaps even others' perceptions of the patient's priorities for the intervention process. A good starting point for the occupational therapist is a careful review of available medical records. The increasing use of electronic medical records makes review of past documentation easier and more efficient. Medical records, in addition to containing pertinent medical history, often contain social and personal information gathered by health care professionals previously involved in the case. Consulted professionals frequently document information from family interviews and conversations. Electronic medical records are usually well organized so information is easy to find. The occupational therapist may find helpful information in physician examination summaries, social work notes, nursing notes, and documentation by the allied health team.

Interviews with family and friends are the primary means for gathering information for an occupational profile. The information gleaned from the medical record review should be used during the interview. Clinicians new to a patient's case must avoid asking families questions they have been asked numerous times before. During the evaluation process, weary families often wonder, "Don't you people ever read each other's notes?" To avoid this situation, the occupational therapist must establish the accuracy of other clinicians' documentation in a manner that precludes repetitively questioning the family. For example, rather than asking how much formal education the patient has, the therapist might instead say, "I understand that your husband completed 4 years of college." The family member can then confirm or correct the statement.

Families and significant others usually have a rich history with the patient and are able to provide vital information regarding the patient's occupational history and life experiences. Depending on the nature and closeness of their relationship, the family member or significant other may be able to provide information about the patient's patterns of daily living, interests, and values. They may even be able to make presumptive comments regarding the patient's priorities for rehabilitation and recovery, although at times families and significant others may seem uncomfortable speculating on these issues. Family members should be asked, however, to share their own goals and priorities for the therapy process. The family's goals provide a beginning point for the intervention process (McNeny, 2007).

Obtaining information from family and friends is not always easy. The family, significant others, and friends may be unaware of the patient's preinjury lifestyle. The patient may physically live some distance from family, with their interaction occurring over the phone, by e-mail, or during visits when normal routines are interrupted. The patient may have few friends intimate enough to know the details of his or her personal life. The family may feel apprehensive about sharing personal information about their loved one. Estrangement between the patient and family members may limit family members' knowledge of details of the patient's lifestyle. Estrangement can also influence family members' perception of the patient's lifestyle and choices.

In addition to interviewing family members and significant others, the occupational therapist can interview nonfamily members. Interviews with ministers or spiritual advisors, sports teammates, work colleagues, or classmates who visit the health care facility may yield additional information. Asking family and friends to share any photos or videos that were taken of the patient before the injury can help the therapist learn about the patient's interaction and communication style and even his or her perception of life goals, priorities, and personal values. Once this information is melded with other interview data, a more coherent portrait of the preinjury occupational profile of the patient may emerge.

The setting for the occupational history interview should be chosen carefully. The therapist should, to the greatest extent possible, select a quiet setting that ensures privacy. Active listening during the interview helps the occupational therapist formulate critical follow-up questions and allows him or her to detect areas of **stress** or unexpressed concerns (Jabri, 1996). A quiet setting can also help families feel more at ease asking questions regarding the patient's injuries and the rehabilitation program.

Sometimes family members and friends are unavailable during the occupational therapist's work hours. Family members' work schedules or family responsibilities may prevent frequent or lengthy visits. The family may not be able to accept phone calls from health care professionals during business hours. If phone calls are not possible, the occupational therapist can use a written family questionnaire left at the bedside to gather information. The questionnaire's purpose as well as an explanation about the manner in which the requested information will be used should be stated clearly on the form. In addition, including the occupational therapist's contact information on the questionnaire allows family members or friends to call if they have questions. Completed questionnaires from several family members and friends often provide a helpful picture of the patient. This task can also support the family's need to be involved in care during the initial stages of recovery when they may be a constant presence by the patient's bedside (Keenan & Joseph, 2010).

Whether the information is gathered from interviews or questionnaires or a combination of the two, the occupational therapist will move from a process of data gathering to data analysis. Through careful analysis, the patient's occupations, the context in which these occupations occur, and the performance skills and client factors required to engage in these occupations are identified. Ongoing conversations with family members and friends during the course of the therapeutic relationship often yield supplementary information while meeting the family's need for ongoing information (Keenan & Joseph, 2010).

The occupational profile provides the foundation for occupational therapy programming. Areas in need of additional investigation become clear as the therapist reviews the data and documents the occupational profile. Once the intervention process begins, the occupational profile provides the framework by which the occupational therapist is able to construct a treatment program of maximal relevancy to the patient.

Occupational Therapy Evaluation and Intervention

The occupational therapy evaluation of the patient with a disorder of consciousness focuses on the patient's level of responsiveness to stimulation as well as on behaviors the patient demonstrates in the absence of clinician-mediated stimulation. The evaluation also includes assessment of specific client factors. Evaluation of performance skills is of particular concern as the patient begins to emerge from coma. The occupational therapy evaluation is conducted at a time and in conditions optimal

The occupational therapy evaluation of the patient with a disorder of consciousness focuses on the patient's level of responsiveness to stimulation as well as on behaviors the patient demonstrates in the absence of clinician-mediated stimulation.

for the patient and in a manner that accommodates the patient's extensive nursing care needs (Antoinette, 1996; Pentland & Whittle, 1999). The nurse and therapist coordinate the timing of the occupational therapy evaluation with necessary nursing intervention to permit a period of rest between the occupational therapy assessment and other required activities.

A review of the patient's medical record will provide information on problems that have arisen during the patient's course of recovery. These problems can include infections accompanied by fever, blood pressure fluctuations, increased intracranial pressure (ICP), **deep vein thrombosis,** seizures, changes in respiratory function, and development of skin breakdown (Giacino, Garber, Katz, & Schiff, 2012; Pentland & Whittle, 1999). The patient may have had surgery or may have other trauma-related injuries, such as fractures, amputations, or wounds. Such injuries can affect functional outcome and length of stay (Englander et al., 1996). The occupational therapist should also determine whether potentially sedating medications are prescribed for the patient because some medications can affect the patient's responsiveness or can result in atypical clinical presentations (Flower & Hellings, 2012; Smith-Gabai, 2011).

Soon after referral, the occupational therapist quietly and, in a formal manner, observes the patient, noting any movement and behavior exhibited by the patient in the absence of stimulation. The therapist determines whether responses seem purposeful or reflexive. During this observation, the therapist closes the door, turns off electronic devices, and asks family to refrain from talking. The occupational therapist specifically looks for spontaneous eye opening, purposeful and voluntary motor responses, and any evidence of visual tracking. Patients still in coma do not open their eyes and exhibit no purposeful movement. Patients in the vegetative state have periods of wakefulness and make some gross responses. Patients transitioning from the vegetative state to the MCS exhibit responses that are more purposeful, localized, and intentional. This formal period of observation provides the occupational therapist with a baseline of the patient's level of responsiveness in a minimally stimulating environment.

Periodic reassessment of the patient's response to sensory stimulation (auditory, visual, motor, oromotor, communication, and arousal functions) and tracking of the patient's responses on a scale such as the CRS–R (Giacino et al., 2004) provide the team with information on changes in the patient's responsiveness. Many scales are intended to be used in serial reassessment of the patient, often on a daily basis to establish response consistency and track changes in consciousness indicating transition from coma to an MCS. Team training in the administration of the selected scale and coordination of the schedule of administration and documentation are crucial to identify changes in consistency and reliability of responses. Analysis of the patient's pattern of responses can support team monitoring, communication, and decision making regarding care. Consistent positive changes in the patient's responsiveness may indicate recovery, and sudden and persistent negative changes may indicate a neurological complication (e.g., increasing ICP) requiring medical intervention.

Influence of the Intensive Care Unit Environment

The ICU environment, which is normally bright and noisy, is a factor in the care of the patient with impaired consciousness. Clients at all three Rancho levels of early recovery can be found in the ICU. Studies have indicated that early mobilization by rehabilitative therapies is beneficial to clients in the early stages of recovery (Hellweg, 2012; Needham, 2008; Nguyen, Thao-Houane, & Warren, 2014; Schweickert et al., 2009).

Overstimulation, however, can result from the cacophony of competing high-volume sound in the ICU as well as from the recurring hands-on care of medical staff, including interventions delivered by the occupational therapist. For this reason, environmental stimulation surrounding the patient should be controlled during occupational therapy sessions. Noise from televisions, radios, and machines should be minimized or eliminated. Extraneous conversation among family and staff should be stopped. If the patient lacks a private ICU cubicle with a door, the bed curtains should be pulled closed to minimize sound and visual stimuli. Extra clothing can be used to warm a patient who appears chilly; a fan can be used to cool a space that feels overly warm. Lighting should be regulated so glare from overhead lights and unshaded windows (to either the nurses' station or outside) is eliminated, if possible. Occupational therapy sessions should be limited to 15 minutes to prevent significant patient fatigue (Golisz, 2009), although one recent study indicated that as much as 90 minutes of rehabilitative therapy per day was beneficial to clients with disorders of consciousness (Seel et al., 2013).

Post–Intensive Care Unit Rehabilitation

Medically stable patients in early recovery may receive rehabilitative services outside of the ICU setting, usually in a rehabilitation program on the acute care unit or rehabilitation services unit. The rehabilitation setting offers a high level of activity, which can be fatiguing and distracting for the patient in early recovery. Therefore, environmental controls should also be applied to the rehabilitation setting to maximize the patient's response to therapeutic interventions. These controls are based on the individual needs of the patient and can include use of a quiet room for treatment, more frequent but shorter therapy sessions, and the incorporation of quiet rest periods into the patient's daily schedule.

Focus on Client Factors

Because disorders of consciousness render people incapable of meaningful, functional performance, the occupational therapist focuses on client factors that, if left unmanaged, could limit or even prohibit functional performance once the patient emerges from unconsciousness. Key client factors that become the emphasis of occupational therapy evaluation and intervention during the period of unconsciousness include mental functions; sensory processing and pain awareness; neuromuscular and movement-related functions; cardiovascular, hematological, immunological, and respiratory system function; and the patient's skin integrity (Golisz, 2009; Turner-Stokes, 2003; Whyte & Nakase-Richardson, 2013).

Alertness and Sensory Processing Function

Alertness and sensory processing are foundational to functional performance but are impaired after severe TBI. The patient in coma has no capacity for sensory awareness or processing. As the patient transitions into the vegetative state, the sleep–wake cycle reemerges, but the patient continues to give no purposeful evidence of awareness of the environment and demonstrates only gross responses to stimuli. Although the patient in the vegetative state may moan or make sounds, he or she has neither understanding of the spoken word nor any ability to communicate meaningfully (Katz et al., 2012).

The patient in the MCS demonstrates inconsistent awareness of self, the environment, and people in the environment. The patient continues to have severely impaired alertness, although he or she is more alert than during the vegetative state. Giacino et al. (2002) reported that demonstration, repeatedly and over time, of two or more of the following responses places a patient in the MCS:

- Follows simple commands
- Gestures in a manner to communicate *yes* or *no*
- Verbalizes in an intelligible manner
- Demonstrates clearly purposeful responses such as reaching for objects or visually tracking an object or person.

The patient in the MCS is able to work in a limited manner on low-level, goal-directed tasks with the occupational therapist.

The patient's awareness of and response to pain are assessed by team members from the earliest hours after TBI. Formal, robust assessment of basic sensory functions such as sight, hearing, taste, smell, touch, **vestibular function,** and temperature sensitivity, as well as early assessment of visual and visual–perceptual function, including evaluation of form and color perception and the ability to visually track an object or person, should be performed only when the patient has reached the MCS (Tipton-Burton, McLaughlin, & Englander, 2013).

Sensory Stimulation Programs

Alertness and sensory processing are challenged during sensory stimulation. *Structured sensory stimulation programs,* also historically labeled *coma arousal protocols,* are focused not on the patient in coma but on patients in the vegetative state or MCS. The theoretical basis for sensory stimulation is centered on the belief that systematically applied stimulation arouses cortical activity and serves to prevent the effects of sensory deprivation. The use of formal sensory stimulation varies from one rehabilitation program to another. Some clinical programs use a uniform sensory stimulation protocol and involve numerous team members in the coordinated administration of stimulation in specific sequences and at set frequencies (Abbate, Trimarchi, Basile, Mazzucchi, & Devalle, 2014). Other programs integrate sensory stimulation into the patient's daily schedule through nursing care and therapy sessions.

A variant of sensory stimulation programming is the sensory regulation approach. Sensory regulation is based on the theory that patients with disorders of consciousness are easily overwhelmed by sensory stimuli because they lack the ability to filter clinician-mediated from environmentally based stimulation. The sensory regulation approach controls and schedules all stimulation provided to the patient, including nursing care, to prevent overstimulation. Structured rest periods are built into the patient's routine and are theorized to be beneficial to the healing brain (Wood, Winkowski, Miller, Tierney, & Goldman, 1992).

In the early history of TBI rehabilitation, sensory stimulation programming was the gold standard of care in many treatment facilities. The clinical value of sensory stimulation programs remains an unsettled area of science, however. Although the use of sensory stimulation does not appear to be harmful, published studies on sensory stimulation have not established its clinical efficacy, nor have they shown that such treatment is detrimental to recovery. Some clinical studies have indicated that improvements in awareness result from structured sensory stimulation (Giacino, 1996; Hirschberg & Giacino, 2011; Wilson, Powell, Elliott, & Thwaites, 1991). Other studies have questioned its efficacy (Abbate et al., 2014; Johnson, Roethig-Johnston, & Richards, 1993; Lombardi, Taricco, De Tanti, Telaro, & Liberati, 2002; Meyer et al., 2010; Wilson, Powell, Brock, & Thwaites, 1996).

No Level I prospective, randomized controlled trials have been completed on sensory stimulation interventions (Giacino et al., 2012). Two systematic reviews of evidence on the topic (Giacino, 1996; Lombardi et al., 2002) concluded that many of the studies have notable flaws in design and analysis. Inconsistencies across studies in the use of appropriate nomenclature to describe the participants' states of unconsciousness make it difficult to compare results. Some studies have concluded that improvements in level of awareness resulted from sensory stimulation, and other studies have found no measurable change or have attributed improvements in arousal to natural recovery (Davis & Gimenez, 2003; Di Stefano, Cortesi, Masotti, Simoncini, & Piperno, 2012; Johnson et al., 1993; Lombardi et al., 2002; Meyer et al., 2010).

Although current evidence does not provide a compelling argument for occupational therapists to use sensory stimulation when patients are in coma, it continues to be used in clinical settings. Sensory stimulation does not appear to have detrimental effects and is low in risk. Giacino (1996) recommended stopping sensory stimulation if the patient's ICP exceeds 20 millimeters of mercury or if the patient demonstrates signs of autonomic dysreflexia or hyperreflexia.

Sensory stimulation is often used as an intervention for patients with altered consciousness, but it can also be used as an ongoing assessment of the patient's responses to stimulation. Monitoring the patient's responses in a consistent and controlled manner may help therapists identify when the patient has emerged naturally from coma (Golisz, 2009). As the patient enters the MCS, the sensory stimulation program may reinforce the patient's voluntary and purposeful responses to environmental stimuli.

To increase the potential relevance to the patient of sensory input, the occupational therapist works with the family to collect personal items to which the patient may respond. These items are used during therapy sessions with the patient. Among the items families can often provide are

- Photo albums or posters of memorable times in the patient's life or of some of the patient's favorite places
- Music the patient enjoys, whether on CD or on an MP3 player
- Objects from the patient's room at home (e.g., posters, stuffed animals, favorite clothes, trophies), particularly items that have a high level of tactile value
- Pictures of the patient's house and car, workplace, favorite actors, movies, sports figures, or hobbies

- Pictures of friends and family labeled with their names
- Favorite grooming products with familiar scents.

Aside from structured sensory stimulation, the patient with a disorder of consciousness experiences stimulation during **passive range of motion** (PROM) and repositioning, during bathing and grooming tasks done by nurses or family caregivers, and during movement from the bed to a chair. These physically oriented activities performed at the start of a therapy session may give the patient warm-up stimulation before other therapeutic tasks are attempted. Regardless of the type of stimulation being offered, a limited number of modes of stimulation should be offered at a time because the patient's sensory processing and attentional skills are limited. The patient should be given adequate time to respond to stimuli, because response delays are common during early recovery from TBI. Clinicians should limit instructions to the patient to coming from one person (Mitchell, Bradley, Welch, & Britton, 1990; Wood et al., 1992).

Team and Family Coordination

Because considerable stimulation occurs during the patient's routine clinical day, the occupational therapist leads the team in controlling sources of stimulation through management of the patient's environment. The occupational therapist helps the team and family identify the perhaps unnoticed sources of environmental stimulation around the patient, such as the TV, lights, visitors' voices, and hallway noise, while providing recommendations about regulating stimulation.

The occupational therapist guides the establishment of a daily routine for the patient. This routine serves as a beginning step for the fuller days of therapy and ADL tasks the patient will experience as he or she improves. This initial daily routine includes the timing of nursing care and therapy services, application and removal of splints and positioners, time in bed and time out of bed, and times of rest when electronics are off, when visitors depart, and when the room is darkened. It also includes times for interaction with family and friends. Family involvement in the rehabilitative program has proven to be an important factor in recovery (Abbasi, Mohammadi, & Sheaykh Rezayi, 2009; Gorji, Araghiyansc, Jafari, Gorgi, & Yazdani, 2014).

The occupational therapist works with the team and family to determine the patient's level of arousal and responsiveness from day to day. Because it is common during early recovery for families to confuse the patient's reflexive responses with intentional responses, the occupational therapist instructs the family in the difference between nonpurposeful and purposeful responses. The occupational therapist also educates the family about the stages of recovery, identifying things they can do to help their loved one as recovery progresses. Providing the family with instructions for providing single stimuli and waiting for the patient's response enables the family to provide intermittent stimulation during evening or weekend hours when the rehabilitation staff are not present.

Neuromuscular and Movement-Related Functions

Patients with a disorder of consciousness usually experience marked **impairment** in neuromuscular function, often marked by **spasticity,** decreased **range of motion** (ROM), and an absence of purposeful movement.

> Regardless of the type of stimulation being offered, a limited number of modes of stimulation should be offered at a time because the patient's sensory processing and attentional skills are limited.

Clinical Assessment of Range of Motion, Spasticity, and Volitional Movement

The patient with a disorder of consciousness is unable to tolerate lengthy evaluations early in recovery and typically requires more than one clinician to assist during movement-related activities. Therefore, the occupational therapist and physical therapist frequently conduct co-evaluations of neuromuscular and movement-related functions such as PROM, muscle tone, reflex function, and postural reactions.

Decreased ROM is a common sequela of TBI and may occur as a result of joint injury, muscle tone abnormality, **contracture,** or **heterotopic ossification** (HO). **Goniometric measurement** provides precise baseline data that permit easy quantification of changes in PROM throughout the recovery period. The purpose of the initial ROM examination is to identify limitations that may be functionally limiting or may result in deformity if left untreated (Gracies, 2001; Hirschberg & Giacino, 2011; Knight, Thornton, & Turner-Stokes, 2003; Lannin, Horsley, Herbert, McCluskey, & Cusick, 2003; Moseley et al., 2008; Mysiw, Fugate, & Clinchot, 2007; Singer, Jegasothy, Singer, Allison, & Dunne, 2004; Stewart, Miller, & Cifu, 1998; Tipton-Burton et al., 2013).

Clinical assessment of neuromuscular and movement function should begin early in the patient's care. The occupational therapist may notice changes in neuromuscular function as the patient transitions through the stages of early recovery. During the evaluation of PROM and muscle tone, the therapist notes the presence of rigidity, resistance, or flaccidity in the extremities as well as the effect of head or trunk position on muscle tone. The presence of abnormal postural reflexes is evaluated as the clinician changes the patient's head or body position (Tipton-Burton et al., 2013).

As the patient transitions to RLA LCF III, the occupational therapist, often with the assistance of another clinician, adds dynamic components to sitting activities to assess the presence and quality of the patient's emerging righting and equilibrium reactions. Using observational skills, the occupational therapist identifies causative factors limiting ROM, such as increased muscle tone, presumed pain, and resistance to passive movement. Patients exhibiting increased muscle tone that inhibits full PROM may need positioning, casting, or splinting (Katalinic, Harvey, & Herbert, 2011; Katalinic et al., 2010).

Maintaining and Restoring Neuromuscular and Movement Functions

Several interventions are available and have proven beneficial for patients with a disorder of consciousness with neuromuscular impairment. Serial casting, positioning, appropriate seating, and management of complications should be the focus of treatment programming.

Serial Casting and Splinting

The use of splints, casts, and extremity positioners must be judiciously considered before implementation. Several studies have indicated that largely short-term improvements in ROM can be achieved through the use of serial casting (Marshall et al., 2007; Moseley et al., 2008). Casting and splinting may be indicated when a patient has increased **tone** that limits movement, when PROM is impaired, and when the potential for joint contracture exists. However, if bed and wheelchair positioning along with a routine PROM program are sufficient to maintain PROM, then casting and splinting may not be necessary (Marshall et al., 2007).

Contractures that result in loss of functional movement are a serious complication of TBI (Gracies, 2001; Moseley et al., 2008; Singer et al., 2004), and the occupational therapist must determine the most appropriate intervention at each point in recovery. Splinting and positioning to prevent secondary complications is often an appropriate path but must be pursued prudently. The appropriate use of stretching, splinting, and positioning early in recovery may help manage potential complications, such as contractures, with casting perhaps showing more efficacy than splints (Lannin et al., 2003; Marshall et al., 2007; Pohl et al., 2002; Whyte, Laborde, & DiPasquale, 1999).

Because of the transient nature of tone during the early days after brain trauma, serial casting is not recommended as a first-line treatment for patients at RLA LCF I and II. In this early stage of recovery, beginning contractures can usually be managed with a vigorous PROM program. However, a review of recent studies indicated a limited long-term benefit from a stretching program in clients at risk for and with contractures (Katalinic et al., 2010). In addition, at least one group of authors has suggested that serial casting may be appropriate if the patient is less active and thus has the potential for loss of ROM (Zablotny, Andric, & Gowland, 1987). Serial casting at this point may prevent the secondary complication of severe PROM limitation, which can impede the patient's readiness for a more intense treatment program centered on aggressive mobility and self-care skills retraining.

Studies of the effectiveness of splints and casts have failed to provide clear protocols for their use. Inhibitory serial casting combines tone-reducing positions with a static positioner worn for a period of time, then removed. Casts are applied and removed in a gradual stretching sequence as PROM improves. Serial casts are constructed of either plastic or fiberglass casting material. Although plaster materials are less expensive, fiberglass material is lighter and more durable, sets more quickly, and is significantly less messy to apply.

When serial casting is begun, the initial joint position should be slightly less than the patient's maximum ROM. If casting is successful, the casted joint angle is then progressively increased with subsequent casts. Evidence from different studies has varied in the recommended duration for each cast application, from a period as short as 4 days to one as long as 7 days showing improvements in ROM (Pohl et al., 2002).

Protection of the patient's skin during serial casting is critical to prevent skin-related complications. If the patient has any persistent reddened areas or open wounds, casting should be deferred until the condition of the skin improves. Even though the entire skin surface being casted is covered heavily with padding material, special gel pads and extra layers of cotton padding are used to cover bony prominences, and casts are kept loose at both ends. Circulation checks of the extremity are done several times throughout the day and evening. A cast saw must be readily available to nurses 24 hours a day for cast removal if the cast appears to have become constrictive.

The objective of the serial casting program has been met when either the desired ROM at the joint has been achieved or no increase in ROM has occurred after the application of two consecutive casts. When the conclusion of the serial casting program is reached, the occupational therapist may choose to use the cast as a night splint. To do this, the final cast is carefully removed, the rough edges are finished off to protect the skin, and straps are attached to provide a secure fit.

These bivalved cast positioners are worn at night to maintain the improved ROM (Tipton-Burton et al., 2013).

Serial casting may be used in conjunction with motor point blocks when spasticity restricts ROM or when the effect of spasticity on joint function is unclear. Motor point injections block innervation of spastic muscles. The physician injects the motor point, after which the occupational therapist applies the initial serial cast. Motor point blocks have been recommended when unconsciousness persists and spasticity becomes chronic (Stewart et al., 1998). However, the evidence to date is limited regarding improvements in ROM through the use of motor point blocks with and without serial casting (Marshall et al., 2007).

Splints commonly used with patients with disorders of consciousness include basic positioning splints such as resting hand splints or foot-drop splints, tone-reducing splints such as the finger abduction resting splint or the neutral forearm positioning splint, and dynamic splints that are progressively adjusted to increase PROM at a joint. Splints are usually recommended for patients who lack active movement (Lannin et al., 2003). Studies on the effectiveness of hand splinting are limited, and no clear protocol has yet been established regarding the use of splints. One study of the use of a functional hand splint with adults who have TBI did not demonstrate any benefit from splinting (Lannin et al., 2003). Additional studies are needed.

Because there is risk of skin breakdown with splinting, therapists typically prescribe a beginning wearing schedule of 2 hours on and 2 hours off, progressing to 4 hours on and 4 hours off as the patient demonstrates improved tolerance for the splint. A regular check of the splint's fit and its impact on skin integrity is critical. The occupational therapist should instruct nurses and interested family members in splint application, the wearing schedule, and skin inspection method.

The use of static positioners such as casts and splints carries potential risks to the patient (Pohl et al., 2002). The risks include discomfort for the patient, self-injury, development of skin breakdown, and facilitation of abnormal tone. In addition, the use of casts and splints complicates nursing care. Occupational therapists contemplating the use of casts or splints must thoughtfully weigh treatment goals against risks that may occur as a result of casting and splinting (Tipton-Burton et al., 2013).

Bed and Wheelchair Positioning

People with disorders of consciousness can present with neuromuscular and movement-related problems resulting from immobility and lack of arousal; abnormal muscle tone; posturing; and concomitant injury to bones, joints, and muscles. Persistent neuromuscular and movement-related problems beyond the stage of early recovery have a significant impact on the patient's ability to return to preferred and necessary occupations (Antoinette, 1996; Blanton, Porter, Smith, & Wolf, 1999; Englander et al., 1996; Hirschberg & Giacino, 2011; Pentland & Whittle, 1999; Sandel, 1996; Whyte et al., 1999). Occupational therapists should work with patients in the early phases of recovery on sound positioning to prevent complications.

Early mobilization during the period of absent or limited consciousness promotes improved respiration and circulation and also provides stimulation to the patient (Schweickert et al., 2009). Mobilization into sitting alters postural tone and changes the position of the extremities, head, and trunk. Pressure on the skin surface is changed. During mobilization, the patient also has the opportunity to engage in dynamic sitting activities that challenge control of the head and trunk.

Early in recovery, when the patient's tolerance for therapy is limited, cotreatment sessions of 15 to 20 minutes by physical and occupational therapy are encouraged. During cotreatment, clinicians work together to move the patient into supported sitting at the edge of the patient's bed (Blanton et al., 1999). Stimulating activities, the use of familiar objects, and low-level functional tasks can be done during cotreatment sessions. Using a photo album of familiar pictures is one tool that can be used at this stage of recovery.

During these early treatment sessions, the occupational therapist needs to monitor the patient's vital signs and motoric responses for signs of distress and responsiveness. Orthostatic hypotension may occur after prolonged bedrest, so blood pressure changes as the patient comes to sitting should be noted (Nguyen et al., 2014). The exertion of sitting may stimulate respiratory changes, requiring monitoring of the patient's oxygen saturation. If the patient is being ventilated, the patency of the ventilator is carefully maintained throughout the session. Changes in ICP must be taken seriously, with therapy activity ceasing if a significant rise occurs. In some centers, the neurosurgeon provides specific parameters for ICP that are helpful to the nursing and allied health staff (Blanton et al., 1999).

Treatment sessions lengthen as the patient's medical stability and tolerance for therapy improve. The patient progresses from sitting briefly and fully supported at the edge of the bed to sitting for longer periods of time in a wheelchair. Care must be taken during transfers to ensure protection of the skin from shearing or bruising. A sufficient number of clinical staff, perhaps using lifting equipment, should be used during transfers to ensure patient safety and comfort. Once seated in an appropriate wheelchair, the patient can also come out of his or her room into other environments that offer additional opportunities for sensory stimulation.

The proper wheelchair for the patient with a disorder of consciousness provides support for the head, arms, and legs. A tilt-in-space wheelchair is beneficial for patients in early recovery because pressure relief and rest of postural muscles may occur while still seated in the wheelchair, eliminating the need for transfers back to bed. Wheelchair cushions that provide proper pressure relief under the buttocks, heels, elbows, and back of head are a necessity because patients in the stages of early recovery will not voluntarily shift their weight. Lap trays, calf and heel straps, and head positioners all benefit the patient who is functioning at a very low level (Blanton et al., 1999). Patients in the vegetative state or the MCS continue to need specialized cushions and wheelchairs with dynamic seat frames such as tilt-in-space, manual recline, and elevating leg rests for pressure relief and prevention of skin breakdown. Attendant-propelled manual wheelchairs are typically used because the patient is dependent on others for mobility. As the minimally conscious patient begins to demonstrate some purposeful movement and is able to follow simple commands, the patient may be switched to a self-propelled manual wheelchair and begin instruction in wheelchair mobility.

A vast amount of specialized seating and wheeled mobility equipment as well as pressure-relieving products are commercially available, with new products and adaptations continually coming on the market. Many rehabilitation programs find it too expensive to keep a stock of wheeled mobility devices suitable for every sort of clinical presentation. Many occupational and physical therapists develop relationships with local durable medical equipment (DME) vendors who rent or loan wheelchairs and reusable positioners to meet patients' specialized needs. These vendors often provide in-house training to staff to help them remain up to date on new products. Seating specialists on staff at DME companies can provide invaluable consultation to busy clinicians as well as follow-up services for patients in early recovery who are in nursing facilities, in specialty programs, or living at home. Occupational therapists must adhere to all rules regarding privacy, conflict of interest, and billing regulations when working with DME vendors.

Facilitating Muscle and Joint Integrity

A program of regular PROM and proper positioning is the beginning step to facilitating purposeful movement. For patients without tonal abnormality, the ROM program consists of moving the extremities through various planes of joint movement at spaced intervals throughout the day. Routine nursing care activities incorporate PROM and supplement the structured PROM program. In addition, interested, involved, and capable family members can be taught simple PROM techniques to carry the program over to evenings and weekends.

Tonal abnormalities, the presence of fractures with associated weight-bearing or positioning restrictions, or the development of HO require precise intervention, including a PROM program. Reflex-inhibiting positions often prove helpful in controlling tonal abnormality. Although research evidence is lacking, many therapists apply theories and observations based on the Bobath method of neurodevelopmental treatment and use key points of control such as the shoulder or pelvis during PROM to help control extensor and flexor posturing by inhibiting or facilitating postures and movement (Bobath, 1978). Controlled stretch of the limb's muscles assists in achieving greater movement through a plane of motion when abnormal tone is present. Because of the influence of abnormal tone, occupational therapists may discover that PROM is easier and more successful in one position over another. The therapist determines the effect of position on PROM by conducting PROM in both sitting and supine as well as when the patient is at rest and in a quiet environment.

Families may find it difficult to learn complex PROM techniques. If possible, therapists identify family members capable of learning at least some of the techniques. A rationale for family involvement in the PROM program is provided in understandable terms. Chunking PROM training for families into small units of instruction facilitates learning. Written or videotaped instructions can supplement individualized instruction, if available. Demonstration of proper technique by family members on multiple occasions ensures that the family is using techniques that promote patient comfort and normalize rather than facilitate abnormal tone.

The patient in the early stages of recovery sometimes presents with limb fractures sustained in the precipitating event. Fractures in patients with TBI have been found to increase length of stay in rehabilitation, with lower-extremity fractures contributing to increased need for assistance with self-care and mobility (Englander et al., 1996). Management of fractures often involves casts and external fixators along with weight-bearing or ROM restrictions. Such restrictions must be incorporated into the treatment program. If the family lacks understanding of the precautions necessary during the healing of orthopedic injuries, they may not be able to competently and safely provide the patient with PROM. The occupational therapist may need to create positioners that allow the patient to lie down and to sit both comfortably and appropriately in the bed or wheelchair while the cast, fixator, or orthopedic device is in place. Foam positioners, lapboards, and slings, sometimes with customized adaptations, are often used for this purpose.

HO, a complication that can occur after TBI, affects joint function. *Heterotopic ossification* is ectopic bone formation in soft tissue or surrounding joints. It occurs most commonly at the large joints of the hip, knee, elbow, and shoulder, with onset 1 to 3 months after injury. Research has not yet identified the mechanism or trigger for the development of HO. The occupational therapist must be continuously alert for the hallmark symptoms of HO: erythema and unusual warmth about the joint, joint swelling, and increasing stiffness at the joint during PROM (Knight et al., 2003; Stewart et al., 1998). A bone scan is used to confirm the diagnosis of HO. HO is very painful, but patients with disorders of consciousness may be unable to indicate the presence of pain during joint movement. Therefore, the occupational therapist must be mindful of the other symptoms.

Medical management of HO includes the administration of medications, radiotherapy, and at times surgery. Therapy management of HO begins conservatively with frequent PROM, although studies have raised questions about how vigorous this PROM program should be (Aubut, Mehta, Cullen, & Teasell, 2011; Knight et al., 2003; Vanden Bossche & Vanderstraeten, 2005). Physician guidance about the frequency and intensity of PROM is critical. In today's health care environment, one discipline alone cannot provide adequate PROM for patients with HO. Therefore, the occupational therapist, physical therapist, and nurse collaborate on a therapeutic regimen to ensure that regular PROM occurs, with family members becoming involved as they are able.

The positioning program for management of HO involves placing the involved extremity in different positions throughout the day to prevent joint deformity. Knees and elbows are alternately placed in extension and flexion, using positioners and splints as needed to maintain positioning. Hip position changes are accomplished by alternating sitting with side-lying and supine positioning at intervals throughout the day. In the side-lying position, foam wedges sometimes successfully maintain hip flexion. In supine, wedges allow for more hip abduction than can be achieved in other positions. The positioning program for HO is very labor intensive and needs to be carefully developed, then communicated fully to all team members to ensure compliance with the schedule of positioning changes and successful maintenance of joint mobility.

HO surrounding lower-extremity joints can interfere with transfers. In such cases, the occupational therapist works with physical therapy to design a technique that minimizes patient discomfort while facilitating the ease and safety of transfers for the patient as well as for the staff. Many facilities follow the recommendations for safe patient handling outlined by the National Institute for Occupational Safety and Health and have no-lift policies requiring therapists to use mechanical lifting devices to ensure safe, effective transfers (Nelson & Baptiste, 2004; Nelson, Harwood, Tracey, & Dunn, 2008). In addition, collaboration may be necessary with nursing staff or family caregivers should barriers to proper hygiene management occur as a result of HO-related joint deformities.

Even with the best intervention program, HO can create a severe joint-function limitation that may require surgical intervention. Surgery is usually delayed until the abnormal bone growth matures in approximately 12 to 18 months postinjury to reduce the probability of redevelopment (Aubut et al., 2011; Ivanhoe, Durand-Sanchez, & Spier, 2012). See Chapter 7 for additional discussion of HO.

Facilitating Occupational Performance

Once the patient with a disorder of consciousness becomes minimally conscious or is at RLA LCF III, the occupational therapist begins to engage the patient, in a limited way, in purposeful activity.

Once the patient with a disorder of consciousness becomes minimally conscious or is at RLA LCF III, the occupational therapist begins to engage the patient, in a limited way, in purposeful activity. Although more aware, the patient at RLA LCF III still exhibits very restricted responses, characterized by delays and inconsistency. Because the patient is unable to interact meaningfully with the environment, the occupational therapist designs interventions that incorporate the patient's occupations and relevant activities as much as possible. The therapist refers back to the occupational profile to understand the patient's preinjury occupations, the contexts in which they occurred, and the performance patterns that supported these occupations. The most elemental of self-care tasks, such as bringing a washcloth to the face or holding a toothbrush, can be used at this stage of recovery. Also, during PROM the occupational therapist can assess the patient's response to simple commands such as "Bend your elbow." The therapist should continually be alert to improvements in the quality, frequency, and accuracy of patient responses.

Appropriate physical assistance and guidance are used with patients at RLA LCF III. Hand-over-hand assist is usually required as the patient attempts to respond to commands or manipulate objects. The occupational therapist notes the manner in which the patient responds to objects presented. The patient's response can provide information to the therapist about specific client factors and help the therapist identify potential problem areas, such as incoordination, visual–perceptual problems, or **apraxia** that may warrant further clinical assessment. Some questions related to patient responses that the occupational therapist should consider while working on purposeful tasks with patients in the MCS are found in Box 5.1.

The minimally responsive patient possesses a limited capacity for performance skills. Higher level elements of performance skills, such as pacing performance, asking for additional information, and organizing tasks, are not reasonably expected of patients in the early stages of recovery. However, the occupational therapist's astute observations of the patient's behavior during therapy may detect improvements in awareness and responsiveness to the environment.

Family Education

Educating and training the family of the patient with a disorder of consciousness is an essential part of the occupational therapy intervention plan. In most cases, families of patients with disorders of consciousness find themselves in a novel and unsettling situation, and therefore they can benefit from professionally planned and delivered information. Distress among families of people with TBI is common (Bond, Draeger, Mandleco, & Donnelly, 2003; Sander, Maestas, Sherer, Malec, & Nakase-Richardson, 2012). Therefore, the occupational therapist strives to establish

---

Box 5.1. Areas of Consideration When Facilitating Purposeful Response in Patients With Disorders of Consciousness

The therapist considers the following questions during occupational therapy sessions to more completely understand the patient's performance skills as well as the influence of context on responsiveness in general.

- Does the patient interact with objects presented? Is the patient able to manipulate the object? Does the patient show any evidence of incoordination or impaired strength as the object is manipulated?
- How does the patient position his or her body in relation to objects presented and manipulated? Is the position chosen and used appropriate to the object?
- How well does the patient attend to the object presented? Is there evidence of fatigue, and at what point in the session did it appear?
- Does the patient recognize the object's purpose? Is the patient doing anything meaningful with the object?
- Is there a difference in the patient's responsiveness as different objects are presented? If the object is placed on a table before the patient, does the patient notice it? Does the patient initiate any action with the object?
- In what ways does the patient demonstrate communicative ability? Does the patient visually orient to the object? Does the patient attempt any verbalizations?
- Does context in any way influence responsiveness? Does the patient interact any differently with familiar objects? Does the patient respond any better when family members or friends present objects or participate in therapy? Is the patient's responsivity any better or worse at particular times of the day?

---

a working alliance with the family. Unmet family needs, including a lack of information from staff, can contribute to conflict between the treatment team and family (McNeny & Wilcox, 1991).

If more than one family member was injured in the accident, the attention of the remaining family members is significantly divided. Family members who were in the same accident as the patient but walked away without significant injury may be troubled by a sense of survivor guilt. Some family members become hypervigilant in the clinical setting, never leaving the bedside and neglecting care of others in the family as well as themselves, while expressing a desire to trade places with the patient (Sander & Kreutzer, 1999). Family members under stress may compulsively and, perhaps irrationally, attempt to manage every detail of their loved one's medical and rehabilitative care, which may at times make the health care team's provision of services more difficult or may create tension with the health care team. Distrust of the health care staff can impair the family's communication with the team.

The patient's trajectory of recovery can also have an impact on the family's overall reaction (Bond et al., 2003). When progress is very slow or nonexistent or if unexpected complications arise, family frustration, anxiety, and anger may surface. Intrafamily fighting and disagreements among friends of the patient may occur. Family members may argue among themselves, blame one another, withhold information from each another or from staff, entangle staff in their conflict, and make development or maintenance of a therapeutic relationship very difficult (Sander & Kreutzer, 1999). These strong emotional responses can at times be directed toward the staff, including the occupational therapist (McNeny & Wilcox, 1991; Sander & Kreutzer, 1999). Displays of hostility and aggression are common among the families of people in coma, although this hostility may be very subtly displayed (Stern, Sazbon, Becker, & Costeff, 1988). Therefore, families in distress need customized, compassionate care from the health care team, despite the pressure on staff for maximized efficiency and productivity that can limit their availability to provide family support.

The occupational therapist faced with a family's distress should not take the family's negative or hostile responses personally. Sometimes staff can defuse family hostility by offering sincere empathy and understanding. When **denial** concerning the realities of the patient's situation is an issue with the family, the occupational therapist should make a concerted effort to gently educate. However, the occupational therapist must resist arguing with the family or displaying evidence to dispute the family's rationales and theories regarding the patient's lack of improvement. If persistent denial leads family members to reject the therapist's advice, the wise clinician can bring another therapist into the case or request a second opinion from an experienced colleague (Godwin et al., 2012; Romano, 1974; Sander & Kreutzer, 1999). A team approach is vital to ensure uniformity of information given to family members.

Grief, worry, fatigue, and shock all affect the family's ability to learn, and yet families frequently express the need to know what is going on and how to assist in the recovery process (Bond et al., 2003). Education and training provided to families should be given in amounts that the family can comprehend and digest without becoming distressed or overwhelmed. The occupational therapist should communicate in a manner that meets the family's best learning style, facilitates comprehension of presented information, and promotes trust.

The occupational therapist can provide suggestions on ways the family can help with the patient's recovery. The family may be asked simply to talk to the patient, using a normal tone of voice. The family should tell the patient who they are and provide orienting information. Families who find it difficult to hold a one-sided conversation can read to the patient from periodicals, spiritual material, cards, letters, and so forth. Family can also provide environmental control and facilitate structured rest. They can be charged with keeping visitors quiet and to a minimum at any one time. The family can do soothing care tasks for the patient, including brushing hair and applying lotion. The therapist can counsel family members in reestablishing their own routines and habits, especially if the period of unconsciousness becomes lengthy. Regaining balance is often difficult for families of patients to do on their own (Godwin et al., 2012).

In addition to helping with PROM and positioning, capable family members can be invited to assist in treatment sessions in small ways, such as holding the wheelchair during transfers, wiping the patient's mouth if drooling occurs during sitting, or handing needed items to the therapist. The occupational therapist monitors family participation, giving ample opportunity for families to ask questions and gain additional information. However, it is important to recognize that not all families are capable of or interested in hands-on participation. In such situations, the therapist should simply give the family permission to visit quietly or observe therapy without providing care.

Occupational therapists work with the interdisciplinary team to meet families' needs. Helping the family maintain a sense of hopefulness regarding their loved one's recovery appears beneficial (Verhaeghe et al., 2007). Formal family conferences, which include the occupational therapist, provide a time during which family concerns can be addressed and information disseminated. Family conferences give the family access to the entire treatment team in one place and provide a forum for asking questions or expressing concerns (Muir, Rosenthal, & Diehl, 1990). These formal meetings help the team determine which areas of function and care are most important to the family. This information is useful in team goal setting and discharge planning. Regardless of which elements of family education the occupational therapist uses, education that is earnestly provided demonstrates the staff's concern, which can facilitate an effective partnership between clinicians and family.

Team Coordination and Collaboration

The occupational therapist documents the findings of the evaluation in the medical record, providing the results of assessments performed as well as recommendations, goals for intervention, and an intervention plan for occupational therapy services. The therapist also informally communicates findings, goals, and plans verbally to others on the interdisciplinary care team or formally during interdisciplinary rounds. Although the format for interdisciplinary rounds varies among facilities, in most facilities the occupational therapist contributes to the development of the team's goals and plan for the patient.

In addition to sharing information with colleagues on the treatment team and with the patient's family, the occupational therapist is often required to communicate with case managers, life care planners, community providers, and other professionals involved in the care of the patient. This communication may be done face to face, by phone, or through the provision of written reports. This communication assists with carryover of intervention strategies as the patient progresses through the continuum of care. Confidentiality standards must be appropriately maintained when information is shared with other professionals providing care to the patient.

When the period of unconsciousness is prolonged, the occupational therapist's role within the treatment team shifts to a more consultative function. With patients who remain in an MCS, the occupational therapist monitors the PROM and positioning program now administered by others on staff. The occupational therapist remains available to provide splint adjustments, consult on positioning, or address changes in joint or muscle function. As discharge approaches, the occupational therapist provides advice on DME needs, adaptation of the discharge environment, and the necessity of continued rehabilitative therapy after discharge.

The occupational therapist's role with the patient also changes when increases in patient responsiveness are noted. According to Giacino, Kezmarsky, DeLuca, and Cicerone (1991), improvements in behavioral responsiveness demonstrated by a client with minimal responsiveness may suggest a positive prognosis. If an assessment of the patient's level of arousal and responsiveness indicates a significant and positive change, an alteration in the occupational therapy treatment program is likely warranted, with an increase in the frequency and intensity of occupational therapy services. Intervention should become more complex and demanding as the patient becomes more capable.

Expected Outcomes

The most desirable outcome for patients experiencing a disorder of consciousness is for unconsciousness to yield to purposeful, intentional responses with eventual resumption of ADLs. Occupational therapy prepares patients for increased

The most desirable outcome for patients experiencing a disorder of consciousness is for unconsciousness to yield to purposeful, intentional responses with eventual resumption of ADLs.

participation in their desired occupations by using measures to prevent disability, which in turn promotes good **quality of life.** By adopting a broader definition of *client* to include family and significant others, the occupational therapist contributes to overall patient satisfaction by providing family education and involving family members in the therapeutic process. The application of client-centered, goal-directed intervention is not only of therapeutic benefit but also enhances the family's understanding of the role and impact of occupational therapy on the ultimate outcome of the rehabilitative process.

Generally speaking, the occupational therapist facilitates a good patient outcome by providing services focused on several key areas:

- Creation of a therapeutic environment that fosters and challenges recovery while avoiding excessive stimulation and fatigue
- Prevention of secondary disability through both remediating and restorative interventions
- Collaboration with the interdisciplinary health care team to facilitate the patient's well-being
- Provision of education and support to the family and significant others
- Involvement in discharge and aftercare planning.

Occupational therapy with patients at RLA LCFs I to III requires patience, perseverance, flexibility, a keen eye for detail, sensitivity, and a long-term perspective. Changes in responsiveness may occur steadily in the days after injury, or the patient's progress may be slow and delayed.

Another positive outcome is for the family to feel competent, involved, and informed as caregivers. Family members need the occupational therapist's expertise and time to help them reach their own goals. Helping family members come to an understanding of the reality of their loved one's injury and prognosis is an ongoing conversation. Communicating realism about the prognosis while maintaining hope is a delicate balance. Dr. Mitchell Rosenthal, a pioneer in rehabilitation of patients with brain injury, once referred to TBI as a puzzle (Rosenthal, 1990). Occupational therapists hold a vital piece of this puzzle—the piece that one hopes will lead to a patient's eventual meaningful and full participation in the occupations of everyday life.

The Case of Diane Archer

Let's revisit the case of Diane Archer, the young woman who sustained a TBI. The case picks up where it left off in Chapter 4.

Chris, the occupational therapist assigned to Diane Archer, went to the ICU the morning after the physician's orders were received to begin evaluating and treating Diane. Chris is a senior occupational therapist who has worked in the regional trauma center since receiving his occupational therapy degree 5 years ago. He has experience treating both orthopedic and neurological populations and has had a nonrotating position on the neurosurgical service for the past 3 years. Another occupational therapist who had extensive experience with the population with TBI had initially mentored Chris when he chose to specialize on this service, and Chris has attended a few continuing education workshops on splinting and serial casting, motor control, and **cognition.**

Chris enjoys the fast-paced trauma floors and the medical aspects of his caseload. He feels confident in his ability to quickly analyze the client factors that require intervention to ensure that his patients have successful outcomes during their ongoing rehabilitation. Sometimes Chris misses being able to engage in true client-centered practice because his patients are often so ill or in coma and are unable to express their goals and desires. Chris feels it is vital to broaden his definition of *client* and engage his patients' families in both the evaluation and the intervention process.

Diane is now 3 days into her coma. Chris's review of Diane's chart showed an unremarkable past medical history. Diane has had only two prior hospitalizations: one at age 16 for an appendectomy and one at age 25 for the birth of her daughter. She drinks socially, does not smoke, and is taking only birth control medication. Her family and social history noted a strong support system that included her husband, parents, siblings and their families, and a tight-knit group of friends.

Her home is a two-story colonial-type house with bathrooms on both floors, but the bedrooms are on the upper floor. There are 3 steps to get into the house and 14 steps to get to the second floor. While reading the chart, Chris noted Diane's physical injuries resulting from the accident, the results of the computed tomography scans, and current vital signs and precautions (i.e., no vestibular stimulation and discontinuation of treatment if blood pressure exceeds 140/90 or oxygen saturation decreases below 90% for more than 15 seconds).

On approaching Diane's bed, Chris observed that family members were present. He introduced himself to Diane's husband, Tom, and her mother and then approached Diane in the hospital bed. Chris noted that Diane was approximately 5 feet, 6 inches tall and weighs 130 pounds. She has dark, shoulder-length hair and fair skin and was wearing the standard hospital gown. She had a tracheostomy tube in her neck and was connected to a ventilator. An intravenous line was in her left arm, and a **nasogastric tube** was taped to her cheek where it exited her left nostril. Diane's eyes were closed, and she appeared unresponsive to her environment. A below-knee fiberglass cast was on her left leg. Chris spent a few minutes explaining occupational therapy and the purpose of his initial visit with Diane to her husband and mother. Chris asked them what they understood about Diane's condition and asked them to tell him a bit about Diane before the accident because she was unable to participate in an occupational profile interview.

To gather additional information for the occupational profile, Chris provided the family with a form that had questions about how Diane spent a typical day, the things she liked and disliked, and her occupation and **leisure** interests (Exhibit 5.1). Although Chris had gathered information from the social worker's chart documentation, he needed to understand other aspects of Diane's life to adequately evaluate and treat her. Chris also provided Tom with a checklist of descriptive words to gain insight into Diane's personality and personal values and suggested items that the family could bring in from home that would be helpful to the rehabilitation team (e.g., photos of family and friends with labels on the back, Diane's favorite perfume, a favorite piece of clothing, an MP3 player with her favorite music).

Because Diane was in a coma and unable to perform any purposeful or occupation-based activities, Chris evaluated the client factors that were affected by Diane's injuries: PROM, muscle tone (documenting the posturing of her right upper extremity), and ability to respond to basic stimulation such as touch and auditory commands (Exhibit 5.2). He monitored her vital signs for any physiological

Exhibit 5.1. Diane Archer's Occupational Profile During the Initial Hospitalization

Previous Areas of Performance
Family reports patient previously performed occupations in the following areas: *ADLs:* Before injury, patient was independent in all ADLs. She preferred showers to baths; dressed casually in the evening and on weekends and professionally for work; ate a relatively healthy diet with little snacking; typically wore light makeup (mascara and lip gloss); slept 6 to 7 hr per night; and enjoyed an intimate relationship with her husband. *IADLs:* Patient was the primary caregiver for her 3-yr-old daughter. Patient drove a car and frequently used public transportation to travel to a nearby city. She was the primary cook in the family and shared interior and exterior home maintenance with her husband. She maintained the family's finances and performed weekly grocery shopping. *Rest and sleep:* Patient typically enjoyed reading before sleeping or used this time to unwind and discuss family issues with her husband. The couple kept a monitor by their bed so they could hear if their daughter called out to them during the night. Patient was not one to nap during the day but enjoyed engaging in cuddle time with her daughter while listening to music. *Education:* Patient was not involved in any formal or informal educational activities at the time of her injury. *Work:* Patient worked as an accountant in a large publishing firm. She worked 37 hr per week and had a good attendance and performance record (according to husband). *Leisure:* Patient engaged in seasonal sports of tennis and skiing as well as hiking and social events. She also enjoyed reading, playing board games, and occasionally watching TV. **Social participation:** Patient interacted frequently with her family and a group of close friends, coworkers, and neighbors. She had a close network of colleagues at her place of employment.

Previous Patterns of Performance
Information gathered from family: *Habits, routines, and rituals:* Patient typically got up at 6:00 a.m. and showered before waking her daughter. Husband made breakfast for family, and all members left the home at 8:00 a.m. Patient typically dropped off daughter at child care and picked her up at 5:30 p.m. Weekday evenings were spent cooking dinner for family, playing with daughter, watching TV with husband, or doing household chores once daughter went to bed. Weekends were spent as a family completing renovation projects (interior and exterior) and day trips for activities with daughter or family (e.g., hiking, visiting family, visiting the zoo). Family celebrations were an important opportunity to gather at either the patient's home or her parents' home with traditional food and activities. *Roles:* Patient's roles included wife, mother, accountant, daughter, sister, aunt, and friend. Husband says patient had established a good balance between the demands of her multiple roles.

Life Contexts and Environments
Cultural: Patient is of third-generation German descent and is reported to have a strong work ethic and belief in loyalty to family and friends. *Physical:* Patient lives in a three-bedroom, two-story house in a suburban neighborhood. Her bedroom is on the second floor. There are full bathrooms located on both floors. The community does not have sidewalks, and local shopping and community buildings are located approximately 3 mi from the home. *Personal:* 28-yr-old wife and mother of 3-yr-old daughter. Middle-class, college-educated accountant. *Temporal:* Patient was engaged in many of the typical behaviors of young adulthood (i.e., establishment of a career and family). *Virtual:* Patient used her smartphone to stay in contact with family and friends via voice and texts. She also used video calls for her parents and siblings to see and speak with her daughter. She used Facebook to connect with family and friends and share updates on family activities. *Social:* Patient was perceived as a social planner by family, friends, and colleagues, often planning gatherings at her home. She also used technological and virtual methods to stay in contact with others.

Values, Beliefs, and Spirituality
Values: Husband says patient believes in marriage as a partnership and that a successful family requires teamwork. *Beliefs:* Patient is described as having a strong sense of ethics and loyalty and values family, friendship, and community. *Spiritual:* Although raised as a Roman Catholic, patient is not a strict observer of organized religion.

Patient's Priorities and Desired Targeted Outcomes (According to Family)
The family expressed their hopes that the patient will be able to eventually resume her roles as a wife and mother and demonstrate the necessary skills to achieve satisfaction and an acceptable quality of life in those roles. They appear overwhelmed at present and unable to express more specific priorities or goals.

Implications for Intervention Planning
Data gathered for the occupational profile will need to be reviewed with the patient later, when she is able to share her priorities for occupational therapy intervention and her desired outcomes for the intervention process.

Note. ADLs = activities of daily living; hr = hours; IADLs = **instrumental activities of daily living;** mi = miles; yr = year.

Exhibit 5.2. Diane Archer's Initial Occupational Therapy Evaluation in the Intensive Care Unit

Performance		
Areas	**Skills**	**Patterns**
The patient is dependent in the performance of all areas of occupation. Information on previous level of function in these areas was collected from the family for the occupational profile.	Unable to evaluate motor skills, process skills, or social interaction skills at present; patient is unable to engage in purposeful and goal-directed behaviors because of coma.	*Habits, routines, and rituals:* Patient's previous habits and routines are nonfunctional. She does not initiate any tasks or activities that were previously part of her daily life. *Roles:* Current roles are not able to be fulfilled. She presently functions in the role of patient. Her lack of responsiveness to her environment prevents her engagement in tasks of her other roles (e.g., wife, daughter, mother).

Client Factors	Context
Spirituality At the patient's mother's request, the local priest comes to the facility every few days to administer a blessing and pray with the family. *Mental Functions* *Global mental functions:* Patient is presently in a coma and minimally responsive to pain. She appears asleep and shows little physiological response to stimulation. *Sensory Functions and Pain* *Seeing:* Patient does not spontaneously open her eyes. Pupillary reactions are sluggish but equal. *Hearing and vestibular functions:* Patient does not respond to sound. *Additional sensory functions:* Patient does not show purposeful or physiological responses to any sensory stimulation at present (e.g., pain, touch, temperature, pressure). *Neuromusculoskeletal and Movement-Related Functions* *Functions of joints and bones:* Patient has full PROM of all joints in both upper limbs. **End feels** of the joint capsules are tight. *Muscle functions:* Patient displays moderate increase in flexor tone in the R UE. L UE displays normal tone. *Movement functions:* Patient postures in **decorticate** position at rest. Although she can be brought into full extension with slow, steady movement and inhibitory techniques, she returns to a flexed position on the removal of these external controls. *Respiratory System Function* Patient is receiving partial assist with her breathing from the endotracheal respirator. *Voice and Speech Functions* Patient is intubated and unable to speak.	*Cultural* The ICU culture is highly technical with an emphasis on survival. Family visiting is restricted to particular lengths of time and particular times of the day. *Physical* Environmental stimuli in the ICU are repetitive in nature (i.e., lighting, sounds, temperature, routines of medical care). The patient's room has a glass wall looking out to the nursing station, thus diminishing any privacy in the room. *Social* Interactions between the staff and family are typically quiet. The patient is not capable of interacting at present, but the nurses speak to her to inform her about the procedures they are performing. They also encourage family to talk with the patient and tell her about events at home. *Personal* Patient is a 28-yr-old married woman who is the mother of a 3-yr-old. She is a college-educated accountant. *Temporal* Early spring.

Implications for Intervention Planning
Patient's current inability to initiate any volitional, purposeful behavior makes participation in occupational therapy intervention initially passive in nature. Intervention will focus on using preparatory methods to prevent secondary physical changes to client factors. The activity and occupational demands during the coma stimulation program will be selected to enhance the potential of eliciting a purposeful, volitional response from the patient. Familiar personal objects, recordings of voices and music, photos, and scents will be used (objects and their properties). The amount of stimulation and potential for habituation of environmental stimuli (e.g., space demands such as lights, mechanical sounds of medical machinery) will be varied to provide novel stimuli that may capture the patient's attention. Although the patient is unable to engage in social interaction, the potential of her responding more to familiar voices and faces will be considered; family will be asked to record some commands to the patient (e.g., "open your eyes," "look at Chris") and encouraged to engage in conversation with the patient during their visits (social demands). Therapy sessions will be conducted 1:1 in settings that enable either greater control of environmental stimuli, especially when response to a command is required, or novel stimuli that may result in an orienting response (e.g., outdoor patio, hospital day room). One-step commands and activities will be selected, and the patient will be given adequate time to respond to stimuli (sequencing or timing). Activities selected for intervention will be as client-centered as possible and will require actions of bilateral UE reaching and grasping, processing skills of attending and appropriately using objects, and interaction skills of gazing and gesturing. Cues or reinforcement will be provided as needed.

Note. ICU = intensive care unit; L = left; PROM = passive range of motion; R = right; UE = upper extremity; yr = year.

changes that might indicate a response to the stimuli or require him to stop the session. He questioned Diane's husband and mother about any particular responses they had seen from Diane because he knew people emerging from coma often respond first to familiar people.

Chris determined at this early phase in Diane's recovery that his occupational therapy intervention approach should focus on using preparatory methods to prevent secondary physical changes, such as tissue contractures and loss of ROM as well as a coma stimulation program (Table 5.3). Chris was familiar with the evidence-based literature on coma stimulation. Although he did not believe he could restore Diane's awareness to her environment, he felt that the consistent monitoring and ongoing evaluation of response to stimulation would provide the team with information on when Diane was naturally awakening from her coma. Following the hospital's TBI service documentation guidelines, Chris charted Diane's responses to the stimulation on the CRS–R (Kalmar & Giacino, 2005). Her initial score on the CRS–R was a 2 out of a possible 23 points because she showed only a flexion withdrawal to noxious stimuli on both upper extremities.

Chris continued to provide twice-daily PROM and sensory stimulation and fitted Diane's right hand for a cloth-covered roll to decrease her fisted position. Chris also used family education as a therapeutic intervention. During his frequent contact with the family, he instructed Tom in how to provide PROM to Diane's limbs

Table 5.3. Sample Activities From Diane Archer's Intervention Plan During the Coma Phase of Recovery

Problems and Goals	Approach	Primary Focus of Intervention	Interventions
Problem: Increased tone in R UE resulting in posturing and potential for decreased ROM *Goal:* Patient will display full PROM in all joints of both UEs. *Goal:* Patient will tolerate wearing a soft splint on R hand for 2-hr on–off schedule to decrease flexor tone and prevent joint and skin contractures. *Goal:* Patient will tolerate wearing serial cast as evidenced by skin integrity, decreased tone, and increased ROM in R elbow and wrist.	• Prevent • Restore	*Client factors:* Structure and functions of joints and bones	*Preparatory methods:* Provide daily PROM to all joints with the use of tone-inhibiting techniques. Provide soft splint for R hand to decrease finger fisting and prevent skin breakdown. Provide serial casting program with cast changes every 4-5 days. Provide proper body alignment in tilt-in-space wheelchair with head rest, lap tray, gel seat cushion, and trunk inserts. *Education:* Instruct patient's husband and mother in the performance of PROM to UEs and the donning and doffing of the hand splint. Provide nursing staff with splint-wearing schedule.
Problem: Decreased response to environmental stimuli *Goal:* Patient will display increased speed and accuracy of responses to sensory stimulation (e.g., will follow 1-step motor response in relation to sensory stimulation within 15 s of request or stimulus).	• Restore	*Client factors:* Mental functions and sensory functions	*Preparatory methods:* Provide daily structured exposure to a variety of sensory stimuli, requesting patient to perform goal-directed behavior. Reinforce positive responses with verbal praise and repetition. *Purposeful activity:* As patient progresses, provide more purposeful activities with expectation of shorter response times (e.g., answer phone, bring washcloth to face). *Education:* Patient's family will perform structured stimulation during evenings and weekends and record responses on provided form.

Note. hr = hours; PROM = passive range of motion; R = right; ROM = range of motion; s = seconds; UE/UEs = upper extremity/extremities.

and how to structure basic coma stimulation techniques. Chris also used his conversations with Tom to educate him about what the next few weeks or months of Diane's recovery might entail. He encouraged Tom to contact the local chapter of the Brain Injury Association for additional information and support.

Throughout the 1st week that Diane was in the ICU, Chris noticed increased responses to sensory stimulation. By the end of the week, Diane would inconsistently track her husband in the room, raise her left arm to touch her husband's or mother's hand, and turn her head toward a recording of her daughter Kate singing a nursery rhyme. Chris charted the frequency and consistency of Diane's responses on the CRS–R grid. Her score had improved to 11 of 23. Diane was gradually weaned off the ventilator, but her tracheal tube was left in place until the team could ensure that she could maintain adequate oxygenation. She continued to receive nutrition through a gastrostomy tube that was placed when the nasogastric tube was removed on Day 5 postinjury. Chris knew that the tube would remain in place until Diane demonstrated the cognitive and physical ability to swallow mechanically altered (i.e., pureed) food.

Acute Rehabilitation Unit of the Trauma Center

During Diane's 2nd week in the ICU, the neurologist and neurosurgeon felt that her status had stabilized. Her GCS was now a 10, her CRS–R was 16 of 23, and the team scored her as a Rancho Level III. Although no longer in coma, Diane was considered minimally responsive. She was breathing without the assistance of the ventilator and showed good oxygen saturation with oxygen delivered via nasal cannulas when her tracheotomy tube was capped.

Diane was transferred to a room on the rehabilitation floor of the trauma center, and Chris continued as her therapist. On admission to the rehab unit, Diane began to show purposeful responses to environmental stimuli with increasing consistency. The team continued to track her progress using the CRS–R. Chris began a serial casting program for Diane's right elbow to try to decrease the flexor tone and her posturing in the decorticate (flexor) position. Chris left the initial cast on for 3 days and then changed the cast every 5 days, consistently gaining approximately 7° to 10° of PROM with each cast change. Diane's husband continued to visit daily for several hours. Now that Diane was out of the ICU, other family members and friends started to visit in the evenings and on the weekends. Although the family felt it was too early to bring daughter Kate to see Diane, recordings of Kate performing simple songs were incorporated into the stimulation program (e.g., Diane was required to press a large switch to activate the devices). At this phase of Diane's recovery, Chris continued to focus the occupational therapy intervention on restoring Diane's underlying client factors (i.e., mental, sensory, neuromusculoskeletal and movement-related functions) and basic skill performance (e.g., gaze, attend, reach, grasp) while preventing further limitations in her motor, process, and interaction skills.

Anya, the physical therapist, and Chris cotreated Diane on many occasions. Both therapists were needed for Diane to sit on a therapy mat and perform simple, purposeful motor acts (e.g., hitting a balloon, reaching for objects, lifting her head to look at her husband, pressing a large switch connected to a recorder to hear Kate singing). They also provided Diane with a tilt-in-space wheelchair with a head rest, lap tray, and inserts to help maintain her trunk balance. During his individual sessions with Diane, Chris tried to incorporate simple purposeful activities, such as picking up a ringing telephone, washing her face, and lifting a cup to her mouth.

Diane now scored a 22 of 23 on the CRS–R, and the team discontinued its use. Chris continued with the serial casting program on Diane's right elbow. A team meeting that included Tom and Diane's parents gave them a report on her status and a plan for discharge to the rehabilitation hospital. Four weeks after her injury, Diane's tracheotomy was removed, and she was transferred to the rehabilitation hospital. She was demonstrating behaviors consistent with Rancho Levels III to IV (agitation).

The case continues at the end of Chapter 6.

References

Abbasi, M., Mohammadi, E., & Sheaykh Rezayi, A. (2009). Effect of a regular family visiting program as an affective, auditory, and tactile stimulation on the consciousness level of comatose patients with a head injury. *Japan Journal of Nursing Science, 6,* 21–26. http://dx.doi.org/10.1111/j.1742-7924.2009.00117.x

Abbate, C., Trimarchi, P. D., Basile, I., Mazzucchi, A., & Devalle, G. (2014). Sensory stimulation for patients with disorders of consciousness: From stimulation to rehabilitation. *Frontiers in Human Neuroscience, 8,* 616. http://dx.doi.org/10.3389/fnhum.2014.00616

American Congress of Rehabilitation Medicine. (1995). Recommendations for use of uniform nomenclature pertinent to patients with severe alterations in consciousness. *Archives of Physical Medicine and Rehabilitation, 76,* 205–209. http://dx.doi.org/10.1016/S0003-9993(95)80031-X

American Congress of Rehabilitation Medicine, Brain Injury-Interdisciplinary Special Interest Group, Disorders of Consciousness Task Force; Seel, R. T., Sherer, M., Whyte, J., Katz, D. I., Giacino, J. T., Rosenbaum, A. M., . . . Zasler, N. (2010). Assessment scales for disorders of consciousness: Evidence-based recommendations for clinical practice and research. *Archives of Physical Medicine and Rehabilitation, 91,* 1795–1813. http://dx.doi.org/10.1016/j.apmr.2010.07.218

Ansell, B. J., & Keenan, J. E. (1989). The Western Neuro Sensory Stimulation Profile: A tool for assessing slow-to-recover head-injured patients. *Archives of Physical Medicine and Rehabilitation, 70,* 104–108.

Antoinette, T. (1996). Rehabilitation nursing management of persons in low level neurologic states. *NeuroRehabilitation, 6,* 33–44. http://dx.doi.org/10.1016/1053-8135(95)00146-8

Aubut, J. A., Mehta, S., Cullen, N., & Teasell, R. W.; ERABI Group; Scire Research Team. (2011). A comparison of heterotopic ossification treatment within the traumatic brain and spinal cord injured population: An evidence based systematic review. *NeuroRehabilitation, 28,* 151–160.

Benzer, A., Mitterschiffthaler, G., Marosi, M., Luef, G., Pühringer, F., De La Renotiere, K., . . . Schmutzhard, E. (1991). Prediction of non-survival after trauma: Innsbruck Coma Scale. *Lancet, 338,* 977–978. http://dx.doi.org/10.1016/0140-6736(91)91840-Q

Blanton, S., Porter, L., Smith, D., & Wolf, S. L. (1999). Strategies to enhance mobility in traumatic brain injured patients. In M. Rosenthal, E. R. Griffith, J. S. Kreutzer, & B. Pentland (Eds.), *Rehabilitation of the adult and child with traumatic brain injury* (3rd ed., pp. 219–241). Philadelphia: F. A. Davis.

Bobath, B. (1978). *Adult hemiplegia: Evaluation and treatment.* London: Churchill Livingstone.

Bond, A. E., Draeger, C. R. L., Mandleco, B., & Donnelly, M. (2003). Needs of family members of patients with severe traumatic brain injury: Implications for evidence-based practice. *Critical Care Nurse, 23,* 63–72.

Borer-Alafi, N., Gil, M., Sazbon, L., & Korn, C. (2002). Loewenstein Communication Scale for the minimally responsive patient. *Brain Injury, 16,* 593–609. http://dx.doi.org/10.1080/02699050110119484

Born, J. D. (1988). The Glasgow-Liège Scale: Prognostic value and evolution of motor response and brain stem reflexes after severe head injury. *Acta Neurochirurgica, 91,* 1–11. http://dx.doi.org/10.1007/BF01400520

Cruse, D., & Chennu, S. (2012). Relationship between etiology and covert cognition in the minimally conscious state. *Neurology, 78,* 816–822. http://dx.doi.org/10.1212/WNL.0b013e318249f764

Davis, A. E., & Gimenez, A. (2003). Cognitive–behavioral recovery in comatose patients following auditory sensory stimulation. *Journal of Neuroscience Nursing, 35,* 202–209, 214. http://dx.doi.org/10.1097/01376517-200308000-00006

Di Stefano, C., Cortesi, A., Masotti, S., Simoncini, L., & Piperno, R. (2012). Increased behavioural responsiveness with complex stimulation in VS and MCS: Preliminary results. *Brain Injury, 26,* 1250–1256. http://dx.doi.org/10.3109/02699052.2012.667588

Edlow, B. L., Takahashi, E., Wu, O., Benner, T., Dai, G., Bu, L., . . . Folkerth, R. D. (2012). Neuroanatomic connectivity of the human ascending arousal system critical to consciousness and its disorders. *Journal of Neuropathology and Experimental Neurology, 71,* 531–546. http://dx.doi.org/10.1097/NEN.0b013e3182588293

Englander, J. S., Cifu, D. X., Wright, J., Zafonte, R., Mann, N., Yablon, S., & Ivanhoe, C. (1996). The impact of acute complications, fractures, and motor deficits on functional outcome and length of stay after traumatic brain injury: A multicenter analysis. *Journal of Head Trauma Rehabilitation, 11,* 15–26. http://dx.doi.org/10.1097/00001199-199610000-00003

Engli, M., & Kirsivali-Farmer, K. (1993). Needs of family members of critically ill patients with and without acute brain injury. *Journal of Neuroscience Nursing, 25,* 78–85. http://dx.doi.org/10.1097/01376517-199304000-00003

Flower, O., & Hellings, S. (2012). Sedation in traumatic brain injury. *Emergency Medicine International, 2012,* 637171. http://dx.doi.org/10.1155/2012/637171

Giacino, J. T. (1996). Sensory stimulation: Theoretical perspectives and the evidence for effectiveness. *NeuroRehabilitation, 6,* 69–78. http://dx.doi.org/10.1016/1053-8135(95)00149-2

Giacino, J. T., Ashwal, S., Childs, N., Cranford, R., Jennett, B., Katz, D. I., . . . Zasler, N. D. (2002). The minimally conscious state: Definition and diagnostic criteria. *Neurology, 58,* 349–353. http://dx.doi.org/10.1212/WNL.58.3.349

Giacino, J. T., Garber, K., Katz, D. I., & Schiff, N. (2012). Assessment and rehabilitative management of individuals with disorders of consciousness. In N. D. Zasler, D. I. Katz, & R. D. Zafonte (Eds.), *Brain injury medicine* (2nd ed., pp. 517–535). New York: Demos.

Giacino, J. T., Kalmar, K., & Whyte, J. (2004). The JFK Coma Recovery Scale–Revised: Measurement characteristics and diagnostic utility. *Archives of Physical Medicine and Rehabilitation, 85,* 2020–2029. http://dx.doi.org/10.1016/j.apmr.2004.02.033

Giacino, J. T., Kezmarsky, M. A., DeLuca, J., & Cicerone, K. D. (1991). Monitoring rate of recovery to predict outcome in minimally responsive patients. *Archives of Physical Medicine and Rehabilitation, 72,* 897–901. http://dx.doi.org/10.1016/0003-9993(91)90008-7

Giacino, J. T., & Smart, C. M. (2007). Recent advances in behavioral assessment of individuals with disorders of consciousness. *Current Opinion in Neurology, 20,* 614–619. http://dx.doi.org/10.1097/WCO.0b013e3282f189ef

Giacino, J. T., Zasler, N. D., Katz, D. I., Kelly, J. P., Rosenberg, J. H., & Filley, C. M. (1997). Development of practice guidelines for assessment and management of the vegetative and minimally conscious states. *Journal of Head Trauma Rehabilitation, 12,* 79–89. http://dx.doi.org/10.1097/00001199-199708000-00008

Gill-Thwaites, H., & Munday, R. (1999). The Sensory Modality Assessment and Rehabilitation Technique (SMART): A comprehensive integrated assessment and treatment protocol for the vegetative state and minimally responsive patient. *Neuropsychological Rehabilitation, 9,* 305–320. http://dx.doi.org/10.1080/096020199389392

Godwin, E. E., Schaat, K. W., & Kreutzer, J. S. (2012). Practical approaches to family assessment and intervention. In N. D. Zasler, D. I. Katz, & R. D. Zafonte (Eds.), *Brain injury medicine* (2nd ed., pp. 1329–1348). New York: Demos.

Golisz, K. M. (2009). *Occupational therapy practice guidelines for adults with traumatic brain injury.* Bethesda, MD: AOTA Press.

Gorji, M. A., Araghiyansc, F., Jafari, H., Gorgi, A. M., & Yazdani, J. (2014). Effect of auditory stimulation on traumatic coma duration in intensive care unit of Medical Sciences University of Mazandarn, Iran. *Saudi Journal of Anaesthesia, 8,* 69–72. http://dx.doi.org/10.4103/1658-354X.125940

Gosseries, O., Bruno, M. A., Chatelle, C., Vanhaudenhuyse, A., Schnakers, C., Soddu, A., & Laureys, S. (2011). Disorders of consciousness: What's in a name? *NeuroRehabilitation, 28,* 3–14. http://dx.doi.org/10.3233/NRE-2011-0625

Gracies, J. M. (2001). Pathophysiology of impairment in patients with spasticity and use of stretch as a treatment of spastic hypertonia. *Physical Medicine and Rehabilitation Clinics of North America, 12,* 747–768, vi.

Hagen, C., Malkmus, D., & Durham, P. (1972). *Levels of Cognitive Functioning*. Downey, CA: Rancho Los Amigos Hospital.

Hellweg, S. (2012). Effectiveness of physiotherapy and occupational therapy after traumatic brain injury in the intensive care unit. *Critical Care Research and Practice, 2012,* 768456. http://dx.doi.org/10.1155/2012/768456

Hirschberg, R., & Giacino, J. T. (2011). The vegetative and minimally conscious states: Diagnosis, prognosis and treatment. *Neurologic Clinics, 29,* 773–786. http://dx.doi.org/10.1016/j.ncl.2011.07.009

Ivanhoe, C. B., Durand-Sanchez, A., & Spier, E. T. (2012). Acute rehabilitation. In N. D. Zasler, D. I. Katz, & R. D. Zafonte (Eds.), *Brain injury medicine* (2nd ed., pp. 385–403). New York: Demos.

Jabri, J. L. (1996). Documentation of occupational therapy services. In L. W. Pedretti (Ed.), *Occupational therapy: Practice skills for physical dysfunction* (4th ed., pp. 55–63). St. Louis: Mosby–Year Book.

Johnson, D. A., Roethig-Johnston, K., & Richards, D. (1993). Biochemical and physiological parameters of recovery in acute severe head injury: Responses to multisensory stimulation. *Brain Injury, 7,* 491–499. http://dx.doi.org/10.3109/02699059309008176

Kalmar, K., & Giacino, J. T. (2005). The JFK Coma Recovery Scale–Revised. *Neuropsychological Rehabilitation, 15,* 454–460. http://dx.doi.org/10.1080/09602010443000425

Katalinic, O. M., Harvey, L. A., & Herbert, R. D. (2011). Effectiveness of stretch for the treatment and prevention of contractures in people with neurological conditions: A systematic review. *Physical Therapy, 91,* 11–24. http://dx.doi.org/10.2522/ptj.20100265

Katalinic, O. M., Harvey, L. A., Herbert, R. D., Moseley, A. M., Lannin, N. A., & Schurr, K. (2010). Stretch for the treatment and prevention of contractures. *Cochrane Database of Systematic Reviews, 2010,* CD007455. http://dx.doi.org/10.1002/14651858.CD007455.pub2

Katz, D. I., & Black, S. E. (1999). Neurological and neuroradiological evaluation. In M. Rosenthal, E. R. Griffith, J. S. Kreutzer, & B. Pentland (Eds.), *Rehabilitation of the adult and child with traumatic brain injury* (3rd ed., pp. 89–116). Philadelphia: F. A. Davis.

Katz, D. I., Polyak, M., Coughlan, D., Nichols, M., & Roche, A. (2009). Natural history of recovery from brain injury after prolonged disorders of consciousness: Outcome of patients admitted to inpatient rehabilitation with 1–4 year follow-up. *Progress in Brain Research, 177,* 73–88. http://dx.doi.org/10.1016/S0079-6123(09)17707-5

Katz, D. I., Zasler, N. D., & Zafonte, R. D. (2012). Clinical continuum of care and natural history. In N. D. Zasler, D. I. Katz, & R. D. Zafonte (Eds.), *Brain injury medicine* (2nd ed., pp. 2–12). New York: Demos.

Keenan, A., & Joseph, L. (2010). The needs of family members of severe traumatic brain injured patients during critical and acute care: A qualitative study. *Canadian Journal of Neuroscience Nursing, 32,* 25–35.

Knight, L. A., Thornton, H. A., & Turner-Stokes, L. (2003). Management of neurogenic heterotopic ossification. *Physiotherapy, 89,* 471–477. http://dx.doi.org/10.1016/S0031-9406(05)60004-1

Kreutzer, J. S., Marwitz, J. H., Godwin, E. E., & Arango-Lasprilla, J. C. (2010). Practical approaches to effective family intervention after brain injury. *Journal of Head Trauma Rehabilitation, 25,* 113–120. http://dx.doi.org/10.1097/HTR.0b013e3181cf0712

Lannin, N. A., Horsley, S. A., Herbert, R., McCluskey, A., & Cusick, A. (2003). Splinting the hand in the functional position after brain impairment: A randomized, controlled trial. *Archives of Physical Medicine and Rehabilitation, 84,* 297–302. http://dx.doi.org/10.1053/apmr.2003.50031

Laureys, S., Celesia, G. G., Cohadon, F., Lavrijsen, J., León-Carrión, J., Sannita, W. G., . . . Dolce, G.; European Task Force on Disorders of Consciousness. (2010). Unresponsive wakefulness syndrome: A new name for the vegetative state or apallic syndrome. *BMC Medicine, 8,* 68. http://dx.doi.org/10.1186/1741-7015-8-68

Lombardi, F., Taricco, M., De Tanti, A., Telaro, E., & Liberati, A. (2002). Sensory stimulation of brain-injured individuals in coma or vegetative state: Results of a Cochrane systematic review. *Clinical Rehabilitation, 16,* 464–472. http://dx.doi.org/10.1191/0269215502cr519oa

Løvstad, M., Frøslie, K. F., Giacino, J. T., Skandsen, T., Anke, A., & Schanke, A. K. (2010). Reliability and diagnostic characteristics of the JFK Coma Recovery Scale–Revised: Exploring the influence of rater's level of experience. *Journal of Head Trauma Rehabilitation, 25,* 349–356. http://dx.doi.org/10.1097/HTR.0b013e3181cec841

Marshall, S., Teasell, R., Bayona, N., Lippert, C., Chundamala, J., Villamere, J., . . . Bayley, M. (2007). Motor impairment rehabilitation post acquired brain injury. *Brain Injury, 21,* 133–160. http://dx.doi.org/10.1080/02699050701201383

McNeny, R. (2007). Therapy for activities of daily living: Theoretical and practical perspectives. In N. D. Zasler, D. I. Katz, & R. D. Zafonte (Eds.), *Brain injury medicine* (pp. 947–959). New York: Demos.

McNeny, R., & Wilcox, P. (1991). Partners by force: The family and the rehabilitation team. *NeuroRehabilitation, 1,* 7–17.

Meyer, M. J., Megyesi, J., Meythaler, J., Murie-Fernandez, M., Aubut, J. A., Foley, N., . . . Teasell, R. (2010). Acute management of acquired brain injury: Part III. An evidence-based review of interventions used to promote arousal from coma. *Brain Injury, 24,* 722–729. http://dx.doi.org/10.3109/02699051003692134

Mitchell, S., Bradley, V. A., Welch, J. L., & Britton, P. G. (1990). Coma arousal procedure: A therapeutic intervention in the treatment of head injury. *Brain Injury, 4,* 273–279. http://dx.doi.org/10.3109/02699059009026177

Model Systems Knowledge Translation Center. (2013). *Resources offered by the MSKTC to support individuals living with traumatic brain injury.* Washington, DC: Author. Retrieved from http://www.msktc.org/lib/docs/Booklet/TBI_Booklet.pdf

Moseley, A. M., Hassett, L. M., Leung, J., Clare, J. S., Herbert, R. D., & Harvey, L. A. (2008). Serial casting versus positioning for the treatment of elbow contractures in adults with traumatic brain injury: A randomized controlled trial. *Clinical Rehabilitation, 22,* 406–417. http://dx.doi.org/10.1177/0269215507083795

Muir, C. A., Rosenthal, M., & Diehl, L. N. (1990). Methods of family intervention. In M. Rosenthal, E. R. Griffith, M. R. Bond, & J. D. Miller (Eds.), *Rehabilitation of the adult and child with traumatic brain injury* (2nd ed., pp. 433–448). Philadelphia: F. A. Davis.

Mysiw, J. W., Fugate, L. P., & Clinchot, D. M. (2007). Assessment, early rehabilitation intervention, and tertiary prevention. In N. D. Zasler, D. I. Katz, & R. D. Zafonte (Eds.), *Brain injury medicine* (pp. 283–301). New York: Demos.

Needham, D. M. (2008). Mobilizing patients in the intensive care unit: Improving neuromuscular weakness and physical function. *JAMA, 300,* 1685–1690. http://dx.doi.org/10.1001/jama.300.14.1685

Nelson, A., & Baptiste, A. S. (2004). Evidence-based practices for safe patient handling and movement. *Online Journal of Issues in Nursing, 9,* 4. Retrieved from http://nursingworld.org/MainMenuCategories/ANAMarketplace/ANAPeriodicals/OJIN/TableofContents/Volume92004/No3Sept04/EvidenceBasedPractices.html

Nelson, A., Harwood, K. J., Tracey, C. A., & Dunn, K. L. (2008). Myths and facts about safe patient handling in rehabilitation. *Rehabilitation Nursing, 33,* 10–17. http://dx.doi.org/10.1002/j.2048-7940.2008.tb00187.x

Nguyen, V., Thao-Houane, T., & Warren, M. L. (2014). Early mobilization: Occupational therapy within the multidisciplinary team approach. *OT Practice, 19*(16), 15–19.

Pape, T. L., Senno, R. G., Guernon, A., & Kelly, J. P. (2005). A measure of neurobehavioral functioning after coma: Part II. Clinical and scientific implementation. *Journal of Rehabilitation Research and Development, 42,* 19–27. http://dx.doi.org/10.1682/JRRD.2004.03.0033

Pentland, B., & Whittle, I. R. (1999). Acute management of brain injury. In M. Rosenthal, E. R. Griffith, J. S. Kreutzer, & B. Pentland (Eds.), *Rehabilitation of the adult and child with traumatic brain injury* (3rd ed., pp. 42–52). Philadelphia: F. A. Davis.

Pohl, M., Rückriem, S., Mehrholz, J., Ritschel, C., Strik, H., & Pause, M. R. (2002). Effectiveness of serial casting in patients with severe cerebral spasticity: A comparison study. *Archives of Physical Medicine and Rehabilitation, 83,* 784–790. http://dx.doi.org/10.1053/apmr.2002.32821

Posner, J. B., Saper, C. B., Schiff, N. D., & Plum, F. (2007). *Plum and Posner's diagnosis of stupor and coma* (4th ed.). Oxford, England: Oxford University Press.

Quality Standards Subcommittee of the American Academy of Neurology. (1995). Practice parameters: Assessment and management of patients in the persistent vegetative state (summary statement). *Neurology, 45,* 1015–1018. http://dx.doi.org/10.1212/WNL.45.5.1015

Rader, M. A., & Ellis, D. W. (1994). The Sensory Stimulation Assessment Measure (SSAM): A tool for early evaluation of severely brain-injured patients. *Brain Injury, 8,* 309–321. http://dx.doi.org/10.3109/02699059409150982

Rappaport, M., Dougherty, A. M., & Kelting, D. L. (1992). Evaluation of coma and vegetative states. *Archives of Physical Medicine and Rehabilitation, 73,* 628–634.

Romano, M. D. (1974). Family response to traumatic head injury. *Scandinavian Journal of Rehabilitation Medicine, 6,* 1–4.

Rosenthal, M. (1990). Preface to the first edition. In M. Rosenthal, E. R. Griffith, M. R. Bond, & J. D. Miller (Eds.), *Rehabilitation of the adult and child with traumatic brain injury* (2nd ed., pp. 433–448). Philadelphia: F. A. Davis.

Sandel, M. E. (1996). Medical management of the comatose, vegetative, or minimally responsive patient. *NeuroRehabilitation, 6,* 9–17. http://dx.doi.org/10.1016/1053-8135(95)00144-1

Sander, A. M., & Kreutzer, J. S. (1999). A holistic approach to family assessment after brain injury. In M. Rosenthal, E. R. Griffith, J. S. Kreutzer, & B. Pentland (Eds.), *Rehabilitation of the adult and child with a traumatic brain injury* (3rd ed., pp. 199–215). Philadelphia: F. A. Davis.

Sander, A. M., Maestas, K. L., Sherer, M., Malec, J. F., & Nakase-Richardson, R. (2012). Relationship of caregiver and family functioning to participation outcomes after postacute rehabilitation for traumatic brain injury: A multicenter investigation. *Archives of Physical Medicine and Rehabilitation, 93,* 842–848. http://dx.doi.org/10.1016/j.apmr.2011.11.031

Schnakers, C., Giacino, J., & Laureys, S. (2010). Detecting signs of consciousness in severely brain injured patients recovering from coma. In Center for International Rehabilitation Research Information and Exchange (Ed.), *International Encyclopedia of Rehabilitation.* Retrieved from http://cirrie.buffalo.edu/encyclopedia/en/article/133/

Schweickert, W. D., Pohlman, M. C., Pohlman, A. S., Nigos, C., Pawlik, A. J., Esbrook, C. L., . . . Kress, J. P. (2009). Early physical and occupational therapy in mechanically ventilated, critically ill patients: A randomised controlled trial. *Lancet, 373,* 1874–1882. http://dx.doi.org/10.1016/S0140-6736(09)60658-9

Seel, R. T., Douglas, J., Dennison, A. C., Heaner, S., Farris, K., & Rogers, C. (2013). Specialized early treatment for persons with disorders of consciousness: Program components and outcomes. *Archives of Physical Medicine and Rehabilitation, 94,* 1908–1923. http://dx.doi.org/10.1016/j.apmr.2012.11.052

Shiel, A., Horn, S. A., Wilson, B. A., Watson, M. J., Campbell, M. J., & McLellan, D. L. (2000). The Wessex Head Injury Matrix (WHIM) main scale: A preliminary report on a scale to assess and monitor patient recovery after severe head injury. *Clinical Rehabilitation, 14,* 408–416. http://dx.doi.org/10.1191/0269215500cr326oa

Silva, S., Alacoque, X., Fourcade, O., Samii, K., Marque, P., Woods, R., . . . Loubinoux, I. (2010). Wakefulness and loss of awareness: Brain and brainstem interaction in the vegetative state. *Neurology, 74,* 313–320. http://dx.doi.org/10.1212/WNL.0b013e3181cbcd96

Singer, B. J., Jegasothy, G. M., Singer, K. P., Allison, G. T., & Dunne, J. W. (2004). Incidence of ankle contracture after moderate to severe acquired brain injury. *Archives of Physical Medicine and Rehabilitation, 85,* 1465–1469. http://dx.doi.org/10.1016/j.apmr.2003.08.103

Smith-Gabai, H. (Ed.). (2011). *Occupational therapy in acute care.* Bethesda, MD: AOTA Press.

Stålhammar, D., & Starmark, J. E. (1986). Assessment of responsiveness in head injury patients: The Glasgow Coma Scale and some comments on alternative methods. *Acta Neurochirurgica, 36,* 91–94.

Stanczak, D. E., White, J. G., III, Gouview, W. D., Moehle, K. A., Daniel, M., Novack, T., & Long, C. J. (1984). Assessment of level of consciousness following severe neurological insult: A comparison of the psychometric qualities of the Glasgow Coma Scale and the Comprehensive Level of Consciousness Scale. *Journal of Neurosurgery, 60,* 955–960. http://dx.doi.org/10.3171/jns.1984.60.5.0955

Stern, J. M., Sazbon, L., Becker, E., & Costeff, H. (1988). Severe behavioural disturbance in families of patients with prolonged coma. *Brain Injury, 2,* 259–262. http://dx.doi.org/10.3109/02699058809150951

Stewart, D. G., Miller, M. A., & Cifu, D. X. (1998). The role of subacute rehabilitation services after brain injury. *NeuroRehabilitation, 10,* 13–23. http://dx.doi.org/10.1016/S1053-8135(97)00041-3

Teasdale, G., & Jennett, B. (1974). Assessment of coma and impaired consciousness: A practical scale. *Lancet, 2,* 81–84. http://dx.doi.org/10.1016/S0140-6736(74)91639-0

Tipton-Burton, M., McLaughlin, R., & Englander, J. (2013). Traumatic brain injury. In H. M. Pendleton & W. Schultz-Krohn (Eds.), *Pedretti's occupational therapy: Practice skills for physical dysfunction* (7th ed., pp. 881–915). St. Louis: Elsevier/Mosby.

Turner-Stokes, L. (Ed.). (2003). *Rehabilitation following acquired brain injury: National clinical guidelines*. London: Royal College of Physicians and British Society of Rehabilitation Medicine. Retrieved from http://bookshop.rcplondon.ac.uk/contents/43986815-4109-4d28-8ce5-ad647dbdbd38.pdf

Vanden Bossche, L., & Vanderstraeten, G. (2005). Heterotopic ossification: A review. *Journal of Rehabilitation Medicine, 37,* 129–136. http://dx.doi.org/10.1080/16501970510027628

Vangel, S. J., Jr., Rapport, L. J., & Hanks, R. A. (2011). Effects of family and caregiver psychosocial functioning on outcomes in persons with traumatic brain injury. *Journal of Head Trauma Rehabilitation, 26,* 20–29. http://dx.doi.org/10.1097/HTR.0b013e318204a70d

Verhaeghe, S. T., van Zuuren, F. J., Defloor, T., Duijnstee, M. S., & Grypdonck, M. H. (2007). The process and the meaning of hope for family members of traumatic coma patients in intensive care. *Qualitative Health Research, 17,* 730–743. http://dx.doi.org/10.1177/1049732307303242

Verhaeghe, S. T., van Zuuren, F. J., Grypdonck, M. H., Duijnstee, M. S., & Defloor, T. (2010a). The focus of family members' functioning in the acute phase of traumatic coma: Part one: The initial battle and protecting life. *Journal of Clinical Nursing, 19,* 574–582. http://dx.doi.org/10.1111/j.1365-2702.2009.02987.x

Verhaeghe, S. T., van Zuuren, F. J., Grypdonck, M. H., Duijnstee, M. S., & Defloor, T. (2010b). The focus of family members' functioning in the acute phase of traumatic coma: Part two: Protecting from suffering and protecting what remains to rebuild life. *Journal of Clinical Nursing, 19,* 583–589. http://dx.doi.org/10.1111/j.1365-2702.2009.02964.x

Whyte, J., Katz, D., Long, D., DiPasquale, M. C., Polansky, M., Kalmar, K., . . . Eifert, B. (2005). Predictors of outcome in prolonged posttraumatic disorders of consciousness and assessment of medication effects: A multicenter study. *Archives of Physical Medicine and Rehabilitation, 86,* 453–462. http://dx.doi.org/10.1016/j.apmr.2004.05.016

Whyte, J., Laborde, A., & DiPasquale, M. C. (1999). Assessment and treatment of the vegetative and minimally conscious patient. In M. Rosenthal, E. R. Griffith, J. S. Kreutzer, & B. Pentland (Eds.), *Rehabilitation of the adult and child with traumatic brain injury* (3rd ed., pp. 435–451). Philadelphia: F. A. Davis.

Whyte, J., & Nakase-Richardson, R. (2013). Disorders of consciousness: Outcomes, comorbidities, and care needs. *Archives of Physical Medicine and Rehabilitation, 94,* 1851–1854. http://dx.doi.org/10.1016/j.apmr.2013.07.003

Wijdicks, E. F. (2006). Clinical scales for comatose patients: The Glasgow Coma Scale in historical context and the new FOUR Score. *Reviews in Neurological Diseases, 3,* 109–117.

Wilson, S. L., Powell, G. E., Brock, D., & Thwaites, H. (1996). Vegetative state and responses to sensory stimulation: An analysis of 24 cases. *Brain Injury, 10,* 807–818. http://dx.doi.org/10.1080/026990596123927

Wilson, S. L., Powell, G. E., Elliott, K., & Thwaites, H. (1991). Sensory stimulation in prolonged coma: Four single case studies. *Brain Injury, 5,* 393–400. http://dx.doi.org/10.3109/02699059109008112

Wood, R. L., Winkowski, T. B., Miller, J. L., Tierney, L., & Goldman, L. (1992). Evaluating sensory regulation as a method to improve awareness in patients with altered states of consciousness: A pilot study. *Brain Injury, 6,* 411–418. http://dx.doi.org/10.3109/02699059209008137

Zablotny, C., Andric, M. F., & Gowland, C. (1987). Serial casting: Clinical applications for adult head-injured patients. *Journal of Head Trauma Rehabilitation, 2,* 46–52. http://dx.doi.org/10.1097/00001199-198706000-00007

CHAPTER 6

The Acute, Inpatient, and Subacute Rehabilitation Phases of Recovery

Marianne H. Mortera, PhD, OTR/L

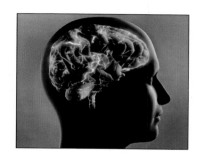

Learning Objectives

After completion of this chapter, readers will be able to

- Identify the issues common to patients at Rancho Los Amigos Levels of Cognitive Functioning (RLA LCF) IV through VI during acute, inpatient, and subacute rehabilitation;
- Identify evidence-based evaluation and intervention approaches to guide best practice for patients at RLA LCF IV through VI during acute, inpatient, and subacute rehabilitation;
- Identify observable behaviors indicating possible underlying impairment and assess activity and participation levels (*International Classification of Functioning, Disability and Health;* World Health Organization, 2001) throughout the patient's length of stay;
- Identify methods for coordinating care and resources with the patient's caregiver and family to enhance support systems for patients at RLA LCF IV through VI; and
- Identify the appropriate course of treatment relative to rehabilitation services along the care continuum.

Key Words

- **activity analysis**
- **activity synthesis**
- **aggression**
- **agitation**
- **behavior management**
- **frames of reference**
- **neurorehabilitation**
- **skilled observation**
- **Structured Functional Cognitive Assessment**
- **treatment principles**
- **underlying impairments**

Introduction

This chapter focuses on adult patients with **traumatic brain injury** (TBI) who are at Rancho Los Amigos Levels of Cognitive Functioning (RLA LCF) IV through VI and who receive occupational therapy in acute, inpatient, and subacute rehabilitation settings. Patients who are transitioning from an intensive care unit or a neurotrauma unit, who are medically stable, or who are emerging from **coma** may, depending on their tolerance for therapy services, be admitted to acute, inpatient, or subacute **rehabilitation**. As patients become more responsive to stimuli, the focus of acute and inpatient rehabilitation is, as much as possible, to enhance the process of neurological recovery. Occupational therapists typically begin working with patients by addressing movement control and basic **activities of daily living** (ADLs). Therapy services address the redevelopment of motor and self-care skills, compensatory training, and caregiver education and training.

To set the stage for an in-depth discussion of occupational therapy for patients in RLA LCF IV through VI, I first present core concepts regarding family needs and discharge planning that transcend Rancho levels. Next, I review the behaviors and functional levels associated with RLA LCF IV through VI. Patients at Level IV require special behavior and environmental management to ensure their safety as they progress toward more active engagement in rehabilitation. Therefore, I discuss the occupational therapy approach to behavior and environmental modification before the more in-depth presentation of occupational therapy evaluation and intervention. The chapter concludes with the continuation of the case example of Diane Archer.

Finally, it is worth noting that TBI rehabilitation services commonly use the language delineated by the *International Classification of Functioning, Disability and Health* (*ICF;* World Health Organization [WHO], 2001). Constantinidou, Wertheimer, Tsanadis, Evans, and Paul (2012) and Gutman, Mortera, Hinojosa, and Kramer (2007) discussed the need for rehabilitation professionals to use the common *ICF* terminology and to not only address impairment-level deficits but also evaluate and then address the ways in which **impairments** affect activity and participation and contextual components of the person's life. Because of their importance to interdisciplinary communication in TBI rehabilitation, I use the *ICF* concepts of *impairment, ability,* and *participation* in this chapter rather than the terminology of the *Occupational Therapy Practice Framework: Domain and Process* (3rd ed.; American Occupational Therapy Association, 2014).

Role of Family, Caregivers, and Significant Others

The effects of TBI go far beyond the patient and can have serious, life-changing consequences for family members, caregivers, or significant others. Family members are often present during the initial hospitalization and throughout rehabilitation, offering both help and support to the patient even as they experience their own grief and **stress.** Because of their essential contribution to the patient's recovery and return to the community, family members' needs are important to occupational therapists throughout the continuum of care. Providing information, resources, and support to the family and caregivers so that they are as well prepared for the future as possible is paramount, and it is a particular challenge under the constraints inherent in shortened lengths of stay, limited resources, and limited staff education and training in how best to work with families and caregivers of patients with TBI. Although therapists' initial concern is helping families deal with their loved one's experience in rehabilitation, concurrently assisting them in postdischarge planning is critical.

Providing sufficient, effective, and efficient family and caregiver education and training regarding the care of a loved one is a challenging task. Rehabilitation professionals can tackle that task by learning about available resources, providing opportunities for participation in the therapy process, and being available to answer questions and provide consistent emotional support. In addition, family

Providing sufficient, effective, and efficient family and caregiver education and training regarding the care of a loved one is a challenging task.

members and caregivers are the best resource for detailed and critical information about the patient's premorbid level of functioning, personality, idiosyncratic **habits** and lifestyle preferences, cultural and social background, and types of relationships before the injury. Information obtained from the family or caregivers should focus on the following considerations:

- The patient's sociocultural and environmental contexts and premorbid status or previous level of functioning
- The patient's role among family and friends
- The patient's education and work history
- The patient's premorbid ability to cope with life stressors and his or her motivation level
- The patient's current support system and who can and will be involved in the patient's immediate care while the patient is in rehabilitation
- Who might participate in the patient's therapy sessions to assist the patient when transitioning out of rehabilitation after discharge
- Available resources for long-term assistance with the patient's care.

In addition, the therapist needs to be acutely aware of how the TBI may be affecting the caregiver's and family's **coping** mechanisms and adaptive or maladaptive processes. The family and caregiver may be a tremendous help and support to the rehabilitation team or, if they are not coping well, may be in dire need of support themselves. Any negative effects that may affect the patient's ability to reach rehabilitation goals should be addressed quickly and in a highly supportive manner to best serve both the patient and the family and caregiver.

Caring for the patient after he or she leaves this phase of rehabilitation is often a source of concern and stress for the family and caregiver. Addressing these concerns and identifying resources for the family and caregiver are often at the forefront of case management. These issues and the process of decision making regarding discharge status depend on how the patient progresses through rehabilitation. Assisting and educating the family and caregiver in how to manage burden-of-care issues at the outset of rehabilitation may help ensure their ability to be present and to cope throughout the recovery process.

Discharge Planning

Discharge planning typically begins on the day of admission to the hospital or rehabilitation unit. Occupational therapists, along with the rest of the rehabilitation team, are always working to prepare the patient and family for optimal functioning and to transition to the next level of care. In acute care, it is often necessary to coordinate discharge plans soon after the initial evaluation process. Discharge planning is a complex decision-making process that involves the consideration of severity-related and socioeconomic factors (Cuthbert et al., 2011). If the patient is not expected to be transferred to either a subacute or an inpatient rehabilitation facility, the patient's anticipated home or discharge environment must be ascertained. The type of environment to which the patient will be discharged may have accessibility and safety challenges or constraints, so it is critical to gather information early in the process from the family or caregiver about the anticipated discharge environment. The necessary durable medical equipment (DME), additional types of adaptive equipment, and possible environmental modifications need to be addressed to ensure the most safe and accessible discharge environment for the patient and family or caregiver.

Discharge concerns will often dovetail with the issue of the patient's health care coverage and personal financial constraints. Typically, patients who are not catastrophically injured or who have a mild to moderate brain injury do not stay in the acute care setting very long, and so they are either sent to rehabilitation or go home to family. However, this situation can be problematic because patients are often discharged with cognitive deficits and may not be safe to be left alone. Coordinating with social services, case managers, and other rehabilitation professionals to plan appropriately for the patient's discharge from the acute care service is beneficial to account for any limitations or lack of resources and any issues regarding long-term care.

Patient Characteristics and Functioning at RLA LCF IV Through VI

In this section, I use the RLA LCF Scale (Hagen, Malkmus, & Durham, 1979) to describe characteristics and needs of patients with TBI who typically receive inpatient rehabilitation, subacute rehabilitation, or both. A revised 10-item version of the RLA LCF Scale (Hagen, 1998) is available at http://www.northeastcenter.com/rancho_los_amigos_revised.htm. However, the 8-item version remains the standard version used in clinical practice and is therefore used here.

Patients at Level III may be able to follow visual stimuli or turn toward or away from loud auditory stimuli but are totally dependent, and their responses are often purposeless or inconsistent (see Chapter 5). Patients at RLA LCF IV may engage in purposeless or unsafe movements and may also demonstrate physical or verbal aggression, confusion, and lack of understanding of their surroundings such that managing unsafe or dysregulated behaviors is an important concern in the acute, inpatient, and subacute phases of rehabilitation. As patients progress into Rancho Levels V and VI, they are increasingly able to respond appropriately to environmental stimuli and follow instructions and, therefore, to fully engage in the therapeutic process.

Patients who are at RLA LCF V (confused, inappropriate, nonagitated) typically present with the ability to attend for only several minutes at a time and are easily distracted (Hagen et al., 1979). They may be able to follow and respond to simple commands but may require cues and often have very low frustration tolerance. Patients may be able to relearn skills that they performed before the injury and engage in simple self-care tasks, but learning new information will be difficult. Patients at this level may need highly structured or step-by-step directions and maximum physical assistance to perform simple or familiar self-care tasks such as washing their face or simple bed mobility such as rolling or supine to sitting. **Attention** may steadily improve, but **memory** is still significantly impaired. Patients may begin to show awareness of self and others.

Increasing consistency of appropriate responses indicates that patients are moving into RLA LCF VI (confused and appropriate). They demonstrate improved ability to pay attention for short periods of time and demonstrate general recall for some events (e.g., a patient may remember that he had visitors this morning) but not for details (e.g., who visited and what was discussed). Patients are increasingly oriented to month and year and may appreciate physical problems but be unaware of problems associated with **cognition** or behavioral control. Patients at RLA LCF VI may be able to initiate simple or familiar self-care tasks such as washing the face or performing bed mobility tasks. Routine self-care tasks may become part of their progression in rehabilitation and may be performed with less structure, less guidance, or fewer cues to complete the tasks. See Table 1.3 in Chapter 1 for full descriptions of the typical behaviors seen at each level of the RLA LCF Scale (Hagen, 1998).

As indicated earlier, patients at RLA LCF IV have distinct rehabilitation needs for managing behavior and the environment to move through this stage as quickly and safely as possible. Management of these issues is discussed in the next section.

Patients at Rancho Los Amigos Levels of Cognitive Functioning IV

Patients at RLA LCF IV (confused, agitated) will typically present with challenging behaviors because they are hypersensitive to internal and environmental stimuli (Hagen et al., 1979). The most typical behaviors include increased agitation, aggression, nonpurposeful motor actions, **mood** swings, incoherent verbalizations, and brief moments of attention (Box 6.1).

Patients with TBI present with many challenges as they progress through the various stages of neurological recovery. The objectives of the occupational therapist and the rehabilitation team are to facilitate the patient's recovery process by (1) providing a positive and safe environment for the patient, caregiver, and staff; (2) minimizing any potential triggers for aggressive or agitated behaviors; and (3) preparing the patient for active participation in the rehabilitation process.

Sandel and Mysiw (1996) defined *posttraumatic agitation* as agitation that occurs during the early stages of recovery from a TBI and that is characterized by delirium and excesses of behavior such as aggression, restlessness, or disinhibition. They found agitation in 86% of patients in the acute setting and in 70% of patients admitted to rehabilitation. Agitation was found to limit the patient's ability to participate in rehabilitation and was associated with lower functional outcomes.

Box 6.1. Rancho Los Amigos Levels of Cognitive Functioning IV (Confused, Agitated)

The following are observable behaviors that describe the patient at Level IV:

- Is alert and in heightened state of activity
- Makes purposeful attempts to remove restraints or tubes or crawl out of bed
- May perform motor activities such as sitting, reaching, and walking but without any apparent purpose or on another's request
- Has very brief and usually nonpurposeful moments of sustained attention and divided attention
- Has absent **short-term memory**
- May cry out or scream out of proportion to stimulus even after its removal
- May exhibit aggressive or flight behavior
- May swing from euphoric to hostile mood with no apparent relationship to environmental events
- Is unable to cooperate with treatment efforts
- Has verbalizations that are frequently incoherent, inappropriate to activity or environment, or both.

The rehabilitation team must focus on several goals with the patient at Rancho Level IV. The primary aims are to continue to assess the patient's ability to respond to stimuli and ensure patient safety. Therapists attempt to actively manage environmental stimuli (i.e., type and level of external stimuli) to decrease the potential for patient distress or behavioral dysregulation.

A longer duration of agitation was associated with a longer length of stay, longer duration of **posttraumatic amnesia** (PTA), and lower functional scores for cognition and motor functions (Sandel & Mysiw, 1996).

Assessing Agitation

Occupational therapists and others use various methods, such as observation, to assess challenging behaviors in patients recovering from TBI, which may involve use of a standardized tool.

Occupational therapists and others use various methods, such as observation, to assess challenging behaviors in patients recovering from TBI, which may involve use of a standardized tool. For example, the Agitated Behavior Scale (Corrigan, 1989) is a normed and standardized observation measure that was developed for use by rehabilitation staff to objectively assess a patient's behaviors in delineated time periods (e.g., a therapist's 30-minute observation period or a nurse's 8-hour shift). It can be used routinely across all shifts to obtain a picture of a patient's performance in all settings and situations on the unit. Disinhibition, aggression, and lability are assessed on a 4-point rating scale. Nott, Chapparo, and Baguley (2006) used documented observations of patient behaviors from health care and rehabilitation staff to develop operational definitions for an extensive list of agitated behaviors. Examples include restlessness or excessive movements, wandering, disinhibition, low tolerance to pain or frustration, combativeness, verbal aggression or screaming, unpredictable **anger,** self-abuse, **emotional lability,** loud or excessive talking, inappropriate gestures or verbalizations, and verbal or motor **perseverations.**

Intervention for Agitation: Behavior Management

Intensive intervention to address agitation requires both therapeutic environments and well-trained rehabilitation staff to protect the health and safety of patients and others (Beaulieu et al., 2008). Environments should be created to minimize agitation and to facilitate the patient's positive or constructive behaviors. However, Beaulieu et al. underscored how difficult it is to implement such an environment. A behavior management training program was provided to rehabilitation staff and then examined for effectiveness with respect to treatment with medication as needed, use of physical restraints, and level of agitation. The training resulted in only a temporary decrease in use of physical restraints. Limitations in how the training program was implemented may have been a factor in the program's limited effectiveness. Beaulieu et al. concluded that the training of rehabilitation staff and the design of therapeutic environments to decrease agitation in patients with TBI are highly complex processes and serious challenges.

As patients show a decrease in agitation behaviors, an intervention such as positive behavior supports (PBS; Ylvisaker, Turkstra, & Coelho, 2005) may be used to address behavioral issues. PBS differs from traditional applied behavioral analysis (ABA). *ABA*, described in detail shortly, involves the use of consequence-based interventions, whereas *PBS* is used to modify patient behavior by providing **antecedent** supports that may influence behavior (Ylvisaker et al., 2005). Another feature of PBS is that it creates a shift from a largely medical, impairment-oriented rehabilitation paradigm to a social participation and support-oriented paradigm (Ylvisaker, Jacobs, & Feeney, 2003), which is congruent with the revisions of WHO's (2001) *ICF.*

The PBS method requires careful recording of behaviors. In the first step of this approach, the team tries to identify what the patient is attempting to communicate.

Although environmental factors may trigger an outburst, the patient's physical state may contribute to challenging behaviors. Is the patient hungry, tired, or in pain? Has he or she been toileted recently? Has his or her personal space inadvertently been violated during routine care? Any of these situations could trigger an agitated or aggressive response. The team, after consideration of possible triggers, then attempts to remove or ameliorate the effects of such triggers whenever possible (i.e., modify the environment). If agitation or aggression persists in the absence of obvious triggers, the team outlines a behavioral program suited to the patient's cognitive ability.

ABA principles are based in the use of positive and negative consequences as a method to deliberately manage behavior. In an ABA approach, the team first identifies patient behaviors to be targeted by the program. Usually, the psychologist or neuropsychologist develops the plan, involving the patient and other caregivers whenever possible. *Positive reinforcers* are often desirable consequences of specific behaviors that increase the frequency of that behavior in the future (e.g., watching a favorite video, listening to favorite music, having a food treat). *Negative reinforcers* are often the removal of something the patient finds undesirable. Methods used to decrease the probability of a given behavior being exhibited again include extinction procedures such as time-outs, which involve the removal of social reinforcement or attention. Other techniques include *negative punishment,* when something desirable to the patient is removed (e.g., loss of TV-viewing or music-listening privileges), or *positive punishment,* when an undesirable consequence follows a behavior. There has been a recent shift away from the use of contingency management strategies typical of the 1980s to more proactive antecedent-focused strategies (Ylvisaker et al., 2007) partly because of the increased evidence that damage to the ventral portions of the **frontal lobe** results in difficulty with consequence-based learning in patients with TBI (Damasio, 1994; Schlund, 2002).

The occupational therapist also needs to consider the effect of the environment on the patient at RLA LCF IV. Creating a safe, albeit prosthetic, environment for patients is of central importance, and many TBI units are designed with this purpose in mind. Surroundings must be reorienting and calming. Patients are provided with an easy-to-understand schedule of activities. Because some patients in this phase present an elopement risk, both PBS and ABA strategies can be incorporated into behavior management. Depending on the state in which facilities are located, it may be possible to house such patients on a locked unit. Where this is not an option, facilities use sensors, typically in the form of a wrist or ankle bracelet, that trigger an alarm if the patient attempts to leave the building. Many centers use a system of around-the-clock, one-to-one companions for patients with challenging behaviors. One-to-one observation, often provided by nursing assistants, means that a staff member accompanies the patient at all times to all activities and is also present at the patient's bedside.

Addressing Orientation as Patients Transition to RLA LCF V

As patients transition from RLA LCF IV to RLA LCF V, they may be less combative and increasingly verbal and yet may continue to be disoriented, wander, and be an inadvertent danger to themselves. **Orientation** generally refers to patients' awareness of time, place, and person and knowledge of their current circumstances and of recent events. Patients at Rancho Level V are likely to be markedly disoriented, and the occupational therapist and rehabilitation team will frequently assess their level of orientation.

The Galveston Orientation and Amnesia Test (Levin, O'Donnell, & Grossman, 1979) is a 10-question test used to assess orientation and PTA in patients with TBI. The items assess orientation to person, place, time, and recall of events both preceding and following the injury. The Confusion Assessment Protocol (Sherer, 2004) is a combination of tests that assess orientation, cognition, and the early stages of confusion in patients with TBI. It assesses seven key symptoms of posttraumatic confusion: (1) disorientation, (2) cognitive impairment, (3) fluctuation of presentation, (4) restlessness, (5) nighttime sleep disturbance, (6) decreased daytime **arousal,** and (7) psychosis-like symptoms.

Yuen and Benzing (1996) suggested a strategy called *cognitive set change through preorientation* that is used to direct a patient to engage in a task of interest if the patient is confused and preoccupied with an event that is not leading to productive performance. For example, a patient may repeatedly state that he just wants to go home and is subsequently not interested in participating in a feeding task. Asking simple questions or providing visual cues about the upcoming task a few minutes ahead of time will help the patient transition from one cognitive set to another. About 5 to 10 minutes before a feeding task, for example, the therapist can use preorientation as a method to gradually change the patient's cognitive set by talking about what they will do during the feeding task and perhaps showing the patient pictures of what the patient will eat. The occupational therapist can then follow up by orienting the patient to the time of 12:00 noon and that lunch will be served shortly. This strategy gradually shifts the patient's thoughts from going home to engaging in the feeding task and can be used to avoid directly confronting a patient. (Further information about assessments that address expected behaviors at RLA LCF V may be found at the Center for Outcome Measurement in Brain Injury website at http://www.tbims.org/combi/list.html.)

Evaluation of Patients With Traumatic Brain Injury in Acute, Inpatient, and Subacute Rehabilitation

Patients recovering from TBI typically do not make dramatic improvements from one RLA level to the next; rather, they demonstrate a great deal of variability hour by hour such that patients often function at more than one RLA level during a given day or week. Therefore, the remainder of this chapter provides guidance for occupational therapy assessment and intervention that generally pertains to patients with TBI at RLA LCF IV to VI in acute medical, inpatient rehabilitation, and subacute rehabilitation settings. After outlining some background considerations, I present information about occupational therapy assessment with a particular emphasis on observation of functional performance, followed by an in-depth discussion of intervention principles and methods.

Initial Concerns and Background Information

A more formalized or standardized evaluation process may be difficult in the acute care stage of recovery given the challenging behavior of patients at RLA LCF IV. The evaluation of such patients must be based on keen observation of responses to stimuli presented to them, and the therapist must also consider environmental conditions and contexts. Patients will have difficulty processing multiple types of environmental stimuli, and their observed responses may or may not be specific or relevant to the type of stimuli.

Early in the assessment process, it is important to identify the patient's pre-TBI and current post-TBI medical status. The therapist should identify injuries that were coincident with the TBI (e.g., fractures, cranial nerve injuries) and any medical conditions associated with the TBI as well as current medications and their potential side effects. Gathering information from the family or caregiver as well as from other rehabilitation staff is critical to the occupational therapy evaluation.

The evaluation of patients at RLA LCF IV must be based on keen observation of responses to stimuli presented to them, and the therapist must also consider environmental conditions and contexts.

Problem Identification

Hinojosa, Kramer, and Crist (2005); Laver-Fawcett (2007); and Mosey (1986) defined the initial *problem identification phase* of any **frame of reference,** or set of guidelines for practice, as the phase in which a patient's status is evaluated using skilled observation of all the areas relative to that patient's unique set of impairments, potential sparing of skills, and how the impairments will affect the patient's ultimate ability to function in his or her sociocultural and environmental contexts. It is important to recognize that at the acute, inpatient, or subacute stage of rehabilitation, evaluation of patients with TBI is not a one-size-fits-all process because the impairments that occur with TBI are highly variable (Hinojosa et al., 2005; Laver-Fawcett, 2007; Toglia & Golisz, 2012). For example, occupational therapists may rely on observation of performance for patients who are not yet able to follow the instructions for formal, standardized assessments. The therapist may use a simple ADL task such as basic bed mobility or face washing as a means of assessing for potential underlying impairments such as decreased **range of motion** (ROM) in the trunk and limbs or poor attention to the task. Subsequently, the therapist may assess the patient at the activity or participation level while considering the patient's contexts to gain a more comprehensive overview of how the patient's underlying impairments affect his or her overall functional status and, ultimately, **quality of life** (Ylvisaker, 2003). As the patient progresses through RLA LCF V and VI, he or she increasingly will be able to participate in more formal or standardized assessment procedures.

Observation Skills

Observation data are highly subjective (Hinojosa et al., 2005; Laver-Fawcett, 2007; Ottenbacher & Tomchek, 1993; Suen & Ary, 1989) and lack reliability. It is important to understand that any observation of behavior contains a degree of subjective bias. When observing a patient at RLA LCF IV or V with significant cognitive impairment, the occupational therapist should present stimuli in a consistent manner to ensure that any changes in how a patient responds to a particular stimulus (e.g., a change in the ability to direct gaze to a visual stimulus or the ability to respond appropriately to a simple command) is a result of a change in the patient's ability, not a change in the way in which the stimulus was presented.

In TBI rehabilitation, especially with patients classified at RLA LCF IV or V, impairments such as abnormal muscle **tone,** poor sitting balance, or poor attention may be operationally defined in terms of observable behaviors. These behaviors are critical in the initial evaluation phase because they can indicate the baseline level of

Improvement or change in observable behavior is interpreted as a manifestation of the change in the underlying impairment that is then documented as the patient progresses.

severity of various underlying impairments. Improvement or change in observable behavior is interpreted as a manifestation of the change in the underlying impairment that is then documented as the patient progresses. Behaviors that may reflect patients' underlying impairment take various forms in terms of what is physically seen, said, heard, or touched by the therapist. Therefore, the therapist should note any patient actions, words, physical signs, or other distinguishing observable behaviors (Mosey, 1986).

For example, the therapist may determine the level of severity of impaired attention by noting the number of seconds or minutes a patient attends to a visual stimulus. A therapist who observes a patient attending to a visual stimulus for 10 seconds on Day 1 and 60 seconds on Day 3 may document the improvement as a change in the level of severity of decreased attention—an objectively defined measure of the behavior that operationally defines *attention*. As another example, a patient may be observed to pull at tubes or lines and loudly yell obscenities—behaviors that are observable and can be clearly documented or noted. The therapist may take these behaviors as an indication that the patient is in a state of agitation or displaying verbal aggression and has a potential impairment in behavioral inhibition. The observation of various behaviors should be noted relative to their duration and the type of environmental stimuli that are present at the time of the behaviors.

The therapist's observation of the behaviors typical of each of the Rancho levels allows for the documentation of progress during rehabilitation. The therapist should determine what specific impairments may be affecting the patient's activity or participation level or functional performance. The patient who progresses from 5 to 10 minutes of unsupported sitting is showing improvement in balance skills, which may then affect his or her ability to show improvement in dressing at the edge of the bed while sitting unsupported. Documenting observable behaviors that indicate improvement in underlying skills that may be affecting functional performance can clarify the patient's progress for the rehabilitation team and family. Structured and objective observations are critical to adequately document a patient's change in status at both the impairment and the activity or participation levels. Later in the chapter, strategies for assessing cognition in the context of observations of functional performance are further discussed.

Assessing Underlying Impairments and Performance Skills

The therapist must first assess TBI-related impairments in the following categories: visual, cognitive–perceptual, motor–physical, sensory, and psychosocial skills, either through informal observation or by means of nonstandardized or standardized assessments at the impairment and activity or participation levels. When assessing impairments that may affect the patient's performance during ADLs, the therapist notes the level of physical or cognitive assistance needed to successfully complete an ADL task. Table 6.1 lists the skills or capacities that are typically assessed in a patient with TBI during the initial evaluation phase of acute rehabilitation and subsequently during inpatient or subacute rehabilitation.

Evaluation of Underlying Impairments

Various assessments are used to determine the patient's baseline status. The assessments described in this section can provide information on the skills and

Table 6.1. Evaluation of Underlying Capacities and Skills

Capacity–Skill Area	Areas to Evaluate
Motor	• ROM • Muscle strength • Muscle tone • Coordination (gross and fine) • Balance and postural reflexes or postural control
Sensory	• Touch • Pain and temperature • **Proprioception** and kinesthesia • Fine discrimination (**stereognosis,** 2-point discrimination, graphesthesia)
Vision	• Oculomotor control (ROM) • Vision reception (acuity) • Visual light reflexes • Visual fields
Perception	• Form constancy • Spatial relationships • Praxis • Figure–ground • Depth perception • Right–left discrimination • Neglect syndromes
Cognition	• Sustained attention • Shifting attention • Concentration • Orientation • Memory (short-term, long-term, retrospective, prospective) • Planning • Organization • Problem solving • Judgment • Insight, awareness of disability • Executive functions
Psychosocial	• Self-concept • Coping skills • Interpersonal skills • Inhibition • Self-control

Note. ROM = range of motion.

capacities discussed in the preceding section. The therapist should establish that the patient is able to understand simple commands and follow simple one- or two-step verbal or demonstrated directions and determine whether the patient is able to participate in the evaluation. Depending on the patient's ability to participate, the therapist will need to determine the extent to which test administration is feasible and how much of each test should be administered given the patient's level of functioning.

Vision Functions

Vision impairments are a frequent consequence of TBI (see Chapter 2). These impairments may include double vision, blurred vision, **visual-field** cuts, or headache resulting from eye strain. Occupational therapists typically screen for vision impairments and refer patients to an ophthalmologist for more definitive evaluation (Gutman & Schonfeld, 2009). *Neuro-ophthalmologists* are ophthalmologists who specialize in the diagnosis and treatment of neurological impairments of the visual system. They understand the medical and surgical support required for problems such as strabismus and are often aware of nonsurgical and pharmacological therapies for **vision rehabilitation.** Optometrists who specialize in vision therapy are trained in the diagnosis and nonsurgical treatment of complex fixation, eye-movement, or *eye-teaming* (i.e., binocular vision) disorders and in perceptual impairments of the visual system. Some optometrists who specialize in low vision evaluation prescribe low vision aids for patients with reduced visual acuity and field expanders for patients with visual-field impairments. Optometrists typically work closely with the occupational therapist or low vision rehabilitation specialist on a vision therapy program, which may include teaching the patient new living and mobility skills to compensate for visual impairments.

Occupational therapists typically assess both the sensory and the motor functions that may affect visual ability. Visual processing can be disrupted because of mechanical damage to the eye and surrounding musculature, damage to the cranial nerves supplying the oculomotor pathways controlling the muscles of the eye, damage to the visual receptive pathway, damage to the visual reflex pathways, disruption of sensory–perceptual function of the eye, or damage to the areas of the cortex responsible for vision functions. Vision sensory assessments start with the visual receptive pathway (cranial nerve II) that carries initial visual receptive information, also known as *acuity,* as well as information or stimuli received from the periphery. These assessments include a basic visual acuity test such as the Snellen test and the confrontation test to evaluate for visual-field deficits in all four visual-field quadrants, incorporating the bilateral, superior, and inferior peripheral areas. Additional vision screens may include a contrast sensitivity test to evaluate for acuity (Gutman & Schonfeld, 2009). It is important that the environment be conducive to valid testing, for example, providing adequate lighting and allowing the patient to use reading glasses when assessing acuity (Gutman & Schonfeld, 2009).

Next, occupational therapists evaluate the vision pathways (cranial nerve III pathways) that mediate the contraction of the pupillary sphincter, resulting in pupillary constriction; the medial recti muscles, resulting in medial eye movement, or **convergence;** and the ciliary muscles of the lens, resulting in **accommodation,** all for the purpose of focusing a near image on the retina (Gutman & Schonfeld, 2009; Nolte, 2009).

The pupillary light reflex response is assessed by noting how quickly and symmetrically the patient's pupils constrict when a penlight is shone into one and then the other eye. The presence of pupillary constriction is first noted in each eye separately. The consensual light reflex response (which results from the bilateral connection of the cranial nerve III reflex pathways for pupillary constriction; Nolte, 2009) is assessed by shining the light into one eye and noting pupillary constriction in the other eye.

The coordinated bilateral adduction of the eyes is important for binocular vision. ***Diplopia*** (i.e., double vision) can result if the extrinsic muscles of one eye are weaker than those of the other eye, resulting in a failure to converge on a single object. Light reflected from the object falls on different areas of the retina, which then activates the visual cortex, and two images are perceived rather than one (Blumenfeld, 2010). While convergence is being tested, the therapist notes the presence of the simultaneous action of the cranial nerve III pathway activating the pupillary sphincter, which causes bilateral pupillary constriction. Occurring simultaneously with convergence and pupillary constriction is accommodation for near focus of the eyes, which is controlled by an additional cranial nerve III pathway to the ciliary body that regulates the lens of the eye for near focus (Nolte, 2009).

The final vision screen assesses the oculomotor pathways for vision (cranial nerves III, IV, and VI). Eye ROM is tested using a target and evaluating whether the patient is able to follow the target with one and then both eyes. Other areas involving eye ROM and strength are tested, such as *visual fixation* (i.e., the ability to hold a stationary gaze), *visual **saccades*** (i.e., the ability to track a target in unpredictable areas of the visual field), and *visual scanning* (i.e., the ability to follow an object in a smooth and continuous path), which allows for skills such as reading (Gutman & Schonfeld, 2009).

A basic vision screen provides the initial evaluation of the foundation visual skills that then form the bases for higher level visual–perceptual skills and cognition. After a basic vision screen, testing of various visual–perceptual areas may be indicated. The Brain Injury Visual Assessment Battery for Adults (biVABA), developed by Mary Warren (1998), consists of standardized assessments that evaluate foundation visual skills (visual acuity, contrast sensitivity, visual fields, pupillary responses, ocular ROM) and visual–perceptual skills. The biVABA is a comprehensive assessment and can be used in treatment planning and determining rehabilitation potential.

Attention Functions

The evaluation of basic attention functions starts with level of alertness and progresses through the ability to perform tasks involving divided attention or high-level **concentration**. The evaluation of attention requires a clear understanding of the theoretical constructs that form the bases for the various types of attention when assessing patients with TBI. Attention testing is often followed by a basic screening of the patient's orientation status or ability to be oriented to person, place, and time. Attention testing is also linked to visual functions because of the attentional system's role in directing a person's visual gaze or visually orienting to a stimulus in the environment (Blumenfeld, 2010).

Attentional impairments may manifest in many ways. Patients may exhibit distractibility, impulsivity, and hypersensitivity to stimuli. Such patients may be distracted by and fail to habituate to external stimuli (i.e., the activities in the intervention area, a noise from outside) or internal stimuli (i.e., the patient's own thoughts, hunger, discomfort), and they may be unable to sustain focus on an activity. Initially, therapy may be provided in a distraction-free environment such as the patient's room or a low-stimulation intervention room, if one is available.

Memory Functions

The evaluation of memory is partially dependent on the patient's ability to attend for even a short period of time. Without adequate attention, information may not be encoded, so what is being assessed is not storage or retrieval ability but rather the failure to encode (i.e., attend). The therapist can tailor the evaluation of retrospective or **prospective memory** functions on the basis of what previously stored information the patient is able to retrieve through the use of strategies or associations. The patient's ability to use strategies to retrieve information should be assessed in terms of how successful the ability to recall information is and why. The patient's use of strategies to recall information becomes just as, if not more, important to the evaluation of memory functions than what the patient actually recalls. For example, information that is meaningful, motivating, familiar, or significant may be more easily recalled than more mundane or less significant personal events. (For a discussion of the various types of memory functions, see Chapter 3.)

Several standardized assessments of memory are available. The Contextual Memory Test (Toglia, 1993a) is extremely useful because it directly assesses the patient's ability to recall 20 objects (in both immediate and delayed conditions) and includes a section designed to evaluate patients' awareness of their memory capacity in which patients are asked to predict how well they will be able to recall the necessary information and estimate how well they actually performed. Another standardized memory test is the Rivermead Behavioural Memory Test–Extended (Wilson, Cockburn, & Baddeley, 1991). The tasks in this test include remembering a name, remembering a hidden belonging, remembering an appointment, and recognizing pictures and faces. It was designed to predict which patients are likely to experience everyday memory problems and is *ecologically valid* (i.e., predictive of a patient's behavior in a variety of real-world settings) and functionally oriented (i.e., test items include functional tasks).

Perceptual Functions

For each patient, the therapist determines whether to formally evaluate perceptual or sensory deficits as well as what approach is most appropriate (which may include the evaluations discussed here). Because perceptual processes are multifaceted and highly integrated, the evaluation of perception is often a challenge. The therapist may start by assessing a patient's ability to perform a simple self-care task; problems observed in a patient's ADL performance may suggest the need for more in-depth perceptual or sensory testing. It is important to bear in mind that if a patient is presenting with difficulty in basic attention or sensory functions, attempts to engage the patient in perceptual testing may be premature. Basic skills such as the initial reception of somatosensory, visual, or auditory stimuli and sustaining a basic level of arousal or attention need to be intact for the patient to process more integrated perceptual skills such as spatial processing, visual–perceptual processing, or visual memory processing (Árnadóttir, 1990; Blumenfeld, 2010).

Perception is the ability to organize sensory input into meaningful patterns that emerge from increasingly integrated levels of processing that form a perceptual whole.

Perception involves the integration of all initial receptive and subsequent integrative processing of sensory modalities—somatosensory, visual, auditory, olfactory, and gustatory senses—starting with primary receptive processing of these basic senses, progressing to the secondary or interpretive modes of processing, and then finally to the tertiary level or integration of all these senses, resulting in a perceptual whole (Árnadóttir, 1990; Blumenfeld, 2010). Therefore, a basic definition of *perception* is the ability to organize sensory input into meaningful patterns that emerge from increasingly integrated levels of processing that form a perceptual whole (Blumenfeld, 2010). Additionally, the integration of meaningful sensory inputs is also affected by other parallel processes such as the influence of the right hemisphere on nonverbal spatial concepts and the influence of the left hemisphere on verbal or language-driven concepts.

Table 6.2. Conceptual Definitions of Perceptual Skills and Impairments

Perceptual Skills	Definitions
Spatial Skills	
Position in space or spatial relations	The ability to distinguish features or position of objects relative to one another and oneself
Right–left discrimination	The ability to distinguish one side from the other and the right from the left
Topographical orientation	The ability to distinguish location of physical landmarks or settings and routes to and from various locations
Visual–Perceptual Skills	
Visual attention	The ability to sustain focus on a visual stimulus
Depth perception	The ability to distinguish relative distances between objects; requires intact binocular vision
Figure–ground discrimination	The ability to distinguish foreground from background
Visual closure	The ability to identify forms or objects from an incomplete array of features or stimuli
Visual–motor integration	The ability to coordinate information from the visual system with body movements during an activity or task
Praxis Skills	
Ideational praxis	The ability to understand motor demands and the characteristics needed to perform a task using motor plans
Ideomotor praxis	The ability to initiate and execute a motor plan from a stored memory engram
Perceptual Impairments	**Definitions**
Right-hemisphere neglect syndromes	The inability to attend to sensory stimuli in the left visual or somatosensory hemispace; manifested as visual neglect, hemisensory neglect syndrome, or left inattention
Agnosia	The inability to attach meaning to stimuli in a single modality (e.g., **prosopagnosia** is the inability to recognize what should be familiar faces)

The pencil-and-paper testing typically used in occupational therapy evaluation of perceptual skills (e.g., form constancy, spatial relationships, praxis, figure–ground, depth perception, right–left discrimination, visual–motor integration, neglect syndromes; see Table 6.2) may not capture how these deficits affect the patient's ability to perform real-world ADL tasks. The following assessments have been developed and tested for the evaluation of a variety of perceptual deficits and are primarily pencil-and-paper or tabletop tests with sound psychometrics.

The Occupational Therapy Adult Perceptual Screening Test (Cooke, McKenna, & Fleming, 2005; Cooke, McKenna, Fleming, & Darnell, 2005) comprises seven subscales in the areas of **agnosia,** visuospatial relations, **unilateral neglect,** constructional skills, **apraxia,** acalculia, and functional skills (Brown & Jäckel, 2007) and has moderate to high interrater reliability and internal consistency ($r = .5–.75$). The Ontario Society of Occupational Therapists Perceptual Evaluation–Revised (Boys, Fisher, & Holzberg, 1991) evaluates sensory and perceptual impairment in areas such as sensory function, scanning, apraxia, spatial awareness, and visual agnosia (Brown & Jäckel, 2007). It was demonstrated to have high interrater reliability ($r = .93$) and internal consistency ($r = .90$; Boys, Fisher, Holzberg, & Reid, 1988).

The **Structured Functional Cognitive Assessment** (SFCA; Mortera, 2004) method is a performance-based and ecologically valid mode of perceptual evaluation and is discussed later in this chapter. This assessment differs from the ones discussed earlier because the focus is to assess the patient during the actual completion of an ADL task rather than with a pencil-and-paper or tabletop task.

Cognitive Self-Awareness

An understanding of the degree to which patients are aware or in **denial** of their disability is crucial in intervention planning and outcome. A significant proportion of adults with TBI demonstrate a lack of awareness of their impairments. The therapist must determine how aware patients are of their impairments and how their self-perceptions match those of their family and clinicians. A lack of awareness may be indicated by behaviors demonstrating that patients are unable to determine whether their disability will have any effect on their ability to perform various ADLs. Denial may be noted when patients appear to be aware of the negative effects of their disability on their performance of ADLs yet continue to say that they can perform them without difficulty. Although patients emerging from Rancho Level IV to Rancho Level V may start to respond to redirection in therapy, they typically lack awareness of what has happened to them and how their functioning has been altered. Because occupational therapists and other team members want to set realistic goals in collaboration with their patients, it is important to get a clear idea of how a lack of self-awareness may affect such an endeavor.

Sherer et al. (2003) examined early predictors of self-awareness after TBI by comparing patient self-ratings to clinician ratings. They found that early impaired self-awareness was predicted by age and functional status (as determined by **FIM™** total score) at admission to inpatient rehabilitation. Clinician, family, and significant other ratings of patient functioning were correlated with each other but were not related to patient self-ratings.

Fisher and Short-DeGraff (1993) examined the relationship among self-awareness, ability to set realistic goals, performance in a cognitive task, and rehabilitation outcome. Self-awareness of patients with brain injuries was measured by direct clinician ratings and the difference between patient and staff ratings on a questionnaire. The study findings indicated that an instrument such as the Canadian Occupational Performance Measure (COPM; Law et al., 2014) may be difficult to use effectively with patients with TBI whose awareness is impaired because the COPM requires a broad awareness of current functioning and how patient performance differs from before the injury.

The 18-item Awareness Questionnaire (Sherer, Bergloff, Boake, High, & Levin, 1998) is a self-report assessment that may also be administered by the family and clinician on which patient and family or clinician scores are compared. The patient's self-awareness is determined by subtracting the family's or clinician's score from the patient's score; this difference ranges from −68 to 68. A difference of more than 20 indicates an impairment in the patient's self-awareness.

Motor Functions

The evaluation of motor function in patients with TBI usually begins by evaluating active and **passive ROM** (PROM). It is also important to grossly assess patients' ability to demonstrate any functional use of the upper extremities such as reaching overhead or to the side, proximal to distal use, bilateral hand use, and functional hand use such as gross grasp and various prehension patterns. Joint integrity and joint alignment are also evaluated to determine whether any biomechanical deficits may need immediate attention, such as soft-tissue tightness, abnormal posturing of a limb, **subluxation,** or pain. If indicated, manual muscle testing can be performed to evaluate muscle strength. Muscle tone is also evaluated relative to how it may affect joint alignment, the quality of any active motion in the trunk or limbs, and whether any resultant **spasticity** is causing pain. The therapist should also assess for pain that may be elicited by other causes. Depending on the extent of motor deficits, patients should be evaluated for any impairment in gross motor or fine motor coordination and speed and dexterity. It is critical to evaluate the patient's balance in several positions and conditions: seated supported, seated unsupported, standing supported, and standing unsupported. Both static and dynamic balance should be evaluated because these skills will affect the patient's safety and performance of ADLs.

Somatosensory Functions

Depending on how well and to what extent patients are able to process and respond to incoming somatosensory stimuli, somatosensory tests should be performed. These tests evaluate patients' reception of tactile senses (light touch, pressure sensitivity, and vibration), pain and temperature, proprioception and kinesthesia, and fine discrimination (stereognosis and graphesthesia). It is important to identify which somatosensory modalities are affected and to what extent. Somatosensory functions are highly integrated and have a significant influence over motor control and motor movement patterns. For example, a patient with impaired lower-extremity proprioception may demonstrate difficulty with stand–pivot transfers or ambulation and may need to use vision to locate the lower limbs in space. Additionally, when impaired proprioception coexists with cognitive impairments in areas such as attention, awareness, or recall, patients' safety may be compromised. Tactile sensory functions, coupled with other sensory modalities, provide the patient with critical information to drive motor output. Obtaining a solid baseline of somatosensory impairments and determining the possible coexistence of other cognitive impairments will assist in planning safe participation in ADLs.

> **Somatosensory functions are highly integrated and have a significant influence over motor control and motor movement patterns.**

Batteries That Assess Multiple Cognitive–Perceptual Domains

Some occupational therapists prefer using assessment batteries that screen for impairments across an array of cognitive and perceptual domains. The Loewenstein Occupational Therapy Cognitive Assessment (Katz, Itzkovich, Averbuch, & Elazar, 1989) is a battery of tests that evaluate the areas of orientation, visual perception, spatial perception, praxis, visuomotor organization, and thinking operations. It has high interrater reliability ($r = .82–.97$) and demonstrated construct, criterion, predictive, and ecological validity (Cooke & Finkelstein, 2007). The Cognitive Assessment of Minnesota (Rustad et al., 1993) comprises 17 subtests ranging from simple to complex that assess a wide range of cognitive skills including attention, memory, visual neglect, mathematics, ability to follow directions, problem solving, and judgment. It has demonstrated internal consistency ($r = .94$) and test–retest reliability ($r = .96$) as well as content and concurrent validity (Cooke & Finkelstein, 2007). The Montreal Cognitive Assessment (Nasreddine et al., 2005) assesses eight cognitive areas: (1) attention and concentration, (2) **executive functions,** (3) memory, (4) language, (5) visuospatial skills, (6) conceptual thinking, (7) calculations, and (8) orientation. It has demonstrated test–retest reliability ($r = .92$) and construct validity ($r = .87$; Cooke & Finkelstein, 2007).

Occupational Therapy Evaluation of Activities of Daily Living

Occupational therapists often use a priori knowledge of what underlying skills—motor, sensory, visual, or cognitive—are required to successfully complete various

ADL tasks. This knowledge stems from performing an activity analysis of ADL tasks and subsequently forming hypotheses about which task components may be associated with underlying impairments that may follow TBI. Therapists then use this assessment to determine what impairments may be interfering with patients' ability to perform an ADL task successfully. Once impairments are identified, therapists may subsequently follow up with more in-depth assessment of those impairment areas if necessary.

Occupational therapists assess basic ADLs both to determine how impairments are affecting functional performance and to assess the patient's functional status and burden of care. Not only can observing the patient perform activities such as washing the face at the bedside be important in evaluation, but this activity may be used as a treatment modality in working on the patient's ability to follow directions, use either an unaffected or affected upper extremity, attend to the functional task, and maintain postural control. The therapeutic use of ADLs as a treatment modality for the purpose of improving an identified impairment may be meaningful to the patient. The ADL areas typically assessed in TBI rehabilitation at the acute, inpatient, and subacute levels of care are listed in Table 6.3.

The FIM is a valid and reliable tool used with inpatient rehabilitation populations including people with TBI (Corrigan, Smith-Knapp, & Granger, 1997; Granger, Hamilton, Linacre, Heinemann, & Wright, 1993; Stineman et al., 1996). The FIM has both motor and cognitive subscales but is typically used to evaluate the patient's degree of independence in basic ADL tasks. It was developed by the Uniform Data System at the State University of New York College at Buffalo as a standardized way for professionals to evaluate patient progress in self-care, functional mobility, communication, cognition, and social interaction. Each area is graded

Table 6.3. Activity of Daily Living Areas Assessed in Acute and Inpatient Settings

Bed mobility	• Bridging • Rolling • Supine to sit • Sit to stand
All functional transfers	• Wheelchair (stand and sit–pivot) • Sliding board • Bathroom—toilet, tub, or shower with or without assistive devices or DME
Mobility	• Mobility via ambulation with or without assistive device • Mobility via manual or power wheelchair
Self-care	• Grooming • Feeding • Dressing • Toileting • Bathing
Beginning meal preparation and simple home management	• Simple cold meal preparation • Basic cleaning and housekeeping • Laundry • Bed making • Shopping • Basic money management
Time management	• Telling time • Use of a calendar • Use of a memory book

Note. DME = durable medical equipment.

on a scale ranging from 1 to 7; a score of 1 indicates *total dependence;* 7 indicates *complete independence.*

Across the United States, occupational therapists use the FIM in the first 3 days after admission to inpatient rehabilitation and during the 3 days leading up to discharge to measure the patient's progress in basic ADLs. Additionally, follow-up is conducted 3 months after the patient's discharge from the inpatient rehabilitation setting. The FIM helps define the level of assistance (typically referred to as the *burden of care*) the patient will need on discharge from inpatient rehabilitation (Granger et al., 1993). In some centers, the FIM is used to monitor weekly progress.

Evaluation of Perception and Cognition During Performance of Activities of Daily Living

The evaluation of perception and cognition within the context of ADL performance is typically necessary with patients at RLA LCF IV through VI whose vision or cognitive deficits interfere with standardized pencil-and-paper assessments. Moreover, it is critical to objectively observe and provide adequate documentation of how these deficits are manifested in the context of ADL performance.

Assessments of perception and cognition should involve the observation of the patient engaged in a familiar routine activity. For example, the patient may be asked to put on or take off a particular piece of clothing, with the therapist observing the behavior and inferring impairments in various perceptual or cognitive processes as they manifest themselves in the patient's performance of the activity (Mortera, 2004). The information gained from informal observation of functional tasks is valuable because the therapist may observe key points at which the patient's ADL performance breaks down (Abreu & Hinojosa, 1992; Baum & Katz, 2010; Dunn, 1993; Hartman-Maeir, Katz, & Baum, 2009; Laver-Fawcett, 2007; Toglia & Golisz, 2012; Vanderploeg, 1994). Dunn (1993) also proposed that observing functional tasks may provide vital feedback that could not otherwise be obtained from contrived tasks. Thus, the therapist and patient are provided with valuable indicators as to how the patient may function despite the presence of cognitive deficits and with or without specific types of assistance in the completion of daily routine activities (Tupper & Cicerone, 1990).

When determining which ADL assessment to use, it is important to remember that those used in inpatient medical rehabilitation usually focus primarily on the evaluation of motor performance. The clinician is thus often unable to determine whether deficits in motor performance or in cognitive processes are interfering with a patient's ability to successfully complete a functional task. Additionally, ADL assessments such as the FIM that primarily provide information about physical assistance may have limitations when determining whether cognitive issues are compromising ADL performance and whether the patient will independently initiate ADLs in the home environment. If a patient is discharged at the level of supervision, the family may not know how much supervision is necessary without a more adequate evaluation of how cognitive deficits interfere with the patient's ability to be independent in performance of ADLs. The patient with a TBI may be discharged at a certain level of supervision but significantly improve in the degree and intensity of supervision needed. Distant supervision is less intense than side-by-side supervision, which requires constant observation and possible cueing in the same room for completion of all tasks. The difference between these two levels of supervision can influence a family's decision to take a patient home.

Structured Functional Cognitive Assessment and Ecologically Valid Evaluation During Activities of Daily Living

The occupational therapist should give special consideration to assessment of the patient's cognitive and perceptual skills during the performance of any functional task (Árnadóttir, 2012; Baum & Katz, 2010; Goverover & Hinojosa, 2002; Hartman-Maeir, Katz, & Baum, 2009; Toglia & Golisz, 2012). Such assessment more completely establishes the burden of care on the basis of the effects that cognitive or perceptual impairments may have on ADL performance. Occupational therapists are responsible for using cognitive assessments that are germane to establishing goals and interventions in the rehabilitation of adults with TBI. Currently, a critical need is the use of ecologically valid cognitive assessments (Acker, 1989; Burgess et al., 2006; Chaytor & Schmitter-Edgecombe, 2003; Chaytor, Schmitter-Edgecombe, & Burr, 2006; Rabin, Burton, & Barr, 2007). Ecologically valid cognitive assessments can aid in the structured observation and documentation of cognitive deficits manifested during ADL performance or performance-based testing.

The ability to more rigorously observe and document underlying perceptual and cognitive impairments during the performance of ADLs by patients at RLA LCF IV who are not able to participate in a more formal or standardized testing situation is critical to the evaluation process. *Structured Functional Cognitive Assessment* (Mortera, 2004, 2012) is a type of performance-based testing that allows the therapist to objectively record perceptual and cognitive deficits during ADL performance. SFCA is a means of documenting baseline functional behaviors to determine realistic goals, plan treatment, and establish burden of care in all areas of dysfunction, and it subsequently allows for adequate reimbursement for rehabilitation services. It encompasses the physical–motor and cognitive impairments that may hinder performance of ADLs and, ultimately, safety and can be used with any ADL task and with patients at any level of functional ability. The following procedures for creating an SFCA are tailored for use by occupational therapists (Benson & Clark, 1982; Benson & Schell, 1997; Cohen & Swerdlik, 1999, 2002; Crocker & Algina, 1986; Mortera, 2004; Mosey, 1996; Murphy & Davidshofer, 1991; Nunnally, 1978; Ottenbacher & Christiansen, 1997).

The therapist completes an activity analysis in which the ADL task is broken down into components and determines the cognitive and perceptual skills needed to complete them (Mortera, 2004). First, though, the therapist must have a thorough understanding of normal cognitive and perceptual skills. This understanding is critical to being able to operationally define the observed behavior and label it (Mosey, 1996). Clearly defined observable behaviors greatly aid in the subsequent documentation of deficit areas in terms of level of severity on the function–dysfunction continuum for patients with cognitive and perceptual impairments.

Clearly defined observable behaviors greatly aid in the subsequent documentation of deficit areas in terms of level of severity on the function–dysfunction continuum for patients with cognitive and perceptual impairments.

To organize this information into an observation schedule to record possible deficits, the therapist first creates a table of specifications (Crocker & Algina, 1986) that details the activity analysis of a selected ADL task and the normal definition of cognitive and perceptual skills elicited by that task (see Table 6.4). This table provides a structure to operationally define observable behaviors by level of

Table 6.4. Table of Specifications for Observation of Behaviors During ADLs

	Cognitive or Perceptual Skill Elicited by Task Component	Observable Behaviors Indicating Function or Dysfunction in Cognitive or Perceptual Skill or Impairment
ADL Task With Task Components in Sequential Order		

Note. ADL/ADLs = activity/activities of daily living.

impairment severity. These operational definitions describe the levels of severity in a scale that is then used in the observation schedule when recording such behaviors.

The observation schedule is used to document the levels of severity in the impairments elicited by the task components (Mortera, 2004). For example, sustained attention during the donning of an upper-body garment may be delineated on the following scale: *Requires no cues to focus on the task of donning upper-body garment/no problem* (0), *requires one to two cues to focus on the task of donning upper-body garment/potential problem* (1), and *requires three or more cues to focus on the task of donning upper-body garment/definite problem* (2). Assessing the possible presence of cognitive impairment during the performance of ADL tasks enables the therapist to understand more clearly how such impairment may potentially affect the patient's current ability to perform ADL tasks and rehabilitation. (Refer to Chapter 3 for additional discussion of performance-based cognitive assessments.)

Intervention Planning Process: Problem Resolution

Occupational therapists strive to provide efficient and cost-effective care that is evidence based and meets the needs of patients with TBI given their limited length of stay in acute, inpatient, and subacute care. To do so, practitioners consider an array of factors in determining intensity, duration, and proposed outcomes of TBI rehabilitation, such as severity of injury, potential for recovery, and nature and extent of social support (Cuthbert et al., 2011). Treatment of the motor, vestibular, sensory, visual, cognitive, perceptual, and psychosocial impairments should be prioritized in terms of their potential impact on the patient's safety and recovery process. Therapists must consider that patients may be in a rapid state of recovery and that the treatment plan will change accordingly. The overarching goals of occupational therapy are to ensure that patients are safe, to prepare patients to be as functional as possible in their ADL performance, and to prepare them for their next level of care or rehabilitation.

Because patients may experience a relatively short length of stay, additional goals would focus on preparing the patient for supervised care at home or for continued outpatient community-based rehabilitation. Patients' family members may also be experiencing stress and will need information to prepare them for their role as primary caregivers. They should especially be aware that people with TBI may demonstrate variability in their functional performance. It is critical that family caregivers know how to manage and respond to the full range of behaviors likely to be demonstrated by the patient with TBI.

The occupational therapist's assessment and intervention process should also take place in an interdisciplinary milieu so that there is a coordinated effort between occupational therapy services and other team members to meet the patient's needs and goals. Although there is no evidence available in this regard, it is reasonable to believe that coordination and consistency between disciplines in patient management and intervention strategies may facilitate learning in both patients and caregivers. For example, when providing care to a patient with agitation, it may be helpful for the staff and caregiver to coordinate the spacing of therapy sessions so as to provide appropriate downtime for rest. Similarly, when therapists are using a journal to assist a patient who has severe memory impairment, the staff and caregiver may be instructed to review journal entries in a consistent manner to maximize the familiarity and reassurance provided by a routine activity and to facilitate the patient's orientation and attention to his or her daily activities.

When determining how to proceed with the intervention planning sequence, it is important to consider the patient's tolerance for treatment activities. The length of the treatment session may need to be reduced and the frequency increased to maximize the patient's participation in treatment activities and minimize the risk for **fatigue,** agitation, or other negative behaviors. Before beginning treatment and throughout the course of the rehabilitation process, the therapist should engage caregivers or family members as much as possible to educate them in the rehabilitation process, for carryover of strategies or skills learned during treatment, and to assist caregivers or family members by addressing their questions or concerns during the rehabilitation process.

Additionally, once the initial baseline observation data used to infer levels of severity in the underlying impairments have been documented, the therapist can then begin the process of creating an initial problem list, setting goals, and planning treatment. This list, which may include impairment-level deficits, can assist the therapist in understanding how the underlying impairments may subsequently affect the patient's activity or participation in certain ADL tasks. The therapist can also use another problem list to identify affected ADLs. Once a list of impairments is created, the therapist will also evaluate the patient's ability to perform various ADLs, if appropriate. The patient who is emerging from coma and is minimally responsive to the environment is not engaging in purposeful activity. For patients who are starting to engage in purposeful activity, the therapist would assess their ability to engage in very simple ADLs as a means of identifying the observable behaviors that indicate the level of severity of the impairments that may be affecting performance of the ADL task.

The therapist should determine whether initially identified impairments, such as the inability to visually track a moving target, sustain attention for 10 minutes, or sit unsupported for 5 minutes, may result in poor balance or may have an impact on performing a basic ADL skill such as washing the face. The therapist should determine which impairments are most critical to address in the initial treatment plan relative to the patient's individual needs and identified problems, the patient's potential for improvement, and patient safety. These impairments will become important baseline criteria when completing an ADL assessment, if and when indicated, because impairments in basic motor functions, sensory functions, and cognitive functions will affect the patient's participation in basic ADL tasks, which is contingent on how much the patient shows return of basic motor, sensory, and cognitive functions. No matter how simple, ADL tasks require intact and integrated body structure components.

The treatment process for patients with TBI requires flexibility and depends on the patient's rate of improvement, any changes in the patient's medical or functional status, caregiver or family member dynamics, and other unforeseen events that may affect the patient's progress. General guidelines can help structure the therapist's approach to the treatment process but allow for flexibility and creativity when designing appropriate treatment conditions or environments. Specific treatment activities are given only as examples that may help the novice therapist understand how to use the guidelines.

Principles Guiding Treatment: Facilitating Occupation-Oriented Intervention

Mosey (1986) defined *treatment principles* as descriptive and prescriptive guidelines that specifically detail the change process during the treatment phase of rehabilitation. The rehabilitation process enables patients to learn new ways to perform previously learned skills that have been disrupted by changes in functioning of the underlying motor, sensory, cognitive, or visual areas. The guidelines for intervention presented in this section are from the neurorehabilitation frame of reference and are based in learning theory principles derived from operant conditioning theory, motor learning theory, and theories on motivation.

The therapist can use these guidelines to set up treatment conditions that enhance practice and repetition and improve patient performance, motivation, and interest. These conditions are critical to ensure positive reinforcement and enhance learning of new skills. The guidelines detail how to design the context and therapist–patient interaction that, when used with an appropriate activity, may enhance the change process. The intent of a specific intervention is to target any one impairment to improve the patient's level of skill and ultimately the patient's functional performance. The guidelines provide the therapist with knowledge of the design of the treatment environment and therapeutic interaction with the patient. They describe the sequence of interaction and nature or quantity and quality of the intervention, not specific activities.

Using activity analysis and activity synthesis, the therapist targets impairments through the selection and set up of specific, appropriately designed activities to meet the goals of the individualized intervention plan. *Activity analysis* is the process by which the task used to facilitate underlying skill areas is broken down into its component parts. *Activity synthesis* is the therapeutic framework in which the component parts or steps are used as a means to an end to improve the underlying skill or address the ADL task performance itself. Activity analysis and activity synthesis incorporate the conditions set forth by the guidelines for intervention, which describe the environmental setup and provide details on the complexity, characteristics, quality, quantity, and sequence of conditions that facilitate or elicit desired behaviors or actions from the patient through his or her participation and interaction in the activity (Mosey, 1986).

Activity synthesis is the therapeutic framework in which the component parts or steps are used as a means to an end to improve the underlying skill or address the ADL task performance itself.

The treatment environment involves arranging the conditions in which skills are facilitated with the goal of improvement in one or more targeted areas or skills. Any changes in the impairments are then assessed relative to their effect on the patient's functional or ADL performance. An improvement in ADL status, particularly in functional areas, is documented evidence of the patient's improvement that can be used to justify continued treatment. This change process is fundamental to the treatment process and describes how the individual patient may best progress given his or her unique set of residual skills, strengths, impairments, and family and sociocultural support systems (Mosey, 1986).

The neurorehabilitation frame of reference consists of general guidelines for intervention, detailed as statements that describe the treatment environment in a more general way relative to how to initially approach and describe the sequence of intervention.

1. *Explain the treatment course so that the patient and caregiver can understand how and why the therapist has selected a certain treatment course, and set up activities that require the patient to increase awareness of postural–motor and perceptual–cognitive deficits, especially during the performance of ADL tasks.* An important goal of occupational therapy is to provide the patient with the opportunity to improve skills through the therapeutic use of ADLs while addressing impairments. If the patient is at RLA LCF IV, the therapist may start by improving the underlying skills that are later integrated to more appropriately engage in ADL or functional tasks. It is important to note that ADL tasks may be the most difficult tasks for the patient to perform because they are often multilevel in terms of task components and require a complex integration of underlying skills. Even a simple task such as washing one's face requires many skills to be integrated into one whole for successful completion. A patient at RLA LCF IV who is just beginning to engage in simple ADLs may be able to do so when the therapist breaks the functional task down into its components and engages the patient in only one or two components until success is achieved. Additional task components are subsequently incorporated until the patient is able to complete the total task.

The therapist may initially use contrived tasks with patients at RLA LCF IV to address more severe impairments. For example, a patient may need assistance from two people to maintain sitting balance on the mat while working on upper-limb reaching activities with simple gross grasp and frequent cues to attend if attention is very poor. Engaging in a dressing task may be too challenging for this patient if he or she is having difficulty working on multiple underlying skills at the same time. Noting how many skills the patient is able to simultaneously and successfully integrate, such as trunk control, upper-limb use, attention, and endurance, will assist the therapist in judging how ready the patient is to engage in the complex steps and activity demands of ADL tasks. Ultimately, the therapist's goal is to use an ADL task for therapeutic purposes (e.g., washing the face at the bedside to improve sitting balance while using the affected upper limb and attending to the task for 5–10 minutes). In terms of functional outcome, using an ADL task to improve underlying skill areas serves the purpose of increasing the patient's actual performance of that ADL task.

It is critical to be able to state to both the patient and the caregiver the what, why, and how of the treatment course so that they are clear, appropriate participation is facilitated, and questions or concerns are addressed. Patients with decreased awareness of their condition must consistently be provided with a rationale in order to adequately participate and benefit from the treatment course. The ability to understand the treatment course may also facilitate the patient's and caregiver's ability to engage in return demonstration of any treatment strategies that may be needed to support progress or rehabilitation potential.

It is also important to educate the family and caregiver in how to assist the patient with ADL performance while fostering an appreciation and understanding for how the patient's impairments affect either separate task components of the ADL or the ADL activity as a whole. Family members will often perform ADL tasks for the patient as acts of kindness and caring and do not fully grasp why the patient needs to do them for himself or herself. Educating the family and caregiver on the therapeutic use of ADLs often aids in their understanding of carryover beyond the therapy session and rehabilitation. The therapist must be sensitive to the family's sociocultural values and bear in mind that they may vary with respect to the notion of independence and interdependence when someone is recovering from an illness or disability. Once the family understands the therapeutic benefits of the patient's doing the tasks, they may be able to refocus their caring behaviors on supporting and encouraging the patient.

In addition, the therapeutic use of ADLs demonstrates to patients how their impairments may affect their ability to perform ADLs and their need for physical and cognitive assistance. Patients who lack awareness of the impact of their deficits on ADL performance may improve their awareness by actually engaging in a task that presents difficulties. They may learn either compensatory strategies or new skills for eventual success with ADL performance.

2. *Set up the human and nonhuman environments to allow or facilitate the change process.* Mosey (1986) stated that both the human and the nonhuman environments are configured together in the treatment session. The *human environment* is defined as those people involved in the treatment course who facilitate the patient's ability to improve the impairments or ADL skills needed to enhance his or her functional status: the rehabilitation staff and caregiver as well as the patient. The *nonhuman environment* is defined as any physical entity that may affect the patient's performance, such as clinic tools or activities, mat, wheelchair, adaptive devices, postural support devices, and ambulation aids, as well as the environmental context, such as furniture, lighting, sounds, or smells. Therapists use the environment to facilitate improvements in the patient's targeted impairments or ADL skills. They design the environment to have a direct effect on the patient's ability to process incoming stimuli and, subsequently, on the patient's actions or responses. The therapist must either upgrade or downgrade environmental conditions to elicit desired actions or responses in the patient that will address impairments and facilitate functional performance. Because the complexity and demands of the environment are critically important, strong skills in activity analysis and activity synthesis can allow the therapist to anchor and direct the treatment course.

The occupational therapist chooses an activity or task on the basis of how it will elicit the specific underlying skills to be addressed and call for the patient to meet the requirements of the environmental setup. For example, two task components inherent in the task of sitting unsupported on the edge of the bed while donning an upper-body garment are pulling the garment over the head and placing the arms into the armholes. A few of the underlying skills addressed with just these two task components are trunk balance, upper-extremity voluntary motion, spatial awareness, and task sequencing. Through activity synthesis, the therapeutic use of this dressing task allows the patient to improve trunk balance, upper-limb use, and cognitive skills while also working on the actual task of donning upper-body garments.

The therapist must be sensitive to the family's sociocultural values and bear in mind that they may vary with respect to the notion of independence and interdependence when someone is recovering from an illness or disability.

The therapist also provides appropriate cues to the patient to address the impairments. For example, the patient who is listing to the weak side while sitting unsupported may be physically cued with a hand on the trunk or shoulder or verbally cued or instructed to correct and maintain his or her center of gravity. The caregiver who is trained in physical, verbal, or tactile cues to facilitate ADL performance may provide assistance as indicated to ensure safe ADL performance.

Training rehabilitation staff, caregivers, and patients in how to observe and interpret patient actions and responses elicited by a particular environmental setup and specific activities or tasks enhances their ability to facilitate skills or ADL performance. Observing and understanding how certain environmental conditions affect patient performance are paramount in subsequently adapting, upgrading, or downgrading the environmental conditions or activity to assist the patient with optimizing his or her performance. Frequent monitoring of patient responses and observable behaviors, while noting the level of severity of each impairment, allows for more accurate and appropriate changes in the environment as needed. Patient actions or responses will vary on the basis of the severity of the impairment, determined from the baseline evaluation findings, interactions with rehabilitation staff and caregivers, interaction with the nonhuman environment, and activity or task demands.

The therapist must first determine the environmental and task demands and how they will facilitate the patient's use of the underlying skill, the therapeutic mode (i.e., use of self) that will support the patient, and how best to instruct caregivers in facilitating patient performance. Setting up the environment begins with the findings of the evaluation and which underlying impairments will be prioritized, based on patient and caregiver needs, patient potential, safety, and feasibility. Once the treatment course has been determined and implemented, ongoing evaluation of the patient's subsequent responses to the environmental setup and making changes as needed will continue until the patient has reached the treatment goals.

Observed changes are those behaviors and actions manifested by improvements in the underlying skill that may affect the patient's ability to perform ADL tasks. These changes are documented in terms of how they affect the patient's functional status in the ADL tasks and whether the patient has met treatment goals. The therapist's ability to record the environmental setup, specific task limitations, level of severity of each impairment, and the overall effects on or change in the patient's ADL or functional status is critical for documenting patient improvements, rehabilitation potential, burden of care, and the need to continue rehabilitation services.

3. *Determine the frames of reference and how to combine or use them sequentially during intervention.* How to determine the treatment course depends on how the therapist uses various frames of reference or guidelines for practice (Mosey, 1986). In occupational therapy, the **top-down approach** is predicated on the use of functional tasks and ways to improve task performance as ends in themselves. ADL training may be compensatory, requiring the use of an adaptive device (e.g., grab bars, wash mitt) for the patient to engage in a desired activity despite impairments. ADL retraining often incorporates practice, repetition, and feedback as methods to teach a patient how to proficiently use various ADL techniques such as one-handed dressing and adaptive devices to improve efficiency and safety. As soon as it is possible, the therapist should incorporate the top-down approach to understand how the patient's identified impairments may be affecting his or her ability to perform ADLs.

The therapist's ability to record the environmental setup, specific task limitations, level of severity of each impairment, and the overall effects on or change in the patient's ADL or functional status is critical for documenting patient improvements, rehabilitation potential, burden of care, and the need to continue rehabilitation services.

The **bottom-up approach** is predicated on addressing underlying skill areas. Graded task activities may be contrived (using materials such as games, pegs, cones, or weights) or functional (using ADL tasks). The use of a bottom-up approach may be indicated if the patient at RLA LCF IV is initially unable to engage in ADLs because they require the integration of multiple skills in multistep tasks, which may be too challenging and difficult during initial treatment sessions. For example, a patient with severe impairments may need to work on basic attentional skills and upright sitting tolerance while seated supported and may not yet be able to engage in a simple grooming task such as washing his or her face while seated in a wheelchair at the sink.

A combination of frames of reference, such as the neurorehabilitation and biomechanical frames of reference, may be necessary to address the needs of the patient with multiple impairments. For example, a patient with severe impairments who is unable to participate in ADLs and who presents with multiple impairments in sensory, motor, perceptual, and cognitive areas may benefit from a bottom-up approach that combines treatment principles and guides the therapist in addressing these multiple impairments during a treatment session. Patients who do not yet show adequate return in the basic postural–motor and perceptual–cognitive foundation skills may need to be provided with brief and simple single-step activities. Patients demonstrating gains in underlying impairments and who can participate in ADLs starting with simple tasks and progressing to more complex tasks can benefit from both bottom-up and top-down approaches. Therapists often use a combination of both bottom-up and top-down approaches to achieve a balance in the provision of services. TBI rehabilitation is complicated and unique to the patient and requires a range of treatment approaches to address complex patient needs.

4. *Set up the selected activity so that the required skills (sensory, postural, motor, perceptual, visual, cognitive) are balanced and graded to achieve challenge and success.* Foundational skills such as sensory and motor skills should be addressed first, and interventions may follow a developmental sequence. Note that the progressive integration of these various skills will also be affected by the patient's ability to meet the task demands and interact with the human and nonhuman environments. When initially determining the treatment course, the therapist should also prioritize those skills that are critical to ensure patient safety. Prioritizing the treatment of specific skills, especially in terms of safety, also determines burden of care and rehabilitation potential. For example, in the inpatient rehabilitation setting, the retraining of gross motor skills focuses on functional mobility: bed mobility (i.e., rolling, bridging, moving up and down the length of the bed, sitting up); sit-to-stand and stand-to-sit from various surfaces; and transfers to and from the bed, wheelchair, toilet, and shower or tub. Early use of the upper limb in functional activities typically falls in the occupational therapist's domain. Depending on how the patient presents, therapy may first focus on use of the upper limb for weight bearing and stabilizing objects, then progress to use of prehension skills.

The initial interventions with the patient should start with the patient in a secure posture, beginning with trunk control and sequentially progressing from supine, sitting, sitting unsupported, standing, and dynamic standing to ambulation with and without assist. Limb use is also incorporated as the patient becomes proficient at each postural milestone. The therapist should note any sensory impairment in the patient's proprioception, visual orientation, and **vestibular functions** and the effect on head control because impairments in these areas may affect the patient's ability to sustain a secure posture, both seated and in standing. Motor demands such as trunk strength, muscle tone imbalance, and any soft-tissue or biomechanical issues will also affect the patient's upright sitting tolerance and ability to sustain proper alignment. The patient's baseline status relative to these skills, determined during the evaluation, informs the therapist regarding the patient's tolerance for therapy targeting each of the impairments.

In addition to the sensory, postural, and motor demands, the therapist should note any impairment in the visual, perceptual, and cognitive skills that may also place additional demands on the patient's ability to sustain upright positioning and use of the trunk and limbs. The ability to tolerate and subsequently process basic sensory input—tactile, auditory, vestibular, and visual stimuli—may affect the ability of the patient at RLA LCF IV to simultaneously sustain basic attention to the task, adequately follow instructions, and maintain motor control.

Initially, intervention may start with activities that challenge the patient's postural or motor capacity before incorporating visual, perceptual, and cognitive demands. For a patient at RLA LCF IV whose ability to sustain attention to the task is limited, the therapist may begin with the patient in a supported upright position with use of the limbs while slowly introducing a simple attentional task. Activities requiring the patient to progress to maintaining dynamic sitting balance or trunk control with limb use, such as with reaching in space, may be more challenging for a patient at RLA LCF IV and may not lend themselves to introducing an additional attentional demand. Any attempt to incorporate cognitive challenges in conjunction with postural and motor demands should be carefully monitored by observing the patient's responses to changes in positioning and demands on trunk control.

The occupational therapist may subsequently have the patient progress through a series of activities that incorporate postural and motor with perceptual and cognitive demands by grading the activities depending on the patient's response to these demands. Head control may need to be addressed for the patient to visually orient to the environment while sustaining verticality of the head and trunk in space. An anterior pelvic tilt and trunk extension may initially be challenging for the patient. Upper-limb use may be another demand if the affected limb is used and effort is needed for upper-limb proximal control combined with distal use (gross grasp or prehension patterns).

If the patient can maintain proper positioning during dynamic reaching tasks, the therapist can challenge the patient by requiring the patient to shift attention between two tasks. Fatigue will be indicated by the breakdown of proper trunk positioning, reduced head or limb control, or decreasing attention to a task; these observations will determine how long the patient should be challenged. Activities at the upper limit of the patient's capacity will require frequent cueing and will initially be sustained only for short periods. If the challenge is set too high, the patient's need for cues may also be very high. Finding the just-right challenge requires ongoing observation of the patient's responses and therapist adjustments to the environment and task demands.

5. Use ***errorless learning*** *to facilitate skill acquisition. Errorless learning is a type* of intervention that is used with patients with severe memory impairment and has

been demonstrated to be effective in teaching patients new information (Cohen, Ylvisaker, Hamilton, Kemp, & Claiman, 2010). Because learning is considered to be dependent on context and relevant cues, the patient is provided with a set of instructions that ensures that errors are not made, resulting in successful performance and, subsequently, a learned skill. For specific examples of the application of errorless learning in treatment, see Chapter 3.

6. *Create an environment that allows for inherently meaningful task engagement and motivation in the patient as well as one that challenges the patient and provides interest.* Occupational therapists should be mindful to select tasks that will seem relevant to the patient. For example, a former athlete or sports enthusiast who sustains a TBI may perceive upper-extremity therapeutic exercises as more meaningful to the rehabilitation process than a task such as folding towels or some other seemingly functional task. Providing the patient with an appropriate rationale or a well-thought-out explanation may engage the patient in a greater variety of meaningful and functional tasks. Therapists need to be careful of any biases or misinterpretation of what patients may deem meaningful or motivating. It is critical that treatment activities reflect what is realistic, necessary, and vital to improving the patient's rehabilitation potential and progress.

Specific Intervention Approaches for Common Impairments

The interventions discussed in this section are paramount when addressing specific needs of the patient with TBI. They provide the means for ensuring that the patient's health and safety are considered first and foremost when delineating the initial and ongoing treatment plans.

Proper Body Alignment and Positioning

Patients recovering from TBI whose ability to hold an upright position is compromised should immediately be provided with a plan to meet their seating needs. The ability to maintain a safe, upright sitting position permits improved head, eye, and upper-extremity movements. It also allows for optimal physiological processes, such as digestion and respiration, and aids in stimulation of cognitive skills through interactions with the external environment. Care must be taken to develop systems that address existing pressure-sore issues and prevent the occurrence of further skin problems.

The occupational therapist must often begin by determining the proper wheelchair, depending on the patient's tolerance for the upright position. If the patient has been confined to bed for any length of time, tolerance to sitting may be minimal from an orthostatic perspective. Patients become rapidly deconditioned after even a few days of bedrest. In such cases, it is wise to mobilize the patient using a recliner wheelchair or a tilt-in-space wheelchair. This approach allows the therapist to put the patient into a recumbent position if his or her blood pressure drops too low when sitting. An abdominal binder and antiembolism compression stockings help avoid orthostatic hypotension at this early stage.

The baseline procedure for assessing the patient's seating needs involves performing a mat evaluation. The goal of the mat evaluation is to determine, through palpation and evaluation of ROM in supine and in seated, whether a neutral position of the pelvis and alignment of the trunk is achievable for seating.

The therapist distinguishes which portions of the anatomy are flexible and which are difficult to align and determines whether fixed deformities are present.

After the mat evaluation, several devices may prove useful in properly positioning the patient for functional seating. Many commercially available cushions can provide positioning devices to accommodate or shift pelvic alignment for a more stable sitting base. In addition, wheelchair backs can be designed with lateral supports to help achieve a midline orientation. Providing a lap tray may further enhance maintenance of a midline position and support weakened upper extremities. Specially designed head supports can be provided for patients who are unable to maintain an upright head position or who have a tendency to tilt the head to one side.

Many pressure-relieving cushions are available to provide proper seating and positioning. Patients at risk for pressure sores require ongoing monitoring while upright, even when using such cushions. The entire team must be engaged in the process of providing adequate pressure relief from the seated position by routinely tilting the chair back for about 30 seconds to allow the area around the patient's ischial tuberosities to revascularize. No cushion by itself will prevent skin breakdown without a frequent and consistent program of pressure relief. In addition, the cushions themselves must be cared for properly to allow them to be as effective as possible.

Impairment of Joint and Bone Functions

Patients with TBI may exhibit decreased muscle length (i.e., ***contracture***) and increased muscle stiffness in their involved extremities, usually as a result of prolonged immobility. The upper-limb muscles that frequently shorten in neurological injuries include shoulder adductors, internal rotators, elbow flexors, forearm pronators, thumb adductors, and long-finger flexors. The negative effects from loss of ROM or disuse are linked to increased muscle stiffness, and contracture is a common occurrence (Moseley et al., 2008).

Contracture alters the resting limb position, thereby affecting the resting length of muscles crossing the joint and the lever–torque angle relationship at the joint (Lieber, 1992). This change, in turn, alters the muscle's force output and can lead to muscle imbalance (Vandervoort, 1999). If patients are not adequately evaluated and monitored closely for potential impairments after TBI, a loss of function may occur such that carrying out routine ADLs becomes extremely difficult.

Patients who can engage in an individualized program of stretching should be trained by the occupational therapist to carry out the exercises on a daily basis. Stretching is excellent preparation for practicing functional activities and can be incorporated directly into practice sessions. Although evidence has not definitively indicated how long stretch should be applied, Harvey and Herbert (2002) found that 30 minutes of prolonged stretch decreased PROM limitations in patients with paraplegia. If the extremity cannot be moved, prolonged passive stretching (i.e., 15–30 minutes) through positioning may also help reduce the tendency toward muscle shortening and stiffness in patients with TBI.

Occupational therapists should focus on stretching the muscle groups that the patient needs to incorporate the upper limb into functional activity. For example, stretching to enhance the ability to bear weight with the involved upper limb allows the uninvolved upper limb to perform fine manipulation tasks. Additionally, prolonged stretch before practicing a functional reaching task may be useful. It is worth noting that a systematic review by Katalinic, Harvey, and Herbert (2011) concluded that the evidence was insufficient or inconclusive for the effectiveness of stretching in people with neurological conditions.

Serial casting with short intervals (i.e., 1–4 days) has been shown to improve ROM with fewer complications and shorter treatment duration (Pohl et al., 2002). Marshall et al.'s (2007) review of the evidence found support for the use of serial casts to increase ROM. Whether increased ROM achieved through serial casting results in improvements in functional task performance is less clear. Mortenson and Eng (2003) concluded that of the three possible outcomes that have been suggested as a rationale for using casting (i.e., increased PROM, decreased spasticity, increased function), only improved PROM has sufficient support to substantiate the use of casts as part of best practice. There is moderate evidence that casting alone is as effective as serial casting and **botulinum toxin** injections in the treatment of plantarflexion contractures resulting from spasticity (Marshall et al., 2007).

The occupational therapist must understand the types of specific physical complications that may further limit joint function. ***Heterotopic ossification*** (HO) is characterized by the formation of excessive bone, which can severely limit ROM in specific joints. The risk for developing HO appears to increase as the severity of the injury, length of immobilization, and duration of coma increase (Varghese, 1992). The condition is referred to as *neurogenic HO* in patients with TBI because the stimulus creating new bone is the cerebral insult. Cullen, Bayley, Bayona, Hilditch, and Aubut (2007) reported that the soft tissue most affected is that of the hips, knees, and elbows. Decreased ROM and pain are the most common problems in patients with HO.

The main treatment options for HO are medications (e.g., ethidronate disodium and nonsteroidal anti-inflammatory drugs), radiation, physical and occupational therapy, and surgery, and these treatment modalities are often used in combination. Most patients can be helped to maintain their ROM through therapies and medicines; a small percentage of patients require surgical excision of the HO when the restrictions in joint mobility, limb positioning, and sitting compromise function. Aubut, Mehta, Cullen, and Teasell (2011) reported that in patients with TBI, surgical excision was found to be an effective means of treatment.

Impairments in Muscle Function

Gracies, Elovic, McGuire, and Simpson (1997) proposed a model for understanding the pathophysiology of impairment after a **central nervous system** (CNS) lesion; they divided muscle overactivity into stretch-related and non–stretch-related categories. In the stretch-related category, spasticity is the most common type of tone abnormality in people with TBI. Lance (1980, cited in Gracies et al., 1997) defined *spasticity* as a motor disorder characterized by a velocity-dependent increase in tonic stretch reflexes (i.e., muscle tone) with exaggerated tendon jerks; it results from hyperexcitability of the stretch reflex and is one component of the upper motor neuron syndrome. Spasticity is noted to predominantly affect flexor groups in the upper extremities and extensor groups in the lower extremities, and it compromises functional use of the limbs. Muscle tone can also be increased in trunk muscles, thereby affecting positioning in bed, sitting upright, standing, and ambulation.

Increased muscle tone can affect head and neck control and further impair function. Spasticity in the pharyngeal and laryngeal muscles can impair phonation, articulation, swallowing, and breathing.

The second type of stretch-related muscle overactivity, described by Denny-Brown (1966, as cited by Gracies et al., 1997), is *spastic dystonia,* a chronic tonic muscle contraction in the absence of phasic stretch or voluntary effort; when present, it is evidenced by sensitivity to tonic stretch in the involved muscles. Gracies et al. (1997) listed the third type of stretch-related muscle overactivity as *spastic cocontraction,* an excessive muscle contraction occurring in the antagonists during a voluntary command on agonists, even in the absence of phasic stretch. For example, when the patient tries to reach forward to grasp an object and extends the wrist to do this, cocontractions of the wrist flexors occur. The wrist flexors and extensors begin working simultaneously, resulting in the wrist contracting first in flexion and then in extension, often repeatedly in succession. The patient is typically unable to inhibit such activity.

It is interesting that, although spasticity is the easiest phenomenon to measure in this model, it is probably the least likely to actually interfere with the patient's ability to regain motor control. The combination of all types of muscle overactivity, along with muscle shortening and paralysis, appears to create the motor problems observed in many patients with TBI. Muscle overactivity, including spasticity, may account for more loss of soft-tissue elasticity, ultimately resulting in contractures and deformities. Other factors contributing to contractures and soft-tissue changes include immobilization, improper positioning, postural malalignment, and flaccidity.

Rigidity, an increase in resistance to passive movement that is independent of velocity, may occur in patients with TBI because of **anoxia** or as a side effect of neuroleptic medications. Rigidity is most prominent in the flexor muscle groups of the upper and lower limbs. *Cogwheel rigidity,* or periodic resistance to passive movement, may result from direct injury to the basal ganglia.

Vision Impairment

One example of an impairment typically requiring intervention during the acute phase of rehabilitation is *diplopia* (i.e., double vision). Diplopia can be caused by damage to cranial nerves II, IV, or VI; fracture to the orbit with eye muscle entrapment; disorders of the extraocular muscles; or disorders of the neuromuscular junction (Blumenfeld, 2002, 2010).

Patients frequently complain about this visual disturbance, which can interfere with recovery of skills. Diplopia can be eliminated by partial visual occlusion. Warren (2011) described a partial occlusion method that requires the application of opaque tape to prescription lenses or to a pair of frames with plain, nonrefractive lenses. The tape is applied to the nasal portion of the eyeglass lens of the nondominant eye to block visual input in the central visual field while leaving the peripheral visual field unobstructed. Using the nondominant eye provides greater comfort to the patient. The tape is applied toward the center of the lens until the patient provides feedback that the diplopia is gone, and the width is adjusted as the **muscle paresis** resolves. Occlusion should not be used with children younger than age 16 without the direction of an ophthalmologist or optometrist. Warren further suggested that, regardless of whether full or partial occlusion is used, daily ROM exercises for the affected eye should be carried out (covering the unaffected eye), including exercises in all directions with the eyes working together (i.e., binocularly). These exercises are important to prevent contracture of the unaffected eye muscles.

Visual-field loss is a common occurrence in patients with TBI. Although vision rehabilitation protocols have been studied, a consensus on a single method has not been achieved, and a variety of methods and techniques are currently being used. Scanning training has been supported as a method to treat visual-field loss (Kingston, Katsaros, Vu, & Goodrich, 2010). Kingston et al. reported the development of a vision rehabilitation method that uses the Neuro Vision Technology (NVT) System (Adelaide, South Australia, Australia; http://www.neurovisiontech.com.au).

The NVT System provides a standardized method to assess and train therapists working with patients specifically with visual-field loss. The NVT System consists of a light panel that elicits the visual stimuli needed for vision scanning and training. Data are recorded using computer software, and the patient's information is stored and can be tracked over time. This reported treatment approach also incorporates compensatory head turning that begins with static exercises during pencil-and-paper tasks and progresses to dynamic exercises in which the patient uses head turning during activities requiring mobility in varied environments. The authors presented a case report in which the patient demonstrated improvements in all visual deficits and increased in self-awareness of his visual deficits as well as of the impact on his functional performance. This method demonstrated clinical effectiveness, but future research on this program is still needed (Kingston et al., 2010). Scanning compensatory therapy is widely used to treat visual-field loss (Bouwmeester, Heutink, & Lucas, 2007; Marshall, 2009; Riggs, Andrews, Roberts, & Gilewski, 2007) and is appropriate for occupational therapists to incorporate in all types of functional activities.

The therapist may teach the patient a strategy to compensate for the visual impairment, but for that strategy to become a habit, the patient must continuously practice it. The therapist engages the patient in tasks ranging from scanning print to scanning the environment for meaningful objects. Scanning exercises may begin with the patient scanning the hospital tray for food or scanning the bathroom for grooming supplies. Scanning must also take place during mobility activities to ensure the patient's safety, whether the patient is using a wheelchair or walking.

The therapist may teach the patient a strategy to compensate for the visual impairment, but for that strategy to become a habit, the patient must continuously practice it.

Scanning exercises present an ideal opportunity to work closely with the physical therapist to ensure that the patient can handle dual visual and physical tasks to negotiate the hospital, home, and community environments. Simulated community tasks such as grocery shopping place demands on multiple systems. The patient must visually scan for items on the store shelf while physically moving in the space and bending or reaching to select the item. Often, the work begins with teaching the patient how to incorporate scanning strategies while moving in the environment. Can the patient successfully locate objects on the walls while moving down the hallway? Can he or she progress to locating moving objects (i.e., people) in this environment? Because many patients with TBI are distractible, careful evaluation of the patient's safety in functional mobility skills must be carried out using the combined expertise of the physical and occupational therapists.

Perceptual Impairment

For patients with a visual neglect syndrome, a systematic approach to retraining visual scanning (i.e., visually searching the environment) is used to improve visual attention to all areas of the environment and thus improve safety and independent functioning. Vision impairment may result from a visual-field deficit (i.e., hemianopsia) or a perceptual–visual neglect syndrome. A visual-field deficit resulting in hemianopsia or some other visual-field loss typically results from damage to cranial nerve II or the visual receptor pathway. Patients are typically aware that they are unable to see stimuli in the affected visual field. Often, they present with excessive head or trunk motion toward the affected side to overcompensate for the inability to receive visual stimuli from the affected visual field.

Patients often manifest perceptual visual neglect or attentional neglect, typically to the left side or hemispace, when damage to the brain occurs, particularly to the right hemisphere (Blumenfeld, 2002). The brain is thought to have an inherent hemispheric asymmetry in which the attention mechanisms of the right hemisphere mediate stimuli from both the right and left hemispaces and the attention mechanisms of the left hemisphere mediate only stimuli from the right hemispace. With lesions to the right hemisphere, patients will still be able to attend to the right side because the left hemisphere is also attending to the right side. However, because damage to the right hemisphere causes little or no attention to the left side, and the left hemisphere attends only to the right side, the result is a left neglect syndrome or visual neglect syndrome to the left hemispace. The difficulty with left visual neglect is that the patient may be unaware of the problem if the visual receptor pathway is intact because the visual fields may not be affected. This unawareness leads to poor attention to the left visual hemispace, and the patient often needs external cues from another person or some physical anchor on the left side to attempt to increase awareness to the left side and, subsequently, attend to visual input from the left side. Right neglect syndromes are possible but rare.

Much of the literature on spatial neglect is focused on understanding the manifestations of neglect syndromes and how to address these deficits in patients with right-hemisphere stroke (Kortte & Hillis, 2009). Although it is possible that a therapist may treat a patient for spatial neglect post-TBI, unilateral neglect is typically not as common a problem for patients with TBI as it is for patients with stroke.

Orientation Remediation

When the patient is at RLA LCF V and VI, intervention begins to focus on the consistent, structured use of compensatory techniques to ascertain orientation information. Occupational therapists may provide orientation groups once or twice per day, at fixed times, to help patients obtain basic information such as the time of year, where they are, what happened to them, and so forth. This process requires teaching patients how to acquire information from the environment, such as from orientation boards, clocks, scenes viewed from the hospital window (e.g., What is the weather like? Are there leaves on the trees?), or the dress of hospital personnel (i.e., white coats and identification badges indicate medical professionals). As patients make progress in retaining basic information, the group leader may then focus on why they are in the hospital. The link is critical to helping patients internalize that they had a TBI. All members of the rehabilitation team reinforce basic orientation information and personally relevant information, from the physicians asking patients questions on morning rounds to each visit by the nurse, physical therapist, speech–language pathologist, and other care providers. Patient intervention sessions are likewise grounded in structure and repetition.

Thomas et al. (2003) and DeGuise, LeBlanc, Feyz, Thomas, and Gusselin (2005) attempted to standardize and assess a program of reality orientation therapy, the North Star Project, which used a standardized approach to materials, environment, and family and staff involvement. The purpose was to increase appropriate patient interaction and reduce PTA. A unique feature was the use of a large Plexiglas footboard for each hospital bed that provided information such as the patient's name, the name of the facility, a clock, and a calendar. DeGuise et al. assessed the effect of this intervention on duration of PTA in 12 patients participating in the North Star Project compared with a control group of 26 patients who were matched on initial **Glasgow Coma Scale** score and age and for whom this approach was not available. The PTA of the participants in the North Star Project was 5 days shorter than that of the control group. Although the finding was not considered statistically significant, the authors nevertheless saw it as clinically relevant.

Attention

The attentional system comprises the major functions of orienting, target **detection,** and tonic arousal. Orienting occurs via the visual system structures of the brain, target detection occurs via the frontal lobe structures, and tonic arousal occurs via the **brainstem** structures. These three functions of the attentional system and their respective neuroanatomical areas are thought to interact with one another.

Attentional interventions focus on building the patient's ability to concentrate (Posner & Petersen, 1990). As always, activity selection should take into consideration the patient's preferences and interests. Patients working on sustained concentration may initially benefit from working with familiar objects in self-care tasks (e.g., washing hands and face, combing hair, brushing teeth, dressing). They may gradually progress to reading and writing activities. If patients have difficulty with focused (selective) concentration, slowly introducing additional stimuli, when patients can tolerate it (i.e., when task performance does not decrease), can help build the ability to focus with competing stimulation. Activities requiring divided and alternating concentration might include the use of simple games involving sorting cards by suit or number and other tasks requiring shifting focus. These exercises should take into account patients' ability to handle mobility tasks simultaneously with distractors in the environment (e.g., walking down a busy corridor). Cicerone et al.'s (2000, 2005, 2011) review of evidence-based cognitive rehabilitation suggested that complex tasks requiring the regulation of attention and an emphasis on strategy training to compensate for attention deficits in functional situations are more effective in postacute rehabilitation than are specific interventions for basic aspects of attention (e.g., reaction time, vigilance).

Memory

A variety of approaches to treating memory dysfunction are available (Toglia, Golisz, & Goverover, 2013). With any approach, the therapist should provide the patient with information on how memory functions in daily life along with strategies to reduce the functional implications of memory impairments. This education can begin in a simple way during the patient's inpatient hospitalization. Depending on the patient's awareness of his or her memory impairment, the therapist may change the focus of the intervention from teaching new strategies to compensate for the memory impairment to reducing the demands on memory by changing the task or environment.

Once patients with TBI begin to have even fleeting awareness of their cognitive problems, memory strategies or tools should be introduced. If the therapist believes that the patient can learn new strategies, he or she may teach the patient a variety of internal strategies to organize the information to assist in recall (e.g., rehearsal, chunking, imagery, retracing events, first-letter cueing, rhymes, story method, face–name associations; Toglia, 1993b). During intervention sessions, the therapist and patient identify the best strategies for recalling information and apply them to a variety of functional tasks, either real or simulated.

In addition to the use of internal memory strategies, the therapist and patient may select a memory aid or cognitive prosthesis (e.g., notebook, appointment book, pill timer, smartphone, other electronic device) to serve as a memory backup, although patients should not use one before they understand the need for and purpose of such tools. Memory books and organizers are compensatory strategies that many patients with TBI need in acute rehabilitation and later in their recovery. In the inpatient rehabilitation setting, memory notebooks are commonly introduced to log the patient's daily tasks and performance.

> **Memory books and organizers are compensatory strategies that many patients with TBI need in acute rehabilitation and later in their recovery.**

It is important to explore memory aids that patients may have used previously, such as smartphone apps, and to remind patients, who are often concerned that the use of such devices will inhibit improvement of their memory, that many people who have not sustained TBI use memory devices. Therapists should explore the feasibility of existing smartphone apps or, if the patient does not have access to or is not familiar with smartphone apps, paper-based notebooks. Intervention sessions can focus on a variety of everyday situations in which the patient needs to either write or retrieve information in the appropriate section of the notebook or enter it into a smartphone calendar.

Dowds et al. (2011) examined the effectiveness of the use of personal digital assistants (PDAs) with patients with TBI in an outpatient and community-based rehabilitation setting. The study incorporated the use of call-in reminders for tasks involving both personal and assigned elements and compared the use of the PDA and paper-based memory aids. The reminder for the PDA was in the form of a written cue with an alarm. Patients using the PDA showed timelier task completion than shown by those using paper-based memory aids. Further research was recommended to examine additional factors, such as individual differences as predictors of outcomes, use of different types of hardware or software, and more ecologically valid assessment of prospective memory and other executive function performance.

Memory aids will prove useful only if the entire team, including significant others (who should be educated in how such tools are to be used with the patient), reinforces their use. To truly make these tools functional after discharge, the therapist needs to identify the types of information that patients might have to maintain while in the community and design a memory aid that will fit their future tasks and lifestyle.

Awareness

To facilitate awareness of impairments in intervention sessions, the occupational therapist should begin therapy by asking the patient to predict how he or she will perform the specific task to be done (Toglia, 2005). Task specificity is important; the therapist may be targeting a cognitive or physical impairment that needs to be brought into the patient's awareness. Once the patient executes the task, the therapist records the patient's performance on the task and asks the patient to self-critique. Did the patient accomplish the task? Did the patient need assistance? Did the results match the patient's expectations? Was the performance or result error free? The therapist compares the patient's responses to these questions with his or her evaluation of the patient's performance, and a conversation about the differences between the therapist's observations and the patient's perceptions serves as a vehicle to heighten the patient's awareness.

Addressing awareness and other cognitive impairments in a group format may prove useful if the patient is able to tolerate activities of this kind. A daily group dealing with awareness could focus the patient on creating realistic goals for the inpatient rehabilitation stay. In addition, as patients are asked to execute a specific task, other group participants can provide feedback on how successfully or unsuccessfully the patient executes the task. Group leaders should encourage and maintain a supportive environment. Ownsworth, McFarland, and Young (2000) found that a group support program was beneficial in improving patients' ability to self-regulate their behavior. Their findings suggested that patients had better awareness of their deficits, were better able to anticipate situations in which they might experience problems, and were able to incorporate strategies into their daily lives.

A systematic review by Schmidt, Lannin, Fleming, and Ownsworth (2011) revealed that studies examining interventions that incorporated some type of feedback intervention improved self-awareness, functional task completion, and satisfaction with performance in patients with brain injury. However, the efficacy of these interventions was not fully determined, and further research was recommended given the difficulty in determining from the studies which form of feedback intervention or protocol was effective. (For a more detailed discussion on general cognitive intervention, see Chapter 3.)

Evaluation and Treatment of Swallowing

Several safety issues are considered when screening patients with severe TBI for **dysphagia,** who may present with respiratory problems, who may have a tracheostomy, or whose breathing may be assisted with a ventilator (Avery, 2008) and who also present with concomitant behavioral and cognitive problems. Before screening, the therapist records the patient's essential medical history, mechanism of trauma, and extent of injury (Alhashemi, 2010) and assesses the patient's head, trunk, and limb control as well as his or her level of arousal, attention, ability to follow commands, and whether the patient has any insight into his or her dysphagia (Avery, 2008). Oral and pharyngeal control, including ROM, muscle tone, strength, reflexes, and sensation are also assessed.

Avery (2008) described two approaches to addressing dysphagia. *Indirect therapy* addresses the underlying skills needed for swallowing such as ROM, strength of the oral and pharyngeal muscles, and coordination. *Direct therapy* addresses the patient's ability to use compensatory swallowing techniques during therapeutic feeding activities. Compensatory strategies are used to modify the size of the bolus, to adapt the texture of foods, and to modify the head and neck position for safer swallowing (Alhashemi, 2010). Addressing both the full evaluation and the treatment of dysphagia in the patient with severe TBI is a complex process, and a referral to either an occupational therapist or a speech–language pathologist who is an expert or specialist in the assessment and treatment of dysphagia should be made after an initial screen.

Special Considerations in Traumatic Brain Injury Rehabilitation

The medical management and rehabilitation of patients with TBI involve specific interventions. It is critical that the occupational therapist have a basic awareness and understanding of the interventions outlined here that may affect the rehabilitation team's overall intervention plans.

Pharmacological Management

Medications can control behavior effectively and allow patients to participate to some degree in their rehabilitation programs, but no specific regimen has been demonstrated to be particularly effective (Deb & Crownshaw, 2004). Methylphenidate (MPH; Ritalin) and dextroamphetamine are the two most commonly used CNS norepinephrine agonists. MPH has been used to target cognitive recovery, particularly in the areas of attention (*vigilance* [i.e., sustained attention], processing speed, distractibility), memory, and motor speed. In the areas of vigilance and sustained attention, several studies found significant improvement or trends in improvement (Evans, Gualtieri, & Patterson, 1987; Mahalick et al., 1998; Whyte et al., 1997).

Kim et al. (2012) noted that MPH has been prescribed for patients with TBI and has been reported to improve their attentional processing. They found that MPH improved attention and speed of processing, specifically reaction time. Their study incorporated the use of perfusion functional magnetic resonance imaging (fMRI) to examine any possible effects with underlying neurocorrelates when patients were given MPH. Kim et al. found that when MPH was administered, there was evidence of a deactivation of activity in the left posterior parietal cortex and the parieto–occipital junction that correlated with an increase in reaction time in patients with TBI. A possible explanation may be that the deactivation of these **parietal lobe** areas allowed for an increase in sustained attention and focus. The parietal lobe functions are thought to be important for stimuli in the peripheral visual fields; perhaps MPH suppresses this function so that focus toward the central visual field is enhanced.

Amantadine is a commonly prescribed medication for patients with disorders of **consciousness.** Giacino et al. (2012) studied the effects of prescribing amantadine in 184 patients with TBI who were **minimally conscious** or in a **vegetative state** 4 to 16 weeks postinjury and who were receiving inpatient rehabilitation. Four weeks of treatment with this medication were provided, and the effect on functional recovery was noted. The group receiving amantadine during this treatment period showed significant improvement in functional behaviors, with consistent responses to commands, intelligible speech, reliable *yes–no* responses, and functional object use.

Medications that are used for treatment of explosive agitation include risperidone (Risperdal), which acts by blocking dopamine and serotonin receptors. This antipsychotic medication has been well researched in psychiatric populations but not in patients with TBI. Risperidone may effectively control challenging behaviors after TBI, but much of this evidence is found in case reports, not randomized controlled trials, which are a higher level of evidence (Schreiber, Klag, Gross, Segman, & Pick, 1998; Silver, Collins, & Zidek, 2003; Temple, 2003). Valproic acid (Depakote) has been used as an anticonvulsant agent in patients with TBI, but it may serve as an effective mood stabilizer for patients who are agitated (Dikmen, Machamer, Winn, Anderson, & Temkin, 2000).

Physicians must take care that medications do not produce further cognitive issues. Patients receiving medications for challenging behaviors must be carefully monitored. In addition, the potential for medication interactions must be fully appreciated. Medical supervision of medications includes awareness of the potential for oversedation, increased seizure activity (Michals, Crismon, Roberts, & Childs, 1993), and chronic overuse that results in permanent side effects, such as tardive dyskinesia and motor restlessness (Fowler, Hertzog, & Wagner, 1995; Silver & Yudofsky, 1993; Wilkinson, Meythaler, & Guin-Renfroe, 1999).

The entire rehabilitation staff should be aware of typical side effects associated with medications and be alert to changes in the patient's medical status, behavior, and cognition. In the inpatient rehabilitation setting, constant communication across all shifts should take place between the physicians and staff about changes made in patients' medications. Ongoing monitoring of agitated behaviors with a formalized scale, such as the Agitated Behavior Scale (Corrigan, 1989), can help determine when pharmacological interventions are working and when they can be stopped. The occupational therapist can provide meaningful feedback about the effectiveness of pharmacological interventions for agitation relative to the patient's ability to engage in functional activities and react appropriately to environmental stimuli.

Transition From Acute, Inpatient, or Subacute Rehabilitation to the Community or Outpatient-Based Care

Toward the end of the patient's acute, inpatient, or subacute care stay, the rehabilitation team will have already prepared for the patient's transition to some other care situation along the care continuum. The team and family or caregiver should already have discussed and determined to where the patient will transition. Discharge needs and concerns include burden of care; type, amount, and duration of caregiver assistance required; DME needs; environmental and home adaptations and recommendations as indicated; and the continuation, type, amount, and duration of rehabilitation services. The rehabilitation team will often provide a justification for continuing rehabilitation services postdischarge if the patient demonstrates good potential for continued recovery as evidenced by steady gains or improvements in both impairments and functional status.

Activities to promote reentry into the community should be integrated into the rehabilitation program as soon as possible while the patient is on the inpatient unit. With the occupational therapist's supervision, patients may practice tasks such as preparing meals, balancing a checkbook, and doing laundry. When it is appropriate, the therapist should take patients into the community to practice a range of activities, including **community mobility,** shopping, and accessing transportation. The patient can make excursions into the community with family or caregivers when the physician (with input from the rehabilitation team) deems it appropriate to do so. Of course, before such an outing the occupational therapist and other team members first work closely with family and caregivers to ensure that they are comfortable and competent with the patient in activities such as wheelchair management, transfers (including car transfers, if applicable), toileting, and supervising self-medication schedules.

At times, it is useful before discharge for patients, family, and caregivers to practice certain skills they will carry out at home. The therapist may work with the patient and his or her family and friends on an independent living experience, which may involve an overnight stay in a model apartment on the unit. The experience allows for a controlled situation in which the patient, family, and caregivers can perform all ADLs as independently as possible, with nursing staff performing checks during the experience. The following day, the therapist meets with the patient and significant others to work out any remaining issues before actual discharge from inpatient rehabilitation.

The occupational therapist, along with other team members, works closely with patients and their family to ensure that all necessary DME and supplies (e.g., wheelchairs, seating systems, commodes, ambulation aids [braces, orthotics, walkers, canes], catheterization supplies) are ordered before discharge. When necessary, training with equipment and supplies should be provided for patients and their family and caregiver.

Rike, Ulleberg, Schultheis, Lundqvist, and Schanke (2014) examined self-regulatory behavior and the impact on driving in people with **acquired brain injury.** They stated that there was no consensus in the literature on the predictive value of neuropsychological testing or on-road driving tests and the incidence of accidents. People's driving behaviors were affected by how well they were able to initiate the self-regulatory skills of modulating attention, inhibition, or other executive functions. Rike et al. recommended that further measures of self-regulatory behavior and its effect on driving should focus on the multidisciplinary assessment, which was seen as more ecologically valid. Archer, Morris, and George (2014) examined physical and cognitive effects in people with multiple sclerosis and their perceptions of the impact of these effects on driving. Findings revealed that the participants experienced a grieving process because of the loss of independence, the need for supportive services as a result of the lack of resources and services for both the participant and family, and a need for more rigorous methods of coordination between health professionals and licensing authorities in serving people with this neurological condition.

Occupational therapists should be aware of how their organization may address the considerations outlined in this section, specific restrictions given patients' current level of functioning, and the concerns that both patients and families may have regarding patients' ability to pursue driving postinjury. Families and patients are often unaware of the impact of the TBI on driving and need to be educated by the rehabilitation team in how to address this issue. Therapists should provide patients and family members with explicit recommendations from the rehabilitation team regarding driver evaluation and training, if appropriate; what specific resources are

Families and patients are often unaware of the impact of the TBI on driving and need to be educated by the rehabilitation team in how to address this issue.

available regarding licensure restrictions; and where they can seek out appropriate or additional resources on transportation needs given the patient's potential inability to drive.

A large part of preparing for community reentry includes learning how to access services and resources. The occupational therapist and other team members work with patients and their family to obtain information on entitlements, supportive services, counseling, and alcohol and drug rehabilitation, if applicable. A valuable source of information is the Brain Injury Association of America (http://www.biausa.org), which has local and state chapters to which people should be referred well before discharge. When feasible, it is ideal to provide patients and their significant others with a mentor who has survived a TBI, is living in the community, and has received specialized training in being a mentor. Mentors can provide relevant support to the patient and family and be a source of advocacy.

People living with TBI will require a multitude of resources and will need to learn how to further enhance their skills from their first experiences with rehabilitation to their transition to outpatient settings or community reintegration. It is paramount that the rehabilitation team use its many resources to provide patients and families with the best and most relevant services to meet their needs during the process of adapting to this significant change in their lives.

The Case of Diane Archer

Let's revisit the case of Diane Archer, the young woman who sustained a TBI. The case picks up where it left off in Chapter 5.

Transfer to the Rehabilitation Hospital

Shortly after admission to the TBI unit of the rehabilitation hospital, Diane was greeted by Lindsey, the occupational therapist assigned to her. Lindsey has more than 8 years of experience working with clients who have experienced strokes and TBI. She worked in acute care and home care before taking her position at the rehab hospital 5 months earlier. She has taken numerous continuing education courses in topics related to stroke and TBI recovery (e.g., motor learning theory, cognitive rehabilitation) and completed a neurodevelopmental treatment–Bobath certificate course in the management and treatment of adults with **hemiplegia.**

Lindsey reviewed the documentation by Chris (the occupational therapist at the trauma center) in the paperwork that accompanied Diane from the trauma center and noted the rehab hospital TBI unit physiatrist's orders in the new chart. When Lindsey first went into Diane's room, she immediately noticed that Diane was restless: Her legs were moving constantly under the blankets, and her left hand was reaching for her husband, pulling the blankets, or grabbing the bed's side rails. Diane's right elbow was in a serial cast, and her right hand, although moving, appeared to have increased flexor tone. Lindsey noted that Diane appeared thin for her height. Diane's long, dark hair was pulled back into a ponytail, and she was wearing a loose-fitting cotton T-shirt and sweatpants. Diane's verbal response to Lindsey's greeting was a loud but monotone, "Hi, who the [expletive] are you? Tom, I want to go home!" Lindsey knew that Diane was entering the agitated phase of recovery (Rancho Level IV).

Lindsey attempted to complete an occupational profile but found that Diane's restlessness and limited ability to attend to requests made gathering information difficult. She knew that her ability to administer formalized assessments would be limited by Diane's agitation. She administered the brief Test of Orientation for Rehabilitation Patients (TORP; Deitz, Beeman, & Thorn, 1993) because it required only verbal responses. Diane was disoriented to personal situation (i.e., previous hospital and cause of hospitalization), time (day of week, time of day, month, year), place (she thought she was at her brother's home), and temporal continuity and had PTA. She was conscious and responsive but forgot all conversations shortly after they occurred.

Because Tom was present, Lindsey used the opportunity to gather background information for the occupational profile. She asked permission to contact Chris to discuss Diane's progress and casting program. Lindsey asked Tom to gather any home videos of Diane so the team could see her normal movement patterns and communication and interaction style. She also asked Tom to provide information about their home by drawing plans of the layout of each room, including the furniture. Tom offered to provide a flash drive with videos of both Diane and their home and yard to help the therapists visualize the rooms and space. Because Tom was planning on returning to work while Diane was in the rehab hospital, they discussed using a logbook with various sections to communicate the activities that Diane completed during intervention and to ask or answer any questions that Tom and the rehab team might have.

The next morning Lindsey and one of the unit nurses performed the self-care portions of the FIM to contribute to the team's total FIM score. Diane required maximal assistance (i.e., scores of 2) for the tasks of dressing, grooming, and toileting. Lindsey felt that Diane's agitation was the primary interfering factor at present. Although Diane showed evidence of impaired motor and cognitive skills, her agitation made it difficult for her to benefit from cueing or adaptive equipment (Exhibit 6.1).

Diane's emerging agitation was monitored by the team using Corrigan's (1989) Agitated Behavior Scale (ABS). The behaviors observed by the team members consisted of distractibility, impulsivity, restlessness, and loud, excessive talking. All behaviors were present to a moderate degree. The period of agitation was especially difficult for Diane's mother, who was concerned that Diane was regressing and that her agitated behaviors were the result of a permanent personality change. Lindsey educated Diane's mother and other family members about the stage of agitation (Table 6.5). She also taught them how to provide cues to redirect Diane's attention and calm her during periods of agitation.

During the 2nd week in the rehab hospital, Diane's agitation began to subside as observed behaviorally and reflected in the ABS scores. Lindsey and the speech–language pathologist conducted a videofluoroscopy exam of Diane's swallowing to ensure that she was not experiencing any episodes of dysphagia. She was cleared to eat all consistencies of food and liquids, so the gastrostomy tube was removed. Lindsey began a feeding program with Diane, and solid foods were gradually introduced. Diane automatically tried to use her right, dominant hand and expressed frustration with its clumsy movement and the cast on her elbow. Diane needed to be monitored during all meals because she impulsively shoved food into her mouth and risked choking and **aspiration.** She scored a 4 (i.e., minimal assistance) on the FIM section related to self-feeding.

Exhibit 6.1. Diane Archer's Initial Occupational Therapy Evaluation in the Rehabilitation Hospital

| Performance | | |
Areas	Skills	Patterns
ADLs: Client able to don overhead shirt and elastic-waist pants with maximal assistance. Totally dependent with more complex clothing and closures. Client requires maximal assistance and cues to bathe, perform grooming activities, and properly cleanse self after toileting. *IADLs, work, and leisure:* Client is unable to perform any of these activities because of agitation and cognitive processing limitations. *Social participation:* Client's current agitated and disinhibited behaviors result in inappropriate social interactions.	*Motor and Praxis Skills* *Motor:* Diane is able to stabilize and align her body to maintain trunk control and sitting balance while performing tasks. During standing activities, contact guard was required because client presented with an ataxic sway. Diane requires the use of a quad cane and moderate assistance of 1 person to walk because of the cast on her L lower leg and her impaired balance. When reaching with her right (dominant) arm, there is evidence of spasticity and only partially isolated movement throughout the elbow and shoulder range. Diane substitutes with trunk movement to reach her goal. She requires contact guard during activities that require trunk bending because she loses her balance and requires assistance to correct her sitting when she reaches to the edge of her range. L UE shows evidence of weakness throughout all muscle groups, resulting in difficulty lifting heavier objects. Diane's ability to move, transport, lift, and grip objects with her R UE is limited, but this limitation appears to be a result of tonal changes rather than underlying muscle strength. Motor endurance is limited. Diane fatigues quickly and requires frequent rest periods. *Praxis:* During ambulation, Diane is unable to follow the cane-and-step sequence because of her agitation and impaired learning. Diane has difficulty coordinating movements of her right extremity to manipulate objects because of the increased tone. Grasp and release, along with flow of movements, are slow, awkward, and occasionally ataxic in nature. Intermittent difficulty calibrating the force of movements is seen in both UEs; the underlying cause appears to be multifaceted (agitation with impulsivity, impaired attention, tonal changes in R UE musculature, evidence of ataxic movement). Cognitive impairments and agitation contribute to her inability to sustain her effort over the course of task performance. *Sensory–Perceptual Skills* Diane's basic sensory skills appear intact, but her attentional impairments limit her ability to appropriately interpret and respond to sensory input. At times, her responses are impulsive, and at other times they are delayed. She requires moderate to maximal cues to position her body to perform safe transfers from the wheelchair or quad cane to the bed and toilet, especially when her need for the toilet is urgent. Diane requires moderate to maximal cues to choose appropriate tools and to use them appropriately (e.g., selecting the spoon rather than the fork to eat pudding). *Emotional Regulation Skills* During periods of agitation or when she experiences pain, Diane makes inappropriate statements (e.g., cursing in public places). She will kiss and hug her husband and parents when they visit, but the behavior appears automatic and **emotion** free. At present, the family has not brought in the client's daughter because of Diane's unpredictable responses and concern for the daughter's reaction to the visible signs of her mother's injury. *Cognitive Skills* Diane shows significant difficulty attending to tasks and maintaining a consistent pace in her performance of simple tasks. She shows impulsivity and distractibility to both internal and external stimuli. Currently, her agitation interferes with her performance of goal-directed tasks and her ability to ask for guidance when confused. Diane's ability to organize task spaces and task objects is difficult to evaluate at present because of her underlying cognitive and attentional impairments. She responds somewhat impulsively to objects in her immediate space but shows no ability to search for needed objects or to gather and organize needed materials (e.g., placement of grooming objects on sink top in bathroom). Diane initiates tasks impulsively without a clear understanding of the task or regard for safety. She requires cues to continue tasks because of attentional impairments and to sequence tasks in logical order (e.g., donning socks before sneakers). Perseveration is noted occasionally, requiring verbal and tactile cues to terminate some actions. Diane's ability to respond to cues (visual, tactile, verbal) is compromised at present. Her ability to learn new ways to perform functional tasks is limited by her inattention and memory impairments. Diane does not notice when she makes errors and thus does not modify her performance or the environment to facilitate her performance. *Communication and Social Skills* Diane is able to articulate the majority of her personal needs (e.g., bathroom), but she has difficulty modulating the volume of her voice when agitated. Her interactions with others show a disregard for social norms and conversational pragmatics.	Information regarding past patterns of performance gathered during acute care hospitalization. *Current habits and routines:* Client is unable to initiate following daily treatment schedule without cues because of memory impairment. *Roles:* Performance of the behavior sets associated with her previous roles is limited by impairments in client factors and performance skill limitations.

(Continued)

Exhibit 6.1. Diane Archer's Initial Occupational Therapy Evaluation in the Rehabilitation Hospital *(cont.)*

Client Factors	Context
Spirituality The local priest continues to come to the facility weekly to pray with the family. Client is able to mouth the words of some familiar prayers but remains restless during these sessions. *Mental Functions* *Global mental functions:* Client is disoriented to time. She shows agitation and disrupted sleep–wake cycles. Impulsivity is noted. *Specific mental functions:* Client displays problems in attention, memory, and higher thought functions. Formal evaluation was unable to be performed because of agitation. Client is unable to sustain attention for more than a few seconds. She does not appear to recognize caregivers, although she does appear to remember family. She is unaware of why she is hospitalized. *Sensory Functions and Pain* *Seeing and related functions:* Client previously wore corrective contacts but is currently wearing her glasses (husband reports the prescription is at least 3 yr old and is unaware of whether her acuity has changed in that time). *Neuromusculoskeletal and Movement-Related Functions* *Functions of joints and bones:* Client has full PROM of all joints in both upper limbs. **End feel** of the joint capsules is tight in R UE. *Muscle functions:* Client displays minimal to moderate increase in flexor tone in the R UE. L UE displays normal tone. *Movement functions:* Client is able to volitionally move R UE, but movement shows evidence of spasticity influenced patterns.	*Cultural* The rehabilitation hospital culture emphasizes the importance of independence and engagement in the therapy process. Families are also encouraged to participate in therapy sessions and continue with selected interventions during evenings and weekends. *Physical* At present, the client is on the TBI Unit in the rehab hospital; environmental stimuli are able to be modulated somewhat by use of different rooms. Dining room appears to be overstimulating, as does the large treatment room. Meals and individualized occupational therapy sessions take place in either the client's room or the small treatment room. The physical structure of the client's room and the community spaces makes it easier to maneuver in a wheelchair. Her room is decorated with some personal items and photos of her family. *Social* Client now has a roommate who is also recovering from a TBI. Client's family visits daily, and client will engage in group activities as her agitation decreases. *Personal* 28-yr-old married woman who is the mother of a toddler. *Temporal* Late spring.
Implications for Intervention Planning	
Client's present state of agitation requires that the occupational therapy intervention be highly structured to monitor the activity demands to ensure that they match the client's current performance skills. Engagement in the intervention process should not increase agitated behavior or outbursts. Familiar personal objects will be used for functional tasks because they may elicit memory for task sequence and performance as well as offer a sense of calm (objects and their properties). Because the amount of stimulation and complexity in the environment (e.g., noise level, number of people, scattered or cluttered surfaces) appears to increase client's distractibility and impulsivity, space demands will be adjusted to match her current mental state. The client is unable to engage in socially appropriate interactions with others and is unable to react appropriately to some of the social norms of the environment (social demands), so her therapy sessions will be conducted 1:1 in private rooms. Activities requiring any form of sequencing or timing between steps will be broken down into 1-step components because of cognitive impairments (e.g., memory, attention, modulation of response speed). Activities selected for intervention will be as client-centered as possible and require actions of balance (sitting and standing); bilateral UE coordination and manipulation; and processing skills of attending, pacing speed of responses, and appropriately initiating and terminating functional tasks involving objects. Cues or task adaptation will be provided as needed.	

Note. ADLs = activities of daily living; IADLs = instrumental activities of daily living; L = left; PROM = passive range of motion; R = right; TBI = traumatic brain injury; UE/UEs = upper extremity/extremities; yr = year/years.

Around her 3rd week in the rehab hospital, Diane's PTA began to clear. Her scores on the TORP improved in all areas. She needed fewer verbal cues to state the correct information and automatically used environmental cues (e.g., wall calendar) to aid her orientation. Diane showed some day-to-day memory but needed multiple cues to recall details of the previous day. Her attention continued to be limited, and Lindsey believed this limitation was significantly affecting Diane's memory. Diane demonstrated retrograde amnesia for approximately 3 months before her injury.

A formalized evaluation of Diane's cognitive and sensory–perceptual skills was initiated during her 3rd week in rehab (see Table 6.5). Lindsey decided to use multiple assessment methods to gain a complete profile of Diane's cognitive performance and rehabilitative needs. Lindsey focused on direct observation and rating of Diane's cognitive skills during functional performance and also evaluated the underlying cognitive impairments that appeared to contribute to Diane's performance.

Table 6.5. Sample Activities From Diane Archer's Intervention Plan During the Acute Rehabilitation Phase of Recovery

Problems and Goals	Approach	Primary Focus of Intervention	Interventions
Problem: Agitation *Goal:* Client will demonstrate decreased agitation as seen in her ability to attend to and participate in simple gross motor and functional activities while modulating her voice volume and amount of talking.	• Establish and restore ability to modulate response to internal and external stimuli	*Client factors:* Global and specific mental functions related to temperament and emotional functions *Performance skills:* Emotion regulation skills, communication and social skills, and cognitive skills (pacing and attending to tasks)	*Preparatory methods:* Minimize environmental stimuli in the client's room. Engage client in any physical activity possible to provide constructive energy release (e.g., gross motor activities). *Purposeful activity:* Engage client in the performance of simple ADL tasks, gross motor activities, and games that the client can complete without increased frustration. Provide physical and cognitive assistance to compensate for impairments; attempt to encourage improved performance only during periods of calm behavior. Vary activities to sustain the client's attention to the tasks. Model desired voice modulation when speaking with or directing client. *Consultation:* Coordinate with nursing staff to develop a therapy schedule for client that balances periods of activity and rest. *Education:* Assist family in understanding why agitation occurs and how to redirect client's attention during episodes.
Problem: Disorientation *Goal:* Client will use environmental cues to provide correct time and place information. *Goal:* Client will require fewer verbal cues to provide correct orientation-related information.	• Establish and restore client's orientation to all spheres • Modify the context to support orientation to time and place	*Client factors:* Global mental functions of orientation	*Preparatory methods:* Hang a large calendar and clock in client's room where they are visible from her bed. When client is not in her room, provide her with verbal cues to correctly identify the day or week, month, date, year, and location. Provide client with a simple logbook with a calendar and schedule of therapy sessions. Have client attempt to recall treatment activities for entry into logbook at the end of sessions. *Purposeful activity:* Have client decorate poster board around calendar with photos of family. Use label maker to create labels to identify family members. Have client cross off previous day on the calendar each morning. Have client engage in a simple orientation-focused board or gross motor game with one or two other clients who also have orientation limitations. *Education:* Educate the family about why disorientation and confusion occur and how to provide orienting information for client.
Problem: Decreased independence in basic ADLs *Goal:* Client will be able to bathe, dress, and groom herself with supervision and minimal verbal cues.	• Establish and restore • Modify	*Performance skills:* Various motor and praxis skills (coordination, manipulation, maintaining balance) and cognitive skills (organizing space and objects, sequencing tasks) *Performance patterns:* Client routine of bathing, dressing, and grooming each morning; institute an ADL program *Areas of occupation:* ADLs of bathing and showering, dressing, personal hygiene, and grooming	*Purposeful activity:* Work with client on creating a list of bathing and grooming items she needs to bring into the shower each morning. Have client create a list of grooming tasks to be completed, and post it on the bathroom mirror. Each afternoon have client select clothing for the next day and hang them on her closet door. *Occupation-based activity:* Engage client in a daily self-care program of showering, dressing, and grooming, providing verbal and physical cues as needed. *Education:* Educate family and nursing staff about any adaptive equipment provided to the client to assist in ADL performance.

(Continued)

Table 6.5. Sample Activities From Diane Archer's Intervention Plan During the Acute Rehabilitation Phase of Recovery *(cont.)*

Problems and Goals	Approach	Primary Focus of Intervention	Interventions
Problem: Increased tone and decreased isolated movement in R UE *Goal:* Client will tolerate wearing serial cast as evidenced by skin integrity, decreased tone, and increased ROM in right elbow and wrist. *Goal:* Client will demonstrate improved quality of isolated movement in R UE.	• Establish and restore normal movement patterns • Prevent decrease in joint ROM and muscle length	*Client factors:* Structure and function of joints and bones; neuromusculoskeletal and movement-related functions *Performance skills:* Motor and praxis skills related to posture, mobility, coordination, reaching and manipulation	*Preparatory methods:* Provide serial casting program with cast changes every 5 days. As client progresses in the casting program, perform cutout over triceps on Day 3 and engage client in a variety of purposeful activities requiring elbow extension (e.g., reaching, weight bearing). Use electrical stimulation to triceps to provide assisted stretch to elbow. Provide AAROM to all joints of both UEs. *Purposeful activity:* Using Gentile's (1987) Taxonomy of Motor Tasks, engage the client in various functional motor tasks (e.g., grooming, self-feeding, object manipulation) with gradual increases in the unpredictability and complexity of the contextual and activity demands. Provide tactile input to guide and normalize movement patterns. *Occupation-based activity:* Encourage normal movement patterns while engaged in all functional and occupation-based activities (e.g., morning grooming).
Problem: Impaired awareness, attention, memory, and executive functions *Goal:* Client will be able to accurately estimate the difficulty of a task and her need to initiate strategies and self-monitor performance during tasks. *Goal:* Client will sustain attention on a given task without evidence of internal or external distractions. *Goal:* Client will be able to successfully use her smartphone to compensate for memory impairments (i.e., identify location to enter information, enter sufficient and accurate detail to assist memory, set alarm to remind).	• Establish and restore cognitive skills; teach client cognitive strategies to improve performance • Modify environment to enhance cognitive capabilities; modify task performance to compensate for cognitive limitations	*Client factors:* Specific mental functions of attention, memory, thought, and higher level cognitive functions *Performance skills:* Cognitive skills related to attention and memory; sequencing and organization of space, objects, and tasks *Performance patterns:* Establishing new routines of entering data into a memory aid	*Preparatory methods:* Have the client estimate task difficulty and her need for strategies and assistance before initiating all treatment tasks. Have client complete short checklist comparing estimate with actual performance. *Purposeful activity:* Using Toglia's (2011) Dynamic Interactional Approach to cognitive rehabilitation, engage the client in various tasks that require the practice of targeted processing strategies in situations that are at the same level of difficulty. Once transfer of the strategy to these new situations is observed, gradually increase the difficulty of the contextual and activity demands. Provide gradually diminishing cues to guide performance and identify methods to enable client to self-cue and monitor performance. *Occupation-based activity:* Have client engage in a variety of activities related to roles, responsibilities, and interests (e.g., financial management, cooking, parenting, gardening, playing simple board games with daughter). *Education:* Educate family and other team members on the use of the smartphone as a memory aid. Ensure that all team members are assisting the client in consistently using the device.

Note. AAROM = active assistive range of motion; ADL/ADLs = activity/activities of daily living; R = right; ROM = range of motion; UE/UEs = upper extremity/extremities.

As part of the cognitive evaluation, Lindsey asked Diane to make lunch using items in the refrigerator. Before initiating the task, Lindsey asked Diane whether she thought she would need any assistance. Diane vaguely identified and described her cognitive and physical difficulties, but she was unable to use this knowledge to anticipate her need for assistance or to judge the difficulty level of the task. Consequently, she overestimated her performance and underestimated her need for assistance. Diane needed Lindsey's assistance to generate the idea of making a sandwich for lunch after staring into the refrigerator for more than 3 minutes. Diane identified the food items she wanted in her sandwich (lettuce, tomato, cheese, lunch meat, mayonnaise) and created a written list of the items with Lindsey's assistance.

Using her wheelchair, Diane had to make several trips to the refrigerator because she forgot all the items she needed to gather. Lindsey assisted Diane with physical components of the task as needed but had Diane complete as much of the task as she could. Diane had difficulty attending to and sequencing the steps of making the sandwich (e.g., she placed mayonnaise on both sides of one piece of bread). She forgot to add the cheese to the sandwich and noted it on the plate only after she had bitten into the sandwich.

Because Diane appeared to demonstrate impairments in attention, memory, high-level reasoning, and executive skills during the functional task, Lindsey decided to specifically assess these underlying skills to better understand how their impairment contributed to Diane's performance. Lindsey administered the Test of Everyday Attention (Robertson, Ward, Ridgeway, & Nimmo-Smith, 1994); Diane demonstrated difficulty with all subtests of the different components of attention (i.e., selective visual and auditory attention, sustained attention, switching attention, divided attention). On the Rivermead Behavioural Memory Test–Extended (Wilson et al., 1991), Diane scored below average in all areas but performed better on tasks that required recognition than on those that required recall. On the Contextual Memory Test (Toglia, 1993a), Diane scored 4 out of 20 on both immediate and delayed recall. She reported that she did not use any particular strategy (e.g., context of the restaurant setting), stating, "I just looked at them." When given recognition cues, she was able to identify 9 of the original 20 items correctly but also gave 4 false-positive responses, selecting items that were not in the original 20.

Over the next few weeks, Diane continued to show steady improvement. Functionally, she was able to perform basic self-care activities with minimal assistance and moderate cues to sequence the clothing and attend to details. During morning self-care activities, Diane made careless errors (e.g., misaligning buttons, putting her shirt on inside out without realizing it, putting on shoes without socks) and occasionally misidentified objects on the bathroom sink (e.g., picked up the shampoo to use as mouthwash). Initially, Lindsey thought Diane might have a perceptual problem, but she believed Diane's errors were related to her impulsivity because Diane could self-correct when cued to slow down and attend to the task.

The cast on Diane's left leg was removed, and she began to walk in physical therapy with a walker and moderate assistance because of her impaired balance and her weak, hemiparetic right arm. Tom and the therapists discussed the possibility of converting their downstairs den into a bedroom until Diane was able to handle the stairs on returning home, but Diane was adamant that she would go up the stairs even if she had to do so sitting on her bottom. The casting program was discontinued after maximal elbow extension range had been achieved. Diane still wore a resting cast at night to maintain her elbow range. She had isolated movement in her right arm, but the movement was slow and clumsy.

Diane was right-hand dominant but had difficulty grasping and manipulating objects during functional tasks because of the underlying tonal changes and spastic quality of movement. During functional tasks, such as brushing her hair or putting on makeup, she frequently switched to using her nondominant left hand out of frustration. Lindsey administered the COPM to identify the things that Diane wanted or needed to be able to do on discharge home (this information was verified

Table 6.6. Diane Archer's Canadian Occupational Performance Measure Results in the Rehabilitation Hospital

Daily Living Concerns	Importance (1 = Low; 10 = High)	Satisfaction (1 = Low; 10 = High)	Ability Level (1 = Low; 10 = High)
Being able to dress and bathe independently	10	3	5
Being able to take care of daughter Kate (i.e., play with her, make her food, help her get dressed)	10	1	3
Being able to cook a simple meal	8	2	3

with Diane's husband because Diane's awareness was still impaired). The results of the COPM are given in Table 6.6.

Diane's daughter, Kate, began making short visits during Diane's 3rd week in the rehab hospital. Although initially awkward with each other, they began to rebuild their relationship. During several of these visits, Lindsey worked with Kate and Diane on tasks that were previously part of Diane's parenting role and were identified in her COPM as being important (e.g., making a sandwich for Kate, playing simple games, and helping Kate put on her shoes and coat). Lindsey also used occupation-based interventions such as making change during simulated shopping, doing laundry, cooking simple meals, and performing simple household cleaning (using the hospital's rehab apartment; Table 6.5). Although Diane was showing improved motor and cognitive skills, she continued to show impaired patterns of performance and needed cues to complete self-care tasks at appropriate times and to establish the performance of these tasks as routine.

For 2 years before her injury, Diane had used her smartphone as a PDA to schedule almost all of her daily activities (e.g., appointments, to-do lists, Kate's play dates, shopping lists), so Lindsey determined that this familiar device might be helpful as a memory aid. To work on retraining Diane with the smartphone apps, Lindsey asked Tom to bring in Diane's phone from home. Lindsey gave Diane various tasks that required her to program the phone and set the alarm (e.g., watch Channel 2 news and note the lead story, ask the head nurse her dog's name, bring your jacket to your next occupational therapy session, ask Tom what he had for lunch today). They also role-played different scenarios in which entering data into the device would be helpful.

Lindsey and the physical therapist performed a home visit to Diane and Tom's home before her discharge to the rehab center's day program. They made several recommendations to ensure Diane's safe movement in the home. Diane's mother would be staying at the house to supervise Diane and to assist in Kate's care until Diane achieved greater independence.

After 5 weeks as an inpatient in the rehab hospital, Diane was transferred to the facility's day program. At the time of discharge, she scored as modified independent (i.e., scores of 6) on the self-care, mobility, and locomotion items of the FIM. She scored as minimal assistance to supervision (i.e., scores of 4–5) on the social adjustment–cooperation, cognitive–problem solving, and communication items. The case of Diane Archer continues at the end of Chapter 7, when Diane returns to the community to continue her recovery.

References

Abreu, B. C., & Hinojosa, J. (1992). The process approach for cognitive–perceptual and postural control dysfunction for adults with brain injuries. In N. Katz (Ed.), *Cognitive rehabilitation: Models for intervention in occupational therapy* (pp. 167–194). Boston: Andover Medical.

Acker, M. B. (1989). A review of the ecological validity of neuropsychological tests. In D. E. Tupper & K. D. Cicerone (Eds.), *The neuropsychology of everyday life: Assessment and basic competencies* (pp. 19–55). Boston: Kluwer.

Alhashemi, H. H. (2010). Dysphagia in severe traumatic brain injury. *Neurosciences, 15,* 231–236.

American Occupational Therapy Association. (2014). Occupational therapy practice framework: Domain and process (3rd ed.). *American Journal of Occupational Therapy, 68*(Suppl. 1), S1–S48. http://dx.doi.org/10.5014/ajot.2014.682006

Archer, C., Morris, L., & George, S. (2014). Assessment and rehabilitation of driver skills: Subjective experiences of people with multiple sclerosis and health professionals. *Disability and Rehabilitation, 36,* 1875–1882. http://dx.doi.org/10.3109/09638288.2013.877089

Árnadóttir, G. (1990). *The brain and behavior: Assessing cortical dysfunction through activities of daily living.* St. Louis: Mosby.

Árnadóttir, G. (2012). Impact of neurobehavioral deficits on activities of daily living. In G. Gillen (Ed.), *Stroke rehabilitation: A function-based approach* (3rd ed., pp. 456–500). St. Louis: Mosby.

Aubut, J. A., Mehta, S., Cullen, N., & Teasell, R. W.; ERABI Group; Scire Research Team. (2011). A comparison of heterotopic ossification treatment within the traumatic brain and spinal cord injured population: An evidence based systematic review. *NeuroRehabilitation, 28,* 151–160. http://dx.doi.org/10.3233/NRE-2011-0643

Avery, W. (2008). Dysphagia. In M. V. Radomski & C. A. Trombly Latham (Eds.), *Occupational therapy for physical dysfunction* (6th ed., pp. 1321–1344). Philadelphia: Lippincott Williams & Wilkins.

Baum, C. M., & Katz, N. (2010). Occupational therapy approach to assessing the relationship between cognition and function. In T. D. Marcotte & I. Grant (Eds.), *Neuropsychology of everyday functioning* (pp. 1–29). New York: Guilford.

Beaulieu, C., Wertheimer, J. C., Pickett, L., Spierre, L., Schnorbus, T., Healy, W., . . . Jones, A. (2008). Behavior management on an acute brain injury unit: Evaluating the effectiveness of an interdisciplinary training program. *Journal of Head Trauma Rehabilitation, 23,* 304–311. http://dx.doi.org/10.1097/01.HTR.0000336843.60961.b7

Benson, J., & Clark, F. (1982). A guide for instrument development and validation. *American Journal of Occupational Therapy, 36,* 789–800. http://dx.doi.org/10.5014/ajot.36.12.789

Benson, J., & Schell, B. A. (1997). Measurement theory: Application to occupational and physical therapy. In J. Van Deusen & D. Brunt (Eds.), *Assessment in occupational therapy and physical therapy* (pp. 3–23). Philadelphia: W. B. Saunders.

Blumenfeld, H. (2002). *Neuroanatomy through clinical cases.* Sunderland, MA: Sinauer Associates.

Blumenfeld, H. (2010). *Neuroanatomy through clinical cases* (2nd ed.). Sunderland, MA: Sinauer Associates.

Bouwmeester, L., Heutink, J., & Lucas, C. (2007). The effect of visual training for patients with visual field defects due to brain damage: A systematic review. *Journal of Neurology, Neurosurgery, and Psychiatry, 78,* 555–564. http://dx.doi.org/10.1136/jnnp.2006.103853

Boys, M., Fisher, P., & Holzberg, C. (1991). *The OSOT Perceptual Evaluation Manual: Revised.* Scarborough, Ontario: Nelson Canada.

Boys, M., Fisher, P., Holzberg, C., & Reid, D. W. (1988). The OSOT Perceptual Evaluation: A research perspective. *American Journal of Occupational Therapy, 42,* 92–98. http://dx.doi.org/10.5014/ajot.42.2.92

Brown, T., & Jäckel, A. L. (2007). Perceptual assessments. In I. E. Asher (Ed.), *Occupational therapy assessment tools: An annotated index* (3rd ed., pp. 353–420). Bethesda, MD: AOTA Press.

Burgess, P. W., Alderman, N., Forbes, C., Costello, A., Coates, L. M., Dawson, D. R., . . . Channon, S. (2006). The case for the development and use of "ecologically valid" measures of executive function in experimental and clinical neuropsychology. *Journal of the International Neuropsychological Society, 12,* 194–209. http://dx.doi.org/10.1017/S1355617706060310

Chaytor, N., & Schmitter-Edgecombe, M. (2003). The ecological validity of neuropsychological tests: A review of the literature on everyday cognitive skills. *Neuropsychology Review, 13,* 181–197. http://dx.doi.org/10.1023/B:NERV.0000009483.91468.fb

Chaytor, N., Schmitter-Edgecombe, M., & Burr, R. (2006). Improving the ecological validity of executive functioning assessment. *Archives of Clinical Neuropsychology, 21,* 217–227. http://dx.doi.org/10.1016/j.acn.2005.12.002

Cicerone, K. D., Dahlberg, C., Kalmar, K., Langenbahn, D. M., Malec, J. F., Bergquist, T. F., . . . Morse, P. A. (2000). Evidence-based cognitive rehabilitation: Recommendations for clinical practice. *Archives of Physical Medicine and Rehabilitation, 81,* 1596–1615. http://dx.doi.org/10.1053/apmr.2000.19240

Cicerone, K. D., Dahlberg, C., Malec, J. F., Langenbahn, D. M., Felicetti, T., Kneipp, S., . . . Catanese, J. (2005). Evidence-based cognitive rehabilitation: Updated review of the literature from 1998 through 2002. *Archives of Physical Medicine and Rehabilitation, 86,* 1681–1692. http://dx.doi.org/10.1016/j.apmr.2005.03.024

Cicerone, K. D., Langenbahn, D. M., Braden, C., Malec, J. F., Kalmar, K., Fraas, M., . . . Ashman, T. (2011). Evidence-based cognitive rehabilitation: Updated review of the literature from 2003 through 2008. *Archives of Physical Medicine and Rehabilitation, 92,* 519–530. http://dx.doi.org/10.1016/j.apmr.2010.11.015

Cohen, M., Ylvisaker, M., Hamilton, J., Kemp, L., & Claiman, B. (2010). Errorless learning of functional life skills in an individual with three aetiologies of severe memory and executive function impairment. *Neuropsychological Rehabilitation, 20,* 355–376. http://dx.doi.org/10.1080/09602010903309401

Cohen, R. J., & Swerdlik, M. E. (1999). *Psychological testing and assessment: An introduction to tests and measurement* (4th ed.). Mountain View, CA: Mayfield.

Cohen, R. J., & Swerdlik, M. E. (2002). *Psychological testing and assessment: An introduction to tests and measurement* (5th ed.). Boston: McGraw-Hill.

Constantinidou, F., Wertheimer, J. C., Tsanadis, J., Evans, C., & Paul, D. R. (2012). Assessment of executive functioning in brain injury: Collaboration between speech–language pathology and neuropsychology for an integrative neuropsychological perspective. *Brain Injury, 26,* 1549–1563. http://dx.doi.org/10.3109/02699052.2012.698786

Cooke, D. M., & Finkelstein, N. (2007). Assessment of process skills and mental functions: Part 1: Cognitive assessments. In I. E. Asher (Ed.), *Occupational therapy assessment tools: An annotated index* (3rd ed., pp. 489–570). Bethesda, MD: AOTA Press.

Cooke, D. M., McKenna, K., & Fleming, J. (2005). Development of a standardized occupational therapy screening tool for visual perception in adults. *Scandinavian Journal of Occupational Therapy, 12,* 59–71. http://dx.doi.org/10.1080/11038120410020683-1

Cooke, D. M., McKenna, K., Fleming, J., & Darnell, R. (2005). The reliability of the Occupational Therapy Adult Perceptual Screening Test (OT–APST). *British Journal of Occupational Therapy, 68,* 509–517. http://dx.doi.org/10.1177/030802260506801105

Corrigan, J. D. (1989). Development of a scale for assessment of agitation following traumatic brain injury. *Journal of Clinical and Experimental Neuropsychology, 11,* 261–277. http://dx.doi.org/10.1080/01688638908400888

Corrigan, J. D., Smith-Knapp, K., & Granger, C. V. (1997). Validity of the Functional Independence Measure for persons with traumatic brain injury. *Archives of Physical Medicine and Rehabilitation, 78,* 828–834. http://dx.doi.org/10.1016/S0003-9993(97)90195-7

Crocker, L., & Algina, J. (1986). *Introduction to classical and modern test theory.* Orlando, FL: Harcourt Brace Jovanovich.

Cullen, N., Bayley, M., Bayona, N., Hilditch, M., & Aubut, J.; ERABI Group. (2007). Management of heterotopic ossification and venous thromboembolism following acquired brain injury. *Brain Injury, 21,* 215–230. http://dx.doi.org/10.1080/02699050701202027

Cuthbert, J. P., Corrigan, J. D., Harrison-Felix, C., Coronado, V., Dijkers, M. P., Heinemann, A. W., & Whiteneck, G. G. (2011). Factors that predict acute hospitalization discharge disposition for adults with moderate to severe traumatic brain injury. *Archives of Physical Medicine and Rehabilitation, 92,* 721–730, e3. http://dx.doi.org/10.1016/j.apmr.2010.12.023

Damasio, A. R. (1994). *Descartes' error: Emotion, reason, and the human brain.* New York: Avon Books.

Deb, S., & Crownshaw, T. (2004). The role of pharmacotherapy in the management of behaviour disorders in traumatic brain injury patients. *Brain Injury, 18,* 1–31. http://dx.doi.org/10.1080/02699050310001110463

DeGuise, E., LeBlanc, J., Feyz, M., Thomas, H., & Gusselin, N. (2005). Effect of an integrated reality orientation programme in acute care on posttraumatic amnesia in patients with traumatic brain injury. *Brain Injury, 19*, 263–269. http://dx.doi.org/10.1080/02699050400004971

Deitz, T., Beeman, C., & Thorn, D. (1993). *Test of Orientation for Rehabilitation Patients.* Tucson, AZ: Therapy Skill Builders.

Denny-Brown, D. (1966). *The cerebral control of movement.* Liverpool, England: Liverpool University Press.

Dikmen, S. S., Machamer, J. E., Winn, H. R., Anderson, G. D., & Temkin, N. R. (2000). Neuropsychological effects of valproate in traumatic brain injury: A randomized trial. *Neurology, 54*, 895–902.

Dowds, M. M., Lee, P. H., Sheer, J. B., O'Neil-Pirozzi, T. M., Xenopoulos-Oddsson, A., Goldstein, R., . . . Glenn, M. B. (2011). Electronic reminding technology following traumatic brain injury: Effects on timely task completion. *Journal of Head Trauma Rehabilitation, 26*, 339–347. http://dx.doi.org/10.1097/HTR.0b013e3181f2bf1d

Dunn, W. (1993). Measurement of function: Actions for the future. *American Journal of Occupational Therapy, 47*, 357–359. http://dx.doi.org/10.5014/ajot.47.4.357

Evans, R. W., Gualtieri, C. T., & Patterson, D. (1987). Treatment of chronic closed head injury with psychostimulant drugs: A controlled case study and an appropriate evaluation procedure. *Journal of Nervous and Mental Disease, 175*, 106–110. http://dx.doi.org/10.1097/00005053-198702000-00007

Fisher, A. G., & Short-DeGraff, M. (1993). Improving functional assessment in occupational therapy: Recommendations and philosophy for change. *American Journal of Occupational Therapy, 47*, 199–201. http://dx.doi.org/10.5014/ajot.47.3.199

Fowler, S. B., Hertzog, J., & Wagner, B. K. (1995). Pharmacological interventions for agitation in head-injured patients in the acute care setting. *Journal of Neuroscience Nursing, 27*, 119–123. http://dx.doi.org/10.1097/01376517-199504000-00011

Gentile, A. M. (1987). Skill acquisition: Action, movement, and neuromotor processes. In J. H. Carr, R. Shepherd, J. Gordon, A. M. Gentile, & J. M. Held (Eds.), *Movement science: Foundations for physical therapy in rehabilitation.* Rockville, MD: Aspen.

Giacino, J. T., Whyte, J., Bagiella, E., Kalmar, K., Childs, N., Khademi, A., . . . Sherer, M. (2012). Placebo-controlled trial of amantadine for severe traumatic brain injury. *New England Journal of Medicine, 366*, 819–826. http://dx.doi.org/10.1056/NEJMoa1102609

Goverover, Y., & Hinojosa, J. (2002). Categorization and deductive reasoning: Predictors of instrumental activities of daily living performance in adults with brain injury. *American Journal of Occupational Therapy, 56*, 509–516. http://dx.doi.org/10.5014/ajot.56.5.509

Gracies, J. M., Elovic, E., McGuire, J., & Simpson, D. M. (1997). Traditional pharmacological treatments for spasticity. Part I: Local treatments. *Muscle and Nerve, 20*(Suppl. 6), 61–91.

Granger, C. V., Hamilton, B. B., Linacre, J. M., Heinemann, A. W., & Wright, B. D. (1993). Performance profiles of the Functional Independence Measures. *American Journal of Physical Medicine and Rehabilitation, 72*, 35–44.

Gutman, S. A., Mortera, M. H., Hinojosa, J., & Kramer, P. (2007). Revision of the *Occupational Therapy Practice Framework. American Journal of Occupational Therapy, 61*, 119–126. http://dx.doi.org/10.5014/ajot.61.1.119

Gutman, S. A., & Schonfeld, A. (2009). *Screening adult neurologic populations: A step-by-step instruction manual* (2nd ed.). Bethesda, MD: AOTA Press.

Hagen, C. (1998). *The Rancho Los Amigos Levels of Cognitive Functioning: The revised levels* (3rd ed.). Downey, CA: Los Amigos Research and Educational Institute.

Hagen, C., Malkmus, D., & Durham, P. (1979). *Levels of cognitive functioning, rehabilitation of the brain-injured adult: Comprehensive physical management.* Downey, CA: Professional Staff Association of Rancho Los Amigos Hospital.

Hartman-Maeir, A., Katz, N., & Baum, C. M. (2009). Cognitive Functional Evaluation (CFE) process for individuals with suspected cognitive disabilities. *Occupational Therapy in Health Care, 23*, 1–23. http://dx.doi.org/10.1080/07380570802455516

Harvey, L. A., & Herbert, R. D. (2002). Muscle stretching for treatment and prevention of contracture in people with spinal cord injury. *Spinal Cord, 40*, 1–9. http://dx.doi.org/10.1038/sj.sc.3101241

Hinojosa, J., Kramer, P., & Crist, P. (Eds.). (2005). *Evaluation: Obtaining and interpreting data* (2nd ed.). Bethesda, MD: AOTA Press.

Katalinic, O. M., Harvey, L. A., & Herbert, R. D. (2011). Effectiveness of stretch for the treatment and prevention of contractures in people with neurological conditions: A systematic review. *Physical Therapy, 91,* 11–24. http://dx.doi.org/10.2522/ptj.20100265

Katz, N., Itzkovich, M., Averbuch, S., & Elazar, B. (1989). Loewenstein Occupational Therapy Cognitive Assessment (LOTCA) battery for brain-injured patients: Reliability and validity. *American Journal of Occupational Therapy, 43,* 184–192. http://dx.doi.org/10.5014/ajot.43.3.184

Kim, J., Whyte, J., Patel, S., Europa, E., Wang, J., Coslett, H. B., & Detre, J. A. (2012). Methylphenidate modulates sustained attention and cortical activation in survivors of traumatic brain injury: A perfusion fMRI study. *Psychopharmacology, 222,* 47–57. http://dx.doi.org/10.1007/s00213-011-2622-8

Kingston, J., Katsaros, J., Vu, Y., & Goodrich, G. L. (2010). Neurological vision rehabilitation: Description and case study. *Journal of Visual Impairment and Blindness, 104,* 603–612.

Kortte, K., & Hillis, A. E. (2009). Recent advances in the understanding of neglect and anosognosia following right hemisphere stroke. *Current Neurology and Neuroscience Reports, 9,* 459–465. http://dx.doi.org/10.1007/s11910-009-0068-8

Lance, J. W. (1980). Symposium synopsis. In R. G. Feldman, R. R. Young, & W. P. Koella (Eds.), *Spasticity: Disordered motor control* (pp. 485–494). Chicago: Yearbook Medical.

Laver-Fawcett, A. J. (2007). *Principles of assessment and outcome measurement for occupational therapists and physiotherapists: Theory, skills, and application.* West Sussex, England: Wiley.

Law, M., Baptiste, S., Carswell, A., McColl, M. A., Polatajko, H., & Pollock, N. (2014). *The Canadian Occupational Performance Measure* (5th ed.). Ottawa, Ontario: CAOT Publications.

Levin, H. S., O'Donnell, V. M., & Grossman, R. G. (1979). The Galveston Orientation and Amnesia Test: A practical scale to assess cognition after head injury. *Journal of Nervous and Mental Disease, 167,* 675–684. http://dx.doi.org/10.1097/00005053-197911000-00004

Lieber, R. L. (1992). *Skeletal muscle and function.* Baltimore: Williams & Wilkins.

Mahalick, D. M., Carmel, P. W., Greenberg, J. P., Molofsky, W., Brown, J. A., Heary, R. F., . . . von der Schmidt, E., III. (1998). Psychopharmacologic treatment of acquired attention disorders in children with brain injury. *Pediatric Neurosurgery, 29,* 121–126. http://dx.doi.org/10.1159/000028705

Marshall, R. S. (2009). Rehabilitation approaches to hemineglect. *Neurologist, 15,* 185–192. http://dx.doi.org/10.1097/NRL.0b013e3181942894

Marshall, S., Teasell, R., Bayona, N., Lippert, C., Chundamala, J., Villamere, J., . . . Bayley, M. (2007). Motor impairment rehabilitation post acquired brain injury. *Brain Injury, 21,* 133–160. http://dx.doi.org/10.1080/02699050701201383

Michals, M. L., Crismon, M. L., Roberts, S., & Childs, A. (1993). Clozapine response and adverse effects in nine brain-injured patients. *Journal of Clinical Pharmacology, 13,* 198–203.

Mortenson, P. A., & Eng, J. J. (2003). The use of casts in the management of joint mobility and hypertonia following brain injury in adults: A systematic review. *Physical Therapy, 83,* 648–658.

Mortera, M. H. (2004). The development of the Cognitive Screening Measure for individuals with brain injury: Initial examination of content validity and interrater reliability (Doctoral dissertation, New York University, 2004). *Dissertation Abstracts International, 65,* 906.

Mortera, M. H. (2012). International Brain Injury Association's 9th World Congress on Brain Injury: Meeting the need for ecologically valid instrument development: Innovation in Structured Functional Cognitive Assessment (SFCA) for individuals with traumatic brain injury. *Brain Injury, 26,* 318.

Moseley, A. M., Hassett, L. M., Leung, J., Clare, J. S., Herbert, R. D., & Harvey, L. A. (2008). Serial casting versus positioning for the treatment of elbow contractures in adults with traumatic brain injury: A randomized controlled trial. *Clinical Rehabilitation, 22,* 406–417. http://dx.doi.org/10.1177/0269215507083795

Mosey, A. C. (1986). *Psychosocial components of occupational therapy.* New York: Raven Press.

Mosey, A. C. (1996). *Applied scientific inquiry in the health professions: An epistemological orientation* (2nd ed.). Bethesda, MD: American Occupational Therapy Association.

Murphy, K. R., & Davidshofer, C. O. (1991). *Psychological testing: Principles and applications* (2nd ed.). Englewood Cliffs, NJ: Prentice-Hall.

Nasreddine, Z. S., Phillips, N. A., Bédirian, V., Charbonneau, S., Whitehead, V., Collin, I., . . . Chertkow, H. (2005). The Montreal Cognitive Assessment, MoCA: A brief screening tool for mild cognitive impairment. *Journal of the American Geriatrics Society, 53,* 695–699. http://dx.doi.org/10.1111/j.1532-5415.2005.53221.x

Nolte, J. (2009). *The human brain: An introduction to its functional anatomy* (6th ed.). St. Louis: Mosby.

Nott, M. T., Chapparo, C., & Baguley, I. J. (2006). Agitation following traumatic brain injury: An Australian sample. *Brain Injury, 20,* 1175–1182. http://dx.doi.org/10.1080/02699050601049114

Nunnally, J. C. (1978). *Psychometric theory* (2nd ed.). New York: McGraw-Hill.

Ottenbacher, K. J., & Christiansen, C. H. (1997). Occupational performance assessment. In C. H. Christiansen & C. M. Baum (Eds.), *Occupational therapy: Enabling function and well-being* (2nd ed., pp. 105–136). Thorofare, NJ: Slack.

Ottenbacher, K. J., & Tomchek, S. D. (1993). Reliability analysis in therapeutic research: Practice and procedures. *American Journal of Occupational Therapy, 47,* 10–16. http://dx.doi.org/10.5014/ajot.47.1.10

Ownsworth, T. L., McFarland, K., & Young, R. M. (2000). Self-awareness and psychosocial functioning following brain injury: An evaluation of a group support programme. *Neuropsychological Rehabilitation, 10,* 465–484. http://dx.doi.org/10.1080/09602010050143559

Pohl, M., Rückriem, S., Mehrholz, J., Ritschel, C., Strik, H., & Pause, M. R. (2002). Effectiveness of serial casting in patients with severe cerebral spasticity: A comparison study. *Archives of Physical Medicine and Rehabilitation, 83,* 784–790. http://dx.doi.org/10.1053/apmr.2002.32821

Posner, M. I., & Petersen, S. E. (1990). The attention system of the human brain. *Annual Review of Neuroscience, 13,* 25–42. http://dx.doi.org/10.1146/annurev.ne.13.030190.000325

Rabin, L. A., Burton, L. A., & Barr, W. B. (2007). Utilization rates of ecologically oriented instruments among clinical neuropsychologists. *Clinical Neuropsychologist, 21,* 727–743. http://dx.doi.org/10.1080/13854040600888776

Riggs, R. V., Andrews, K., Roberts, P., & Gilewski, M. (2007). Visual deficit interventions in adult stroke and brain injury: A systematic review. *American Journal of Physical Medicine and Rehabilitation, 86,* 853–860. http://dx.doi.org/10.1097/PHM.0b013e318151f907

Rike, P. O., Ulleberg, P., Schultheis, M. T., Lundqvist, A., & Schanke, A. K. (2014). Behavioural ratings of self-regulatory mechanisms and driving behaviour after an acquired brain injury. *Brain Injury, 28,* 1687–1699. http://dx.doi.org/10.3109/02699052.2014.947632

Robertson, I. H., Ward, T., Ridgeway, V., & Nimmo-Smith, I. (1994). *The Test of Everyday Attention (TEA).* Bury St. Edmunds, England: Thames Valley Test Co.

Rustad, R. A., DeGroot, T. L., Jungkunz, M. L., Freeberg, K. S., Borowick, L. G., & Wanttie, A. M. (1993). *Cognitive Assessment of Minnesota (CAM).* San Antonio: Therapy Skill Builders.

Sandel, M. E., & Mysiw, W. J. (1996). The agitated brain injured patient. Part 1: Definitions, differential diagnosis, and assessment. *Archives of Physical Medicine and Rehabilitation, 77,* 617–623. http://dx.doi.org/10.1016/S0003-9993(96)90306-8

Schlund, M. W. (2002). Effects of acquired brain injury on adaptive choice and the role of reduced sensitivity to contingencies. *Brain Injury, 16,* 527–535. http://dx.doi.org/10.1080/02699050110113679

Schmidt, J., Lannin, N., Fleming, J., & Ownsworth, T. (2011). Feedback interventions for impaired self-awareness following brain injury: A systematic review. *Journal of Rehabilitation Medicine, 43,* 673–680. http://dx.doi.org/10.2340/16501977-0846

Schreiber, S., Klag, E., Gross, Y., Segman, R. H., & Pick, C. G. (1998). Beneficial effect of risperidone on sleep disturbance and psychosis following traumatic brain injury. *International Clinical Psychopharmacology, 13,* 273–275. http://dx.doi.org/10.1097/00004850-199811000-00006

Sherer, M. (2004). *Introduction to the Confusion Assessment Protocol.* Retrieved November 3, 2014, from http://www.tbims.org/combi/cap

Sherer, M., Bergloff, P., Boake, C., High, W., Jr., & Levin, E. (1998). The Awareness Questionnaire: Factor structure and internal consistency. *Brain Injury, 12,* 63–68. http://dx.doi.org/10.1080/026990598122863

Sherer, M., Hart, T., Nick, T. G., Whyte, J., Thompson, R. N., & Yablon, S. A. (2003). Early impaired self-awareness after traumatic brain injury. *Archives of Physical Medicine and Rehabilitation, 84,* 168–176. http://dx.doi.org/10.1053/apmr.2003.50045

Silver, B. V., Collins, L., & Zidek, K. A. (2003). Risperidone treatment of motor restlessness following anoxic brain injury. *Brain Injury, 17,* 237–244. http://dx.doi.org/10.1080/0269905021000013192

Silver, J. M., & Yudofsky, S. C. (1993). Pharmacologic treatment of neuropsychiatric disorders. *NeuroRehabilitation, 3,* 15–25.

Stineman, M. G., Shea, J. A., Jette, A., Tassoni, C. J., Ottenbacher, K. J., Fiedler, R., & Granger, C. V. (1996). The Functional Independence Measure: Tests of scaling assumptions, structure, and reliability across 20 diverse impairment categories. *Archives of Physical Medicine and Rehabilitation, 77,* 1101–1108. http://dx.doi.org/10.1016/S0003-9993(96)90130-6

Suen, H. K., & Ary, D. (1989). *Analyzing quantitative behavioral observation data.* Hillsdale, NJ: Erlbaum.

Temple, M. J. (2003). Use of atypical anti-psychotics in the management of post-traumatic confusional states in traumatic brain injury. *Journal of the Royal Army Medical Corps, 149,* 54–55. http://dx.doi.org/10.1136/jramc-149-01-10

Thomas, H., Feyz, M., LeBlanc, J., Brosseau, J., Champoux, M. C., Christopher, A., . . . Lin, H. (2003). North Star Project: Reality orientation in an acute care setting for patients with traumatic brain injuries. *Journal of Head Trauma Rehabilitation, 18,* 292–302. http://dx.doi.org/10.1097/00001199-200305000-00007

Toglia, J. P. (1993a). *The Contextual Memory Test.* Tucson, AZ: Therapy Skill Builders.

Toglia, J. P. (1993b). Lesson 4: Attention and memory. In C. B. Royeen (Ed.), *Cognitive rehabilitation* (pp. 4–72). Bethesda, MD: American Occupational Therapy Association.

Toglia, J. (2005). A dynamic interactional approach to cognitive rehabilitation. In N. Katz (Ed.), *Cognition and occupation across the life span: Models for intervention in occupational therapy* (2nd ed., pp. 29–72). Bethesda, MD: AOTA Press.

Toglia, J. P. (2011). The Dynamic Interactional Model of cognition in cognitive rehabilitation. In N. Katz (Ed.), *Cognition, occupation, and participation across the life span: Neuroscience, neurorehabilitation, and models of intervention in occupational therapy* (3rd ed., pp. 161–201). Bethesda, MD: AOTA Press.

Toglia, J. P., & Golisz, K. M. (2012). Therapy for activities of daily living: Theoretical and practical perspectives. In N. D. Zasler, D. I. Katz, & R. D. Zafonte (Eds.), *Brain injury medicine* (2nd ed., pp. 1162–1177). New York: Demos.

Toglia, J. P., Golisz, K. M., & Goverover, Y. (2013). Evaluation and intervention for cognitive perceptual impairments. In B. A. Boyt Schell, G. Gillen, M. Scaffa, & E. S. Cohn (Eds.), *Willard and Spackman's occupational therapy* (12th ed., pp. 779–815). Philadelphia: Lippincott Williams & Wilkins.

Tupper, D. E., & Cicerone, K. D. (1990). *The neuropsychology of everyday life: Assessment and basic competencies.* Boston: Kluwer.

Vanderploeg, R. D. (1994). *Clinician's guide to neuropsychological assessment.* Hillsdale, NJ: Erlbaum.

Vandervoort, A. A. (1999). Ankle mobility and postural stability. *Physiotherapy Theory and Practice, 15,* 91–103. http://dx.doi.org/10.1080/095939899307793

Varghese, G. (1992). Heterotopic ossification. *Physical Rehabilitation Clinics of North America, 3,* 407–415.

Warren, M. (1998). *Brain Injury Visual Assessment Battery for Adults.* Lenexa, KS: visABILITIES Rehab Services.

Warren, M. (2011). Intervention for adults with vision impairment from acquired brain injury. In M. Warren & E. A. Barstow (Eds.), *Occupational therapy interventions for adults with low vision* (pp. 403–448). Bethesda, MD: AOTA Press.

Whyte, J., Hart, T., Schuster, K., Fleming, M., Polansky, M., & Coslett, H. B. (1997). Effects of methylphenidate on attentional function after traumatic brain injury. A randomized, placebo-controlled trial. *American Journal of Physical Medicine and Rehabilitation, 76,* 440–450. http://dx.doi.org/10.1097/00002060-199711000-00002

Wilkinson, R., Meythaler, J. M., & Guin-Renfroe, S. (1999). Neuroleptic malignant syndrome induced by haloperidol following traumatic brain injury. *Brain Injury, 13,* 1025–1031. http://dx.doi.org/10.1080/026990599121034

Wilson, B., Cockburn, J., & Baddeley, A. (1991). *RBMT–E—The Rivermead Behavioural Memory Test–Extended.* London: Thames Valley Test Co.

World Health Organization. (2001). *International classification of functioning, disability and health (short version).* Geneva: Author.

Ylvisaker, M. (2003). Context-sensitive cognitive rehabilitation: Theory and practice. *Brain Impairment, 4,* 1–16. http://dx.doi.org/10.1375/brim.4.1.1.27031

Ylvisaker, M., Jacobs, H. E., & Feeney, T. (2003). Positive supports for people who experience behavioral and cognitive disability after brain injury: A review. *Journal of Head Trauma Rehabilitation, 18*, 7–32. http://dx.doi.org/10.1097/00001199-200301000-00005

Ylvisaker, M., Turkstra, L. S., & Coelho, C. (2005). Behavioral and social interventions for individuals with traumatic brain injury: A summary of the research with clinical implications. *Seminars in Speech and Language, 26*, 256–267. http://dx.doi.org/10.1055/s-2005-922104

Ylvisaker, M., Turkstra, L., Coehlo, C., Yorkston, K., Kennedy, M., Sohlberg, M., & Avery, J. (2007). Behavioral interventions for individuals with behavior disorders after TBI: A systematic review of the evidence. *Brain Injury, 21*, 769–805. http://dx.doi.org/10.1080/02699050701482470

Yuen, H. K., & Benzing, P. (1996). Treatment methodology: Guiding of behaviour through redirection in brain injury rehabilitation. *Brain Injury, 10*, 229–238. http://dx.doi.org/10.1080/026990596124548

CHAPTER 7

Community Recovery and Participation

Steven Wheeler, PhD, OTR/L, CBIS

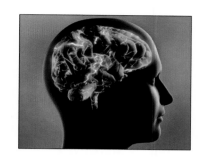

Learning Objectives

After completion of this chapter, readers will be able to

- Differentiate among the cognitive, behavioral, and functional sequelae of **traumatic brain injury** (TBI) in people at the community level of recovery;
- Identify the client factors and performance skills influencing the occupational performance of people with TBI at the community level of recovery;
- Select assessments to evaluate the client with TBI at the community level of recovery;
- Identify evidence-based interventions to promote the resumption of occupational roles and facilitate social participation for people with TBI;
- Identify possible community-based intervention settings for the client recovering from TBI; and
- Recognize the importance of the outcomes process and the need for evidence of effectiveness of care for the client with TBI at the community level of recovery.

Key Words

- **community reintegration**
- **coping skills**
- **executive functions**
- **goal setting**
- **life satisfaction**
- **participation**
- **self-awareness**

Introduction

The community phase of recovery after traumatic brain injury (TBI), with its focus on community participation, represents a distinct phase of TBI **rehabilitation.** Clients at this point in the recovery process are typically functioning at higher cognitive and physical levels than during the early stages of recovery, but in many cases this level is inadequate for their successful return to preinjury occupations and roles. The challenges of community reentry amid residual TBI-related **impairment** contribute to new, and often unexpected, psychosocial and emotional difficulties for clients and their family. Additionally, client performance in the structured hospital setting may not equate to similar success in natural environments.

Occupational therapy plays an important role in the transition from hospital to community for people with TBI. The scope of the occupational therapy profession is considerable, and the training of occupational therapy practitioners is diverse and well suited to understanding the range of factors that affect **community integration** after TBI.

As the average length of hospital stay after TBI continues to decrease and the limitations of inpatient rehabilitation to completely prepare clients for community living are increasingly recognized, the transition from the hospital to the community continues to gain attention as an important stage of the rehabilitation continuum.

As the average length of hospital stay after TBI continues to decrease and the limitations of inpatient rehabilitation to completely prepare clients for community living are increasingly recognized, the transition from the hospital to the community continues to gain attention as an important stage of the rehabilitation continuum (Golisz, 2009). This trend has the potential to create exciting opportunities for occupational therapy. By supporting occupation-based assessment and intervention in natural environments, services at this stage are consistent with occupational therapy's commitment to client-centered practice and community participation. The community stage of rehabilitation is also a challenging one for the occupational therapist. Community-based assessment and intervention can be complex, unpredictable, and long term. Functional treatment gains may facilitate the client's progression to new life challenges and, frequently, the emergence of previously unrecognized difficulties for both clients and their families.

Community-based assessment and intervention after TBI provide valuable contributions to optimizing functional independence and **quality of life** (QoL). The struggles encountered by many people with TBI and their families after hospital discharge have been well documented in the literature (Blake, 2008; Kalechstein, Newton, & van Gorp, 2003; Ponsford, Draper, & Schönberger, 2008). The vast majority of people seen in rehabilitation after TBI return to the community with some residual cognitive, psychosocial, behavioral, or physical impairment (Kersel, Marsh, Havill, & Sleigh, 2001; Testa, Malec, Moessner, & Brown, 2006). People with moderate to severe TBI living in the community have been found to be less likely to live independently; less likely to be fully employed; and less likely to participate successfully in housekeeping, parenting, and **leisure** activities (Ponsford et al., 2008; Turner, Fleming, Cornwell, Haines, & Ownsworth, 2009).

These situations, combined with social isolation and relationship difficulties, are estimated to contribute to 80% of the lifetime costs to society of TBI because of their impact on long-term care needs, burden of disease, and lost productivity (Faul, Wald, Rutland-Brown, Sullivent, & Sattin, 2007). The excitement and optimism of many people with TBI and their loved ones at the time of hospital discharge can develop into feelings of frustration and despair (Ponsford, Olver, Ponsford, & Nelms, 2003).

The aim of this chapter is to prepare occupational therapy practitioners to work effectively with people with TBI who are residing in the community. Although a discussion of more traditional assessments and interventions is important to this process, expertise at this phase of rehabilitation can be attained only through a thorough understanding of the many issues contributing to successful community reentry, including the client's occupations, roles, and environments and the effects of larger societal factors. The primary emphasis of this chapter is on the community phase of rehabilitation for adults after moderate to severe TBI, defined by a **Glasgow Coma Scale** score of 12 or less (Orman, Kraus, Zaloshnja, & Miller, 2011), which generally involves loss of **consciousness** and a period of hospitalization. Although much of the information presented in this chapter is applicable to younger populations, a full description of TBI in childhood and adolescence, and the dynamics associated with it, is beyond the scope of this chapter.

The Person With Traumatic Brain Injury at the Community Stage of Recovery

Most people with TBI discharged home or to some form of community-based rehabilitation setting have regained basic self-care, mobility, and communication skills. However, long-term residual cognitive, physical, psychosocial, emotional, or behavioral deficits are common and diverse, complicating the transition to the community (Lefebvre, Cloutier, & Josée Levert, 2008). In this section, I address the specific types of TBI-related deficits commonly observed during this phase of recovery.

Cognitive Impairments

People with TBI attempting community reintegration typically present at Rancho Los Amigos Levels of Cognitive Functioning (RLA LCF) VII and VIII of the original scale, and at Levels IX and X of the modified version of this scale (presented in Chapter 1; Hagen, 1998). The modified version attempts to capture higher level cognitive abilities, known as *executive functions,* that have a significant impact on adult role performance at the community stage of recovery (Hagen, 1998). Executive functions, described in Table 7.1, include self-monitoring, self-awareness, initiation, and social competence.

The pace and extent of progression through the higher Rancho levels are unique to each person, and complete resolution of cognitive symptoms is not typical after moderate to severe TBI. Residual cognitive deficits, along with changes in behavior and personality, have been found to have a greater impact on post-TBI functional performance and QoL than do physical disabilities (Khan, Baguley, & Cameron, 2003; Tsaousides & Gordon, 2009). The person functioning at Rancho VII could be independent with many aspects of basic self-care and meet many demands of a more structured daily routine but is likely to experience considerable difficulty attaining similar success with more complex and unpredictable home and community tasks such as meal preparation, driving, and child care that rely heavily on executive functions. Executive functions are essential to adult role participation, supporting the ability to engage in independent, purposeful occupations and to initiate, plan, set goals, monitor performance, anticipate consequences, and respond flexibly and adaptively (Strauss, Sherman, & Spreen, 2006). Sometimes referred to as *executive dysfunction* or *dysexecutive syndrome,* these impairments are best suited to assessment and interventions involving real-life tasks in natural settings (Novakovic-Agopian et al., 2014).

Accurate self-awareness of deficits and limitations after TBI has been associated with more intact cognitive, behavioral, and affective functioning, as well as more functional independence after TBI (Noé et al., 2005). Conversely, decreased self-awareness of cognitive, emotional, and behavioral impairments is one of the greatest obstacles in TBI rehabilitation (Kelley et al., 2014). For the occupational therapist, the process of setting client-centered goals can be challenging with a client who denies or minimizes the existence of impairments, functional limitations, or the need for rehabilitation. Researchers and clinicians agree that a significant factor mediating therapeutic success after TBI is the client's ability to

Table 7.1. Definitions of Executive Functions

Term	Definition
Initiation	The ability to start an activity. Deficits in this area include lacking spontaneity, being slow to respond, or lacking initiative. Deficits may be misinterpreted as lack of motivation or drive and can be a considerable source of frustration for both client and family.
Planning	The ability to organize the steps to complete an action, weigh alternatives, develop a framework for carrying out the plan, prepare for setbacks in carrying out the plan, assemble the needed materials, and possess the skills necessary to carry out the plan (McDonald et al., 2002). Deficits impair the ability to perform adult home, academic, or vocational roles.
Problem solving and decision making	The ability to integrate several cognitive skills, including attention, initiation, impulse control, organization, categorization, mental flexibility, and reasoning skills, and the ability to self-evaluate. Deficits affect the ability to select among various options to make a decision (Parente & Hermann, 2003).
Mental flexibility	The ability to initiate, stop, and switch actions depending on feedback from the environment during goal-oriented task performance (Goverover & Hinojosa, 2002). Deficits result in behavior that appears **perseverative** and concrete with limited ability to generalize current information for future problem solving. Tasks such as meal preparation, driving, and financial planning and many **instrumental activities of daily living** are affected.
Goal setting	The ability to determine what one wants and to foresee the future realization of those needs. Goal attainment involves estimating task difficulty and self-evaluating performance so that adjustments can be made, both of which are affected by impaired self-awareness of deficits or abilities.
Self-awareness	The ability to accurately recognize one's abilities and limitations. It is influenced by many factors, including memory, decreased sensory or perceptual abilities, impulsivity, and inability to plan for the future. Deficits affect the ability to accept feedback from others related to limitations and the ability to benefit from rehabilitation (Fischer et al., 2004). Impaired self-awareness also affects social interactions, including difficulties with personal boundaries, managing arguments and anger, and adjusting to unexpected changes (McDonald et al., 2002).
Self-monitoring and self-correction	The ability to evaluate and regulate the quality and quantity of one's behavior to allow identification and correction of incorrect responses. Deficits affect a person's ability to manage his or her own learning and apply correct strategies to accomplish goals.
Concept formation and abstraction	The ability to make inferences from information. Deficits contribute to limited imagination, problems generalizing from individual events, failing to plan ahead, and difficulty explaining ideas (Parente & Hermann, 2003). Information is viewed in a concrete manner, contributing to a rigid approach to thinking (Golisz & Toglia, 2003).
Categorization	The ability to find commonalities among large amounts of information and assign objects and events into groups (Parente & Hermann, 2003). Deficits affect all cognitive skills and abilities (Ashley, 2004).
Generalization	The ability to use a newly learned strategy in novel situations. Deficits affect the ability to learn a skill in one setting and apply it elsewhere.

Source. Zoltan (2007).

recognize deficits and motivation to change or adapt to the environment. Trudel, Tryon, and Purdum (1998) found a direct relationship between unawareness of impairments and poorer recovery 7 years postinjury, and Kelley et al. (2014) had similar findings 5 years postinjury. Koskinen (1998) reported that impaired awareness of deficits was strongly correlated with a decrease in family well-being 10 years after TBI.

Attention and **memory** impairment, typically addressed throughout the rehabilitation process, can further complicate rehabilitation at the community stage. These impairments can limit generalization and the application of learned information to novel contexts (Parente & Anderson-Parente, 1989), contributing to reduced rehabilitation benefit, and they affect the person's ability to function socially, perform home management tasks (Powell, Temkin, Machamer, & Dikmen, 2007), and fulfill employment and academic potential (Ponsford et al., 2008).

Physical Impairments

The impact of residual sensorimotor impairments can play a considerable role in the success of the transition from the hospital to the community setting. Although considered less of a determinant of community success than cognitive and behavioral sequelae, physical problems, coupled with cognitive, behavioral, and social deficits, can severely affect a client's ability to achieve work, school, and community goals in addition to causing an overall decrease in his or her functional activity level. Poor coordination, weakness, **spasticity, ataxia,** and **vestibular problems** may be present to varying degrees, particularly in people with a history of severe TBI.

As with many TBI-related impairments, managing physical deficits can be a lifelong process. In a study of neuromotor recovery after TBI, Walker and Pickett (2007) found a general pattern of recovery that slowed at 6-month follow-up. In their cohort of 102 participants, more than one-third showed at least one neuromotor abnormality 2 years after inpatient rehabilitation. More than one-quarter of participants had gait abnormalities, which may reduce the ability to engage in work, school, and volunteer activities (Perry, Woollard, Little, & Shroyer, 2014). Basford et al. (2003) indicated that vestibular dysfunction was a common long-term contributor to postural instability and functional gait problems after TBI. Impairments to the vestibular system may result from damage to the vestibular nerve as it passes through the internal acoustic meatus that is caused by shearing and the acceleration–deceleration forces commonly experienced during TBI (Basford et al., 2003). In a sample of clients with TBI, Jury and Flynn (2001) also found frequent vestibular impairment that affected balance reactions and safety during functional mobility. Balance reaction impairments have been linked to safety during basic **activities of daily living** (ADLs), work tasks, **community mobility,** and sports (Gottshall, Drake, Gray, McDonald, & Hoffer, 2003).

Improved medical stability, physical endurance, and cognitive functioning of people at the community stage of TBI rehabilitation may result in recommendations for surgical and other interventions that may have been contraindicated or of lesser priority during acute care. Additionally, spasticity, impaired muscle control, and weakness lead to muscle imbalance and, over time, soft-tissue shortening and static **contracture.** Such deformities in the trunk, upper extremities, and lower extremities contribute to impaired volitional movements and significant functional difficulties (Namdari, Alosh, Baldwin, Mehta, & Keenan, 2012).

Although nonoperative treatment methods such as medications, nerve blocks, **botulinum toxin** injections, and serial casting are generally considered preferred options for managing spasticity that may lead to static contractures, surgical procedures to address contractures may be recommended for people with whom such approaches are unsuccessful. Such procedures for the upper extremity, such as selective shoulder tendon lengthening, were found to decrease subjective pain and improve active **range of motion** (ROM) and **passive range of motion** (PROM) and self-care (Namdari, Alosh, et al., 2012). Surgical release of contracted muscles was found to reduce subjective pain, decrease spasticity, and improve PROM (Namdari, Horneff, Baldwin, & Keenan, 2012). Clients with TBI who have completed their initial rehabilitation may need an additional period of rehabilitation after surgery to address new physical challenges and the potential functional improvements offered by the intervention.

It is estimated that 10% to 20% of people with TBI develop ***heterotopic ossification*** (HO), a condition characterized by periarticular formation of bone in soft-tissue structures (such as skin and skeletal muscle) where bone does not normally exist (Hosalkar, Pandya, Hsu, Kamath, & Keenan, 2010). Observable signs of HO include joint swelling or warmth, joint pain, decreased ROM at the affected joint, and a palpable mass (Pape, Marsh, Morley, Krettek, & Giannoudis, 2004). HO identified in the early stages may be addressed with gentle ROM exercises, terminal resistance training through a pain-free ROM, nonsteroidal anti-inflammatories, or radiation therapy (Hosalkar et al., 2010). When surgical removal of HO is indicated, Garland and Varpetian (2003) recommended having the procedure at 18 months postinjury in cases involving TBI to ensure that the bone tissue has matured and to reduce the likelihood of recurrence. Preoperative ROM exercises and strengthening may prevent muscle atrophy and preserve joint motion. Postoperative rehabilitation also involves ROM exercises along with an emphasis on edema control, scar management, and infection prevention (Casavant & Hastings, 2006).

Constraint-induced movement therapy (CIMT) is an intervention to facilitate motor recovery in cases of upper-extremity spastic hemiparesis. CIMT involves the restraint of the less affected upper limb accompanied by the shaping and repetitive task-oriented training of the more affected upper limb (Taub & Wolfe, 1997). CIMT attempts to counteract the negative functional impact of **learned nonuse,** which can occur when a person progressively avoids using the more affected arm in favor of the nonparetic arm because of unsuccessful movements during the acute and subacute stages of recovery. When this occurs, **plasticity** becomes maladaptive, responding to nonuse and abnormal movements with patterns of circuitry reorganization that actually interfere with functional gains (Chen, Epstein, & Stern, 2010; Taub, Uswatte, & Elbert, 2002).

The typical protocol for CIMT involves restraint of the unaffected upper extremity during 90% of waking hours and, at the same time, repeated and intensive practice with the more affected upper extremity for 6 hours or more per day (Page, Levine, Leonard, Szaflarski, & Kissela, 2008). Although the majority of evidence supporting CIMT has been drawn from the stroke population, Shaw et al. (2005) found improved upper-extremity function after a 2-week period of the intervention with a sample of 22 participants with TBI onset of more than 1 year. The physical and cognitive demands of CIMT, along with the necessary level of compliance, may limit its clinical feasibility with some people with TBI. Modified CIMT protocols have been used, involving significantly shortened training and immobilization periods, and have produced positive functional outcomes for people with **cerebrovascular accident** (Shi, Tian, Yang, & Zhao, 2011; Souza, Conforto, Orsini, Stern, & Andre, 2015). Because CIMT focuses on remediation of hemiparesis, the vast majority of studies investigating CIMT have used participants with stroke. Variations of CIMT protocols with adults with TBI and the outcomes of CIMT programs in the population with TBI have not been specifically investigated.

Psychological and Emotional Functioning

For many clients, the consequences of TBI are debilitating and persistent and can include considerable neuropsychiatric difficulties at the community stage of rehabilitation. Major depression is one of the most frequently reported neurobehavioral sequelae after TBI and has been found to occur in 12% to 60% of the population (Bryant et al., 2010). In a multicenter study involving 666 nonacute participants with moderate to severe TBI, **fatigue** (29%), distractibility (28%), **anger** and irritability (28%), and rumination (25%) were identified as the most common depressive symptoms (Seel et al., 2003). Theories attempting to explain the nature of the relationship between TBI and depression have proposed preinjury depression, preinjury personality type, social integration after injury, family support, neurochemical imbalances, and site of anatomical damage as contributing factors (Jean-Bay, 2000; Ownsworth & Oei, 1998; Rosenthal, Christensen, & Ross, 1998).

Depression complicates the process of recovery and rehabilitation because increased effort in **information processing** is required in the context of depression, and motivation toward rehabilitation goals is impaired (Jean-Bay, 2000). As a result, treatment goals to reestablish meaningful social and occupational roles may be compromised. In a study looking at insight and readiness to engage in therapy after TBI, O'Callaghan, McAllister, and Wilson (2012) found that all 16 participants in the study mentioned "surviving depression" at some point in their rehabilitation.

> **Depression complicates the process of recovery and rehabilitation because increased effort in information processing is required in the context of depression, and motivation toward rehabilitation goals is impaired.**

As the client's confusion clears and self-awareness improves, the structure and support of inpatient rehabilitation is withdrawn, and the client faces the challenges of community living, creating a period of vulnerability. Unemployment, social isolation, and emotional distress, combined with reduced cognitive resources for **coping,** increase the susceptibility of people with TBI to contemplate suicide and engage in suicidal behavior (Simpson & Tate, 2007; Tsaousides, Cantor, & Gordon, 2011). The presence of suicidal ideation after TBI is estimated to be approximately 18% to 28% (Kishi, Robinson, & Kosier, 2001; Simpson & Tate, 2007; Tsaousides et al., 2011) compared with approximately 3% in the general population (Kessler, Berglund, Borges, Nock, & Wang, 2005).

Simpson and Tate (2002) identified four preinjury risk factors associated with suicidal ideation for people with TBI: (1) suicide attempts, (2) alcohol abuse, (3) drug abuse, and (4) emotional or psychiatric disturbance. Although research has suggested that there is no critical period postinjury during which suicidal ideation is more likely to occur (Simpson & Tate, 2007), it is recognized that as **cognition** improves and insight into residual deficits increases, survivors of TBI are at greater risk for depression (Malec, Testa, Rush, Brown, & Moessner, 2007). The role of TBI-related impairment of executive functions in suicidal behavior has not been firmly established. Impulsivity has been identified as a main dimension of suicidality in people with depression (Corruble, Benyamina, Bayle, Falissard, & Hardy, 2003), but the role of impulsivity in suicide has not been studied in people with TBI.

The strongest and most significant predictor of suicidal ideation in a study of 356 community-dwelling people with TBI was impaired psychosocial functioning, including perceptions of health, QoL, and social support (Tsaousides et al., 2011). Other studies have reported a relationship between suicidal ideation and poor vocational outcomes (Seel et al., 2003). Currently, no evidence has supported a relationship between gender differences or injury severity and suicidal ideation (Simpson & Tate, 2002).

Self-esteem refers to a person's self-assessment of his or her worth and is often adversely affected by TBI. Typically, the more aware people with TBI are of their postinjury limitations, the more likely they are to have changes in self-esteem. Building self-esteem through success-oriented experiences is a critical but challenging component of the rehabilitation process. People with low self-esteem tend to avoid challenging tasks, not invest in relationships, or sabotage an important event to avoid the possibility of failure or rejection.

Occupational therapists can use strategies such as therapeutic relationship building, client-centered goal setting, family and caregiver education, and supportive **group interventions** to create an environment conducive to functional risk taking and an opportunity for the experiences necessary to build self-esteem to the level necessary for goal achievement and satisfying life experiences (Hadas-Lidor, Weiss, & Kozulin, 2011). Selecting treatment goals and outcomes in collaboration with the person with TBI and the caregiver has been demonstrated to have a positive impact on the therapy process and to facilitate better clinical outcomes (Doig, Fleming, Kuipers, & Cornwell, 2010; Wressle, Eeg-Olofsson, Marcusson, & Henriksson, 2002).

Sleep Disturbance and Fatigue

Sleep disturbance is one of the most common yet least studied sequelae of TBI. Although more often referenced in regard to mild TBI, 30% to 70% of people with moderate to severe TBI experience some form of postinjury sleep disturbance (Ouellet, Savard, & Morin, 2004). This finding is not surprising given that brain regions and systems regulating **arousal,** alertness, attention, and sleep are vulnerable to TBI. Cohen, Oksenberg, Snir, Stern, and Groswasser (1992) reported that difficulty initiating and maintaining sleep was most common among hospitalized patients, and *daytime somnolence* (i.e., excessive daytime sleepiness) was most common among discharged patients. Sleep disturbances can affect attention, problem solving, memory, and judgment, impeding rehabilitation and contributing to greater functional difficulties and poorer occupational outcomes (Masel, Scheibel, Kimbark, & Kuna, 2001; Ouellet et al., 2004).

Fatigue, a complex experience involving a decreased capacity for physical and mental activity because of the reduced availability of the physiological and psychological resources necessary to perform the activity (Aaronson et al., 1999; Ponsford, Schönberger, & Rajaratnam, 2015), is reported by more than 60% of people with moderate to severe TBI at least 12 months postinjury (Cantor et al., 2008). Fatigue may be the consequence of the direct effects of the TBI as well as the cause of **anxiety,** depression, and daytime sleepiness (Bushnik, Englander, & Wright, 2008), which can, in turn, exacerbate fatigue through their impact on cognitive functioning and sleep or through the additional physical or mental effort required to perform tasks that were performed with little or no effort before injury (Kohl, Wylie, Genova, Hillary, & DeLuca, 2009; Ponsford et al., 2012, 2015).

TBI-related fatigue has been postulated to be the direct result of mechanical disruption to the brain resulting in **diffuse axonal injury,** impaired excitability of the motor cortex, and hypopituitarism (Bushnik et al., 2008). TBI-related fatigue may also be a consequence of pain, depression, and anxiety, all relatively common after TBI (Bushnik et al., 2008). Physical functioning, attention and **concentration,** memory, and communication can be adversely affected by fatigue, creating difficulties with participating in daily occupations, decreasing the quality of task performance, and creating possible safety risks.

Community Participation After Traumatic Brain Injury

Successful and satisfying community integration has come to be recognized as a primary goal of rehabilitation for people with TBI (McCabe et al., 2007; Sander, Clark, & Pappadis, 2010). Described as "having something to do, somewhere to live, and someone to love" (McColl et al., 1998, p. 16), *community integration* is a multidimensional concept involving various aspects of human functioning that are known to be affected by TBI (McCabe et al., 2007). McCabe et al. described the five areas of the community integration stage of the rehabilitation process as (1) independence and social integration, (2) satisfaction and QoL, (3) productivity, (4) return to driving, and (5) caregiver burden. To competently address the challenges facing people with TBI who are being discharged to the community, occupational therapy practitioners must fully appreciate the complexities of a community as well as what it means to successfully participate in one.

According to Mallinson and Hammel (2010), community participation occurs "at the intersection of what the person can do, wants to do, has the opportunity or affordances to do, and is not prevented from doing by the world in which the person lives and seeks to participate" (p. S30). Moore (1996) defined *community* as "the setting in which, from one generation to the next, human beings learn how to be fully human" (p. 96) and noted that community membership contributes to a person's self-identity and provides a sense of meaning and direction to a person's daily routine. In short, community membership is important to people's QoL regardless of disability. In a series of focus groups conducted with people after TBI, McColl et al. (1998) reported that all participants expressed the importance of meeting new people and making new friends. Similar studies have also identified the importance of social interactions as well as the need to feel like part of the community (Sander, Pappadis, Clark, & Struchen, 2011). Unfortunately, *social isolation* (the absence of a sense of community participation) is among the most profound and distressing changes after TBI (Ponsford, 2003).

McColl (1998) described successful community integration as incorporating clients into communities in which they are both happy and productive. Occupational therapy assessment and intervention at the community stage moves beyond a focus on specific symptoms to gaining an appreciation of the client's desired communities and facilitating both productive occupation in meaningful roles and satisfaction with life within those roles and contexts. Primary considerations include factors within and outside the person influencing participation in social, familial, educational, vocational, and other roles. According to McColl and Bickenbach (1998),

> When we move away from the purely biomechanical understanding of disability and adopt the perspective of a person with a disability living in society, it is no longer possible to abstract disability from the social and environmental context in which people live. We cannot ignore the world, in short, because the way the world is organized to a considerable extent determines what it means to have a disability. The consequences of disability are the result of an interaction between the individual, his or her physical or mental abilities, and the physical and social context in which that person lives. (p. 131)

This description is consistent with the World Health Organization's (WHO's) description of participation, a concept embraced by the profession of occupational

To competently address the challenges facing people with TBI who are being discharged to the community, occupational therapy practitioners must fully appreciate the complexities of a community as well as what it means to successfully participate in one.

therapy. *Participation* is defined in WHO's (2001) *International Classification of Functioning, Disability and Health (ICF)* as "involvement in life situations" (p. 123) and has been used in numerous studies related to TBI recovery, yet how participation is operationalized varies widely on the basis of how it is measured. The *ICF* model (presented in Figure 7.1) demonstrates the relationship among a person's impairments (body functions and structure), ability to execute a task or action (activity), and performance in life roles or situations (participation). Additionally, it delineates the contributions to participation of environmental supports and barriers (environmental factors) and of the factors associated with the person with the disability (personal factors).

Although intended to represent all disabling conditions, the *ICF* model has gained worldwide acceptance and boosted attention to participation outcomes in disability policy and research. The *ICF* serves as a useful guide for occupational therapy research, assessment, and intervention at the community stage, placing the ultimate rehabilitation focus on community participation over remediation of impairment (Sloan, Winkler, & Callaway, 2004).

Participation-focused assessment requires a **top-down approach,** starting with gathering information on what the person wants to do, followed by an analysis of the person as he or she performs the desired occupations (see Table 7.2 for selected participation-level assessments). Consideration of the challenges affecting participation, including client factors, is the final stage of the process (Simmons & Griswold, 2010). For example, the inability to drive may significantly compromise participation in social, vocational, and leisure roles. On gaining an appreciation of the decreased or lost participation and the client's perspective, the therapist would investigate laws related to driving after TBI, impairments contributing to driving difficulties, personal factors such as the client's preinjury driving experience and age, and any environmental barriers or supports, including the availability of public transportation to meet community involvement.

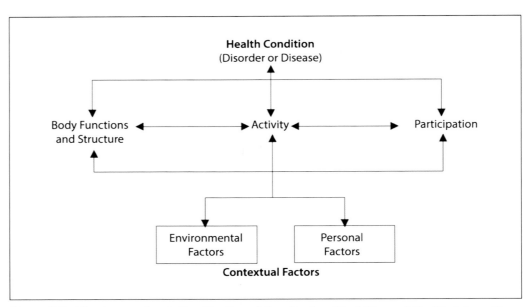

Figure 7.1. The *International Classification of Functioning, Disability and Health*: Interactions Among Components.

Source. World Health Organization (2001, p. 18).

Table 7.2. Selected Community Integration, Participation, and Instrumental Activities of Daily Living Assessments

Assessment	Description	Comments (Reliability and Validity)
Activity Measure for Post Acute Care (Haley et al., 2004)	Functional outcomes system assessing *ICF* activity limitations. Can be used across postacute care settings and consists of a comprehensive list of 240 functional activities. Item bank includes 101 Basic Mobility items, 70 Daily Activity items, and 69 Applied Cognitive items. Assesses multiple aspects (i.e., difficulty, assistance, limitations) of a person's ability to perform specific daily activities. Instrument can be administered by using direct patient responses, by professional judgment, or by proxy report.	Using computer adaptive testing, items that will be administered to a specific patient are preselected on the basis of responses to previous items, reducing the time it takes to complete the assessment. Research has shown acceptable test–retest, internal consistency, and subject–proxy reliability.
Árnadóttir OT-ADL Neurobehavioral Evaluation (Árnadóttir, 1990)	Uses activity analysis to relate the results of OT-ADL evaluation to specific neurobehavioral impairments and to generate hypotheses about the localization of cerebral dysfunction. Impairment Scale with 2 subscales. Uses independent ordinal scale for each of the ADL areas assessed on the Functional Independence Scale, with higher scores indicating greater independence.	Good interrater reliability has been established. Limited ability to differentiate between left- and right-hemisphere lesions in a study on the assessment's construct validity attributed to hypothesis that both hemispheres contribute important and necessary functions to the completion of ADL tasks (Gardarsdóttir & Kaplan, 2002).
Assessment of Motor and Process Skills (Fisher & Jones, 2012, 2014)	Observational measure of the quality of a person's performance of functional tasks. The quality of the person's ADL performance is assessed by rating the effort, efficiency, safety, and independence of 16 motor and 20 process skill items. More than 100 standardized ADL tasks can be selected to assess. Requires therapist certification to administer.	Reliability and validity have been proven in many studies. Selecting from the more than 100 calibrated ADL tasks enables selection of culturally relevant and appropriately challenging ADL tasks.
Brain Injury Community Rehabilitation Outcome–39 (BICRO–39; Powell et al., 1998)	39 items structured into 8 domains (personal care, mobility, self-organization, partner–child contact, parent–sibling contact, socializing, productive employment, psychological well-being). All items are rated on a 6-point scale, with some domains rating frequency and other domains rating degree of assistance. Total scores range from 0 to 195, with lower scores representing better outcome.	Test–retest reliability of the BICRO–39 scales was sound, and several studies have provided evidence of construct validity.
Canadian Occupational Performance Measure (COPM; Law et al., 2014)	Client-centered, occupation-based assessment in which the client identifies personal goals in areas of occupation (self-care, productivity, leisure), rating his or her perceived performance on and satisfaction with each occupation on a scale ranging from 1 to 10.	Numerous studies have supported the reliability, validity, and clinical utility of the COPM. Impaired self-awareness may limit use of the COPM in clients with TBI (Jenkinson et al., 2007).
Community Integration Measure (McColl et al., 2001)	Brief client-centered 10-item checklist consisting of 4 categories: assimilation (conformity, orientation, acceptance), social support (close and diffuse relationships), occupation (leisure, productivity), and independent living (personal independence, satisfaction with living arrangement). Focused on subjective experiences rather than on objective or observable aspects of integration. Respondents rate statements on a 5-point Likert scale noting the degree of agreement with the statement.	Strong internal consistency reliability. Content, discriminant, construct, and criterion validity were all supported.
Community Integration Questionnaire (CIQ; Willer et al., 1994), CIQ–II (Johnston et al., 2005)	Developed for the TBI Model Systems program, this 15-item questionnaire assesses home integration, social integration, and productivity in employment, volunteer work, or school. It can be administered in person or via telephone to either the person with TBI or a proxy. The CIQ–II expands the original CIQ to 48 items (24 each in functional–instrumental activities and social–recreational activities). Responses describe frequency, level, or type of community activity or status/role. Each CIQ–II question is supplemented with 3 additional ratings that include satisfaction with activity, desire for change, and importance of change.	The CIQ has acceptable interrater reliability but a lower intraclass correlation coefficient. No formal content or face validity studies. Some activities on the CIQ–II were found to have low or little relevance to satisfaction of people 12 mo after TBI. Content validity showed excellent relationship between PART–O and CIQ–II.

(Continued)

Table 7.2. Selected Community Integration, Participation, and Instrumental Activities of Daily Living Assessments *(cont.)*

Assessment	Description	Comments (Reliability and Validity)
Craig Handicap Assessment and Reporting Technique (CHART; Mellick et al., 1999; Whiteneck et al., 1992)	32 items measure the degree to which impairments and disabilities result in handicaps in the years after initial rehabilitation in the areas of physical independence, cognitive independence, mobility, occupation, social integration, and economic self-sufficiency. Multiple measurements over time can provide insight into adaptation and adjustment to the TBI. A 19-item short form (CHART–SF) is also available.	Established as a reliable and valid assessment. Although initially developed to assess handicap resulting from physical disabilities, a cognitive subscale extended the usefulness of the scale to clients with cognitive impairments.
Craig Hospital Inventory of Environmental Factors (CHIEF; Whiteneck et al., 2004)	25-item inventory (or 12-item short form, CHIEF–SF) that assesses frequency and magnitude of the impact that physical, social, and political environments have as barriers or facilitators to full participation in the community. Domains are policies, physical and structural, work and school, attitudes and support, and services and assistance. Multiple assessments over time can provide insights into adaptation to TBI and changes in environmental barriers.	High test–retest reliability demonstrated, but lower participant–proxy agreement suggests that proxies may not be able to accurately predict how their disabled family members perceive the impact of the environment on themselves. Hence, use of proxies is not recommended. Reliability of the scale's overall internal consistency is good.
Functional Assessment Measure (FAM; Hall, 1997)	An expansion of the **FIM™** to include 12 items related to community functioning (e.g., car transfers, employability, adjustment to limitations, swallowing function). Used in conjunction with the FIM.	Reported to add sensitivity beyond the FIM. Reliability of FAM established to the extent that staff can be trained to administer it with an accuracy of 80% or better (Donaghy & Wass, 1998).
IADL Profile (Bottari et al., 2009)	Performance-based measure of independence in IADLs based on executive functioning. Administered in a client's home and community environment. Establishes whether observed difficulties are related to goal formulation, planning, carrying out the task, or attaining the initial task goal.	Moderate to good interrater agreement and criterion-related validity in relation to TBI injury severity, education, and executive function measures of planning and **working memory.** Evaluator training and observation of clients in numerous situations (8 tasks) over an extended period (about 3 hr) increased the reliability and generalizability of the profile (Bottari et al., 2010).
Mayo–Portland Adaptability Inventory (MPAI–4; Malec, 2005)	35-item inventory designed to assist in the evaluation of people during the community phase of recovery from TBI. Items representing typically experienced physical, cognitive, emotional, behavioral, and social problems after TBI are analyzed on 3 indices: ability, adjustment, and participation. The Participation Index (M2PI) consists of an 8-item subset of the MPAI–4 that correlates highly with the entire inventory. Raters evaluate the degree of limitations in areas of initiation, self-care, social contact, recreation, employment, transportation, household management, and financial management.	Reliability and validity have been studied extensively. The M2PI correlates well with the entire MPAI–4.
Participation Assessment With Recombined Tools–Objective (PART–O; Whiteneck et al., 2011)	24-item assessment based on 3 legacy instruments of participation: CIQ–II, POPS, and CHART. Objective data on frequency of engagement in activities related to 6 of the 9 areas of the *ICF* (domestic life, interpersonal interactions and relationships, major life areas, and community, social, and civic life).	Strong concurrent validity with other participation and functional measures. Test–retest and participant–proxy agreement have not been established yet. Development of a subjective measure of participation to complement the PART–O is planned.
Participation Objective, Participation Subjective (POPS; Brown et al., 2004)	The 26 items are sorted into 5 categories: domestic life; major life activities; transportation; interpersonal interactions and relationships; and community, recreational, and civic life. Client rates frequency and satisfaction with participation.	Because the instrument provides objective descriptive data as well as subjective data, reliability and validity are complex. Acceptable levels of test–retest reliability were found in those measures expected to be more stable. Validity has not been evaluated.

(Continued)

Table 7.2. Selected Community Integration, Participation, and Instrumental Activities of Daily Living Assessments *(cont.)*

Assessment	Description	Comments (Reliability and Validity)
Participation Profile (PAR-PRO; Ostir et al., 2006)	Measures frequency of participation with 20 items selected from the *ICF* domains of participation (e.g., domestic life, interpersonal interactions and relationships, and major life areas such as work or education) using a 5-point scale. Data are collected at 3 points in time (admission, discharge, and follow-up). Preinjury data used as benchmark for follow-up.	Good internal consistency. Further research needed on equivalency of client vs. proxy respondent ratings.

Source. From *Occupational Therapy Practice Guidelines for Adults With Traumatic Brain Injury* (pp. 22–26), by K. Golisz, 2009, Bethesda, MD: AOTA Press. Copyright © 2009 by the American Occupational Therapy Association. Adapted with permission.

Note. ADL/ADLs = activity/activities of daily living; hr = hours; IADL/IADLs = instrumental activity/activities of daily living; ICF = *International Classification of Functioning, Disability and Health* (World Health Organization, 2001); mo = months; OT = occupational therapy; TBI = traumatic brain injury.

In an effort to better understand community participation for people with moderate to severe TBI, McColl et al. (1998) conducted structured interviews. Participants identified the following themes:

- *General integration*—understanding the rules and knowing how to fit in, feeling accepted, and knowing one's way around the community
- *Social support*—intimate relationships (e.g., spouse, significant other, parent, close friend) and diffuse relationships (e.g., neighbors, workers in community stores)
- *Occupation*—paid work, volunteer work, and leisure activities
- *Independent living*—living situation, such as with whom they live, and self-determination (the ability to freely choose activities).

These themes help link participation to community, connecting the importance of personally meaningful productive activity within the community with the need for acceptance by members of the community. By gaining an appreciation of these important factors, the occupational therapist is ideally positioned not only to conduct a comprehensive evaluation at the community stage but also to interpret findings and observations in a manner necessary for community-based treatment planning.

Life Satisfaction at the Community Stage of Rehabilitation

Fuhrer (1994) asserted that evaluations of rehabilitation outcome are incomplete if they ignore the subjective well-being of the person being served. This notion is supported in the *ICF*, which described participation as "involvement in a life situation or as 'the lived experiences' of people in the actual contexts in which they live" (WHO, 2001, pp. 14–15). Profound psychosocial disability and social isolation after TBI often contribute to decreased **life satisfaction** (Hagen, 2003; Sloan et al., 2004). Successful community participation is more than simply doing things in the community. It also involves a sense of belonging and feeling accepted and satisfied with one's life.

Occupational therapists must understand issues related to life satisfaction after TBI and include measures that take into account the client's perspective on participation, sense of well-being, and general life satisfaction. Instruments such as the Participation Objective, Participation Subjective (POPS) explore both the frequency with which a person engages in home and community activities and his or her subjective view, based on how important and salient the activity is to the person (Brown et al., 2004). The multidimensional and individualized nature of community integration may necessitate the use of multiple assessment strategies and approaches to capture both client performance and client perspective (Wheeler, Lane, & McMahon, 2007).

Occupational therapists must understand issues related to life satisfaction after TBI and include measures that take into account the client's perspective on participation, sense of well-being, and general life satisfaction.

Are people with TBI living in the community generally satisfied with their lives? Research has produced varied results but has facilitated a better understanding of factors that may contribute to life satisfaction after TBI (Burleigh, Farber, & Gillard, 1998; Corrigan, 2001). In a sample of people with TBI 1 to 2 years postinjury, Corrigan (2001) reported motor independence at rehabilitation discharge, not having a preinjury history of substance abuse, absence of depressed **mood,** social integration, and having gainful employment to be associated with higher self-reported life satisfaction. Other researchers (Warren, Wrigley, Yoels, & Fine, 1996) have reported a positive association between life satisfaction and employment, functional memory capacity, bowel independence, marital status, and family satisfaction. Burleigh et al. (1998) examined the relationship between community integration, as measured by the Community Integration Questionnaire, and life satisfaction among 30 adults with TBI who were at least 8 years postinjury. Findings from the study indicated a significant relationship between life satisfaction and social integration, which includes social interactions with friends and family, leisure pursuits with others, and involvement in community activities.

These findings are similar to those of Wheeler's (2012) study of a group of people with severe TBI in a community-based **residential rehabilitation** program, and they support Hagen's (2003) notion that a sense of belonging among friends, family, and community is critical to experiencing life satisfaction. Other studies have identified positive relationships between life satisfaction and returning to meaningful work (Melamed, Groswasser, & Stern, 1992; Underhill et al., 2003), whereas Johansson and Bernspång (2001) found low levels of life satisfaction after TBI regardless of whether a person was working at the time of evaluation. In contrast, Koskinen (1998) reported that 70% of a sample of people with severe TBI identified being satisfied or rather satisfied with life 10 years postinjury.

It appears that life satisfaction, much like other constructs being measured at the community stage of rehabilitation, is complex and multidimensional. In Wheeler's (2012) study of 40 people with severe TBI enrolled in a community-based residential rehabilitation program, a statistically significant decrease in overall self-reported life satisfaction was found at 90-day follow-up. This decrease occurred despite an increase in community integration as measured by improved independence in home management, **social participation,** and productive activity. At 1-year follow-up, however, a return to baseline (i.e., before-intervention) levels of self-reported life satisfaction was found, and a positive relationship between life satisfaction and community participation was observed. The initial decrease in life satisfaction may be attributable to increasing self-awareness during involvement in intensive individual skills training and group therapy.

According to Toglia and Kirk (2000), self-awareness increases through participation in different types of tasks. It is possible that in Wheeler's study, the process of working on challenging tasks and receiving staff and other client feedback on performance resulted in clients becoming increasingly dissatisfied as they became more aware of the extent of their injury-related difficulties. The development of self-awareness after TBI is generally considered to be a gradual process that involves comparing performance on functional tasks in a familiar setting with people's premorbid functional level (Dirette & Plaisier, 2007) and "coming to terms with their new selves" (O'Callaghan et al., 2012, p. 1607). It is possible that an initial decrease in life satisfaction may be a necessary component of treatment for those people whose awareness deficits are impeding successful community participation.

Intervention Settings

The community phase of TBI recovery generally begins on discharge from an inpatient facility. From there, the path to recovery becomes less predictable, influenced by factors such as injury severity, family and client expectations, ability to pay for needed professional and nonprofessional supports, and transportation to various types of services (Katz, Zasler, & Zafonte, 2007). The complexity of services and relationships between them are outlined in Figure 7.2.

Outpatient Rehabilitation Programs

Outpatient services generally involve the recipient of services living at home and coming to a rehabilitation setting for structured therapy programming (Senelick & Dougherty, 2001). Through interactions with the real-world home environment after hospital discharge, the person involved in outpatient rehabilitation is reintroduced to the challenges of community living with the support of the outpatient rehabilitation team. Outpatient programs provide multidiscipline or single-discipline therapy, depending on the needs of the client, and involve client-centered interventions that target those residual deficits negatively affecting the capacity for successful community participation. Wheelchair and equipment clinics, driving evaluations, and augmentative communication clinics are components of many outpatient programs. Opportunities to provide therapy in home and community settings are generally very limited during outpatient rehabilitation as a result of therapist time limitations and productivity standards.

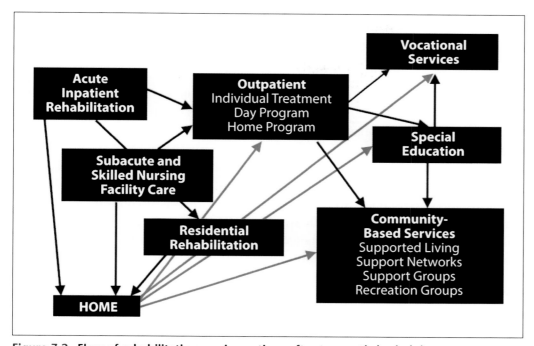

Figure 7.2. Flow of rehabilitation service options after traumatic brain injury.

Source. Adapted from "Clinical Continuum of Care and Natural History," by D. I. Katz, N. D. Zasler, & R. D. Zafonte, in *Brain Injury Medicine: Principles and Practice* (p. 6), by N. D. Zasler, D. I. Katz, & R. D. Zafonte (Eds.), 2007, New York: Demos. Copyright © 2007 by Demos Medical Publishing. Used with permission.

Note. Black arrows represent traditional flow of service options following traumatic brain injury; red arrows represent possible service options while living at home.

As such, outpatient programs often rely heavily on caregiver training and home-work activities.

Evidence for the effectiveness of outpatient TBI rehabilitation is mixed. Many outpatient rehabilitation programs are hospital based. Poor generalization of skills from the structured hospital setting to the community has been identified as a key reason for poor community integration after TBI (Feeney, Ylvisaker, Rosen, & Greene, 2001; Hayden, Moreault, LeBlanc, & Plenger, 2000). However, evidence has supported occupation-based outpatient occupational therapy as a means of improv-ing occupational performance and QoL (Trombly, Radomski, Trexel, & Burnet-Smith, 2002). Simulation of real-life activities, use of homework, and family and caregiver education have all been associated with improved generalization of skills (Trombly et al., 2002). Evidence has also supported the benefits of outpatient exer-cise programs to improve mood and QoL for people living in the community (Wise, Hoffman, Powell, Bombardier, & Bell, 2012).

Day Treatment Programs

Facility-based **day treatment programs** provide rehabilitation during the day so that the person can return home at night. Services are generally provided for 4 to 8 hours in a structured format. Day treatment programs generally include compo-nents for vocational and community reentry using group interventions and often involve traditional rehabilitation therapies, including individual and group occu-pational therapy to address residual physical, cognitive, and social impairments (Altman, Swick, Parrot, & Malec, 2010). These multidisciplinary programs build on skills training performed in the clinical setting through regular community activities (i.e., restaurant trips, shopping, grocery shopping, community events), social skills training, vocational training, and cognitive interventions. As is the case with other settings during the community recovery phase, the degree of involvement of occu-pational therapy is often influenced by both client-specific needs and reimburse-ment regulations and eligibility (Katz et al., 2007; Wheeler, 2014).

Numerous studies have reported client benefits from participation in day treat-ment programs (Geurtsen, van Heugten, Martina, & Geurts, 2010; Hashimoto, Okamoto, Watanabe, & Ohashi, 2006; Malec, 2001). Geurtsen et al. (2010) conducted a systematic review of the effectiveness of comprehensive TBI rehabilitation programs for adults in the chronic phase of recovery. These authors reviewed a total of 13 pro-grams and concluded that day treatment programs had the highest level of evidence. Simmons and Griswold (2010) used structured and unstructured group activities as part of an outpatient day program and found significant improvements in social skills over an 8-week period. A detailed discussion of specific interventions used in these and other postacute rehabilitation programs is provided later in this chapter.

Transitional Living Programs

Nonmedical residential programs that teach skills for community living are labeled *transitional living programs*. These programs may be offered in a house, group of apartments, campus setting, or ranch where the survivor lives in a structured environment in which necessary therapies are provided. The goal is to foster the client's independence, but supervision, safety, and support are always available. Individual treatment programs can range from focusing on basic self-care skills to vocational and educational activities, depending on the needs of the client (Geurtsen et al., 2011; Senelick & Dougherty, 2001; Wheeler, 2012). Training and education related to community interaction; prevocational and vocational training; and cognitive, speech, and behavior therapies structured to meet clients' individual needs are also offered. The setting aims to provide a naturalistic environment for social interaction in which clients can work on improving their social skills.

People with severe TBI can achieve significant improvements in home management, social participation, and productive activity through participation in daily residential transitional living programs (Geurtsen et al., 2011, 2012). Community-based transitional living programs have a positive effect on independent living skills, social competence, socially appropriate behavior, and employment (Geurtsen et al., 2012; Harrick, Krefting, Johnston, Carlson, & Minnes, 1994; Wheeler, 2012).

Geurtsen et al. (2011) reported improvements in independent living, societal participation, emotional well-being, and QoL after clients participated in a 3-month multidisciplinary residential community reintegration program. Outcomes from their study included an increase in the number of people able to live independently from 25% before treatment to 72% after treatment and 66% at 1-year follow-up. Their program involved three modules: (1) independent living, focusing on home management activities; (2) social–emotional, providing training in coping strategies and education in brain injury and its functional consequences; and (3) vocational, addressing skills and participation in work (supported or paid, volunteer, or sheltered) and leisure. The program combined group (approximately 10% of the time) and individual (approximately 90% of the time) interventions. A 3-year follow-up by these researchers found that the gains achieved at 1 year remained stable over time (Geurtsen et al., 2012).

Wheeler (2012) described a similar program combining individual skills coaching, structured and unstructured group activities, and multidisciplinary rehabilitation services including occupational therapy. Improved participation in home management, social interactions, and productive activity was reported at 1-year follow-up. Although these results are promising, funding for such programs by commercial insurance remains limited, reducing access to people eligible through state Medicaid waiver programs and other sources (Katz et al., 2007; Wheeler, 2014).

Supported Employment Programs and Vocational Rehabilitation

Vocational and prevocational programs for people with TBI address work behaviors and provide advocacy with the goal of productive employment. A return to meaningful employment is a commonly used measure of successful community reentry and rehabilitation program effectiveness (Kelley et al., 2014). Literature on TBI rehabilitation equates return to work after TBI with other important outcomes such as improved QoL and social integration (Wehman, Targett, West, & Kregel, 2005), improved self-esteem, reduced substance abuse, and reduced disability (Johansson & Tham, 2006). The existence of residual social and behavioral impairments plays a crucial role in successful return to employment, and attention to these and other problematic impairments will generally precede placement in a work site. Topics in prevocational skills training may include communication skills, time management, organizational skills, and computer skills. Volunteer work may serve as a preparatory step toward the return-to-work goal or may become an end goal for those whose severity of impairments and long-term deficits prevent the option of a return to paid employment.

Supported employment services prepare, place, train, and maintain gainful employment in the community for people with TBI. Essential elements of the supported employment model include

- Pay for real work
- Integration into the workplace with nondisabled workers
- Long-term ongoing supportive services to facilitate job retention
- Job placement of people with severe handicapping conditions
- Interagency cooperation and funding of these services.

Research on supported employment validates the model as an effective means of **vocational rehabilitation** after TBI (O'Brien, 2007; Vandiver, Johnson, & Christofero-Snider, 2003; Wehman et al., 2003). Return-to-work outcomes are most likely to be achieved when using a client-centered approach, combining staff expertise in TBI with skilled assessment and training in actual workplace settings (O'Brien, 2007). The success of a supported employment program is influenced by the degree of staff commitment to and training in the unique needs of the population with TBI (Wehman et al., 2003). Many comprehensive postacute rehabilitation programs include vocational training and supported employment (Geurtsen et al., 2011; Wheeler, 2012).

> Return-to-work outcomes are most likely to be achieved when using a client-centered approach, combining staff expertise in TBI with skilled assessment and training in actual workplace settings.

School Reentry Programs

Specialized school reentry programs seek to prepare students with TBI to return to academic life by coaching them to use various strategies to facilitate academic success, including how to develop study habits. School reentry programs can be associated with a particular educational institution, can be a private service, or can be a component of a larger community reentry program (Phipps, 2006). TBI may affect the way a student thinks, speaks, and behaves in the classroom environment (Burkhardt & Rotatori, 2010). Common TBI-related impairments that can have an impact on school performance include inattention to task, memory impairments, executive dysfunction (e.g., impulsivity; decreased self-awareness; organization, planning, and sequencing difficulties), issues with sensory overload, language problems, and difficulty with written and oral communication. Independent living issues and social participation in the school environment can also be major barriers to student success, especially for students who reside in college housing.

TBI was established as a disability category under the Individuals With Disabilities Education Act of 1990 (Pub. L. 101–476), which means that students who are high school age and younger can utilize the services of the school-based interdisciplinary team. Goals for intervention are established in the individualized education program. The needs of students with TBI can challenge educators, who typically lack the educational training specific to TBI-related impairments. A report by Mohr and Bullock (2005) outlined potential issues related to teacher preparedness for students with TBI that include a lack of teacher awareness regarding TBI impairments and the course of recovery, poorly defined educational goals, and few specific accommodations for students with TBI. Provision of support by occupational therapists and other rehabilitation professionals to teachers through collaboration and in-service education is a necessary step in ensuring continuity between therapy interventions and classroom implementation (Glang, Tyler, Pearson, Todis, & Morvant, 2004).

Students who are injured while in high school may need to acquire new skills and coping strategies when moving from the supportive home environment to a college communal living setting. Peer mentoring and life coaching models may be of particular importance here, especially when supports and training are provided in the classroom, campus, and community environments (Wheeler, 2014). Such models support a long-term client-centered focus that emphasizes training approaches suited to the specific needs of the client (Sloan et al., 2004). Return to school is often categorized with other productive outcome measures of community reentry, such as work and volunteer activities (Malec, 2005; Willer, Ottenbacher, & Coad, 1994).

Home-Based Programs

The client's home is the ideal setting to address specific home management issues for people with TBI after hospital discharge. Unfortunately, many people who might benefit from functional occupational therapy interventions in their homes do not receive them. Reimbursement eligibility for home-based services typically depends on the person's physical functional level. For example, Medicare guidelines and some Medicaid waiver programs require the person to be homebound (i.e., leaving the home requires considerable and taxing effort), leaving services unfunded for physically mobile clients whose occupational performance deficits stem from cognitive problems. Additionally, occupational therapy does not currently qualify for initiation of care or services for Medicare beneficiaries, meaning that another service such as nursing, physical therapy, or speech therapy must be initially required for a patient to be eligible for occupational therapy. Once services are initiated, occupational therapy can continue care when other skilled services have been discontinued (Marrelli & Krulish, 1999). Advocacy efforts continue at the federal level to change legislation to enable occupational therapists to initiate home care services under Medicare.

Health care practitioners have explored approaches to home-based intervention beyond traditional home health direct care services to meet the needs of people with TBI. For example, Warden et al. (2000) evaluated the effectiveness of a home-based telerehabilitation educational and counseling program for people with moderate to severe TBI discharged from an inpatient rehabilitation program. The home program included 30-minute weekly telephone support and education. The researchers reported that participants' cognitive and behavioral functioning was similar to that of a comparison group participating in a hospital-based cognitive rehabilitation program over the evaluation period and concluded that home interventions "may provide effective care at a lower cost" (p. 1101). Expansion of the telerehabilitation service delivery model to Internet-based formats holds promise for people with TBI (Warden et al., 2000).

Resumption of Life Roles and Managing Life Transitions

The transition from hospital to community after TBI is typically a time of adjustment during which people with TBI and their family members try to reorganize their daily routines and occupational roles (Turner, Fleming, Ownsworth, & Cornwell, 2011). In this section, I discuss specific adjustment challenges characterizing the process of community reentry after TBI and tools that can assist occupational therapists in evaluating these areas. Through an understanding of transition challenges and methods for evaluating them, the occupational therapist lays the groundwork for the planning and implementation of client-centered intervention to foster community participation.

Changes in Family Dynamics

Optimal community participation for the person with TBI cannot be achieved without consideration of the role of the family and family dynamics. Studies have shown that the strongest predictor of emotional distress for people with TBI is life satisfaction (Vangel, Rapport, & Hanks, 2011). **Stress** and strain within the family system after TBI influence the ultimate outcome for the family member with TBI. The significant strain placed on family members caring for injured relatives has a negative impact on their physical health, contributes to emotional distress, and increases the likelihood of depression (Connolly & O'Dowd, 2001; Knight, Devereux, & Godfrey, 1998; Leathem, Heath, & Woolley, 1996). Unfortunately, many family caregivers and significant others report that 10 years after the TBI, they still manage all of their family member's ADLs and instrumental activities of daily living (IADLs) and that they are exhausted by their caregiving responsibilities (Lefebvre et al., 2008). Research has suggested that the well-being of the person with TBI affects the well-being of the family, and the well-being of the family affects the well-being of the person with TBI (Vangel et al., 2011).

The marital relationship can be particularly prone to disruption after TBI. Studies have highlighted the challenges spouses face coping with their partner's emotional unpredictability, dependency, self-centeredness, and childlike behaviors after TBI (Marsh, Kersel, Havill, & Sleigh, 1998). In particular, high levels of behavioral and cognitive problems have been linked to increased caregiver distress and unhealthy family functioning (Anderson, Parmenter, & Mok, 2002). Couples are more likely to describe their spousal relationship positively when they receive support from family and friends; had a strong relationship before the injury; had previous knowledge or experience relevant to disability; and had positive communication and coping skills such as spirituality, humor, and the ability to accept change (Gill, Sander, Robins, Mazzei, & Struchen, 2011). The availability of community resources and supports has also been found to contribute positively to the well-being and community integration of both individuals and couples (Hanks, Rapport, Wertheimer, & Koviak, 2012).

The effects of TBI can significantly challenge physical and emotional intimacy within a marriage. Female caregivers have reported that their partner seemed like a stranger after the TBI (Gosling & Oddy, 1999). Couples interviewed after one partner sustained a TBI reported that caregiver responsibilities and role changes in the marital relationship left the uninjured partner with reduced energy to devote to emotional or physical intimacy (Gill et al., 2011). Physical and emotional intimacy can be disrupted by changes in brain function after TBI in addition to sensorimotor impairments, cognitive impairments, depression, and anxiety (Downing, Stolwyk, & Ponsford, 2013; Hanks, Sander, Millis, Hammond, & Maestas, 2013; Ponsford, Downing, & Stolwyk, 2013). In a study of 862 participants with moderate to severe TBI, Downing et al. (2013) reported that fatigue was the most common cause of sexual changes postinjury, followed by higher levels of depression and anxiety and lower self-esteem. For men, impaired sexual arousal can result in the inability to

Couples are more likely to describe their spousal relationship positively when they receive support from family and friends; had a strong relationship before the injury; had previous knowledge or experience relevant to disability; and had positive communication and coping skills such as spirituality, humor, and the ability to accept change.

obtain or maintain an erection (Ponsford, 2003). Men also report decreased sexual desire, decreased ability to achieve orgasm, decreased frequency of sexual activity, and overall decreased quality of and satisfaction with sexual experiences (Kreuter, Dahllöf, Gudjonsson, Sullivan, & Siösteen, 1998; Ponsford, 2003). Women may experience decreased vaginal lubrication, decreased sexual arousal, decreased ability to achieve orgasm, and pain during sexual activity (Hibbard, Gordon, Flanagan, Haddad, & Labinsky, 2000).

Despite the impact of TBI on family functioning, changes in family roles, and elevated levels of psychological distress among caregivers (Gan & Schuller, 2002), investigations of marital breakdown after TBI have produced widely varying findings (Wood & Rutterford, 2006). Studies that have included marital stability as part of the overall client postinjury profile have indicated divorce and separation rates ranging from as low as 15% at 17 years postinjury (Wood & Rutterford, 2006) to as high as 45% at 10 years postinjury (Jacobsson, Westerberg, Söderberg, & Lexell, 2009). Kreutzer, Marwitz, Hsu, Williams, and Riddick (2007) found marital stability among people with TBI, reporting a divorce rate of 17% and separation rate of 8% in a group of people 30 to 96 months postinjury. They concluded that these findings "do not support contentions that persons with brain injury are at greater risk for divorce relative to the general population. Nor do findings suggest that males are more likely to leave injured female partners" (p. 53). These researchers did find that older people were less likely to divorce and that couples married longer before injury were more likely to stay together. When marital breakdown does occur, additional challenges to community participation may arise as a consequence of changes in living situations and loss of levels of emotional and functional support.

Comprehensive occupational therapy at the community stage requires, when possible, a thorough appreciation of caregiver issues and family dynamics. People without a supportive and stable family are at a disadvantage in their efforts to reestablish successful and satisfying community participation. Including family and caregivers in the treatment process along with ongoing reevaluation of their stress level can yield important insights into the client's support system, an important element of functional recovery. Additionally, occupational therapists can work with members of the multidisciplinary treatment team to seek out and identify community supports to provide information, respite, assistance, and encouragement for both the survivor and family.

Coping and Community Supports for Clients and Families

Difficulties with community reintegration after TBI require considerable adaptation by both survivors and family members and are often associated with increased emotional disturbance (Ruttan, Martin, Liu, Colella, & Green, 2008). *Coping* has been defined as the ability to change cognitive and behavioral efforts to manage specific internal and external demands that are appraised as exceeding the resources of the individual (Lazarus & Folkman, 1984). Coping is an essential and necessary aspect of catastrophic loss and change and can have adaptive or maladaptive styles. Occupational therapists must have a thorough understanding of coping because a client's selected coping strategies can negatively affect his or her ability to cope with life stressors and degree of progress in occupational therapy (Gage, 1992;

Regardless of how psychologically well adjusted a person is before injury, TBI is associated with increased emotional disturbance and often represents a fundamental challenge to the person's beliefs about the self and the nature of the world.

Wood & Doughty, 2013). Regardless of how psychologically well adjusted a person is before injury, TBI is associated with increased emotional disturbance and often represents a fundamental challenge to the person's beliefs about the self and the nature of the world (Sloan et al., 2004; Spitz, Schönberger, & Ponsford, 2013). Levy (2006) emphasized that, given the relationship between clients' psychological and emotional responses to their injury and their functional recovery, interventions related to coping should be central to the occupational therapy process.

Coping strategies are commonly defined as either emotion focused or problem focused (Spitz et al., 2013). *Problem-focused coping* is characterized by the use of strategies to deal with the problem. *Emotion-focused coping,* including techniques such as suppression, wishful thinking, and drug use, attempts to modulate the person's emotional response to the stressful event (Spitz et al., 2013). A person's personal resources, such as level of cognitive functioning, beliefs, and traits, along with environmental factors, are thought to influence coping strategies during stressful situations (Kendall & Terry, 1996). Awareness of deficits has been associated with level of emotional distress experienced, with greater awareness linked to higher rates of depression and anxiety (Wallace & Bogner, 2000). The cognitive sequelae of TBI, including attention, memory, and problem-solving deficits, may reduce a person's available resources to implement adaptive coping strategies (Bryant, Marosszeky, Crooks, Baguley, & Gurka, 2000). People with TBI tend to display a reduction in the use of active, problem-focused coping and an increase in maladaptive passive emotional coping (Kendall, Shum, Lack, Bull, & Fee, 2001; Kortte, Wegener, & Chwalisz, 2003). Additionally, the largest single category of people who sustain TBI are young men, who may not have had the opportunity to develop adaptive coping strategies before their injury (Anson & Ponsford, 2006).

The use of cognitive–behavioral therapy coping skills group interventions has a positive influence on the development of effective coping styles in people with TBI (Anson & Ponsford, 2006). Analyzing the relationship among cognitive impairment, coping style, and emotional adjustment after TBI, Spitz et al. (2013) reported greater levels of self-reported depression and anxiety among people demonstrating poorer performance on various cognitive measures, including memory, attention, executive functions, and information processing. These authors recommended combining cognitive rehabilitation and coping skills interventions to facilitate the use of more active, solution-focused strategies for managing adjustment issues.

When discussing coping after TBI, it is important to make a distinction between organic self-awareness deficits (i.e., **anosognosia**) and psychological **denial,** a psychological **defense mechanism** (Toglia & Kirk, 2000). *Psychological denial,* in this respect, is an involuntary and useful coping strategy during the early stages of recovery after a traumatic event. When the nature of the stressful event exceeds the person's capacity to cope, denying that the event has occurred allows the person to consciously maintain a sense of competence instead of overwhelming depression and anxiety. However, continued nonacceptance of the TBI beyond the acute stages of recovery is associated with poorer life outcomes (Curran, Ponsford, & Crowe, 2000; Moore & Stambrook, 1995). People in denial of their disability have partial knowledge of their impairments and struggle to accept and deal with this new information (Prigatano & Klonoff, 1998). In these situations, clients' resistance to feedback about TBI impairments is common and may elicit an angry response from them. It has been suggested that postacute rehabilitation should incorporate interventions to decrease denial while teaching clients about physical, cognitive, emotional, psychological, and behavioral deficits (Dyer, Bell, McCann, & Rauch, 2006; Moore & Stambrook, 1995).

The coping process after TBI extends well beyond the person with TBI. After TBI, the disruption of the normal life course is considerable for both injured people and their families (Anderson, Simpson, & Morey, 2013; Dikmen, Machamer, Powell, & Temkin, 2003). Support systems are a key determinant of postinjury caregiver distress and family adjustment (Ergh, Rapport, Coleman, & Hanks, 2002). Research on social support after TBI has indicated that, over time, both caregivers and people with TBI become isolated from their support networks, which can result in caregiver distress (Anderson et al., 2013; Temkin, Corrigan, Dikmen, & Machamer, 2009). Ergh et al. (2002) examined family dysfunction and caregiver distress among 60 pairs of people with TBI and their caregivers. They concluded that, in the absence of adequate social support, caregiver distress increased with longer time since injury, cognitive dysfunction, and lack of awareness of deficits in care recipients. Caregiving family members with little support are consequently at risk for burnout and less effective partners in the rehabilitation process (Brown et al., 1999).

An important distinction in the social support literature involves the difference between *enacted support* (i.e., specific help received from others) and *perceived support* (i.e., the generalized belief that people value you and would be there for you in a time of need; Ergh et al., 2002). A support serves its intended purpose only if it is perceived as being a support by the caregiver. Caregivers with perceived social support fare better in many ways than those who do not perceive themselves to be supported (Ergh et al., 2002). As such, it is important for occupational therapy practitioners, along with other rehabilitation clinicians, to consider family members as essential partners in the ongoing rehabilitation process and strive to assist all concerned in achieving successful long-term adjustment (Brown et al., 1999). Evaluation of caregiver supports, using instruments such as the Family Needs Questionnaire–Revised (Kreutzer & Marwitz, 2008), Caregiver Strain Index (Robinson, 1983), or Service Obstacles Scale (Marwitz & Kreutzer, 1996), can yield valuable insights into the existence and quality of perceived supports.

Brain injury support groups generally provide face-to-face interactions among people whose lives have been affected by brain injury. Many groups are operated through volunteer organizations, meet at regular intervals, and provide opportunities for information sharing and companionship. Although the value of such groups is widely recognized, research to identify the impact of such programs on the various aspects of families' community participation and caregiver functioning has been sparse (Brown et al., 1999). Brown et al. (1999) compared caregivers participating in traditional on-site caregiver support groups ($n = 39$) with caregivers from rural communities participating in a similar support program but via teleconference. Both programs involved weekly meetings for 9 to 10 weeks. They found statistically significant improvements in both groups in regard to caregiver burden and family functioning. Social media afford additional forums for communication and support for people who are unable to access more traditional, face-to-face support groups.

Continued research is needed to identify the specific benefits of different types of support programs, particularly those heavily using Internet-based education and support.

Returning to Work After Traumatic Brain Injury

People with TBI often experience difficulty securing or returning to competitive employment after injury and fail to maintain employment because of cognitive deficits, impaired psychosocial functioning, and physical and sensory disabilities (Ponsford & Spitz, 2014). Estimates of the employment rate for people with TBI range from 20% to 50% depending on the severity of injury; the person's prior work experience; and demographic characteristics such as age, education, and socioeconomic status (Keyser-Marcus et al., 2002).

Being employed has consistently been associated with better post-TBI QoL (Nalder et al., 2012) and is an important occupational therapy outcome. Many assessments used by occupational therapists at the level of participation include items relating to vocational participation (e.g., competitive employment, school, volunteer work; see Table 7.2). Work contributes to a person's self-esteem and gives a person a sense of control over his or her life and economic independence and provides a structured daily routine. A person's work influences his or her self-perceptions, values, and thinking as the person negotiates the demands of various challenges and expectations of the job. Additionally, work affords social opportunities and contributes higher self-reported QoL and independent living (Temkin et al., 2009). The transition from hospital to home is often associated with increased idle time and feelings of boredom (Rittman et al., 2004). Unemployed people with moderate to severe TBI report higher levels of depression, anxiety, and fatigue, and experience a variety of other symptoms compared with their employed counterparts, despite equivalent levels of cognitive functioning and preinjury job satisfaction (Franulic, Carbonell, Pinto, & Sepulveda, 2004; McCrimmon & Oddy, 2006).

Positive factors influencing the capacity to return to work after TBI include younger age, a higher level of education, better postinjury cognitive abilities, and the absence of psychiatric disorder or substance abuse. Findings of links between injury severity and return to work have been inconsistent but, generally speaking, more severe injuries have a more negative impact on return to work, in part because of greater cognitive impairment and injury-related physical impairment (McCrimmon & Oddy, 2006; Ponsford & Spitz, 2014; Tsaousides, Ashman, & Seter, 2008). The type of preinjury work is also important, with manual workers who have residual physical impairments being less likely to return to work (Walker, Marwitz, Kreutzer, Hart, & Novack, 2006). Adequate self-awareness and acceptance of disabilities have also been identified as essential requirements for return to work and education (Kelley et al., 2014; Trudel et al., 1998; Wehman et al., 2005). Similarly, severity of injury, cognitive impairments, and physical impairments have also been linked to employment stability, evaluated by the ability to remain in a job over time. Ponsford et al. (2015) found that, among people with moderate to severe TBI who returned to work postinjury, only 44% remained employed 3 years after injury.

Beyond the well-documented benefits of a successful return to paid employment (Franulic et al., 2004; McCrimmon & Oddy, 2006), engaging in a productive volunteer activity may also promote self-awareness, acceptance, and psychological well-being. For example, volunteer work allows people with TBI to test their limits and abilities, to explore new avenues of work, to develop new interests, or to discover new sets of capacities that may lead to productive activity despite existing limitations (Ouellet, Morin, & Lavoie, 2009). Despite having a larger proportion of more severely injured people receiving long-term disability benefits, which might be associated with higher levels of psychological distress, a group of people with TBI who engaged in volunteer work did not differ significantly in their psychological adjustment from a group of people with TBI who were either competitively employed or engaged in academic pursuits (Ouellet et al., 2009). For clients with severe injuries who are unable to return to competitive employment, volunteer work should be considered to support their social roles.

Misconceptions about TBI among the general public, including employers, can have negative consequences in the return-to-work process. Research has suggested that people with visible injuries and disability suffer stigma, are less often offered employment, and are avoided by people. Employers and coworkers may have unrealistic expectations of people whose injuries and disabilities are not visible, as is often the case with TBI. Potential employers may misattribute an applicant's irregular work history to the applicant's personality rather than to poor support or work task incompatibility (Martz, 2003).

Although getting clients back to meaningful work activities is a challenge for the occupational therapist, research has supported the value of vocational rehabilitation, even for people with severe injuries (Fadyl & McPherson, 2009; Malec & Moessner, 2006). Fadyl and McPherson (2009) described three categories of vocational rehabilitation for people with TBI:

1. *Program-based vocational rehabilitation,* involving intensive individualized rehabilitation of work skills in a structured environment, guided work trials, and assisted job placement with transitional job support
2. *Supported employment,* including job placement, on-the-job training, and long-term support and job skills reinforcement
3. *Case coordination,* involving a holistic rehabilitation approach that is individualized to suit the client's specific needs.

Resource facilitation is a means of providing support that considers potential environmental barriers to the return-to-work transition. Engaging employers in return-to-work plans and providing TBI-related employer education are key areas of focus in resource facilitation (Trexler, Trexler, Malec, Klyce, & Parrott, 2010). Other aspects of resource facilitation include assisting the client with public transit options, promoting access to trained job supports and mental health services, promoting family education, and assisting with access to various state agencies (Trexler et al., 2010). Trexler et al. concluded that a 6-month program of resource facilitation as a means of promoting access to and coordination of services improves community participation and return to work, particularly if initiated soon after discharge from acute rehabilitation.

Engaging employers in return-to-work plans and providing TBI-related employer education are key areas of focus in resource facilitation.

Research continues on the effectiveness of the various models of vocational rehabilitation in response to the high number of people with TBI on long-term or permanent disability and government assistance programs, even after intensive vocational rehabilitation (Fadyl & McPherson, 2009). Some people with TBI-related long-term unemployment may find ways to remain active and productive, for example, through volunteer work, but many do not, with potentially important repercussions for their psychological and physical well-being (Corrigan, 2001).

Returning to School After Traumatic Brain Injury

Young adulthood is a period in which many people are engaged in a structured academic program such as high school or college. It also marks the period (ages 15–24 years) in which the risk of injury is highest (Corrigan, Selassie, & Orman, 2010). On discharge from the inpatient rehabilitation setting, students with TBI often aim to return to their academic pursuits but may be unprepared for the challenges they face and may be at increased risk of failure. Attention, memory, learning, and social–emotional impairments, coupled with executive function and self-regulation impairments, place these young adults at unique risk for failure, particularly at the college level (Kennedy & Krause, 2011). The National Longitudinal Transition Study–2 reported that students with TBI whose injuries occurred before the onset of postsecondary education demonstrated significantly lower college graduation rates than their nondisabled peers (Wagner, Newman, Cameto, Garza, & Levine, 2005).

Many students with TBI enter or reenter the classroom without visible disabilities and are often placed in the classroom without consideration of the need for accommodations. Taylor et al. (2002) noted that, after returning to the classroom after TBI, students may continue to function in the normal range for months or years depending on their preinjury level and degree of assistance from teachers and family. However, academic failure and the emergence of behavioral and social difficulties are commonplace (Max, 2005). If residual cognitive and social impairments remain unidentified by the academic institution, the student may not be offered needed accommodations and supports. These students are at greater risk for frustration, failure, social rejection, and placement in special education settings with students with dissimilar learning and social issues (Deaton, 1990). Students injured late in high school frequently struggle with more problems in college, where the level of special services and TBI awareness are often even lower than in high school (Kennedy, Krause, & Turkstra, 2008).

Kennedy and Krause (2011) described the application of a dynamic coaching model of supported education, involving self-regulated learning, with two college students with severe TBI. The intervention involved

1. Guided conversations about strengths and weaknesses based on assessment test results;
2. Establishment of academic and other specific goals around themes of studying and learning, time management, and relating to others;
3. Discussion of skills related to studying and time management—useful approaches versus ineffective approaches for each course;
4. Identification of human supports such as friends, family, disability service counselors, and vocational rehabilitation counselors;
5. Identification of, and plan to use, academic accommodations;
6. Direct individualized coaching, including direct instruction on agreed-on strategies and evaluation of the effectiveness of such strategies (i.e., what is working and what is not) related to assignment and test performance; and

7. End-of-semester portfolio preparation, in which students outline relative strengths and weaknesses, along with descriptions of various study and learning strategies and time management tools that were beneficial throughout the academic year.

Kennedy and Krause reported that the approach yielded positive results for both students as measured by improved performance on tests and assignments, good academic standing, completion of the majority of credits attempted, and positive academic decision making. Occupational therapists working in higher education settings may be afforded opportunities to work with college students who have sustained TBI. Systematic documentation of the strategies used to support the students' academic and college life success can contribute to the limited literature in this area of practice.

Leisure Participation After Traumatic Brain Injury

Recognition of the importance of participation in leisure activities as a component of occupational engagement is part of the philosophical foundations of occupational therapy and may also be regarded as a key rehabilitation outcome (Bier, Dutil, & Couture, 2009). **Leisure participation** makes a valuable contribution to all aspects of health—psychological, social, physical, and spiritual—and has both short- and long-term benefits (Caldwell & Smith, 1988; Suto, 1998). For people with TBI, one determinant of satisfaction with life in general is the resumption of leisure activities and, more specifically, involvement in activities with friends and family outside the home (Anke & Fugl-Meyer, 2003). Studies have shown a disruption in leisure engagement after TBI, with changes in the frequency of socialization, time spent on leisure-type activities, and the types of activities done compared with before the TBI (Kersel et al., 2001; Ponsford, Olver, & Curran, 1995).

Occupational therapists should be cognizant of the benefits of leisure participation after TBI and ensure inclusion of leisure in the assessment and treatment plan. Leisure facilitates awareness of deficits and fosters the development of skills to deal with environmental influences, increases social interaction, and enhances skills that can be transferred to other ADLs (Bier et al., 2009). Over time, the successes derived from leisure participation can help build self-esteem. According to Prigatano (1989), leisure allows people with TBI to "be in contact with experiences that maintain a sense of old identity while at the same time helping them face the changes following brain injury" (p. 428). Involvement in leisure activities helps to create a broader social network while providing respite or additional social opportunities for family and friends. Additionally, leisure is an occupation through which therapeutic goals can be achieved (Blacker, Broadhurst, & Teixeira, 2008) and provides an opportunity for physical and cognitive rehabilitation whereby the person with TBI can find meaning and enjoyment in life while testing identity changes in a setting that is often less threatening than that of nonleisure home and community activities (Lyons, 1993; Malley, Cooper, & Cope, 2008).

Physical activity after TBI has been directly associated with improving cognitive, physical, and psychosocial health (Driver & Ede, 2009; Grealy, Johnson, & Rushton, 1999; Pawlowski, Dixon-Ibarra, & Driver, 2013). Improved mood, cardiovascular fitness, and self-esteem were reported among a group of people with TBI who participated in a 12-week aerobic exercise program of three 30-minute sessions per week

> Involvement in leisure activities helps to create a broader social network while providing respite or additional social opportunities for family and friends. Additionally, leisure is an occupation through which therapeutic goals can be achieved.

(Schwandt et al., 2012). A variety of approaches to exercise were used to accommodate client deficits and improve client participation and interest in the program.

Despite its obvious importance, leisure is rarely incorporated into rehabilitation programs, and therapeutic recreation is viewed as a nonessential service (Bier et al., 2009). Clinicians often consider the inclusion of leisure in rehabilitation as a luxury in comparison to functional or work-related goals, a finding attributable in part to payer reimbursement and client priorities (Turner, Chapman, McSherry, Krishnagiri, & Watts, 2000). Bier et al. (2009) found that many people with TBI were less concerned about a decline in leisure activity involvement than they were about a decline in other activities. They suggested that many people with TBI report greater self-actualization through work and that as a result these people may be more focused on return to work or school than on reengaging in previous leisure activities.

Community Mobility and Driving Skills

For many people after TBI, driving is an enabling activity that is highly connected to societal participation and the resumption of a satisfying lifestyle. Driving is rated among the most desired activities that people with TBI could not perform postinjury (Johnston, Goverover, & Dijkers, 2005), and driving cessation among this group is linked to lower rates of community integration and life satisfaction (Johnston et al., 2005; Klonoff et al., 2006).

Residual cognitive, behavioral, and physical sequelae of TBI may compromise the ability to resume driving safely (Labbe, Vance, Wadley, & Novack, 2014; Lundqvist, Alinder, & Rönnberg, 2008). The following impairments associated with TBI have been linked to unsafe driving:

- Impaired attention and memory (Mathias & Wheaton, 2007; Vakil, Kraus, Bor, & Groswasser, 2002)
- Impaired executive functions (i.e., deficits in flexibility, inhibition, planning, reasoning, awareness; Hart, Seignourel, & Sherer, 2009; McDonald, Flashman, & Saykin, 2002; Rapport, Bryer, & Hanks, 2008)
- Decreased information processing speed (Mathias & Wheaton, 2007)
- Impaired cognitive control (the ability to orchestrate thought and action in accordance with internal goals; Larson, Perlstein, Demery, & Stigge-Kaufman, 2006)
- Emotional instability (aggression, impulsiveness, irritability, **apathy;** Greve et al., 2001)
- Impaired muscle **tone,** decreased balance, and ataxia (Marcotte et al., 2008).

Although these difficulties may compromise fitness to drive after moderate to severe TBI, reported rates of return to driving range from 40% to 80% (Novack et al., 2010). Among these people, almost two-thirds never have their driving skills formally tested (Fisk, Schneider, & Novack, 1998).

Driving is a dynamic and complex activity. Ortoleva, Brugger, Van der Linden, and Walder (2012) conducted a comprehensive review of predictors of the ability to return to driving after TBI. They concluded that, based on the existing studies, no single assessment adequately predicts driving capacity after TBI. People with severe TBI who resume driving and are involved in a vehicle crash are more than twice as likely as people without TBI to be the at-fault party (Bivona et al., 2012). The increased risk after TBI is typically attributable to two areas of impairment:

1. *Neuropsychological skills*—attention, concentration, memory, and executive functions
2. *Neuropsychiatric problems*—anxiety, impulsiveness, or inability to evaluate the consequences of unwise behavior.

Impaired self-awareness together with sensorimotor and neuropsychiatric impairments may result in increased risk of involvement in vehicle crashes resulting from unsafe driving behavior (Rapport et al., 2008). For example, Lundqvist and Alinder (2007) studied people with brain injuries who passed and failed driving tests and found that, unlike those who passed on-road evaluations, those who failed overestimated their driving ability. They proposed that more accurate self-assessment enabled people to modify behavior and adapt to residual deficits and hence optimize their driving performance. In a study of driving behavior of adults after TBI, Labbe et al. (2014) concluded that young men may be particularly at risk with regard to driving in that they are more likely to return to driving and less likely to modify driving behavior after their injury.

Decisions made by family members and caregivers are cited as the most common reason for limiting driving among those who want to do so after TBI (Rapport, Hanks, & Bryer, 2006). However, a study by Coleman et al. (2002) found that perceptions of driving fitness held by significant others are only moderately correlated with actual ability to drive. This finding suggests that although some people who resume driving with impaired skills after TBI may pose a risk to both themselves and the public, those people inaccurately considered unsafe to drive may be unnecessarily limited in independence, community access, and social opportunities.

An understanding of the relationship among person, occupation, and environment uniquely positions occupational therapists to provide valued and evidence-based services that promote driving as an occupation (Dickerson, Reistetter, Schold Davis, & Monahan, 2011). Table 7.3 details common elements of a driving evaluation. Several commercially available driving simulators can provide qualitative and quantitative information on

A study by Coleman et al. (2002) found that perceptions of driving fitness held by significant others are only moderately correlated with actual ability to drive.

Table 7.3. Common Considerations in the Assessment of Specific Driving-Related Skills

Skill Category	Specific Skill Requirements
Visuospatial skills	• Visual acuity and the need for corrective lenses • Visual attention, visual memory, and ability to attend and maintain concentration to relevant tasks • Peripheral vision
Physical skills	• Ability to steer, brake within a reasonable amount of time, and control speed • Reaction time • Need for assistive devices or vehicle modifications • Ability to get into and out of the car
Perceptual skills	• Ability to judge distances between cars while driving on the roads and while parking • Ability to recognize shape and color of traffic signs • Ability to perceive and attend to the entire **visual field;** absence of visual neglect and tendency to drift to one side of road • Ability to interpret complex visual information, maps, intersections, and traffic issues
Judgment	• Adequate decision-making skills in emergency situations • Self-awareness of strengths and weaknesses

driving-related skills while avoiding putting the client and others in danger. Although use of simulators with people after TBI has been described as a means of supplementing assessment findings and assisting with treatment recommendations, the evidence is limited supporting the ability to predict behind-the-wheel performance on the basis of simulator driving performance (D'apolito, Massonneau, Paillat, & Azouvi, 2013).

Occupational therapists may pursue specialized training in driving assessment and rehabilitation through advanced certification programs such as those of the Association for Driver Rehabilitation Specialists. Certified driver rehabilitation specialists provide driver evaluation, driver training, vehicle consultation, vehicle modification recommendations, adaptive equipment instruction, and on-the-road training. Additionally, they make recommendations for safe driving to the referring physician, state licensing agency, or both. Evidence is limited supporting the effectiveness of such recommendations or specific driver rehabilitation programs.

Use of Everyday Technology

The use of electrical, technical, and mechanical equipment is common in U.S. homes and community settings. Everyday technology has been developed to make life easier, safer, and more efficient, improving the ability to perform complex occupations, such as shopping, managing finances, locating places, and learning new tasks—activities frequently described as difficult for people with TBI. Most everyday technology was developed for people without disabilities and may pose access challenges for people with cognitive, physical, and psychological impairments.

The rapid development of technology has the potential to significantly support community participation after TBI. In particular, the emergence of hand-held computers has expanded the use of computer technology to allow access to computer technology outside the home. Research in the first decade of the 21st century demonstrated the potential benefits of hand-held computers, also known as *personal digital assistants* (PDAs), to facilitate **prospective memory** involved in everyday tasks such as taking medications, planning and organizing schedules, and keeping appointments (Gentry, Wallace, Kvarfordt, & Lynch, 2008). A client's preinjury familiarity with computers and the extent of cognitive deficits are contributing factors to the successful use of PDAs in everyday activities (Gentry et al., 2008).

Engström, Lexell, and Lund (2010) studied issues surrounding access to everyday technology among people with TBI. Numerous themes characterized the challenges related to the use of everyday technology and contributing to difficulties with performing occupations and participating in life situations. Difficulties were mostly related to advanced technology, such as computers and mobile phones, used to support social, educational, and vocational participation. Cognitive impairments were most often described as interfering with the successful use of technology, even if participants were proficient in its use before their TBI. Problems related to difficulties with everyday technology included

- Following sequences and steps required to use technology;
- Using manuals and learning to use the new technology;
- Recognizing, finding, remembering, and using technology functions;
- Experiencing fatigue and other impairments during efforts to learn and use technology; and
- Feeling pressure from others regarding the use of technology.

Technology use is a central feature of everyday community participation. As such, occupational therapists should assess the use of everyday technology at the community stage. Gentry, Wallace, Kvarfordt, and Lynch (2010) developed the Functional Assessment Tool for Cognitive Assistive Technology (FATCAT), an easy-to-administer questionnaire for assessing assistive technology needs and abilities. Proficiency in the use of assistive technology for various aspects of home and community management (i.e., medication reminders, learning new information, performing cooking tasks), as well as for vocational tasks, is rated on a scale ranging from 1 to 10. The FATCAT also includes a section to list applications, training strategies, and follow-up for each device identified.

The growing number of apps for smartphones has promise to facilitate functional performance and community participation while maintaining the ability of the person with TBI to blend in with peers using similar apps. Therapists need to review and select apps that are appropriate for their clients' needs, that are easy to learn, and that can adapt as the client improves or assumes new life roles and tasks.

Reestablishing or Developing Relationships

Social isolation is perhaps the most profound life change for persons with TBI (Conneeley, 2002). A decrease in the number and depth of social relationships over time has been documented as a long-term problem for people with TBI. Poor communication skills after TBI can result in reduced participation in social activities and decreased life satisfaction (Dahlberg et al., 2007). Two years postinjury, many people with moderate to severe TBI continue to experience difficulties with social skills, which often leads to social isolation and depression (Engberg & Teasdale, 2004). Personality or behavior changes, motor and sensory impairments, and unemployment are also among the factors contributing to unsatisfying social relationships after TBI. According to Rowlands (2001), social relationships may increase in number over time but tend to be superficial, contributing to the common complaint of loneliness. Opportunities to develop new relationships are limited, further reducing self-esteem and contributing to a sense of isolation and depression (Rowlands, 2001).

Social competence has been emphasized as a significant factor in the successful reintegration into home, work, and school after TBI because it supports the formation of new friendships and the maintenance of preexisting social relationships. Successful social communication involves a complex interaction of factors including cognitive abilities, awareness of social rules, speech, language and conversation skills, emotional control, and self-monitoring (Dahlberg et al., 2007). When compared with neurologically healthy control participants, people with severe TBI have been found to have impaired social competence (Galski, Tompkins, & Johnston, 1998; McDonald & Flanagan, 2004; Sale, Revell, West, & Kregel, 1992).

Using qualitative interviews with employers, Sale et al. (1992) found that the most common causes of job separation in people with TBI were interpersonal difficulties, social cue misinterpretation, and inappropriate verbalizations. Impaired conversation turn-taking, ability to initiate and sustain meaningful conversation, ability to express thoughts in an organized manner, self-monitoring ability, disinhibition, and social perception have been reported also (Galski et al., 1998; McDonald

& Flanagan, 2004). Occupational therapists use individual and group interventions to support social skill development, which are detailed later in this chapter.

Aggression is a possible neurobehavioral sequela of TBI (Dyer et al., 2006; Vaishnavi, Rao, & Fann, 2009). Although not the most common psychological symptom experienced after TBI, few symptoms are more debilitating than aggression from the standpoint of relationships and rehabilitation (Cusimano, Holmes, Sawicki, & Topolovec-Vranic, 2014). A variety of theoretical mechanisms have been proposed to explain the link between TBI and aggression (Grafman et al., 1996; Greve et al., 2001). Verbal aggression and anger have been identified as principal aggressive symptoms after TBI, with physical aggression less frequent (Dyer et al., 2006).

Many factors are likely to contribute to postinjury aggression. Anatomically, the **frontal** and **temporal lobes** of the brain are particularly susceptible to damage given their proximity to bony structures at the base of the skull (Ashley, 2010). The disinhibition of aggression commonly occurs after damage to the orbitofrontal cortex, which impairs the ability to regulate impulses and social behavior, whereas injury to the temporal lobes can result in emotional instability and poorly directed outbursts of anger (Dyer et al., 2006; Greve et al., 2001). Postinjury psychosocial stressors such as unemployment, boredom, frustration, depression, and difficulty coping with postinjury physical and cognitive decline may also contribute to aggressive behavior (Baguley, Cooper, & Felmingham, 2006).

Regardless of its cause, the ultimate impact of postinjury anger and aggression can be devastating for people with TBI and their families. Consequently, the management of these behaviors is a commonly cited rehabilitation goal (Lazaro, Butler, & Felmingham, 2000). Treatment of aggressive behavior after TBI includes behavior therapy, which involves reinforcing desirable behaviors and attempting to assist the client in eliminating unwanted or undesirable ones (Ducharme, 2000). Teaching adaptive behaviors (i.e., communicative, social, or cognitive skills) facilitates the development of alternative, more socially acceptable behavior strategies.

Occupational Therapy Assessment and Treatment at the Community Stage of Rehabilitation

In this section, I detail specific strategies that occupational therapists can use to work with people with TBI at the community stage of rehabilitation. The top-down assessment approach, beginning with the occupational profile, allows the therapist to gain an understanding of the client's concerns and identify those activities that are most important in the person's everyday life. Such assessment involves collecting information on the client's previous lifestyle, functioning, daily routine, and cultural beliefs (Toglia & Golisz, 2012). Areas to address in this process include the person's preinjury home, work, and community environments; social supports; roles; interests; and activities.

When current goals and occupational performance levels have been established, the therapist determines specific causes of unsuccessful and dissatisfying performance. Table 7.2 lists assessment instruments that can be used by the occupational therapist to collect data in a more standardized manner to supplement clinical observations made during the community stage. Many assessments tap constructs across domains (participation, activity, impairments, environmental barriers, client personal factors) and hence are suitable for use at various points in the assessment process.

The ultimate objective of the community stage of rehabilitation—fostering community participation—begins with a thorough assessment of the person's functioning.

General Assessment and Treatment Issues

Participation is difficult to measure because its quality and quantity are influenced by environmental and personal characteristics (Heinemann, 2010). This person–environment interaction is multidimensional, affected by what the person can do and wants to do as well as by what the **social environment** enables or permits the person to do. Researchers have agreed that no single measure is likely to fully describe the complex interactions between people and the environments that affect participation (Heinemann, 2010).

Evaluation begins by gathering information on the client and what he or she wants to do and is then followed by an analysis of the person performing desired occupations. Client and environmental factors that support or hinder performance and participation are considered throughout the process. Table 7.2 provides a list of participation-level assessments occupational therapists can use to assess role performance along with the interaction among physical, cultural, and social barriers to participation.

Additionally, many assessment tools look at cognitive, physical, social, emotional, and behavioral deficits that may contribute to reduced societal participation. These instruments assist in the collection of data and quantification of progress but do not replace clinical observation and activity analysis. The scope of community-based participation after TBI exceeds the content of any one measure or assessment approach. With a deep appreciation of how clients define satisfying community participation, occupational therapists can apply clinical reasoning skills to accurately select and interpret assessments and plan and implement client-centered interventions.

Specific assessments that occupational therapists select at the community stage can be as diverse as the participation barriers, activity restrictions, and impairments that affect community reentry after TBI. A discussion of specific assessment and treatment approaches to common impairments and activities that affect community participation is included later in this section. First, I present general challenges that occupational therapists may face when working with the client with TBI and family or caregivers at the community stage.

Impact of Self-Awareness Deficit on Occupational Therapy Assessment

Anosognosia, the physiologically based unawareness of one's deficits resulting from disability, is among the most common cognitive impairments observed in adults after TBI (Sherer, Bergloff, Boake, High, & Levin, 1998). It is generally accepted that for adults with TBI to effectively engage in the therapy process, they must be aware of their impairments and be willing to actively address these impairments in therapy (O'Callaghan et al., 2012). Impaired self-awareness is particularly challenging for rehabilitation professionals because it affects not only people's belief about their cognitive and physical impairments but also their ability to benefit from rehabilitation (Kelley et al., 2014; Trahan, Pépin, & Hopps, 2006). Only by attaining some level of intellectual awareness is the client in a position to participate in a client-centered goal-setting and treatment-planning process.

In a study involving people with TBI and people with spinal cord injury, Trahan et al. (2006) found that, compared with clinician ratings, people with TBI tended to underestimate their emotional, behavioral, and cognitive disabilities, whereas

No single measure is likely to fully describe the complex interactions between people and the environments that affect participation.

people with spinal cord injury accurately assessed their disabilities in all spheres. This finding points to the existence of impaired self-awareness. Clients who manifested an accurate perception of themselves as well as a greater willingness to change performed better than did clients who inaccurately perceived their limitations (Flashman & McAllister, 2002; Kelley et al., 2014).

Table 7.4 highlights instruments that the occupational therapist can use to evaluate a client's level of self-awareness. Many of these instruments involve evaluating the difference between client self-report and the ratings of people familiar with the client on items related to impairments and functional limitations (e.g., discrepancy ratings). Barco, Crosson, Bolesta, Werts, and Stout (1991) identified three levels of awareness:

1. *Intellectual awareness*—the capacity to understand to some degree that a particular function is diminished from premorbid levels
2. *Emergent awareness*—the ability to recognize a problem when it is actually happening
3. *Anticipatory awareness*—the ability to anticipate that a problem is going to happen because of some deficit.

Barco et al. proposed that these levels of awareness are hierarchical in nature, in that some degree of intellectual awareness is required for both emergent and anticipatory awareness. Toglia and Kirk (2000) questioned the uniformity of the hierarchy across performance areas, suggesting instead that anticipatory and emergent awareness may be evident in some situations but not in others, depending on a person's knowledge, beliefs, and affective states. For example, a person may recognize memory problems but at the same time be unaware of deficits in social situations or everyday problem solving.

The Toglia and Kirk model emphasizes the importance of perceived ***self-efficacy,*** or the person's inner sense of control, and emphasizes examining the person's perception of ability within the context of a task or situation as part of the assessment of awareness. Low self-efficacy is associated with reduced motivation, lack of persistence, poor coping skills, and emotional distress (Bandura, 1997).

Table 7.4. Selected Assessments for Establishing Client Self-Awareness

Assessment and Category	Description
Awareness Questionnaire (Sherer et al., 1998)	Client and family member or significant other and a clinician independently compare the ability of the client with TBI to perform various tasks using a 5-point rating scale. Differences in ratings represent degree of client awareness of deficit.
Neurobehavioral Functioning Inventory (Kreutzer et al., 1999)	A 76-item inventory with identical client and caregiver versions that collects information on behaviors and symptoms associated with TBI. Includes Depression, Somatic Complaints, Memory/Attention, Communication, Aggression, and Motor subscales. Comparison of client and caregiver forms allows evaluation of differing perceptions of symptom severity. Often used to evaluate health-related QoL after TBI.
Self-Awareness of Deficits Interview (Fleming et al., 1996)	Interviewer-rated semistructured interview developed to assess a client's level of awareness at 3 levels (1) awareness of brain injury–related deficits, (2) awareness of functional implications of deficits on everyday life, and (3) ability to set realistic goals and predict one's future.
Patient Competency Rating Scale (Prigatano & Altman, 1990)	A 30-item self-report scale developed to evaluate lack of insight through independent client and caregiver ratings of how easy or difficult it is for client to carry out various activities. Discrepancies between client and caregiver ratings indicate impaired self-awareness.

Source. From *Occupational Therapy Practice Guidelines for Adults With Traumatic Brain Injury* (pp. 22–26), by K. Golisz, 2009, Bethesda, MD: AOTA Press. Copyright © 2009 by the American Occupational Therapy Association. Adapted with permission.

Note. QoL = quality of life; TBI = traumatic brain injury.

Toglia and Kirk suggested using **metacognition** and metamemory paradigms to evaluate self-efficacy and self-monitoring during task performance. This process involves having clients estimate or judge learning or performance before performing a task and then comparing their predictions with actual performance. In this context, the use of functional activities by occupational therapy practitioners serves as a means of both assessment and intervention.

Assessment at the community stage of recovery is distinct from that at previous stages of TBI rehabilitation in that the degree of a client's cognitive impairments may not be fully evident until he or she is discharged to the home and community and faces complex daily activities in natural and often unpredictable environments (Golisz, 2009). In this respect, it can appear to the client or family that impairments are getting worse when, in fact, challenges in the environment are illuminating problems that were not evident in the structured hospital setting. This is particularly likely with executive functions, many of which do not present in the absence of unstructured daily social and activity demands.

Goal Setting and Treatment Planning to Facilitate Community Participation

Client-centered goal setting is central to occupational therapy practice and is well suited to the challenges of community-based TBI rehabilitation (American Occupational Therapy Association, 2014; Barnes & Ward, 2000; Law & Baptiste, 2002). Powell et al. (2007) emphasized that accurate information about the client's abilities and experiences before injury is essential to assessing the client's abilities postinjury. In their study of the extent to which home management activities were being performed a year after TBI, these researchers found that a relatively high percentage of participants not doing common home management tasks when evaluated also reported not performing these tasks before their injury.

Goal-based measures, such as the Canadian Occupational Performance Measure (COPM; Law et al., 2014) and **Goal Attainment Scaling** (GAS), have been used effectively by occupational therapists to facilitate a sense of goal ownership with clients and to measure client progress over time. People who generate their own goals, including clients with TBI, are more likely to want to work on the goals and to report that the goals are important to them (Doig et al., 2010).

Studies using the COPM in a variety of TBI rehabilitation settings have found that it is sensitive to change and that its use provides a sense of satisfaction with progress in both clients with TBI and their significant others (Doig, Fleming, Cornwell, & Kuipers, 2009). GAS can be used to translate the broad client-centered goals from the COPM into specific behavioral actions. In a study combining use of the COPM and GAS with both people with TBI and caregivers, Doig et al. (2010) concluded that the measures were sensitive to change for people with TBI. They noted, however, that in some clients with moderate to severe awareness deficits, client ratings on the COPM did not reflect positive change even though objective assessment and significant-other ratings indicated otherwise. By receiving feedback about performance during the therapy and GAS process, the clients' self-awareness improved over time, and postintervention COPM ratings became more realistic (Doig et al., 2010).

GAS can be used to motivate participants, foster awareness of deficits, and provide a structured means to gauge progress. In GAS, progress on each goal is evaluated on a scale ranging from -2 to $+2$, with a weighting of zero indicating no change.

Assessment at the community stage of recovery is distinct from that at previous stages of TBI rehabilitation in that the degree of a client's cognitive impairments may not be fully evident until he or she is discharged to the home and community and faces complex daily activities in natural and often unpredictable environments.

Pluses and minuses on the scale represent more or less favorable outcomes, respectively. Dahlberg et al. (2007) described a social communication skills training program in which goals were developed with input from participants and scaled into five steps with progress evaluated by the clients themselves, the group leaders, and a significant other. An example of a cognitive social goal from this study is as follows:

GOAL: I will interrupt less during a 15-minute conversation.
−2 = I will interrupt less than 4 or more times during a 15-minute conversation with 1 prompt.
−1 = I will interrupt less than 4 times during a 15-minute conversation.
  0 = I will interrupt less than 2 times during a 15-minute conversation.
+1 = I will interrupt only 1 time during a 15-minute conversation.
+2 = I will not interrupt during a 15-minute conversation.

Goals focused on numerous aspects of social communication, including self-awareness (i.e., "I will be able to name my social skill strengths and weaknesses"), speech (i.e., "I will speak slowly enough to be understood 90% of the time"), and interpersonal communication (i.e., "I will be able to name three places to meet new people, and I will visit one of those places").

It is important to note that client-centered goal setting is not synonymous with relinquishing total decision making to the client or doing whatever treatment the client believes is worthwhile (Law & Baptiste, 2002). Therapists are responsible for determining whether situations place clients at risk, are fiscally irresponsible, or have ethical or legal implications and for assisting clients with examining and understanding such issues. The enormous growth of research related to postacute TBI rehabilitation over the past 20 years has greatly enhanced occupational therapists' ability to base clinical decision making on evidence to provide best practice.

Turner, Ownsworth, Turpin, Fleming, and Griffin (2008) developed a framework for classifying self-identified goals after TBI that can be used by occupational therapists in community-based rehabilitation to monitor the scope of a client's treatment plan. The categories focusing on common community reintegration problems after TBI are as follows:

1. Relationships (e.g., family, interpersonal relationships, friendships, social activities)
2. Work and education (e.g., returning to previous employment or school, seeking new employment, considering new educational pursuits or training, volunteer activities)
3. Injury rehabilitation
4. Health and leisure
5. Daily life management
6. General life and personal goals.

Interventions to improve self-awareness after moderate to severe TBI support the premise that life experiences relevant to a person's goals may increase his or her understanding of the implications of the injury, leading to more realistic expectations about future outcomes.

These researchers found that when engaged in goal setting, clients with TBI at the community stage of recovery tended to focus more on injury goals consistent with the physical aspects of recovery than on goals addressing cognitive, social, and emotional difficulties.

Interventions to improve self-awareness after moderate to severe TBI support the premise that life experiences relevant to a person's goals may increase his or her understanding of the implications of the injury, leading to more realistic expectations about future outcomes. Goverover, Johnston, Toglia, and Deluca (2007) used self-awareness training during IADL tasks. The program involved having participants define the goals of the task, predict task performance, anticipate and preplan for any obstacles that they felt they would encounter during task performance, choose a strategy to circumvent such difficulties, and anticipate the amount of assistance they felt they would need to successfully perform the task. Then, after performing the IADL task, participants completed a self-evaluation of the task, engaged in a discussion with the therapist regarding task performance and their performance relative to pretask questions, received feedback from the therapist regarding observed performance, and, finally, wrote about the experience in a journal. Although improvements were observed in specific task awareness, self-regulation, and functional performance, improvements were not observed in general awareness and community integration, a finding that is consistent with Toglia and Kirk's (2000) conjecture regarding the specificity of the development of self-awareness.

Interventions to Facilitate Community Participation

Research to support interventions facilitating success and satisfying community participation after TBI continues to evolve. Given the complexity of issues involved in treatment at the community stage, therapists must consider numerous factors in deciding how to provide treatment. These factors include

- Use of individual or group interventions
- Anticipated role of the family
- Frequency and duration of sessions
- Insurance and reimbursement issues
- Transportation barriers affecting program participation
- Intervention setting—clinic, simulated environments, real environments
- Caseload issues and therapist availability
- Safety issues (e.g., potential for aggressive behavior, liability issues involved with transporting clients, availability of support staff).

Such considerations are influenced by therapist, client, program, financial, and other factors. As a result of the constraints that these factors place on the therapist's design of services, real-world interventions are rarely ideal, and therapists must be creative in the optimal use of available options for each client. Although evidence has supported treatment throughout the continuum of recovery, Golisz (2009) noted that the chronic, complex, and continuously evolving nature of recovery from TBI makes it very difficult to determine the optimal and most cost-effective amount of intervention for any particular client.

Regardless of the approach, frequency, and setting, therapists facilitating the transition to the community after TBI can benefit from the guiding principles established in Willer and Corrigan's (1994) Whatever It Takes approach. Their model is based on the following principles:

1. No two people with **acquired brain injury** are alike.
2. Skills are more likely to generalize when they are taught in the environment in which they can be used.

3. Environments are easier to change than people.
4. Community integration should be holistic.
5. Life is a place-and-train venture.
6. Natural supports last longer than professionals.
7. Interventions must not do more harm than good.
8. The service system presents many barriers to community integration.
9. Respect for the person is paramount.
10. People's needs last a lifetime; so should their resources.

Intervention at the community phase of recovery is dynamic and ever changing. Hence, once the treatment plan is initiated, there are no clearly defined borders among evaluation, treatment, and follow-up.

Priority 1: Therapeutic Relationship Building

Therapeutic relationship building is at the core of the art of occupational therapy practice.

Therapeutic relationship building is at the core of the art of occupational therapy practice. Mosey (1981) wrote, "The capacity to establish rapport, to empathize, and to guide others to know how to make use of their potential as participants in a community illustrates the art of occupational therapy" (p. 4).

Intervention at the community stage of rehabilitation carries tremendous possibilities for a client at an unpredictable stage of recovery. Shopping for and preparing a meal, resuming social and leisure interests, engaging in parenting or spousal roles, or perhaps even returning to work or school are exciting possibilities after TBI that, unfortunately, become increasingly uncertain in the face of residual impairments, fears, and environmental barriers. The consequences of clients' unsuccessful efforts to return to their preinjury life can have a negative impact on self-esteem and limit their willingness to engage in challenging tasks for fear of failure. Facing challenges is necessary to reach postinjury potential, build self-esteem, and enhance QoL.

Central to the success of community-based rehabilitation is the foundation of a supportive, therapeutic relationship so that clients understand that they can fail at a task or make mistakes without losing the occupational therapist's support. Participation-level goal attainment often involves working outside a client's comfort zone, improving self-awareness of deficits, which may at the same time increase the client's susceptibility to depression and anxiety and initially reduced life satisfaction. Such a process of "restructuring of self-knowledge" (Ownsworth & Clare, 2006, p. 792) can represent a potential threat to self-esteem, personal control, and independence, so the therapist must closely monitor clients' coping strategies and emotional reactions.

Clients may test a therapist's commitment to the therapeutic relationship by sabotaging tasks or presenting with defiant, aggressive, or insulting behavior. If the therapist understands such actions and behaviors as a component of the relationship-building process, then the client's behaviors can be interpreted as aspects of recovery as opposed to noncompliance or the need for a staffing change. Approaches to fostering the therapeutic relationship include negotiating to achieve a common understanding, validating the client's perspective, fostering self-advocacy, and providing encouragement and feedback (Sloan et al., 2004). The trusting and collaborative nature of the therapist–client relationship can foster a milieu that rewards effort and builds self-esteem through goal attainment. The strength of the relationship is established over time through shared experiences.

Individualized Skills Training to Facilitate Community Participation

Most community reintegration models and interventions include components of individual skill building that involve the client and the therapist. Such one-on-one approaches are well suited to specific functional IADL skills training but have limitations, especially with respect to elements of social behavior. Many intervention models in occupational therapy and psychology involve the therapist coaching the client with TBI in clinic and community settings.

Sloan et al. (2004) described skills development after TBI in a community approach to participation. They detailed the use of the approach in an occupational therapy treatment program, emphasizing the following components:

- Address skills that are related to the client's goals: The top-down approach is based on the notion that clients are more motivated when there is an explicit link between the skill and the desired goal.
- Simplify and structure the task in which the skills are to be learned: Tasks should be simplified to increase the likelihood of success. Strategies may be used to compensate for impairments. Self-confidence and skill level increase as the interventions progress and the client becomes better able to meet everyday challenges.
- Build on strengths: Observing the client allows the therapist to identify personal strengths and skills that can serve as a positive platform for skill development. Pursuing preinjury activities may facilitate success, based on the notion that it is easier to relearn an old skill than learn a new one.
- Develop routines: The goal of skill development is automatic performance within the context of the client's daily routine. Routines provide opportunities for repeated, consistent practice, and contexts provide natural cues and prompts.

Skills training in basic ADLs and IADLs meets both short- and long-term needs of the person with TBI. Clients at the community stage of recovery can present with varying degrees of residual impairment, so functional training can range from basic self-care activities to higher level prevocational, leisure, or community occupations. Achieving independence in basic self-care and some advanced living skills provides the ideal foundation for community participation. Clients increasingly use compensatory strategies as they increasingly recognize their long-term residual impairments.

Research to support the use of individualized skills training by occupational therapy practitioners continues to evolve. Wheeler et al. (2007) reported significant improvements in home integration and community integration but not in social participation, as measured with the Community Integration Questionnaire in people with moderate to severe TBI after a 90-day period in an interdisciplinary community reentry program. In this program, occupational therapy practitioners accompanied clients to home, work, school, and various community sites and assisted clients in learning and attending to the tasks required for success in that setting.

Gentry et al. (2008) reported positive functional outcomes from a training program using a PDA. During an 8-week training period that included one-on-one home-based training, participants were instructed in using the PDA to assist with everyday tasks. Participants were taught how to enter appointments into the PDA as well as how to use the address book, schedule medication, and use alarm features for reminders. Participants were also trained in additional features of interest, such as gaming features, use of the camera, and so forth. Findings from the study supported the training program as evidenced by improved self-ratings in everyday life tasks.

Vocational skill building has been a central feature of return-to-work programs after TBI. According to Braveman (2012), the extent to which a disability may interfere with occupational performance and challenge a worker's occupational identity, competence, and adaptation depends on the following factors:

- Has the person previously developed a strong sense of occupational identity as a worker on which he or she can draw?
- At what level can the challenge of occupational performance be characterized—impairment, activity, or participation?
- Does the person anticipate the impairment or disability to be temporary or permanent, and does he or she expect increased participation in the future?
- How severe an impact on occupational performance does the person perceive the impairment or disability to have?
- Are there adequate social and environmental supports on which the person can draw to remediate or adapt to limitations to facilitate improved occupational performance?

Analysis of these questions helps to clarify many of the challenges associated with returning to work after TBI. As discussed throughout this chapter, people with moderate to severe TBI often undergo some degree of personality change, may have diverse impairments that can significantly affect participation in vocational tasks, and, in cases of impaired self-awareness, have difficulty making accurate appraisals of the impact of deficits on work performance. Kelley et al. (2014) examined neurobehavioral outcomes 5 years or more after moderate to severe TBI and concluded that people were more likely to gain employment when they were aware of their cognitive deficits and abilities.

For many people with TBI, return to work is one of the ultimate symbols of success in regard to transition back to the community. According to Wehman, Gentry, West, and Arango-Lasprilla (2009), the basic principle of return-to-work services for people with TBI is that "everyone is employable when provided the right type, level, and intensity of support and when efforts are made to help them locate workplaces and positions in which they will be valued and accommodated" (p. 915).

Return-to-work interventions generally reflect a combination of skills training addressing the needs of the person with TBI and support within that person's vocational, social, and economic environments (Kowalske, Plenger, Lusby, & Hayden, 2000; Wehman et al., 2009). Work-related skills training might involve locating job opportunities, completing applications, rehearsing interviewing skills, getting to work on time, learning job skills, and communicating on the job, with the nature of services dependent on each client's desires, abilities, and needed supports (Wehman et al., 2009).

The provision of support is central to the supported employment model, which involves coaching in job search strategies as well as training in compensatory skills to facilitate success while on the job. As proficiency improves, the coach gradually fades his or her presence on the job while maintaining contact with both employee and employer on an as-needed basis.

Developing Skills to Facilitate Social Participation

Occupational therapy offers a unique and valuable contribution to the facilitation of social participation after TBI. Interventions to address social competence and social participation are a critical element of any TBI rehabilitation program at the community stage. The effect of impaired social skills manifests in virtually every important domain of community-based TBI outcome—family relationships, friendships, employment, school, and leisure (Dahlberg et al., 2006; Doble, Bonnell, & Magill-Evans, 1991). For example, although most adults with TBI remember how to do their preinjury job and, at some point, may be able to return to work, their success tends to be unstable because of interpersonal difficulties, especially in the presence of deficits in executive cognitive functioning (Arlinghaus, Shoaib, & Price, 2005).

Occupational therapists must consider all skills required for occupational engagement to adequately address clients' participation needs (Simmons & Griswold, 2010). Social skills include both basic competencies and situation-relevant behaviors that enable a person to be accepted and liked in valued social settings (Dahlberg et al., 2006; Feeney et al., 2001). Socially skilled people are capable of influencing others in a positive manner and with their intended effect. In addition, they are able to be affected positively by others in the way that others would like to affect them.

Ylvisaker and Feeney (1998) conceptualized the qualities of socially skilled people as including

- *Cognition:* social cognition (i.e., knowledge of relevant social rules, roles, and routines and ability to effectively perceive and interpret the social behavior of others), general cognition, and decision making
- *Communication (i.e., language and nonlanguage behavior):* effective communication of intentions in ways that are considered situationally appropriate by others; knowing how to enter into an interaction with others, comfortably maintaining that interaction, and negotiating conflicts
- *Self:* awareness of interactive strengths and weaknesses, being reasonably comfortable with self as a social agent
- *Support for interaction:* dressing and grooming self in ways considered appropriate in the person's social milieu and understood and accepted by members of the social groups with which they choose to affiliate.

Similarly, Hawley and Newman (2006) described social skills as including communicating needs and thoughts, listening and understanding others, giving and interpreting nonverbal communication, regulating **emotions** during social interactions, being assertive, working with others to solve problems, and following social boundaries and rules.

The Occupational Therapy Intervention Process Model (OTIPM) is a practice model in which occupation is central. It emphasizes assessment and intervention directed to the person's performance of motor, process, and social interaction skills during an occupational task in the natural context (Fisher, 2009). The most critical step in this top-down approach is observing the person performing desired and challenging tasks and completing a performance analysis to determine skills that are effective or ineffective in supporting the person's performance of the tasks. A performance analysis involves observing a person engage in relevant tasks in the natural context as well as a critical analysis of the goal-directed actions observed. Only after the analysis

> Interventions to address social competence and social participation are a critical element of any TBI rehabilitation program at the community stage. The effect of impaired social skills manifests in virtually every important domain of community-based TBI outcome—family relationships, friendships, employment, school, and leisure.

does the occupational therapist consider the cause of the performance difficulties (e.g., person factors including body function, task demands, environmental influence). The OTIPM further guides occupational therapists to establish goals with the person on the basis of the performance analysis and desired occupational engagement. The performance analysis is central to determining intervention approaches to support occupational performance associated with the person's goals (Fisher, 2009).

The Evaluation of Social Interaction (ESI; Fisher & Griswold, 2014) was designed to assess a client's quality of interaction as he or she engages in real interactions with client-specified intended purposes and with social partners with whom the person would typically need or want to interact. The client is observed in the natural context to (1) establish his or her baseline level of performance, (2) plan occupational therapy services, and (3) measure progress or change over time, including the effectiveness of occupational therapy services. The skills evaluated in the assessment provide a useful structure for a detailed social skills training curriculum. A description of these skills and the specific subskills required for competent performance is provided in Table 7.5.

Using the ESI approach enables the client and occupational therapist to focus on social interaction in a structured way to support a skill area that had previously been unaddressed. Simmons and Griswold (2010) noted that occupational therapists do not need to create separate or special social skills programs but rather can add strategies to support existing social interaction in naturally occurring contexts. This inclusive approach provides opportunities to better address client needs beyond traditional rehabilitation structures and time frames. Adapting the social and physical environment

Table 7.5. Social Interaction Skills Assessed in the Evaluation of Social Interaction

Area of Social Interaction	Specific Social Interaction Skills
Initiating and terminating social interaction	• Approaches/Starts—greeting or initiating interaction • Concludes/Disengages—ending interaction
Producing social interaction	• Produces Speech—communicating using speech or signed or augmentative messages, speaking clearly, not mumbling • Gesticulates—using gestures to communicate • Speaks Fluently—speaking not too fast, slow, or uneven; pausing during messages; stuttering
Physically supporting social interaction	• Turns Toward—turning body and face toward social partner • Looks—looking at and making eye contact • Places Self—keeping personal space and distance from social partner; positioning too close or too far from social partner • Touches—making physical contact with social partner, avoiding touch • Regulates—controlling impulses and behaviors
Shaping content of social interaction	• Questions—requesting information or opinion • Replies—providing relevant responses with appropriate detail to social partner's messages • Discloses—revealing opinions, feelings, or private information about oneself or others; defaming or insulting others • Expresses Emotion—displaying affect and emotions, using sarcasm • Disagrees—disagreeing with social partner's suggestion or opinion, whining when disagreeing • Thanks—acknowledging information, compliments, help, or material objects
Maintaining flow of social interaction	• Transitions—changing topic of conversation • Times Response—responding too soon or too late, interrupting • Times Duration—sending messages that are too long or too short • Takes Turns—dominating, being dominated, "interrogating"
Verbally supporting social interaction	• Matches Language—using tone of voice, dialect, jargon, and level of language appropriate for social partner; whining • Clarifies—making sure social partner follows conversation • Acknowledges/Encourages—responding to social partner, encouraging participation in social interaction, encouraging continued interaction • Emphasizes—supporting social partner's feelings and experiences
Adapting social interaction	• Heeds—keeping the plot, heeding intended purpose of the social exchange • Accommodates—changing method of social interaction or asking for help • Benefits—demonstrating social interaction skill problems that recur or persist, repeating messages

Source. From *Evaluation of Social Interaction* (3rd ed.), by A. G. Fisher and L. A. Griswold, 2014, Fort Collins, CO: Three Star Press. Copyright © 2014 by Three Star Press. Reprinted with permission.

to foster social interaction promotes opportunities to practice social interaction skills, and social interaction supports existing program activities. Many treatment programs use group interventions, in whole or in part, which are discussed in the next section.

Group Interventions to Build Social Skills and Social Participation

Clients with TBI who have communication impairments or who experience social isolation and limited participation in their communities may benefit from group intervention (Golisz, 2009). As a social microcosm, therapy groups provide an ideal setting for interpersonal learning, social skills development, and interpersonal relationships that can exert a powerful influence on the client (Yalom, 1995). Group interventions provide important social feedback from other group members, both positive and negative, allowing the client to address problematic social behaviors within the supportive structure of the group. Although group topics can provide information to enhance social skills, it is through group dynamics and the therapeutic community that behavior changes occur (Yalom, 1995). According to Yalom, therapeutic communities rely on group pressure and interdependence to encourage reality testing and to instill a sense of individual responsibility toward the group. Therapist group leaders need to ensure that group structures are flexible enough to allow relationship building among participants so that the group serves to reinforce desirable social behavior and extinguish undesirable behaviors.

> As a social microcosm, therapy groups provide an ideal setting for interpersonal learning, social skills development, and interpersonal relationships that can exert a powerful influence on the client.

Schwartzberg, Howe, and Barnes (2008) discussed the functional group model, a task-oriented approach that encourages active participation among members to achieve common group goals. Basic assumptions of the model are as follows:

1. The goal of the functional group is not the product of the group, even though the group may have a meaningful product, but rather the learning process that occurs through active participation.
2. Functional groups nurture interpersonal and intrapersonal development through activity choice, climate, and goals.
3. Functional groups make use of both the human and the nonhuman environment and **object relations,** and attention is directed to attachments to people and objects, separations from people and objects, and the symbolic nature of attachment.
4. Functional group leaders are cognizant of clients' need for self-motivation and desire for mastery and guide the activity of the group accordingly.

Although specific research investigating the efficacy of the functional group model with people with TBI is lacking, the model is well suited to addressing the severity and depth of social difficulties commonly seen in this population. After TBI, people may demonstrate poor social competence and an apparent indifference to social feedback that impairs their ability to anticipate social consequences. They may demonstrate a lack of concern for social norms and appropriateness, an indifference to social cues, a lack of appreciation of social stimulus value, or a lack of awareness of their effect on others. Process-oriented group therapy provides a powerful opportunity for participants to form relationships with other people with TBI, relationships that can potentially influence specific behaviors to a much greater degree than interactions within the larger society.

Groups can be integrated into various community-based TBI treatment settings. Simmons and Griswold (2010) implemented a group intervention as part of a community-based day program in an effort to empower members and improve their occupational performance. The program involved both casual interactions and skills-training groups pertaining to areas such as computer use, social groups, current events, or movie discussions. Structured group sessions focused on areas that were creative, emotional–spiritual, functional, vocational, recreational–leisure, and related to physical fitness. Using the ESI, based on the OTIPM, to guide intervention related to social skills performance during daily occupations, the researchers found significant improvements over an 8-week period. The findings supported group interventions and occupational therapy services provided in a community-based program context for those living with TBI.

Therapists can benefit from resources that detail topics and strategies for group interventions for people with TBI. Dahlberg et al. (2007) conducted a 12-week social communication skills group (1.5-hour weekly sessions) that significantly improved both communication skills and self-reported life satisfaction. The topics of the group sessions followed the program described in *Social Skills and Traumatic Brain Injury* (Hawley & Newman, 2006) and were arranged as follows:

1. Group overview: learning the skills of a good communicator
2. Self-assessment and setting goals
3. Presenting yourself successfully and starting conversations
4. Developing conversation strategies and using feedback
5. Being assertive and solving problems
6. Practice in the community
7. Developing self-confidence through positive self-talk
8. Setting and respecting social boundaries
9. Videotaping and problem solving
10. Video review and feedback
11. Conflict resolution
12. Closure and celebration.

The program used a group coleader, which allowed two clinician perspectives and two role models. Emphasis was placed on facilitating self-awareness, progressing to individual goal setting that used GAS. The group process was used to foster interaction among group members, creating an environment conducive to feedback, problem solving, social support, and awareness that one is not alone. Finally, the group involved family and friends and included homework assignments to facilitate generalization of skills to home and community environments. At each session, participants were provided with time to discuss events from the previous week, time in the middle of the session for an unstructured break, and time toward the conclusion of each session to summarize the meeting and plan for the following week.

Group interventions are often conducted in conjunction with individual therapy sessions. Ownsworth, Little, Turner, Hawkes, and Shum (2008) conducted a randomized controlled trial comparing participants in one of three conditions: (1) group-based support, (2) individual occupation-based support, and (3) a combined group and individual support. The group intervention involved one 3-hour session per week over 8 weeks and used **psychoeducation,** group feedback, and goal setting and evaluation. Group topics included understanding and managing cognitive impairment, social skills and communication, emotional changes and coping, and motivation. The individual intervention focused on client-centered goals and occupation-based activity performed for 3 hours per week over 8 weeks in the context of the client's home and community (Ownsworth et al., 2008). The combined group and individual intervention provided 12 hours of individual occupation-based sessions and 12 hours of group work, an amount of therapy time equivalent to that of the other two conditions. Outcomes were based on COPM ratings and scores on the Patient Competency Rating Scale (Prigatano & Altman, 1990) and the Brain Injury Community Rehabilitation Outcome–39 scales (Powell, Beckers, & Greenwood, 1998).

Findings from the study supported that the individualized intervention was most effective in goal attainment at postintervention assessment but that it was not sufficient to maintain these changes at 3-month follow-up. Greater satisfaction with goal attainment was most likely to occur and be maintained at 3-month follow-up after the combined intervention and was most notable in the areas of behavioral competency and psychological well-being (Ownsworth et al., 2008).

Occupational therapy practitioners can use numerous themes in therapeutic group settings. These themes might include setting goals for independence, managing anger, managing memory difficulties, coping with loneliness, self-esteem and self-efficacy, family issues, community access, and other issues relevant to the group. Therapist group leaders can use their position to gauge group process and adjust the degree of direction provided on the basis of the group's developmental stage and the extent and severity of cognitive deficits among group members.

Outcomes and Lifelong Needs

Improving community participation outcomes after TBI involves a long-term perspective and an appreciation of the fact that although impairments may plateau over time, activity and participation levels generally fluctuate throughout the life span (Sloan et al., 2004; Ylvisaker, 2003). The effect of TBI on independence, employment, leisure, family life, and psychosocial functioning has been documented throughout this chapter. At a societal level, the effect of TBI is enormous, with annual TBI-related direct and indirect medical costs in the United States estimated at almost $76 billion (Brain Injury Association of America, 2014).

Marwitz, Cifu, Englander, and High (2001) analyzed the incidence of rehospitalizations in a large cohort over a 5-year period after TBI. The incidence of rehospitalizations ranged from 22.9% at 1 year after injury to 17% at 5 years. The majority of rehospitalizations in the first 3 years were for orthopedic and reconstructive surgeries; by Year 5, rehospitalizations were increasingly for urgent or nonelective reasons including seizures and psychiatric problems.

The various outcome-based studies presented throughout this chapter have supported the ability of occupation-based programs to bridge the gap from hospital to community. However, implementation of comprehensive services has been slow to change on a national level, and access to them remains a major barrier for many. The third-party reimbursement system has been slow to adopt community-based TBI rehabilitation as a necessary phase of the recovery process. Kerkhoff (2009) noted,

> Healthcare and long-term support services for individuals with cognitive impairment have traditionally varied significantly across states, calling into question the concept that "best practices" are universally adopted solely based upon the premise that their effectiveness and efficiency have been demonstrated. (p. 476)

Implementation of comprehensive services has been slow to change on a national level, and access to them remains a major barrier for many.

Funding issues are commonly cited as a major obstacle to program implementation at the community level. Providing cost-effective and efficient services at a time when clients can identify their problems, develop personal goals, consider their own options, and make their own choices is most conducive to the optimal use of limited resources. Kerkhoff (2009) challenged rehabilitation and mental health professionals to work together to "craft a workable, accessible, inclusive, and integrated healthcare plan" (p. 476) so that people with legitimate rehabilitation needs have the opportunity to benefit from quality services. Recent studies supporting individual and group models to facilitate participation at the community stage have established an important foundation on which such a best-practice framework can be established.

The Case of Diane Archer

Let's revisit the case of Diane Archer, the young woman who sustained a TBI. The case picks up where we left off at the end of Chapter 6.

The Day Hospital and Outpatient Programs

Diane was assigned a new occupational therapist, Carmen, on her discharge to the day hospital. Carmen was a relatively new occupational therapist—she had only 2 years of experience—but this was her second career after having taught special education high school classes for 10 years. Carmen was drawn to the occupational therapy profession after working with several students who had sustained brain injury. Carmen was the mother of a 10-year-old but could recall parenting a toddler.

On Diane's first morning in the day program, her mother drove Diane and her daughter Kate to the facility. Carmen met them in the day room and noted that Kate was sitting on her grandmother's lap while Diane sat next to them. Diane wore a pair of jeans and a long-sleeved shirt. She wore her long hair down, and she was not wearing makeup. Diane responded to questions her mother asked, but she did not appear to initiate conversation with her mother or Kate. Carmen introduced herself and arranged to meet Diane's mother and daughter back in the same room at the end of the day.

Carmen had completed a comprehensive review of Diane's medical history and had several assessments she wanted to administer to understand Diane's present occupational performance. They spent a few hours on her first day completing the COPM and used the Assessment of Motor and Process Skills (Fisher & Jones, 2012, 2014) to analyze Diane's process and motor skills while she prepared a simple lunch for the two of them. They discussed Diane's goals for her occupational therapy sessions and the strategies she had learned from Lindsey, her occupational therapist in the rehabilitation hospital. The results of the COPM are listed in Table 7.6.

Carmen also performed an evaluation of client factors in the areas of cognitive (mental function), sensory, and motor skills. She administered several assessments of executive function, including the Executive Function Performance Test (Baum, Morrison, Hahn, & Edwards, 2008) and the Modified Multiple Errands Test (Shallice & Burgess, 1991; see Exhibit 7.1). These assessments required Diane to plan, initiate, and prioritize in novel, unstructured tasks, such as those frequently encountered in the community (e.g., complete a series of errands in an unfamiliar small shopping area while spending as little money and time as possible). Because Diane reported memory as a concern, Carmen used the Everyday Memory Questionnaire

Table 7.6. Diane Archer's Canadian Occupational Performance Measure Results in the Community Day Program

Daily Living Concerns	Importance (1 = *low;* 10 = *high*)	Satisfaction (1 = *low;* 10 = *high*)	Ability Level (1 = *low;* 10 = *high*)
Keep track of daily schedule and tasks Diane wants or needs to complete (e.g., play dates for daughter Kate, medical appointments).	10	1	5
Structure Kate's time and engage in simple games with her.	10	2	3
Plan and shop for weekly meals without assistance from her mother.	8	2	3
Manage the household budget (i.e., balance checkbook, pay monthly bills).	8	2	2
Relearn computerized accounting system she was familiar with at previous employment.	6	2	2
Perform basic work skills to return to job as an accountant.	6	2	2

(Sunderland & Harris, 1994) to explore Diane's perception of the everyday situations in which her memory failed. Carmen gave Diane a copy of this questionnaire and asked her to have her husband, Tom, complete it so she could compare their responses. Carmen asked Diane to complete a variety of memory tasks that were either time based (e.g., check the pot on the stove in 5 minutes) or event based (e.g., mail the letter when you pass the mailbox) to evaluate Diane's prospective memory, an important type of memory for community functioning.

Carmen had read in the chart that Diane had used her smartphone as a memory aid in the rehab setting, so she asked Diane how the phone was functioning as a memory aid since her discharge home; they agreed to keep working on making it functional for her transition to home. Diane mentioned that Tom and she thought her tablet computer might also be helpful. She had tended to keep it set up in the kitchen before her accident and checked it frequently throughout the day. Diane kept recipes and the family schedule on the tablet. Carmen promised to explore some tablet apps that might help Diane structure her daily tasks independently.

Carmen and the entire rehabilitation team used several assessments to gather initial data on Diane's functioning within her home and community, the FIM™ (Granger, Hamilton, Linacre, Heinemann, & Wright, 1993) and the Functional Assessment Measure (FAM; Hall, 1997) and the Mayo–Portland Adaptability Inventory (Malec & Thompson, 1994). The assessments showed that although Diane was now independent in all self-care, mobility, and locomotion activities, she needed moderate assistance for community access and employability and scored as modified independent in attention and safety judgment. The team also used the POPS assessment (Brown et al., 2004) to identify the home and community tasks Diane rated as important along with her perception of her current and desired activity levels. Diane's self-identified priorities fell within the subscales related to domestic life and interpersonal interactions and relationships (Exhibit 7.2).

Over the course of the next month, Diane and Carmen focused the occupational therapy intervention on Diane's ability to resume the roles of mother, homemaker, friend, and worker (Table 7.7). They set weekly goals for Diane to assume increasing responsibilities in her home and decrease her reliance on her mother. They also explored social networking as a means for Diane to reconnect with friends. As Carmen used occupation-based interventions with Diane, her client gradually grew

Exhibit 7.1. Diane Archer's Initial Occupational Therapy Evaluation in the Community Day Program

Performance		
Areas	**Skills**	**Patterns**
ADLs: Client is independent in all basic self-care. Client is able to don and doff her contact lenses independently. *IADLs:* Client is supervised by her husband or mother in caregiving activities for her 3.5-yr-old daughter. Client does not drive. She performs simple household chores and activities with cues and assistance. Activities of shopping, banking, meal planning, and financial management are performed by her husband or mother. *Education:* Client was not involved in any formal or informal educational activities at the time of her injury. *Work:* Client is not working. *Leisure:* Client participates in playing simple board games with her daughter and occasionally watches TV. *Social participation:* Client is able to participate in small social gatherings of 2–3 people but tends to respond to, more than initiate, conversation. Her present social circle is limited to family and 2 close friends.	*Motor and Praxis Skills* *Motor:* Diane is able to stabilize, align, and position her body appropriately to given tasks. She walks without an assistive device, but ataxia is observed when walking at faster speeds. Client reports impaired balance with occasional falls in her yard on uneven surfaces. She is able to reach and bend in all directions but needs to maintain one arm in contact with a stable surface to prevent a loss of balance when reaching near the end of her range. Diane is able to coordinate movements of her right (dominant) extremity and manipulate objects with only occasional evidence of slow or awkward movements. She is able to move, transport, lift, and grip objects with either or both hands (e.g., cooking pot filled with water). She appropriately uses surfaces to slide heavier items to prevent loss of balance. Motor endurance is still limited. Diane fatigues quickly and requires daily rest periods each afternoon. She retires to bed earlier than before her injury. *Cognitive Skills* Diane shows difficulty attending to tasks as the complexity of the task or the environmental distractions increase. Diane does not seek additional information or clarification when uncertain of the task requirements. She needs cues to initiate tasks and to maintain a consistent pace in her performance. At times her responses are delayed and at other times impulsive. Once started in a task, she is able to appropriately sequence and terminate actions. Diane's ability to organize task spaces and task objects is influenced by her difficulty with initiation. She can verbalize organizational structure of space and objects but needs cues to search for needed objects, gather and organize needed materials, and restore materials to their appropriate places (e.g., placement of grooming objects on sink top in bathroom). Diane is responsive to cues (i.e., visual, tactile, verbal), but repeated experiences are needed when learning new material because of her memory impairments. Diane does not consistently anticipate how her limitations will influence her task performance, but she does notice her errors and attempts to accommodate or adjust her performance or the environment when errors or problems occur. *Communication and Social Skills* Diane is able to articulate her needs and engage in conversation. Her cognitive limitations influence all aspects of Diane's verbal and nonverbal communication and interaction skills. Her interactions with others, although not socially inappropriate, are more as a responder than as an initiator of conversations.	*Current* **habits** *and routines:* Client typically gets up at 7:00 a.m. and showers before waking her daughter. Client then makes breakfast for daughter and herself (usually cold cereal and juice). Husband leaves for work around 8:00 a.m. when client's mother comes to spend the day. Client's day is typically spent in therapy until 3:00 p.m., when she takes a half-hour nap before going with her mother to pick up her daughter from child care. She helps her mother prepare dinner around 5:30 p.m. Weekday evenings are spent taking walks with daughter in stroller, playing with daughter, watching TV, or doing household chores with husband once daughter goes to bed. Weekends are spent together as a family, or client and her daughter go to her mother's home while her husband has to work. Occasional family outings are taken with either her husband or her parents. Client requires structure and verbal cueing to initiate many of her daily routines but is able to carry out the tasks with distant supervision. She attempts to carry out new useful habits using the cognitive strategies learned in the acute rehabilitation setting (e.g., use of smartphone for memory) but needs further experience to translate the functional application of these strategies to the community. *Roles:* Client is gradually resuming some of her previous roles as wife and mother, but her independence in the tasks of these roles is altered.

Client Factors	Context

Spirituality
 Client states that her family, particularly her daughter, inspires and motivates her to improve and continue in therapy even on days when she wants to give up.
 Mental Functions
    Global mental functions: Client is oriented to person, place, and time. Energy and drive appear limited: Client does not initiate conversations or activities independently.
    Specific mental functions: Client displays problems in attention, memory, and higher thought functions as determined by observation and performance on specific assessments. Client has difficulty concentrating in noisier environments, and her performance (speed and accuracy) decreases. She has difficulty with day-to-day memory and prospective memory. She can perform basic calculation functions but is unable to independently complete complex calculations, which she was highly familiar with in her previous role as an accountant.
	Cultural
	 The day program is a community of people recovering from severe neurological injuries. This culture emphasizes self-determination of intervention priorities and collective responsibility for the environment. Clients and families are encouraged to participate in meetings of the local Brain Injury Association.
	 Physical
	 The day program is located in a separate facility on the grounds of the rehabilitation hospital. It has several small rooms for individual client sessions and a large living room, dining room, and kitchen for group-based activities. Client is now living at home in her 2-story house with her husband and 3.5-yr-old daughter. She is able to access all rooms of the house and has returned to sleeping in the upstairs bedroom with her husband.

(Continued)

Exhibit 7.1. Diane Archer's Initial Occupational Therapy Evaluation in the Community Day Program *(cont.)*

Performance	
Client Factors	**Context**

Sensory Functions and Pain
  Seeing and related functions: All sensory functions are intact.
Neuromusculoskeletal and Movement-Related Functions
  Functions of joints and bones: Client has full PROM of all joints in both upper limbs.
  Muscle functions: Client displays minimal increase in flexor tone in the R UE when fatigued or stressed. L UE displays normal tone.
  Movement functions: Client is able to volitionally move R UE without evidence of spasticity, but movements are slower. Her gait pattern shows evidence of ataxia when walking at a faster speed.
	Social
	Within the day program, the client responds to questions asked but does not initiate conversation with her therapist or other clients. The client and family report that she tends to avoid larger social functions and limits her interactions to family members and a few close friends seen 1:1. Client reports dissatisfaction with the social perception of herself as an injured person.
	Personal
	28-yr-old woman who is a wife and a mother to a toddler.
	Temporal
	Early summer; participants attend the day program between 9:00 a.m. and 3:00 p.m.
	Virtual
	The client does not participate in chat rooms or e-mail communication.

Implications for Intervention Planning	
Client's occupational therapy intervention will focus on continued areas of decreased occupational performance in her life roles of wife, mother, homemaker, and worker as identified in the COPM. Engagement in client-centered occupation-based activities will focus on diminishing the functional effect of the client's impairments in memory and executive functions while improving her independence in IADLs, ability to engage in remunerative employment, and participation in social and leisure activities within her community. The activity demands (objects, space, social, sequencing and timing, required actions) of tasks used in intervention will be manipulated to address cognitive skills by providing opportunities for the client to use strategies to improve performance.	

Note. ADLs = activities of daily living; COPM = Canadian Occupational Performance Measure; IADLs = instrumental activities of daily living; L = left; PROM = passive range of motion; R = right; UE = upper extremity; yr = year.

more confident in her abilities to incorporate cognitive-based strategies to accomplish the tasks that she needed and wanted to complete.

Diane participated in a twice-weekly group intervention session as well as in individualized sessions with Carmen. The group focused on higher level IADL and community-based activities that involved social pragmatics. Weekly meals planned by the group, and community outings for shopping and leisure activities, were used to work on Diane's individual goals as well as social skills.

After 3 months as a day program client, Diane was switched to outpatient status (i.e., individualized occupational therapy sessions twice a week) for an additional 3 months, until her insurance company denied further services. During the outpatient program, Diane and Carmen explored vocational issues. Diane expressed awareness that her present difficulties in processing speed might make returning to her previous employer (a fast-paced setting) unrealistic. She participated in the volunteer program at the hospital and worked with the volunteer program's treasurer on reviewing the accounts and preparing a draft of the annual financial report that the program prepared for the hospital. She also performed accounting reviews and reports of the sales receipts from the volunteer-run gift shop. Carmen and Diane used these tasks in their sessions as a realistic activity to work on Diane's remaining cognitive processing limitations. They also explored the possibility of Diane's returning to work as an accountant in a part-time position in a slower paced setting that offered more potential to modify her work tasks and environment to accommodate her cognitive impairments. Carmen assisted Diane in contacting the State Office of Vocational Rehabilitation to identify the resources they could offer to support her goal to return to gainful employment.

Exhibit 7.2. Diane Archer's Responses on the Initial Participation Objective, Participation Subjective Assessment

	Activity	Current Activity Level						Desired Activity Level					How Important						
		All	Most	Some	None	NA	DK	More	Less	Same	NA	DK	Most	Very	Mod	Little	Not	NA	DK
1	Shopping for groceries, drugs, other necessities	3	2	1	**0**		9	**1**	2	3		9	**4**	3	2	1	0		9
2	Preparing meals, cooking	3	2	**1**	0		9	**1**	2	3		9	**4**	3	2	1	0		9
4	Caring for and supervising children or dependent adults	3	2	**1**	0	7	9	**1**	2	3	7	9	**4**	3	2	1	0	7	9

		Current Activity Level					Desired Activity Level				How Important					
		Hours	Per:	Day	Week	Month	More	Less	Same	DK	Most	Very	Mod	Little	Not	DK
9	Work for pay	0		O	O	●	**1**	2	3	9	4	**3**	2	1	0	9
12	Drive or ride in a car	0		O	O	●	**1**	2	3	9	**4**	3	2	1	0	9

		Current Activity Level					Desired Activity Level				How Important					
		Times	Per:	Day	Week	Month	More	Less	Same	DK	Most	Very	Mod	Little	Not	DK
14	Socialize with friends, by phone or at home	1		O	O	●	**1**	2	3	9	**4**	3	2	1	0	9
17	Go out to visit friends or family, social events and occasions	1		O	O	●	**1**	2	3	9	**4**	3	2	1	0	9
24	Go shopping	0		O	O	●	**1**	2	3	9	**4**	3	2	1	0	9

Note. Bold/shaded cells show the client's selections on this sample response score sheet. DK = don't know; Mod = moderately; NA = not applicable.

Diane participated in a rehabilitative driving evaluation and training program with one of the occupational therapists at the rehab facility and successfully passed the state retesting program. During her last week as an outpatient, Diane achieved her goal of having the confidence to drive independently to the hospital for her intervention sessions.

At her discharge from the outpatient program, several of the outcome measures administered at admission were rescored. On the Mayo–Portland Adaptability Inventory, Diane rated her abilities, emotions, and behaviors as only mild problems that did not interfere with activities; she rated use of her hands, memory, and balance as interfering with activities 5% to 24% of the time. In the category of social and community participation, Diane scored herself as mildly impaired in leisure and recreational activities and work activities. She did not identify any severe behavior problems. Carmen and the team were pleased that Diane's awareness of her current abilities matched their perception of her capabilities.

Table 7.7. Sample Activities From Diane Archer's Intervention Plan During the Community Phase of Recovery

Problems and Goals	Approach	Primary Focus of Intervention	Interventions
Continued goals from the inpatient rehabilitation phase of recovery *Problem:* Impaired memory and executive functions *Goal:* Client will be able to accurately estimate the difficulty of a task and her need to initiate strategies and self-monitor performance during tasks. *Goal:* Client will be able to successfully use her smartphone to compensate for memory impairments (i.e., identify location to enter information, enter sufficient and accurate detail to assist memory, set alarm to remind).	• Establish and restore cognitive skills; teach client cognitive strategies to improve performance • Modify environment to enhance cognitive capabilities; modify task performance to compensate for cognitive limitations	*Client factors:* Specific mental functions of memory, thought, and higher level cognitive functions *Performance skills:* Cognitive skills of attention and memory, multitasking, executive functions, organizing space and objects, and awareness and self-monitoring of performance *Performance patterns:* Translation of new routines for use of the smartphone as a memory aid into client's home and community living	*Preparatory methods:* Have the client estimate task difficulty and her need for strategies and assistance before initiating all treatment tasks. Have client complete short checklist comparing estimation with actual performance. *Purposeful activity:* Continue using Toglia's (2011) Dynamic Interactional Approach to engage the client in various tasks that require targeted processing strategies in situations that are within the same level of difficulty; the difficulty level of the activity demands is higher than what could be achieved on an inpatient basis. Client's need for external cues is significantly decreased, and she continues to work on identifying methods to self-cue and monitor performance. *Occupation-based activity:* Use client-centered occupation-based activities related to roles, responsibilities, and interests (e.g., financial management, cooking, parenting, gardening, playing simple board games with daughter).
Problem: Decreased independence in IADLs *Goal:* Client will be able to perform monthly budget and bill-paying activity. *Goal:* Client will be able to plan, shop, and cook basic meals for herself and her family. *Goal:* Client will be able to participate in a driving assessment and rehabilitation program to return to independent community driving. *Goal:* Client will be able to structure her daughter's time and engage in simple games and constructive activities, giving appropriate feedback, instruction, and encouragement.	• Establish and restore cognitive skills; teach client cognitive strategies to improve performance • Maintain performance capabilities regained to support occupational performance • Modify environment to enhance cognitive capabilities; modify task performance to compensate for cognitive limitations	*Client factors:* Specific mental functions of memory, thought, and high-level cognitive functions *Performance skills:* Cognitive skills of attention and memory, multitasking, executive functions, organizing space and objects, and awareness and self-monitoring of performance; motor skills of coordination and endurance *Areas of occupation:* IADLs (child rearing, community mobility, financial management, home establishment and management, meal preparation and cleanup, safety procedures and emergency responses, shopping)	*Purposeful activity:* Do sample menu planning, sample budgeting activities (on paper and computer), and planning simple craft and art activities appropriate for toddler. Review simple computer CD-ROM activities for preschool-age child and rewrite instructions to be able to guide daughter. Write shopping list of craft activity materials needed. *Occupation-based activity:* Have client bring in monthly bills to perform monthly financial activity using her online banking account. Have client grocery shop and cook simple meals in individual and group settings. Participate in driving rehabilitation program. *Consultation:* Collaborate with client on the analysis of existing performance difficulties and generation of possible solutions. Provide client with a feedback log to track usefulness of new strategies and techniques in her home and community. *Education:* Keep client's husband and mother informed about any new strategies or techniques used to increase client's independence so they can apply these strategies in the home environment.

(Continued)

Table 7.7. Sample Activities From Diane Archer's Intervention Plan During the Community Phase of Recovery *(cont.)*

Problems and Goals	Approach	Primary Focus of Intervention	Interventions
Problem: Decreased ability to engage in remunerative employment *Goal:* Client will demonstrate the ability to perform basic accounting and bookkeeping tasks (balance sheets, monthly summary of income and expenses, etc.) for hospital volunteer services.	• Establish and restore cognitive skills; teach client cognitive strategies to improve performance • Maintain performance capabilities regained to support occupational performance • Modify environment to enhance cognitive capabilities; modify task performance to compensate for cognitive limitations	*Client factors:* Specific mental functions (attention and memory functions, higher level cognitive functions, calculation functions) *Performance skills:* Cognitive skills of attention and memory, multitasking, executive functions, organizing space and objects, and awareness and self-monitoring of performance *Performance patterns:* Habits to ensure accuracy of work (e.g., separate piles of receipts, check work completed, monitor accuracy) *Areas of occupation:* Work (employment interests and pursuits, **job performance**)	*Purposeful activity:* Have client complete a detailed job description and analysis of her current capabilities to perform the job tasks. Identify possible modifications to tasks to accommodate for client's current limitations and environmental modifications that enhance cognitive performance. Have client use self-cueing strategies to check and correct her work. *Occupation-based activity:* Working with director of volunteer services and treasurer of volunteer program, have client perform monthly bookkeeping activities. *Consultation:* Collaborate with client on contacting the State Office of Vocational Rehabilitation.
Problem: Decreased participation in social and leisure activities *Goal:* Client will plan and complete 1 community outing per week with her husband, daughter, or a friend (e.g., going to library or a local cultural or sporting event, having lunch or shopping with friend).	• Establish and restore cognitive skills; teach client cognitive strategies to improve performance • Maintain performance capabilities regained to support occupational performance • Modify environment to enhance cognitive capabilities; modify task performance to compensate for cognitive limitations	*Performance skills:* Cognitive skills of attention and memory, executive functions, sequencing, and awareness and self-monitoring of performance; communication and social skills of information exchange and relationship maintenance *Performance patterns:* New routines to fulfill roles of parent, partner, and friend *Areas of occupation:* Social participation (community, family, and friends); leisure participation	*Purposeful activity:* Gather information on possible leisure and social activities (e.g., phone calls, searches of newspaper and Internet sites for local activities). Have client plan time sequence for events, financial needs, and hypothetical problem solving of emergency situations. Practice social pragmatics in group activities and through role playing. *Occupation-based activity:* Engage client in community outings with groups during therapy sessions. Have client engage in community outings with family and friends and provide feedback to therapist on success of task.

Note. IADLs = instrumental activities of daily living.

Diane's Continued Recovery in the Community

It has been a year since Diane sustained her TBI, a year of changes in almost all contexts of her life. At a recent follow-up appointment with the TBI rehabilitation team, Diane completed the POPS again to review her current level of community participation (Exhibit 7.3).

Diane is now safe to be home alone with Kate, although her mother and Tom frequently check in with her during the day via Skype and phone calls. She limits her driving trips to within her community (e.g., shopping, local library, visits to her parents' home) because Kate's chattering during the trips makes Diane anxious. Diane's balance remains impaired, and she has taken a few scary falls while running after Kate. Diane began swimming and working out with weights weekly at the local health club to increase her strength and stamina. She has not taken any of the aerobic classes offered at the club because she is fearful of falling. Diane has volunteered in her daughter's preschool program a few afternoons, but she finds the number of

Exhibit 7.3. Diane Archer's Responses on the Participation Objective, Participation Subjective Assessment 1 Year Postinjury

	Activity	Current Activity Level						Desired Activity Level					How Important						
		All	Most	Some	None	NA	DK	More	Less	Same	NA	DK	Most	Very	Mod	Little	Not	NA	DK
1	Shopping for groceries, drugs, other necessities	3	2	**1**	0		9	**1**	2	3		9	4	**3**	2	1	0		9
2	Preparing meals, cooking	3	**2**	1	0		9	1	2	**3**		9	4	**3**	2	1	0		9
4	Caring for and supervising children or dependent adults	3	**2**	1	0	7	9	**1**	2	3	7	9	**4**	3	2	1	0	7	9

		Current Activity Level					Desired Activity Level				How Important					
		Hours	Per:	Day	Week	Month	More	Less	Same	DK	Most	Very	Mod	Little	Not	DK
9	Work for pay	12		O	●	O	**1**	2	3	9	4	**3**	2	1	0	9
12	Drive or ride in a car	5		O	●	O	**1**	2	3	9	**4**	3	2	1	0	9

		Current Activity Level					Desired Activity Level				How Important					
		Times	Per:	Day	Week	Month	More	Less	Same	DK	Most	Very	Mod	Little	Not	DK
14	Socialize with friends, by phone or at home	3		O	●	O	1	2	**3**	9	**4**	3	2	1	0	9
17	Go out to visit friends or family, social events and occasions	1–2		O	●	O	1	2	**3**	9	**4**	3	2	1	0	9
24	Go shopping	1–2		O	O	●	**1**	2	3	9	**4**	3	2	1	0	9

Note. Bold/shaded cells show the client's selections on this sample response score sheet. DK = don't know; Mod = moderately; NA = not applicable.

children overstimulating and leaves feeling mentally and physically fatigued. She is able to organize simple play activities when Kate has a play date with one friend.

Diane continues to use apps on her smartphone to help manage her memory impairments and organize her daily tasks. Each evening after Kate has gone to bed, Diane plans activities she wants to accomplish the following day and schedules them into the calendar on her phone. She also downloads meal ideas for the next day to the tablet computer and updates the weekly shopping list. This quiet time is also an opportunity for Tom and her to discuss plans and strategies for future family activities.

Diane recently obtained a part-time job as a bookkeeper for a small business owned by a family friend who is aware of Diane's limitations. She works three mornings each week and enjoys the job and social contacts she has made. The job itself is not time pressured. She shares a private office with another bookkeeper and has been able to modify the environmental stimuli to enhance her cognitive skills. Diane hopes to gradually increase the complexity of job tasks that she can accomplish and hopes to increase her hours over the next few months.

Tom and Diane sought psychological couple counseling about 8 months after her injury to explore the effect the injury had on their relationships and roles.

Tom reports that Diane's personality is changed from before the injury. Previously, she tended to be energetic and quick to laugh; she now takes less initiative in most situations. Her previous proficiency at multitasking is no longer observed. Each task needs to be done with great attention to detail and without distraction, not an easy task with a toddler at home. Tom and Diane's social life has also changed. Tom believes some of their friends feel awkward around them, and Diane's balance problems limit their ability to participate in some of the group sporting activities they used to enjoy (e.g., skiing, tennis). Although Tom states he misses aspects of the old Diane, he is grateful that Kate and he still have her in their lives. Tom had to get a part-time second job to cover the family expenses, medical bills, and Diane's reduced income. Tom and Diane have found support and practical life strategies through their network of friends from the local Brain Injury Association. Diane regularly attends the association's support group, and Tom joins the family group periodically.

On the anniversary of her accident, Diane and Tom reflected on their difficult past year. They also discussed the future and the goals that Diane wants to achieve: driving greater distances (e.g., to friends' homes), taking a refresher course in accounting at the local community college, and returning to work full-time as an accountant. Although Diane's insurance will no longer pay for services, Tom and the family have agreed to hire a private home-based occupational therapist to consult and help Diane reach her goals.

References

Aaronson, L. S., Teel, C. S., Cassmeyer, V., Neuberger, G. B., Pallikkathayil, L., Pierce, J., . . . Wingate, A. (1999). Defining and measuring fatigue. *Image: The Journal of Nursing Scholarship, 31,* 45–50. http://dx.doi.org/10.1111/j.1547-5069.1999.tb00420.x

Altman, I. M., Swick, S., Parrot, D., & Malec, J. F. (2010). Effectiveness of community-based rehabilitation after traumatic brain injury for 489 program completers compared with those precipitously discharged. *Archives of Physical Medicine and Rehabilitation, 91,* 1697–1704. http://dx.doi.org/10.1016/j.apmr.2010.08.001

American Occupational Therapy Association. (2014). Occupational therapy practice framework: Domain and process (3rd ed.). *American Journal of Occupational Therapy, 68*(Suppl.1), S1–S48. http://dx.doi.org/10.5014/ajot.2014.682006

Anderson, M. I., Parmenter, T. R., & Mok, M. (2002). The relationship between neurobehavioural problems of severe traumatic brain injury (TBI), family functioning and the psychological well-being of the spouse/caregiver: Path model analysis. *Brain Injury, 16,* 743–757. http://dx.doi.org/10.1080/02699050210128906

Anderson, M. I., Simpson, G. K., & Morey, P. J. (2013). The impact of neurobehavioral impairment on family functioning and the psychological well-being of male versus female caregivers of relatives with severe traumatic brain injury: Multigroup analysis. *Journal of Head Trauma Rehabilitation, 28,* 453–463. http://dx.doi.org/10.1097/HTR.0b013e31825d6087

Anke, A. G., & Fugl-Meyer, A. R. (2003). Life satisfaction several years after severe multiple trauma: A retrospective investigation. *Clinical Rehabilitation, 17,* 431–442. http://dx.doi.org/10.1191/0269215503cr629oa

Anson, K., & Ponsford, J. (2006). Coping and emotional adjustment following traumatic brain injury. *Journal of Head Trauma Rehabilitation, 21,* 248–259. http://dx.doi.org/10.1097/00001199-200605000-00005

Arlinghaus, K., Shoaib, A., & Price, T. (2005). Neuropsychiatric assessment. In J. M. Silver, T. W. McAllister, & S. C. Yudofsky (Eds.), *Textbook of traumatic brain injury* (pp. 59–78). Washington, DC: American Psychiatric Publishing.

Árnadóttir, G. (1990). *The brain and behavior: Assessing cortical function through activities of daily living.* St. Louis: Mosby.

Ashley, M. (2004). Evaluation of traumatic brain injury following acute rehabilitation. In M. Ashley (Ed.), *Traumatic brain injury: Rehabilitative treatment and case management* (2nd ed., pp. 613–640). Boca Raton, FL: CRC Press.

Ashley, M. (Ed.). (2010). *Traumatic brain injury: Rehabilitation, treatment, and case management.* Boca Raton, FL: CRC Press.

Baguley, I. J., Cooper, J., & Felmingham, K. (2006). Aggressive behavior following traumatic brain injury: How common is common? *Journal of Head Trauma Rehabilitation, 21,* 45–56. http://dx.doi.org/10.1097/00001199-200601000-00005

Bandura, A. (1997). *Self-efficacy: The exercise of control.* New York: W. H. Freeman.

Barco, P., Crosson, B., Bolesta, M., Werts, D., & Stout, R. (1991). Training awareness and compensation in postacute head injury rehabilitation. In J. Kreutzer & P. Wehman (Eds.), *Cognitive rehabilitation for persons with traumatic brain injury: A functional approach* (pp. 129–146). Baltimore: Paul H. Brookes.

Barnes, M., & Ward, A. (2000). *Textbook of rehabilitation medicine.* Oxford, England: Oxford University Press.

Basford, J. R., Chou, L. S., Kaufman, K. R., Brey, R. H., Walker, A., Malec, J. F., . . . Brown, A. W. (2003). An assessment of gait and balance deficits after traumatic brain injury. *Archives of Physical Medicine and Rehabilitation, 84,* 343–349. http://dx.doi.org/10.1053/apmr.2003.50034

Baum, C. M., Morrison, T., Hahn, M., & Edwards, D. F. (2008). *Test manual: Executive Function Performance Test.* St. Louis: Washington University.

Bier, N., Dutil, E., & Couture, M. (2009). Factors affecting leisure participation after a traumatic brain injury: An exploratory study. *Journal of Head Trauma Rehabilitation, 24,* 187–194. http://dx.doi.org/10.1097/HTR.0b013e3181a0b15a

Bivona, U., D'Ippolito, M., Giustini, M., Vignally, P., Longo, E., Taggi, F., & Formisano, R. (2012). Return to driving after severe traumatic brain injury: Increased risk of traffic accidents and personal responsibility. *Journal of Head Trauma Rehabilitation, 27,* 210–215. http://dx.doi.org/10.1097/HTR.0b013e31822178a9

Blacker, D., Broadhurst, L., & Teixeira, L. (2008). The role of occupational therapy in leisure adaptation with complex neurological disability: A discussion using two case study examples. *NeuroRehabilitation, 23,* 313–319.

Blake, H. (2008). Caregiver stress in traumatic brain injury. *International Journal of Therapy and Rehabilitation, 15,* 263–271. http://dx.doi.org/10.12968/ijtr.2008.15.6.29878

Bottari, C., Dassa, C., Rainville, C., & Dutil, E. (2009). The criterion-related validity of the IADL Profile with measures of executive functions, indices of trauma severity and sociodemographic characteristics. *Brain Injury, 23,* 322–335. http://dx.doi.org/10.1080/02699050902788436

Bottari, C., Dassa, C., Rainville, C., & Dutil, E. (2010). A generalizability study of the Instrumental Activities of Daily Living Profile. *Archives of Physical Medicine and Rehabilitation, 91,* 734–742. http://dx.doi.org/10.1016/j.apmr.2009.12.023

Brain Injury Association of America. (2014). *Brain injury statistics.* Retrieved from http://www.biausa.org/glossary.htm

Braveman, B. (2012). Development of the worker role and worker identity. In B. Braveman & J. Page (Eds.), *Work: Promoting participation and productivity through occupational therapy* (pp. 28–51). Philadelphia: F. A. Davis.

Brown, M., Dijkers, M. P., Gordon, W. A., Ashman, T., Charatz, H., & Cheng, Z. (2004). Participation Objective, Participation Subjective: A measure of participation combining outsider and insider perspectives. *Journal of Head Trauma Rehabilitation, 19,* 459–481. http://dx.doi.org/10.1097/00001199-200411000-00004

Brown, R., Pain, K., Berwald, C., Hirschi, P., Delehanty, R., & Miller, H. (1999). Distance education and caregiver support groups: Comparison of traditional and telephone groups. *Journal of Head Trauma Rehabilitation, 14,* 257–268. http://dx.doi.org/10.1097/00001199-199906000-00006

Bryant, R., Creamer, M., O'Donnell, M., Silove, D., Clark, C., & McFarlane, A. (2010). The psychological sequelae of traumatic brain injury. *American Journal of Psychiatry, 167,* 312–320. http://dx.doi.org/10.1176/appi.ajp.2009.09050617

Bryant, R., Marosszeky, J. E., Crooks, J., Baguley, I., & Gurka, J. (2000). Coping style and post-traumatic stress disorder following severe traumatic brain injury. *Brain Injury, 14,* 175–180. http://dx.doi.org/10.1080/026990500120826

Burkhardt, S., & Rotatori, A. (2010). Educating students with traumatic brain injury. In P. Peterson, E. Baker, & B. McGaw (Eds.), *International encyclopedia of education* (3rd ed., pp. 695–700). Oxford, England: Elsevier.

Burleigh, S. A., Farber, R. S., & Gillard, M. (1998). Community integration and life satisfaction after traumatic brain injury: Long-term findings. *American Journal of Occupational Therapy, 52,* 45–52. http://dx.doi.org/10.5014/ajot.52.1.45

Bushnik, T., Englander, J., & Wright, J. (2008). Patterns of fatigue and its correlates over the first 2 years after traumatic brain injury. *Journal of Head Trauma Rehabilitation, 23,* 25–32. http://dx.doi.org/10.1097/01.HTR.0000308718.88214.bb

Caldwell, L. L., & Smith, E. A. (1988). Leisure: An overlooked component of health promotion. *Canadian Journal of Public Health, 79,* S44–S48.

Cantor, J., Ashman, T., Gordon, W., Ginsberg, A., Engmann, C., Egan, M., . . . & Flanagan, S. (2008). Fatigue after traumatic brain injury and its impact on participation and quality of life. *Journal of Head Trauma Rehabilitation, 23,* 41–51. http://dx.doi.org/10.1097/01.HTR.0000308720.70288.af

Casavant, A., & Hastings, H. (2006). Heterotopic ossification about the elbow: A therapist's guide to evaluation and management. *Journal of Hand Therapy, 19,* 255–266.

Chen, H., Epstein, J., & Stern, E. (2010). Neural plasticity after acquired brain injury: Evidence from functional neuroimaging. *PM&R: The Journal of Injury, Function, and Rehabilitation, 2*(Suppl. 2), S306–S312. http://dx.doi.org/10.1016/j.pmrj.2010.10.006

Cohen, M., Oksenberg, A., Snir, D., Stern, M. J., & Groswasser, Z. (1992). Temporally related changes of sleep complaints in traumatic brain injured patients. *Journal of Neurology, Neurosurgery, and Psychiatry, 55,* 313–315. http://dx.doi.org/10.1136/jnnp.55.4.313

Coleman, R. D., Rapport, L. J., Ergh, T. C., Hanks, R. A., Ricker, J. H., & Millis, S. R. (2002). Predictors of driving outcome after traumatic brain injury. *Archives of Physical Medicine and Rehabilitation, 83,* 1415–1422. http://dx.doi.org/10.1053/apmr.2002.35111

Conneeley, A. (2002). Social integration following traumatic brain injury and rehabilitation. *British Journal of Occupational Therapy, 65,* 356–362. http://dx.doi.org/10.1177/030802260206500802

Connolly, D., & O'Dowd, T. (2001). The impact of different disabilities arising from head injury on the primary caregiver. *British Journal of Occupational Therapy, 64,* 41–46. http://dx.doi.org/10.1177/030802260106400108

Corrigan, J. D. (2001). Conducting statewide needs assessments for persons with traumatic brain injury. *Journal of Head Trauma Rehabilitation, 16,* 1–19. http://dx.doi.org/10.1097/00001199-200102000-00004

Corrigan, J. D., Selassie, A. W., & Orman, J. A. (2010). The epidemiology of traumatic brain injury. *Journal of Head Trauma Rehabilitation, 25,* 72–80. http://dx.doi.org/10.1097/HTR.0b013e3181ccc8b4

Corruble, E., Benyamina, A., Bayle, F., Falissard, B., & Hardy, P. (2003). Understanding impulsivity in severe depression? A psychometrical contribution. *Progress in Neuro-Psychopharmacology and Biological Psychiatry, 27,* 829–833. http://dx.doi.org/10.1016/S0278-5846(03)00115-5

Curran, C. A., Ponsford, J. L., & Crowe, S. (2000). Coping strategies and emotional outcome following traumatic brain injury: A comparison with orthopedic patients. *Journal of Head Trauma Rehabilitation, 15,* 1256–1274. http://dx.doi.org/10.1097/00001199-200012000-00006

Cusimano, M. D., Holmes, S. A., Sawicki, C., & Topolovec-Vranic, J. (2014). Assessing aggression following traumatic brain injury: A systematic review of validated aggression scales. *Journal of Head Trauma Rehabilitation, 29,* 172–184. http://dx.doi.org/10.1097/HTR.0b013e31827c7d15

Dahlberg, C. A., Cusick, C. P., Hawley, L. A., Newman, J. K., Morey, C. E., Harrison-Felix, C. L., & Whiteneck, G. G. (2007). Treatment efficacy of social communication skills training after traumatic brain injury: A randomized treatment and deferred treatment controlled trial. *Archives of Physical Medicine and Rehabilitation, 88,* 1561–1573. http://dx.doi.org/10.1016/j.apmr.2007.07.033

Dahlberg, C., Hawley, L., Morey, C., Newman, J., Cusick, C. P., & Harrison-Felix, C. (2006). Social communication skills in persons with post-acute traumatic brain injury: Three perspectives. *Brain Injury, 20,* 425–435. http://dx.doi.org/10.1080/02699050600664574

D'apolito, A. C., Massonneau, A., Paillat, C., & Azouvi, P. (2013). Impact of brain injury on driving skills. *Annals of Physical and Rehabilitation Medicine, 56,* 63–80. http://dx.doi.org/10.1016/j.rehab.2012.12.002

Deaton, A. (1990). Behavior change strategies for children and adolescents with traumatic brain injury. In E. D. Bigler (Ed.), *Traumatic brain injury* (pp. 231–249). Austin, TX: PRO-ED.

Dickerson, A., Reistetter, T., Schold Davis, E., & Monahan, M. (2011). Evaluating driving as a valued instrumental activity of daily living. *American Journal of Occupational Therapy, 65,* 64–75. http://dx.doi.org/10.5014/ajot.2011.09052

Dikmen, S., Machamer, J., Powell, J., & Temkin, N. (2003). Outcome 3 to 5 years following traumatic brain injury. *Archives of Physical Medicine and Rehabilitation, 84,* 1449–1457. http://dx.doi.org/10.1016/s0003-9993(03)00287-9

Dirette, D. K., & Plaisier, B. R. (2007). The development of self-awareness of deficits from 1 week to 1 year after traumatic brain injury: Preliminary findings. *Brain Injury, 21,* 1131–1136. http://dx.doi.org/10.1080/02699050701687326

Doble, S. E., Bonnell, J. E., & Magill-Evans, J. (1991). Evaluation of social skills: A survey of current practice. *Canadian Journal of Occupational Therapy, 58,* 241–249. http://dx.doi.org/10.1177/000841749105800506

Doig, E., Fleming, J., Cornwell, P. L., & Kuipers, P. (2009). Qualitative exploration of a client-centered, goal-directed approach to community-based occupational therapy for adults with traumatic brain injury. *American Journal of Occupational Therapy, 63,* 559–568. http://dx.doi.org/10.5014/ajot.63.5.559

Doig, E., Fleming, J., Kuipers, P., & Cornwell, P. L. (2010). Clinical utility of the combined use of the Canadian Occupational Performance Measure and Goal Attainment Scaling. *American Journal of Occupational Therapy, 64,* 904–914. http://dx.doi.org/10.5014/ajot.2010.08156

Donaghy, S., & Wass, P. J. (1998). Interrater reliability of the Functional Assessment Measure in a brain injury rehabilitation program. *Archives of Physical Medicine and Rehabilitation, 79,* 1231–1236. http://dx.doi.org/10.1016/S0003-9993(98)90267-2

Downing, M. G., Stolwyk, R., & Ponsford, J. L. (2013). Sexual changes in individuals with traumatic brain injury: A control comparison. *Journal of Head Trauma Rehabilitation, 28,* 171–178. http://dx.doi.org/10.1097/HTR.0b013e31828b4f63

Driver, S., & Ede, A. (2009). Impact of physical activity on mood after TBI. *Brain Injury, 23,* 203–212. http://dx.doi.org/10.1080/02699050802695574

Ducharme, J. M. (2000). Treatment of maladaptive behavior in acquired brain injury: Remedial approaches in postacute settings. *Clinical Psychology Review, 20,* 405–426. http://dx.doi.org/10.1016/S0272-7358(98)00102-0

Dyer, K. F., Bell, R., McCann, J., & Rauch, R. (2006). Aggression after traumatic brain injury: Analysing socially desirable responses and the nature of aggressive traits. *Brain Injury, 20,* 1163–1173. http://dx.doi.org/10.1080/02699050601049312

Engberg, A. W., & Teasdale, T. W. (2004). Psychosocial outcome following traumatic brain injury in adults: A long-term population-based follow-up. *Brain Injury, 18,* 533–545. http://dx.doi.org/10.1080/02699050310001645829

Engström, A. L., Lexell, J., & Lund, M. L. (2010). Difficulties in using everyday technology after acquired brain injury: A qualitative analysis. *Scandinavian Journal of Occupational Therapy, 17,* 233–243. http://dx.doi.org/10.3109/11038120903191806

Ergh, T. C., Rapport, L. J., Coleman, R. D., & Hanks, R. A. (2002). Predictors of caregiver and family functioning following traumatic brain injury: Social support moderates caregiver distress. *Journal of Head Trauma Rehabilitation, 17,* 155–174. http://dx.doi.org/10.1097/00001199-200204000-00006

Fadyl, J. K., & McPherson, K. M. (2009). Approaches to vocational rehabilitation after traumatic brain injury: A review of the evidence. *Journal of Head Trauma Rehabilitation, 24,* 195–212. http://dx.doi.org/10.1097/HTR.0b013e3181a0d458

Faul, M., Wald, M. M., Rutland-Brown, W., Sullivent, E. E., & Sattin, R. W. (2007). Using a cost–benefit analysis to estimate outcomes of a clinical treatment guideline: Testing the Brain Trauma Foundation guidelines for the treatment of severe traumatic brain injury. *Journal of Trauma, 63,* 1271–1278. http://dx.doi.org/10.1097/TA.0b013e3181493080

Feeney, T. J., Ylvisaker, M., Rosen, B. H., & Greene, P. (2001). Community supports for individuals with challenging behavior after brain injury: An analysis of the New York State Behavioral Resource Project. *Journal of Head Trauma Rehabilitation, 16,* 61–75. http://dx.doi.org/10.1097/00001199-200102000-00008

Fischer, S., Trexler, L. E., & Gauggel, S. (2004). Awareness of activity limitations and prediction of performance in patients with brain injuries and orthopedic disorders. *Journal of the International Neuropsychological Society, 10,* 190–199. http://dx.doi.org/10.1017/S1355617704102051

Fisher, A. G. (2009). *Occupational Therapy Intervention Process Model: A model for planning and implementing top-down, client-centered, and occupation-based interventions.* Fort Collins, CO: Three Star Press.

Fisher, A. G., & Griswold, L. A. (2014). *Evaluation of Social Interaction* (3rd ed.). Fort Collins, CO: Three Star Press.

Fisher, A. G., & Jones, K. B. (2012). *Assessment of Motor and Process Skills. Vol. 1: Development, standardization, and administration manual* (rev. 7th ed.). Fort Collins, CO: Three Star Press.

Fisher, A. G., & Jones, K. B. (2014). *Assessment of Motor and Process Skills. Vol. 2: User manual* (8th ed.). Fort Collins, CO: Three Star Press.

Fisk, G. D., Schneider, J. J., & Novack, T. A. (1998). Driving following traumatic brain injury: Prevalence, exposure, advice, and evaluations. *Brain Injury, 12,* 683–695. http://dx.doi.org/10.1080/026990598122241

Flashman, L. A., & McAllister, T. W. (2002). Lack of awareness and its impact in traumatic brain injury. *NeuroRehabilitation, 17,* 285–296.

Fleming, J. M., Strong, J., & Ashton, R. (1996). Self-awareness of deficits in adults with traumatic brain injury: How best to measure? *Brain Injury, 10,* 1–15. http://dx.doi.org/10.1080/026990596124674

Franulic, A., Carbonell, C. G., Pinto, P., & Sepulveda, I. (2004). Psychosocial adjustment and employment outcome 2, 5 and 10 years after TBI. *Brain Injury, 18,* 119–129. http://dx.doi.org/10.1080/0269905031000149515

Fuhrer, M. J. (1994). Subjective well-being: Implications for medical rehabilitation outcomes and models of disablement. *American Journal of Physical Medicine and Rehabilitation, 73,* 358–364. http://dx.doi.org/10.1097/00002060-199409000-00010

Gage, M. (1992). The appraisal model of coping: An assessment and intervention model for occupational therapy. *American Journal of Occupational Therapy, 46,* 353–362. http://dx.doi.org/10.5014/ajot.46.4.353

Galski, T., Tompkins, C., & Johnston, M. V. (1998). Competence in discourse as a measure of social integration and quality of life in persons with traumatic brain injury. *Brain Injury, 12,* 769–782. http://dx.doi.org/10.1080/026990598122160

Gan, C., & Schuller, R. (2002). Family system outcome following acquired brain injury: Clinical and research perspectives. *Brain Injury, 16,* 311–322.

Gardarsdóttir, S., & Kaplan, S. (2002). Validity of the Árnadóttir OT-ADL Neurobehavioral Evaluation (A-ONE): Performance in activities of daily living and neurobehavioral impairments of persons with left and right hemisphere damage. *American Journal of Occupational Therapy, 56,* 499–508. http://dx.doi.org/10.5014/ajot.56.5.499

Garland, D., & Varpetian, A. (2003). Heterotopic ossification in traumatic brain injury. In M. Ashley (Ed.), *Traumatic brain injury rehabilitative treatment and case management* (2nd ed., pp. 119–132). Boca Raton, FL: CRC Press.

Gentry, T., Wallace, J., Kvarfordt, C., & Lynch, K. B. (2008). Personal digital assistants as cognitive aids for individuals with severe traumatic brain injury: A community-based trial. *Brain Injury, 22,* 19–24. http://dx.doi.org/10.1080/02699050701810688

Gentry, T., Wallace, J., Kvarfordt, C., & Lynch, K. B. (2010). Personal digital assistants as cognitive aids for high school students with autism: Results of a community-based trial. *Journal of Vocational Rehabilitation, 32,* 101–107. http://dx.doi.org/10.3233/JVR-2010-0499

Geurtsen, G. J., van Heugten, C. M., Martina, J. D., & Geurts, A. C. (2010). Comprehensive rehabilitation programmes in the chronic phase after severe brain injury: A systematic review. *Journal of Rehabilitation Medicine, 42,* 97–110. http://dx.doi.org/10.2340/16501977-0508

Geurtsen, G. J., van Heugten, C. M., Martina, J. D., Rietveld, A. C., Meijer, R., & Geurts, A. C. (2011). A prospective study to evaluate a residential community reintegration program for patients with chronic acquired brain injury. *Archives of Physical Medicine and Rehabilitation, 92,* 696–704. http://dx.doi.org/10.1016/j.apmr.2010.12.022

Geurtsen, G. J., van Heugten, C. M., Martina, J. D., Rietveld, A. C., Meijer, R., & Geurts, A. C. (2012). Three-year follow-up results of a residential community reintegration program for patients with chronic acquired brain injury. *Archives of Physical Medicine and Rehabilitation, 93,* 908–911. http://dx.doi.org/10.1016/j.apmr.2011.12.008

Gill, C. J., Sander, A. M., Robins, N., Mazzei, D. K., & Struchen, M. A. (2011). Exploring experiences of intimacy from the viewpoint of individuals with traumatic brain injury and their partners. *Journal of Head Trauma Rehabilitation, 26,* 56–68. http://dx.doi.org/10.1097/HTR.0b013e3182048ee9

Glang, A., Tyler, J., Pearson, S., Todis, B., & Morvant, M. (2004). Improving educational services for students with TBI through statewide consulting teams. *NeuroRehabilitation, 19,* 219–231.

Golisz, K. (2009). *Occupational therapy practice guidelines for adults with traumatic brain injury.* Bethesda, MD: AOTA Press.

Golisz, K., & Toglia, J. (2003). Perception and cognition. In E. B. Crepeau, E. S. Cohn, & B. A. Boyt Schell (Eds.), *Willard and Spackman's occupational therapy* (10th ed., pp. 395–416). Philadelphia: Lippincott Williams & Wilkins.

Gosling, J., & Oddy, M. (1999). Rearranged marriages: Marital relationships after head injury. *Brain Injury, 13,* 785–796. http://dx.doi.org/10.1080/026990599121179

Gottshall, K., Drake, A., Gray, N., McDonald, E., & Hoffer, M. E. (2003). Objective vestibular tests as outcome measures in head injury patients. *Laryngoscope, 113,* 1746–1750. http://dx.doi.org/10.1097/00005537-200310000-00016

Goverover, Y., & Hinojosa, J. (2002). Categorization and deductive reasoning: Predictors of instrumental activities of daily living performance in adults with brain injury. *American Journal of Occupational Therapy, 56,* 509–516. http://dx.doi.org/10.5014/ajot.56.5.509

Goverover, Y., Johnston, M. V., Toglia, J., & Deluca, J. (2007). Treatment to improve self-awareness in persons with acquired brain injury. *Brain Injury, 21,* 913–923. http://dx.doi.org/10.1080/02699050701553205

Grafman, J., Schwab, K., Warden, D., Pridgen, A., Brown, H. R., & Salazar, A. M. (1996). Frontal lobe injuries, violence, and aggression: A report of the Vietnam Head Injury Study. *Neurology, 46,* 1231–1238. http://dx.doi.org/10.1212/WNL.46.5.1231

Granger, C. V., Hamilton, B. B., Linacre, J. M., Heinemann, A. W., & Wright, B. D. (1993). Performance profiles of the Functional Independence Measure. *American Journal of Physical Medicine and Rehabilitation, 72,* 35–44.

Grealy, M. A., Johnson, D. A., & Rushton, S. K. (1999). Improving cognitive function after brain injury: The use of exercise and virtual reality. *Archives of Physical Medicine and Rehabilitation, 80,* 661–667. http://dx.doi.org/10.1016/S0003-9993(99)90169-7

Greve, K. W., Sherwin, E., Stanford, M. S., Mathias, C., Love, J., & Ramzinski, P. (2001). Personality and neurocognitive correlates of impulsive aggression in long-term survivors of severe traumatic brain injury. *Brain Injury, 15,* 255–262. http://dx.doi.org/10.1080/026990501300005695

Hadas-Lidor, N., Weiss, P., & Kozulin, A. (2011). Dynamic cognitive intervention: Application in occupational therapy. In N. Katz (Ed.), *Cognition, occupation, and participation across the life span: Neuroscience, neurorehabilitation, and models of intervention in occupational therapy* (3rd ed; 323–350). Bethesda, MD: AOTA Press.

Hagen, C. (1998). *The Rancho Los Amigos Levels of Cognitive Functioning: The revised levels* (3rd ed.). Downey, CA: Los Amigos Research & Educational Institute.

Hagen, C. (2003). *Traumatic brain injury: A team approach to rehabilitation for children and adults.* Atlanta: Presentation for the Continuing Education Programs of America.

Haley, S., Andres, P., Coster, W., Kosinski, M., Ni, P., & Jette, A. (2004). Short-form activity measure for post-acute care. *Archives of Physical Medicine and Rehabilitation, 85,* 649–660.

Hall, K. (1997). The Functional Assessment Measure. *Journal of Rehabilitation Outcomes, 1,* 63–65.

Hanks, R. A., Rapport, L. J., Wertheimer, J., & Koviak, C. (2012). Randomized controlled trial of peer mentoring for individuals with traumatic brain injury and their significant others. *Archives of Physical Medicine and Rehabilitation, 93,* 1297–1304. http://dx.doi.org/10.1016/j.apmr.2012.04.027

Hanks, R. A., Sander, A. M., Millis, S. R., Hammond, F. M., & Maestas, K. L. (2013). Changes in sexual functioning from 6 to 12 months following traumatic brain injury: A prospective TBI model system multicenter study. *Journal of Head Trauma Rehabilitation, 28,* 179–185. http://dx.doi.org/10.1097/HTR.0b013e31828b4fae

Harrick, L., Krefting, L., Johnston, J., Carlson, P., & Minnes, P. (1994). Stability of functional outcomes following transitional living programme participation: 3-year follow-up. *Brain Injury, 8,* 439–447. http://dx.doi.org/10.3109/02699059409150995

Hart, T., Seignourel, P. J., & Sherer, M. (2009). A longitudinal study of awareness of deficit after moderate to severe traumatic brain injury. *Neuropsychological Rehabilitation, 19*, 161–176. http://dx.doi.org/10.1080/09602010802188393

Hashimoto, K., Okamoto, T., Watanabe, S., & Ohashi, M. (2006). Effectiveness of a comprehensive day treatment program for rehabilitation of patients with acquired brain injury in Japan. *Journal of Rehabilitation Medicine, 38*, 20–25. http://dx.doi.org/10.1080/16501970510038573

Hawley, L., & Newman, J. (2006). *Social skills and traumatic brain injury: A workbook for group treatment*. Denver: Authors.

Hayden, M. E., Moreault, A. M., LeBlanc, J., & Plenger, P. M. (2000). Reducing level of handicap in traumatic brain injury: An environmentally based model of treatment. *Journal of Head Trauma Rehabilitation, 15*, 1000–1021. http://dx.doi.org/10.1097/00001199-200008000-00004

Heinemann, A. W. (2010). Measurement of participation in rehabilitation research. *Archives of Physical Medicine and Rehabilitation, 91*(Suppl.), S1–S4. http://dx.doi.org/10.1016/j.apmr.2009.08.155

Hibbard, M., Gordon, W., Flanagan, S., Haddad, L., & Labinsky, E. (2000). Sexual dysfunction after traumatic brain injury. *NeuroRehabilitation, 15*, 107–120.

Hosalkar, H., Pandya, N. K., Hsu, J. E., Kamath, A. F., & Keenan, M. A. (2010). What's new in orthopaedic rehabilitation. *Journal of Bone and Joint Surgery, 92*, 1805–1812. http://dx.doi.org/10.2106/JBJS.J.00335

Individuals With Disabilities Education Act of 1990, Pub. L. 101–476, renamed the Individuals With Disabilities Education Improvement Act, codified at 20 U.S.C. §§ 1400-1482.

Jacobsson, L. J., Westerberg, M., Söderberg, S., & Lexell, J. (2009). Functioning and disability 6–15 years after traumatic brain injuries in northern Sweden. *Acta Neurologica Scandinavica, 120*, 389–395. http://dx.doi.org/10.1111/j.1600-0404.2009.01238.x

Jean-Bay, E. (2000). The biobehavioral correlates of post-traumatic brain injury depression. *Journal of Neuroscience Nursing, 32*, 169–176. http://dx.doi.org/10.1097/01376517-200006000-00009

Jenkinson, N., Ownsworth, T., & Shum, D. (2007). Utility of the Canadian Occupational Performance Measure in community-based brain injury rehabilitation. *Brain Injury, 21*, 1283–1294. http://dx.doi.org/10.1080/02699050701739531

Johansson, U., & Bernspång, B. (2001). Predicting return to work after brain injury using occupational therapy assessments. *Disability and Rehabilitation, 23*, 474–480. http://dx.doi.org/10.1080/09638280010010688

Johansson, U., & Tham, K. (2006). The meaning of work after acquired brain injury. *American Journal of Occupational Therapy, 60*, 60–69. http://dx.doi.org/10.5014/ajot.60.1.60

Johnston, M. V., Goverover, Y., & Dijkers, M. (2005). Community activities and individuals' satisfaction with them: Quality of life in the first year after traumatic brain injury. *Archives of Physical Medicine and Rehabilitation, 86*, 735–745. http://dx.doi.org/10.1016/j.apmr.2004.10.031

Jury, M. A., & Flynn, M. C. (2001). Auditory and vestibular sequelae to traumatic brain injury: A pilot study. *New Zealand Medical Journal, 114*, 286–288.

Kalechstein, A. D., Newton, T. F., & van Gorp, W. G. (2003). Neurocognitive functioning is associated with employment status: A quantitative review. *Journal of Clinical and Experimental Neuropsychology, 25*, 1186–1191. http://dx.doi.org/10.1076/jcen.25.8.1186.16723

Katz, D. I., Zasler, N. D., & Zafonte, R. D. (2007). Clinical continuum of care and natural history. In N. D. Zasler, D. I. Katz, & R. D. Zafonte (Eds.), *Brain injury medicine: Principles and practice* (pp. 1–13). New York: Demos.

Kelley, E., Sullivan, C., Loughlin, J. K., Hutson, L., Dahdah, M. N., Long, M. K., . . . Poole, J. H. (2014). Self-awareness and neurobehavioral outcomes, 5 years or more after moderate to severe brain injury. *Journal of Head Trauma Rehabilitation, 29*, 147–152. http://dx.doi.org/10.1097/HTR.0b013e31826db6b9

Kendall, E., Shum, D., Lack, B., Bull, S., & Fee, C. (2001). Coping following traumatic brain injury: The need for contextually sensitive assessment. *Brain Impairment, 2*, 81–96. http://dx.doi.org/10.1375/brim.2.2.81

Kendall, E., & Terry, D. (1996). Psychosocial adjustment following closed head injury: A model for understanding individual differences and predicting outcome. *Neuropsychological Rehabilitation, 6*, 101–132. http://dx.doi.org/10.1080/713755502

Kennedy, M. R., & Krause, M. O. (2011). Self-regulated learning in a dynamic coaching model for supporting college students with traumatic brain injury: Two case reports. *Journal of Head Trauma Rehabilitation, 26,* 212–223. http://dx.doi.org/10.1097/HTR.0b013e318218dd0e

Kennedy, M. R., Krause, M. O., & Turkstra, L. S. (2008). An electronic survey about college experiences after traumatic brain injury. *NeuroRehabilitation, 23,* 511–520.

Kerkhoff, T. R. (2009). Ethics and healthcare reform: Can we afford the status quo? *Journal of Head Trauma Rehabilitation, 24,* 475–477. http://dx.doi.org/10.1097/HTR.0b013e3181c4cd75

Kersel, D. A., Marsh, N. V., Havill, J. H., & Sleigh, J. W. (2001). Psychosocial functioning during the year following severe traumatic brain injury. *Brain Injury, 15,* 683–696. http://dx.doi.org/10.1080/02699050010013662

Kessler, R. C., Berglund, P., Borges, G., Nock, M., & Wang, P. S. (2005). Trends in suicide ideation, plans, gestures, and attempts in the United States, 1990–1992 to 2001–2003. *JAMA, 293,* 2487–2495. http://dx.doi.org/10.1001/jama.293.20.2487

Keyser-Marcus, L. A., Bricout, J. C., Wehman, P., Campbell, L. R., Cifu, D. X., Englander, J., . . . Zafonte, R. D. (2002). Acute predictors of return to employment after traumatic brain injury: A longitudinal follow-up. *Archives of Physical Medicine and Rehabilitation, 83,* 635–641. http://dx.doi.org/10.1053/apmr.2002.31605

Khan, F., Baguley, I. J., & Cameron, I. D. (2003). Rehabilitation after traumatic brain injury. *Medical Journal of Australia, 178,* 290–295.

Kishi, Y., Robinson, R. G., & Kosier, J. T. (2001). Suicidal ideation among patients during the rehabilitation period after life-threatening physical illness. *Journal of Nervous and Mental Disease, 189,* 623–628. http://dx.doi.org/10.1097/00005053-200109000-00009

Klonoff, P. S., Watt, L. M., Dawson, L. K., Henderson, S. W., Gehrels, J. A., & Wethe, J. V. (2006). Psychosocial outcomes 1–7 years after comprehensive milieu-oriented neurorehabilitation: The role of pre-injury status. *Brain Injury, 20,* 601–612. http://dx.doi.org/10.1080/02699050600744301

Knight, R. G., Devereux, R., & Godfrey, H. P. (1998). Caring for a family member with a traumatic brain injury. *Brain Injury, 12,* 467–481. http://dx.doi.org/10.1080/026990598122430

Kohl, A. D., Wylie, G. R., Genova, H. M., Hillary, F. G., & DeLuca, J. (2009). The neural correlates of cognitive fatigue in traumatic brain injury using functional MRI. *Brain Injury, 23,* 420–432. http://dx.doi.org/10.1080/02699050902788519

Kortte, K., Wegener, S., & Chwalisz, K. (2003). Anosognosia and denial: Their relationship to coping and depression in acquired brain injury. *Rehabilitation Psychology, 48,* 131–136. http://dx.doi.org/10.1037/0090-5550.48.3.131

Koskinen, S. (1998). Quality of life 10 years after a very severe traumatic brain injury (TBI): The perspective of the injured and the closest relative. *Brain Injury, 12,* 631–648. http://dx.doi.org/10.1080/026990598122205

Kowalske, K., Plenger, P. M., Lusby, B., & Hayden, M. E. (2000). Vocational reentry following TBI: An enablement model. *Journal of Head Trauma Rehabilitation, 15,* 989–999. http://dx.doi.org/10.1097/00001199-200008000-00003

Kreuter, M., Dahllöf, A. G., Gudjonsson, G., Sullivan, M., & Siösteen, A. (1998). Sexual adjustment and its predictors after traumatic brain injury. *Brain Injury, 12,* 349–368. http://dx.doi.org/10.1080/026990598122494

Kreutzer, J., & Marwitz, J. (2008). *The Family Needs Questionnaire–Revised.* Richmond, VA: National Resource Center for Traumatic Brain Injury.

Kreutzer, J., Marwitz, J., Hsu, N., Williams, K., & Riddick, A. (2007). Marital stability after brain injury: An investigation and analysis. *NeuroRehabilitation, 22,* 53–59.

Kreutzer, J., Seel, R., & Marwitz, J. (1999). *The Neurobehavioral Functioning Inventory.* San Antonio: Psychological Corporation.

Labbe, D. R., Vance, D. E., Wadley, V., & Novack, T. A. (2014). Predictors of driving avoidance and exposure following traumatic brain injury. *Journal of Head Trauma Rehabilitation, 29,* 185–192. http://dx.doi.org/10.1097/HTR.0b013e3182795211

Larson, M. J., Perlstein, W. M., Demery, J. A., & Stigge-Kaufman, D. A. (2006). Cognitive control impairments in traumatic brain injury. *Journal of Clinical and Experimental Neuropsychology, 28,* 968–986. http://dx.doi.org/10.1080/13803390600646860

Law, M., & Baptiste, S. (2002). Working in partnerships with our clients. In M. Law, C. Baum, & S. Baptiste (Eds.), *Occupation-based practice: Fostering performance and participation* (pp. 17–25). Thorofare, NJ: Slack.

Law, M., Baptiste, S., Carswell, A., McColl, M. A., Polatajko, H., & Pollock, N. (2014). *The Canadian Occupational Performance Measure* (5th ed.). Ottawa, Ontario: CAOT Publications.

Lazaro, F., Butler, R., & Felmingham, S. (2000). In-patient neuropsychiatric brain injury rehabilitation. *Psychiatric Bulletin, 24,* 264–266. http://dx.doi.org/10.1192/pb.24.7.264

Lazarus, R., & Folkman, S. (1984). *Stress, appraisal, and coping.* New York: Springer.

Leathem, J., Heath, E., & Woolley, C. (1996). Relatives' perceptions of role change, social support and stress after traumatic brain injury. *Brain Injury, 10,* 27–38. http://dx.doi.org/10.1080/026990596124692

Lefebvre, H., Cloutier, G., & Josée Levert, M. (2008). Perspectives of survivors of traumatic brain injury and their caregivers on long-term social integration. *Brain Injury, 22,* 535–543. http://dx.doi.org/10.1080/02699050802158243

Levy, L. (2006). Psychosocial practice essentials in neurorehabilitation: Stress, coping, and adaptation. In G. Giles (Ed.), *Core concepts in neurorehabilitation* (Neurorehabilitation Self-Paced Clinical Course Series, pp. 91–122). Bethesda, MD: American Occupational Therapy Association.

Lundqvist, A., & Alinder, J. (2007). Driving after brain injury: Self-awareness and coping at the tactical level of control. *Brain Injury, 21,* 1109–1117. http://dx.doi.org/10.1080/02699050701651660

Lundqvist, A., Alinder, J., & Rönnberg, J. (2008). Factors influencing driving 10 years after brain injury. *Brain Injury, 22,* 295–304. http://dx.doi.org/10.1080/02699050801966133

Lyons, R. (1993). Meaningful activity and disability: Capitalizing upon the potential of outreach recreation networks in Canada. *Canadian Journal of Rehabilitation, 6,* 256–265.

Malec, J. F. (2001). Impact of comprehensive day treatment on societal participation for persons with acquired brain injury. *Archives of Physical Medicine and Rehabilitation, 82,* 885–895. http://dx.doi.org/10.1053/apmr.2001.23895

Malec, J. F. (2005). *Introduction to the Mayo–Portland Adaptability Inventory.* Retrieved from http://www.tbims.org/combi/mpai

Malec, J. F., & Moessner, A. M. (2006). Replicated positive results for the VCC Model of vocational intervention after ABI within the social model of disability. *Brain Injury, 20,* 227–236. http://dx.doi.org/10.1080/02699050500488124

Malec, J. F., Testa, J. A., Rush, B. K., Brown, A. W., & Moessner, A. M. (2007). Self-assessment of impairment, impaired self-awareness, and depression after traumatic brain injury. *Journal of Head Trauma Rehabilitation, 22,* 156–166. http://dx.doi.org/10.1097/01.HTR.0000271116.12028.af

Malec, J. F., & Thompson, J. M. (1994). Relationship of the Mayo–Portland Adaptability Inventory to functional outcome and cognitive performance measures. *Journal of Head Trauma Rehabilitation, 9,* 1–15.

Malley, D., Cooper, J., & Cope, J. (2008). Adapting leisure activity for adults with neuropsychological deficits following acquired brain injury. *NeuroRehabilitation, 23,* 329–334.

Mallinson, T., & Hammel, J. (2010). Measurement of participation: Intersecting person, task, and environment. *Archives of Physical Medicine and Rehabilitation, 91*(Suppl.), S29–S33. http://dx.doi.org/10.1016/j.apmr.2010.04.027

Marcotte, T. D., Rosenthal, T. J., Roberts, E., Lampinen, S., Scott, J. C., Allen, R. W., & Corey-Bloom, J. (2008). The contribution of cognition and spasticity to driving performance in multiple sclerosis. *Archives of Physical Medicine and Rehabilitation, 89,* 1753–1758. http://dx.doi.org/10.1016/j.apmr.2007.12.049

Marrelli, T., & Krulish, L. (1999). *Home care therapy: Quality, documentation, and reimbursement.* Boca Grande, FL: Marrelli & Associates.

Marsh, N. V., Kersel, D. A., Havill, J. H., & Sleigh, J. W. (1998). Caregiver burden at 6 months following severe traumatic brain injury. *Brain Injury, 12,* 225–238. http://dx.doi.org/10.1080/026990598122700

Martz, E. (2003). Invisibility of disability and work experience as predictors of employment among community college students with disabilities. *Journal of Vocational Rehabilitation, 18,* 153–161.

Marwitz, J., Cifu, D. X., Englander, J., & High, W. M., Jr. (2001). A multi-center analysis of rehospitalizations five years after brain injury. *Journal of Head Trauma Rehabilitation, 16,* 307–317. http://dx.doi.org/10.1097/00001199-200108000-00002

Marwitz, J., & Kreutzer, J. (1996). *The Service Obstacles Scale (SOS).* Richmond: Medical College of Virginia of Virginia Commonwealth University.

Masel, B. E., Scheibel, R. S., Kimbark, T., & Kuna, S. T. (2001). Excessive daytime sleepiness in adults with brain injuries. *Archives of Physical Medicine and Rehabilitation, 82,* 1526–1532. http://dx.doi.org/10.1053/apmr.2001.26093

Mathias, J. L., & Wheaton, P. (2007). Changes in attention and information-processing speed following severe traumatic brain injury: A meta-analytic review. *Neuropsychology, 21,* 212–223. http://dx.doi.org/10.1037/0894-4105.21.2.212

Max, J. (2005). Children and adolescents. In J. M. Silver, T. W. McAllister, & S. C. Yudofsky (Eds.), *Textbook of traumatic brain injury* (pp. 477–494). Washington, DC: American Psychiatric Publishing.

McCabe, P., Lippert, C., Weiser, M., Hilditch, M., Hartridge, C., & Villamere, J.; ERABI Group. (2007). Community reintegration following acquired brain injury. *Brain Injury, 21,* 231–257. http://dx.doi.org/10.1080/02699050701201631

McColl, M. A. (1998). What do we need to know to practice occupational therapy in the community? *American Journal of Occupational Therapy, 52,* 11–18. http://dx.doi.org/10.5014/ajot.52.1.11

McColl, M. A., & Bickenbach, J. (1998). Consequences of disability. In M. A. McColl & J. Bickenbach (Eds.), *Introduction to disability* (pp. 131–133). Philadelphia: W. B. Saunders.

McColl, M. A., Carlson, P., Johnston, J., Minnes, P., Shue, K., Davies, D., & Karlovits, T. (1998). The definition of community integration: Perspectives of people with brain injuries. *Brain Injury, 12,* 15–30. http://dx.doi.org/10.1080/026990598122827

McColl, M. A., Davies, D., Carlson, P., Johnston, J., & Minnes, P. (2001). The Community Integration Measure: Development and preliminary validation. *Archives of Physical Medicine and Rehabilitation, 82,* 429–434. http://dx.doi.org/10.1053/apmr.2001.22195

McCrimmon, S., & Oddy, M. (2006). Return to work following moderate-to-severe traumatic brain injury. *Brain Injury, 20,* 1037–1046. http://dx.doi.org/10.1080/02699050600909656

McDonald, B. C., Flashman, L. A., & Saykin, A. J. (2002). Executive dysfunction following traumatic brain injury: Neural substrates and treatment strategies. *NeuroRehabilitation, 17,* 333–344.

McDonald, S., & Flanagan, S. (2004). Social perception deficits after traumatic brain injury: Interaction between emotion recognition, mentalizing ability, and social communication. *Neuropsychology, 18,* 572–579. http://dx.doi.org/10.1037/0894-4105.18.3.572

Melamed, S., Groswasser, Z., & Stern, M. J. (1992). Acceptance of disability, work involvement and subjective rehabilitation status of traumatic brain-injured (TBI) patients. *Brain Injury, 6,* 233–243. http://dx.doi.org/10.3109/02699059209029665

Mellick, D., Walker, N., Brooks, C., & Whiteneck, G. (1999). Incorporating the cognitive independence domain into CHART. *Journal of Rehabilitation Outcomes Measurement, 3,* 12–21.

Mohr, J., & Bullock, L. (2005). Traumatic brain injury: Perspectives from educational professionals. *Preventing School Failure, 49,* 53–57. http://dx.doi.org/10.3200/PSFL.49.4.53-57

Moore, A. (1996). The band community: Synchronizing human activity cycles for group cooperation. In R. Zemke & F. Clark (Eds.), *Occupational science: The evolving discipline* (pp. 95–106). Philadelphia: F. A. Davis.

Moore, A. D., & Stambrook, M. (1995). Cognitive moderators of outcome following traumatic brain injury: A conceptual model and implications for rehabilitation. *Brain Injury, 9,* 109–130. http://dx.doi.org/10.3109/02699059509008185

Mosey, A. (1981). *Occupational therapy: Configuration of a profession.* New York: Raven Press.

Nalder, E., Fleming, J., Foster, M., Cornwell, P., Shields, C., & Khan, A. (2012). Identifying factors associated with perceived success in the transition from hospital to home after brain injury. *Journal of Head Trauma Rehabilitation, 27,* 143–153. http://dx.doi.org/10.1097/HTR.0b013e3182168fb1

Namdari, S., Alosh, H., Baldwin, K., Mehta, S., & Keenan, M. A. (2012). Outcomes of tendon fractional lengthenings to improve shoulder function in patients with spastic hemiparesis. *Journal of Shoulder and Elbow Surgery, 21,* 691–698. http://dx.doi.org/10.1016/j.jse.2011.03.026

Namdari, S., Horneff, J. G., Baldwin, K., & Keenan, M. A. (2012). Muscle releases to improve passive motion and relieve pain in patients with spastic hemiplegia and elbow flexion contractures. *Journal of Shoulder and Elbow Surgery, 21,* 1357–1362. http://dx.doi.org/10.1016/j.jse.2011.09.029

Noé, E., Ferri, J., Caballero, M. C., Villodre, R., Sanchez, A., & Chirivella, J. (2005). Self-awareness after acquired brain injury: Predictors and rehabilitation. *Journal of Neurology, 252,* 168–175. http://dx.doi.org/10.1007/s00415-005-0625-2

Novack, T., Labbe, D., Grote, M., Carlson, N., Sherer, M., Hart, T., . . . Seel, R. (2010). Return to driving within 5 years of moderate to severe traumatic brain injury. *Brain Injury, 24,* 464–471. http://dx.doi.org/10.3109/02699051003601713

Novakovic-Agopian, T., Chen, A. J., Rome, S., Rossi, A., Abrams, G., D' Esposito, M., . . . Castelli, H. (2014). Assessment of subcomponents of executive functioning in ecologically valid settings: The Goal Processing Scale. *Journal of Head Trauma Rehabilitation, 29,* 136–146. http://dx.doi.org/10.1097/HTR.0b013e3182691b15

O'Brien, L. (2007). Achieving a successful and sustainable return to the workforce after ABI: A client-centered approach. *Brain Injury, 21,* 465–478. http://dx.doi.org/10.1080/02699050701315134

O'Callaghan, A., McAllister, L., & Wilson, L. (2012). Insight vs readiness: Factors affecting engagement in therapy from the perspectives of adults with TBI and their significant others. *Brain Injury, 26,* 1599–1610. http://dx.doi.org/10.3109/02699052.2012.698788

Orman, J. A. L., Kraus, J. F., Zaloshnja, E., & Miller, T. (2011). Epidemiology. In J. M. Silver, T. W. McAllister, & S. C. Yudofsky (Eds.), *Textbook of traumatic brain injury* (2nd ed., pp. 3–22). Washington, DC: American Psychiatric Publishing.

Ortoleva, C., Brugger, C., Van der Linden, M., & Walder, B. (2012). Prediction of driving capacity after traumatic brain injury: A systematic review. *Journal of Head Trauma Rehabilitation, 27,* 302–313. http://dx.doi.org/10.1097/HTR.0b013e3182236299

Ostir, G. V., Granger, C. V., Black, T., Roberts, P., Burgos, L., Martinkewiz, P., & Ottenbacher, K. J. (2006). Preliminary results for the PAR-PRO: A measure of home and community participation. *Archives of Physical Medicine and Rehabilitation, 87,* 1043–1051. http://dx.doi.org/10.1016/j.apmr.2006.04.024

Ouellet, M. C., Morin, C. M., & Lavoie, A. (2009). Volunteer work and psychological health following traumatic brain injury. *Journal of Head Trauma Rehabilitation, 24,* 262–271. http://dx.doi.org/10.1097/HTR.0b013e3181a68b73

Ouellet, M. C., Savard, J., & Morin, C. M. (2004). Insomnia following traumatic brain injury: A review. *Neurorehabilitation and Neural Repair, 18,* 187–198. http://dx.doi.org/10.1177/1545968304271405

Ownsworth, T., & Clare, L. (2006). The association between awareness deficits and rehabilitation outcome following acquired brain injury. *Clinical Psychology Review, 26,* 783–795. http://dx.doi.org/10.1016/j.cpr.2006.05.003

Ownsworth, T., Little, T., Turner, B., Hawkes, A., & Shum, D. (2008). Assessing emotional status following acquired brain injury: The clinical potential of the Depression, Anxiety and Stress Scales. *Brain Injury, 22,* 858–869. http://dx.doi.org/10.1080/02699050802446697

Ownsworth, T. L., & Oei, T. P. (1998). Depression after traumatic brain injury: Conceptualization and treatment considerations. *Brain Injury, 12,* 735–751. http://dx.doi.org/10.1080/026990598122133

Page, S. J., Levine, P., Leonard, A., Szaflarski, J. P., & Kissela, B. M. (2008). Modified constraint-induced therapy in chronic stroke: Results of a single-blinded randomized controlled trial. *Physical Therapy, 88,* 333–340. http://dx.doi.org/10.2522/ptj.20060029

Pape, H. C., Marsh, S., Morley, J. R., Krettek, C., & Giannoudis, P. V. (2004). Current concepts in the development of heterotopic ossification. *Journal of Bone and Joint Surgery, 86,* 783–787. http://dx.doi.org/10.1302/0301-620X.86B6.15356

Parente, R., & Anderson-Parente, J. (1989). Retraining memory: Theory and application. *Journal of Head Trauma Rehabilitation, 4,* 55–65. http://dx.doi.org/10.1097/00001199-198909000-00009

Parente, R., & Hermann, D. (2003). *Retraining cognition: Techniques and applications* (2nd ed.). Austin, TX: PRO-ED.

Pawlowski, J., Dixon-Ibarra, A., & Driver, S. (2013). Review of the status of physical activity research for individuals with traumatic brain injury. *Archives of Physical Medicine and Rehabilitation, 94,* 1184–1189. http://dx.doi.org/10.1016/j.apmr.2013.01.005

Perry, S. B., Woollard, J., Little, S., & Shroyer, K. (2014). Relationships among measures of balance, gait, and community integration in people with brain injury. *Journal of Head Trauma Rehabilitation, 29,* 117–124. http://dx.doi.org/10.1097/HTR.0b013e3182864f2f

Phipps, S. (2006). Community participation. In K. Golisz (Ed.) & G. M. Giles (Series Ed.), *Neurorehabilitation for traumatic brain injury* (Neurorehabilitation Self-Paced Clinical Course Series, pp. 93–134). Bethesda, MD: American Occupational Therapy Association.

Ponsford, J. (2003). Sexual changes associated with traumatic brain injury. *Neuropsychological Rehabilitation, 13,* 275–289. http://dx.doi.org/10.1080/09602010244000363

Ponsford, J., Downing, M. G., & Stolwyk, R. (2013). Factors associated with sexuality following traumatic brain injury. *Journal of Head Trauma Rehabilitation, 28,* 195–201. http://dx.doi.org/10.1097/HTR.0b013e31828b4f7b

Ponsford, J., Draper, K., & Schönberger, M. (2008). Functional outcome 10 years after traumatic brain injury: Its relationship with demographic, injury severity, and cognitive and emotional status. *Journal of the International Neuropsychological Society, 14,* 233–242. http://dx.doi.org/10.1017/S1355617708080272

Ponsford, J., Olver, J., & Curran, C. (1995). A profile of outcome: 2 years after traumatic brain injury. *Brain Injury, 9,* 1–10. http://dx.doi.org/10.3109/02699059509004565

Ponsford, J., Olver, J., Ponsford, M., & Nelms, R. (2003). Long-term adjustment of families following traumatic brain injury where comprehensive rehabilitation has been provided. *Brain Injury, 17,* 453–468. http://dx.doi.org/10.1080/0269905031000070143

Ponsford, J., Schönberger, M., & Rajaratnam, S. M. W. (2015). A model of fatigue following traumatic brain injury. *Journal of Head Trauma Rehabilitation, 30,* 277–282. http://dx.doi.org/10.1097/HTR.0000000000000049

Ponsford, J., & Spitz, G. (2014). Stability of employment over the first 3 years following traumatic brain injury. *Journal of Head Trauma Rehabilitation, 30,* E1–E11. http://dx.doi.org/10.1097/HTR.0000000000000033

Ponsford, J., Ziino, C., Parcell, D. L., Shekleton, J. A., Roper, M., Redman, J. R., . . . Rajaratnam, S. M. (2012). Fatigue and sleep disturbance following traumatic brain injury: Their nature, causes, and potential treatments. *Journal of Head Trauma Rehabilitation, 27,* 224–233. http://dx.doi.org/10.1097/HTR.0b013e31824ee1a8

Powell, J., Beckers, K., & Greenwood, R. (1998). Measuring progress and outcome in rehabilitation after brain injury with a new assessment instrument—The BICRO–39 scales. Brain Injury Community Rehabilitation Outcome. *Archives of Physical Medicine and Rehabilitation, 79,* 1213–1225.

Powell, J. M., Temkin, N. R., Machamer, J. E., & Dikmen, S. S. (2007). Gaining insight into patients' perspectives on participation in home management activities after traumatic brain injury. *American Journal of Occupational Therapy, 61,* 269–279. http://dx.doi.org/10.5014/ajot.61.3.269

Prigatano, G. P. (1989). Work, love, and play after brain injury. *Bulletin of the Menninger Clinic, 53,* 414–431.

Prigatano, G. P., & Altman, I. M. (1990). Impaired awareness of behavioral limitations after traumatic brain injury. *Archives of Physical Medicine and Rehabilitation, 71,* 1058–1064.

Prigatano, G. P., & Klonoff, P. (1998). A clinician's rating scale for evaluating impaired self-awareness and denial of disability after brain injury. *Clinical Neuropsychologist, 12,* 56–67. http://dx.doi.org/10.1076/clin.12.1.56.1721

Rapport, L. J., Bryer, R. C., & Hanks, R. A. (2008). Driving and community integration after traumatic brain injury. *Archives of Physical Medicine and Rehabilitation, 89,* 922–930. http://dx.doi.org/10.1016/j.apmr.2008.01.009

Rapport, L. J., Hanks, R. A., & Bryer, R. C. (2006). Barriers to driving and community integration after traumatic brain injury. *Journal of Head Trauma Rehabilitation, 21,* 34–44. http://dx.doi.org/10.1097/00001199-200601000-00004

Rittman, M., Faircloth, C., Boylstein, C., Gubrium, J. F., Williams, C., Van Puymbroeck, M., & Ellis, C. (2004). The experience of time in the transition from hospital to home following stroke. *Journal of Rehabilitation Research and Development, 41,* 259–268. http://dx.doi.org/10.1682/JRRD.2003.06.0099

Robinson, B. C. (1983). Validation of a Caregiver Strain Index. *Journal of Gerontology, 38,* 344–348. http://dx.doi.org/10.1093/geronj/38.3.344

Rosenthal, M., Christensen, B. K., & Ross, T. P. (1998). Depression following traumatic brain injury. *Archives of Physical Medicine and Rehabilitation, 79,* 90–103. http://dx.doi.org/10.1016/S0003-9993(98)90215-5

Rowlands, A. (2001). Ability or disability? Strength-based practice in the area of traumatic brain injury. *Families in Society, 82,* 273–286. http://dx.doi.org/10.1606/1044-3894.201

Ruttan, L., Martin, K., Liu, A., Colella, B., & Green, R. E. (2008). Long-term cognitive out-come in moderate to severe traumatic brain injury: A meta-analysis examining timed and untimed tests at 1 and 4.5 or more years after injury. *Archives of Physical Medicine and Rehabilitation, 89*(Suppl.), S69–S76. http://dx.doi.org/10.1016/j.apmr.2008.07.007

Sale, P., Revell, W., West, M., & Kregel, J. (1992). Achievements and challenges II: A five-year analysis of supported employment expenditures. *Journal of the Association for Persons With Severe Handicaps, 17,* 236–246.

Sander, A. M., Clark, A., & Pappadis, M. R. (2010). What is community integration anyway? Defining meaning following traumatic brain injury. *Journal of Head Trauma Rehabilitation, 25,* 121–127. http://dx.doi.org/10.1097/HTR.0b013e3181cd1635

Sander, A. M., Pappadis, M. R., Clark, A. N., & Struchen, M. A. (2011). Perceptions of com-munity integration in an ethnically diverse sample. *Journal of Head Trauma Rehabilitation, 26,* 158–169. http://dx.doi.org/10.1097/HTR.0b013e3181e7537e

Schwandt, M., Harris, J. E., Thomas, S., Keightley, M., Snaiderman, A., & Colantonio, A. (2012). Feasibility and effect of aerobic exercise for lowering depressive symptoms among individuals with traumatic brain injury: A pilot study. *Journal of Head Trauma Rehabilita-tion, 27,* 99–103. http://dx.doi.org/10.1097/HTR.0b013e31820e6858

Schwartzberg, S., Howe, M., & Barnes, M. A. (2008). *Groups: Applying the functional group model.* Philadelphia: F. A. Davis.

Seel, R. T., Kreutzer, J. S., Rosenthal, M., Hammond, F. M., Corrigan, J. D., & Black, K. (2003). Depression after traumatic brain injury: A National Institute on Disability and Rehabilita-tion Research Model Systems multicenter investigation. *Archives of Physical Medicine and Rehabilitation, 84,* 177–184. http://dx.doi.org/10.1053/apmr.2003.50106

Senelick, R., & Dougherty, K. (2001). *Living with brain injury: A guide for families.* Birmingham, AL: Healthsouth Press.

Shallice, T., & Burgess, P. W. (1991). Deficits in strategy application following frontal lobe damage in man. *Brain, 114,* 727–741.

Shaw, S. E., Morris, D. M., Uswatte, G., McKay, S., Meythaler, J. M., & Taub, E. (2005). Constraint-induced movement therapy for recovery of upper-limb function following traumatic brain injury. *Journal of Rehabilitation Research and Development, 42,* 769–778. http://dx.doi.org/10.1682/JRRD.2005.06.0094

Sherer, M., Bergloff, P., Boake, C., High, W., Jr., & Levin, E. (1998). The Awareness Question-naire: Factor structure and internal consistency. *Brain Injury, 12,* 63–68. http://dx.doi.org/10.1080/026990598122863

Shi, Y. X., Tian, J. H., Yang, K. H., & Zhao, Y. (2011). Modified constraint-induced movement therapy versus traditional rehabilitation in patients with upper-extremity dysfunction after stroke: A systematic review and meta-analysis. *Archives of Physical Medicine and Reha-bilitation, 92,* 972–982. http://dx.doi.org/10.1016/j.apmr.2010.12.036

Simmons, C. D., & Griswold, L. A. (2010). Using the Evaluation of Social Interaction in a community-based program for persons with traumatic brain injury. *Scandinavian Journal of Occupational Therapy, 17,* 49–56. http://dx.doi.org/10.3109/11038120903350303

Simpson, G., & Tate, R. (2002). Suicidality after traumatic brain injury: Demographic, injury and clinical correlates. *Psychological Medicine, 32,* 687–697.

Simpson, G., & Tate, R. (2007). Suicidality in people surviving a traumatic brain injury: Preva-lence, risk factors and implications for clinical management. *Brain Injury, 21,* 1335–1351. http://dx.doi.org/10.1080/02699050701785542

Sloan, S., Winkler, D., & Callaway, L. (2004). Community integration following severe trau-matic brain injury: Outcomes and best practice. *Brain Impairment, 5,* 12–29. http://dx.doi.org/10.1375/brim.5.1.12.35399

Souza, W., Conforto, A., Orsini, M., Stern, A., & Andre, C. (2015). Similar effects of two modified constraint-induced therapy protocols on motor impairment, motor func-tion, and quality of life in patients with chronic stroke. *Neurology International, 7,* 5430. http://dx.doi.org/10.4081/ni.2015.5430

Spitz, G., Schönberger, M., & Ponsford, J. (2013). The relations among cognitive impairment, coping style, and emotional adjustment following traumatic brain injury. *Journal of Head Trauma Rehabilitation, 28,* 116–125. http://dx.doi.org/10.1097/HTR.0b013e3182452f4f

Strauss, E., Sherman, E., & Spreen, O. (2006). *A compendium of neuropsychological tests.* New York: Oxford University Press.

Sunderland, A., & Harris, J. (1994). Memory failures in everyday life following severe head injury. *Journal of Clinical Neuropsychology, 6,* 127–142.

Suto, M. (1998). Leisure in occupational therapy. *Canadian Journal of Occupational Therapy, 65,* 271–278. http://dx.doi.org/10.1177/000841749806500504

Taub, E., Uswatte, G., & Elbert, T. (2002). New treatments in neurorehabilitation founded on basic research. *Nature Reviews Neuroscience, 3,* 228–236. http://dx.doi.org/10.1038/nrn754

Taub, E., & Wolfe, S. (1997). Constraint-induced movement techniques to facilitate upper extremity use in stroke patients. *Topics in Stroke Rehabilitation, 3,* 38–61.

Taylor, H. G., Yeates, K. O., Wade, S. L., Drotar, D., Stancin, T., & Minich, N. (2002). A prospective study of short- and long-term outcomes after traumatic brain injury in children: Behavior and achievement. *Neuropsychology, 16,* 15–27. http://dx.doi.org/10.1037/0894-4105.16.1.15

Temkin, N., Corrigan, J., Dikmen, S., & Machamer, J. (2009). Social functioning after traumatic brain injury. *Journal of Head Trauma Rehabilitation, 24,* 460–467. http://dx.doi.org/10.1097/HTR.0b013e318c13413

Testa, J. A., Malec, J. F., Moessner, A. M., & Brown, A. W. (2006). Predicting family functioning after TBI: Impact of neurobehavioral factors. *Journal of Head Trauma Rehabilitation, 21,* 236–247. http://dx.doi.org/10.1097/00001199-200605000-00004

Toglia, J. P. (2011). The Dynamic Interactional Model of cognition in cognitive rehabilitation. In N. Katz (Ed.), *Cognition, occupation, and participation across the life span: Neuroscience, neurorehabilitation, and models of intervention in occupational therapy* (3rd ed., pp. 161–201). Bethesda, MD: AOTA Press.

Toglia, J. P., & Golisz, K. M. (2012). Therapy for activities of daily living: Theoretical and practical perspectives. In N. D. Zasler, D. I. Katz, & R. D. Zafonte (Eds.), *Brain injury medicine: Principles and practice* (2nd ed., pp. 1162–1177). New York: Demos.

Toglia, J. P., & Kirk, U. (2000). Understanding awareness deficits following brain injury. *Neuro-Rehabilitation, 15,* 57–70.

Trahan, E., Pépin, M., & Hopps, S. (2006). Impaired awareness of deficits and treatment adherence among people with traumatic brain injury or spinal cord injury. *Journal of Head Trauma Rehabilitation, 21,* 226–235. http://dx.doi.org/10.1097/00001199-200605000-00003

Trexler, L. E., Trexler, L. C., Malec, J. F., Klyce, D., & Parrott, D. (2010). Prospective randomized controlled trial of resource facilitation on community participation and vocational outcome following brain injury. *Journal of Head Trauma Rehabilitation, 25,* 440–446. http://dx.doi.org/10.1097/HTR.0b013e3181d41139

Trombly, C. A., Radomski, M. V., Trexel, C., & Burnet-Smith, S. E. (2002). Occupational therapy and achievement of self-identified goals by adults with acquired brain injury: Phase II. *American Journal of Occupational Therapy, 56,* 489–498. http://dx.doi.org/10.5014/ajot.56.5.489

Trudel, T., Tryon, W., & Purdum, C. (1998). Awareness of disability and long-term outcome after traumatic brain injury. *Rehabilitation Psychology, 43,* 267–281. http://dx.doi.org/10.1037/0090-5550.43.4.267

Tsaousides, T., Ashman, T., & Seter, C. (2008). The psychological effects of employment after traumatic brain injury: Objective and subjective indicators. *Rehabilitation Psychology, 53,* 456–463. http://dx.doi.org/10.1037/a0012579

Tsaousides, T., Cantor, J. B., & Gordon, W. A. (2011). Suicidal ideation following traumatic brain injury: Prevalence rates and correlates in adults living in the community. *Journal of Head Trauma Rehabilitation, 26,* 265–275. http://dx.doi.org/10.1097/HTR.0b013e3182225271

Tsaousides, T., & Gordon, W. A. (2009). Cognitive rehabilitation following traumatic brain injury: Assessment to treatment. *Mount Sinai Journal of Medicine, 76,* 173–181. http://dx.doi.org/10.1002/msj.20099

Turner, B., Fleming, J., Cornwell, P., Haines, T., & Ownsworth, T. (2009). Profiling early outcomes during the transition from hospital to home after brain injury. *Brain Injury, 23,* 51–60. http://dx.doi.org/10.1080/02699050802635257

Turner, B., Fleming, J., Ownsworth, T., & Cornwell, P. (2011). Perceptions of recovery during the early transition phase from hospital to home following acquired brain injury: A journey of discovery. *Neuropsychological Rehabilitation, 21,* 64–91. http://dx.doi.org/10.1080/09602011.2010.527747

Turner, B., Ownsworth, T., Turpin, M., Fleming, J., & Griffin, J. (2008). Self-identified goals and the ability to set realistic goals following acquired brain injury: A classified framework. *Australian Journal of Occupational Therapy, 55,* 96–107. http://dx.doi.org/10.1111/j.1440-1630.2007.00660.x

Turner, H., Chapman, S., McSherry, A., Krishnagiri, S., & Watts, J. (2000). Leisure assessment in occupational therapy: An exploratory study. *Occupational Therapy in Health Care, 12,* 73–85. http://dx.doi.org/10.1080/J003v12n02_05

Underhill, A. T., Lobello, S. G., Stroud, T. P., Terry, K. S., Devivo, M. J., & Fine, P. R. (2003). Depression and life satisfaction in patients with traumatic brain injury: A longitudinal study. *Brain Injury, 17,* 973–982. http://dx.doi.org/10.1080/0269905031000110418

Vaishnavi, S., Rao, V., & Fann, J. R. (2009). Neuropsychiatric problems after traumatic brain injury: Unraveling the silent epidemic. *Psychosomatics, 50,* 198–205. http://dx.doi.org/10.1176/appi.psy.50.3.198

Vakil, E., Kraus, A., Bor, B., & Groswasser, Z. (2002). Impaired skill learning in patients with severe closed-head injury as demonstrated by the serial reaction time (SRT) task. *Brain and Cognition, 50,* 304–315. http://dx.doi.org/10.1016/S0278-2626(02)00515-8

Vandiver, V. L., Johnson, J., & Christofero-Snider, C. (2003). Supporting employment for adults with acquired brain injury: A conceptual model. *Journal of Head Trauma Rehabilitation, 18,* 457–463. http://dx.doi.org/10.1097/00001199-200309000-00007

Vangel, S. J., Jr., Rapport, L. J., & Hanks, R. A. (2011). Effects of family and caregiver psychosocial functioning on outcomes in persons with traumatic brain injury. *Journal of Head Trauma Rehabilitation, 26,* 20–29. http://dx.doi.org/10.1097/HTR.0b013e318204a70d

Wagner, M., Newman, L., Cameto, R., Garza, N., & Levine, P. (2005). *After high school: A first look at the postschool experiences of youth with disabilities: A report from the National Longitudinal Transition Study–2 (NLTS–2).* Menlo Park, CA: SRI International. Retrieved from http://www.nlts2.org/reports/2005_04/nlts2_report_2005_04_execsum.pdf

Walker, W. C., Marwitz, J. H., Kreutzer, J. S., Hart, T., & Novack, T. A. (2006). Occupational categories and return to work after traumatic brain injury: A multicenter study. *Archives of Physical Medicine and Rehabilitation, 87,* 1576–1582. http://dx.doi.org/10.1016/j.apmr.2006.08.335

Walker, W. C., & Pickett, T. C. (2007). Motor impairment after severe traumatic brain injury: A longitudinal multicenter study. *Journal of Rehabilitation Research and Development, 44,* 975–982. http://dx.doi.org/10.1682/JRRD.2006.12.0158

Wallace, C. A., & Bogner, J. (2000). Awareness of deficits: Emotional implications for persons with brain injury and their significant others. *Brain Injury, 14,* 549–562. http://dx.doi.org/10.1080/026990500120457

Warden, D. L., Salazar, A. M., Martin, E. M., Schwab, K. A., Coyle, M., & Walter, J.; DVHIP Study Group. (2000). A home program of rehabilitation for moderately severe traumatic brain injury patients. *Journal of Head Trauma Rehabilitation, 15,* 1092–1102. http://dx.doi.org/10.1097/00001199-200010000-00003

Warren, L., Wrigley, J. M., Yoels, W. C., & Fine, P. R. (1996). Factors associated with life satisfaction among a sample of persons with neurotrauma. *Journal of Rehabilitation Research and Development, 33,* 404–408.

Wehman, P., Gentry, T., West, M., & Arango-Lasprilla, J. C. (2009). Community integration: Current issues in cognitive and vocational rehabilitation for individuals with ABI. *Journal of Rehabilitation Research and Development, 46,* 909–918. http://dx.doi.org/10.1682/JRRD.2008.08.0105

Wehman, P., Kregel, J., Keyser-Marcus, L., Sherron-Targett, P., Campbell, L., West, M., & Cifu, D. X. (2003). Supported employment for persons with traumatic brain injury: A preliminary investigation of long-term follow-up costs and program efficiency. *Archives of Physical Medicine and Rehabilitation, 84,* 192–196. http://dx.doi.org/10.1053/apmr.2003.50027

Wehman, P., Targett, P., West, M., & Kregel, J. (2005). Productive work and employment for persons with traumatic brain injury: What have we learned after 20 years? *Journal of Head Trauma Rehabilitation, 20,* 115–127. http://dx.doi.org/10.1097/00001199-200503000-00001

Wheeler, S. (2012). The impact of intensive community-based rehabilitation on community participation and life satisfaction following severe traumatic brain injury. In A. Agriwal (Ed.), *Brain injury: Functional aspects, rehabilitation, and prevention* (pp. 95–120). Rijeka, Croatia: Intech.

Wheeler, S. (2014). Providing occupational therapy for individuals with traumatic brain injury. In B. A. Boyt Schell, G. Gillen, M. E. Scaffa, & E. S. Cohn (Eds.), *Willard and Spackman's occupational therapy* (12th ed., pp. 925–935). Philadelphia: Lippincott Williams & Wilkins.

Wheeler, S., Lane, S., & McMahon, B. (2007). Community participation and life satisfaction following intensive community-based rehabilitation using a life skills training approach. *OTJR: Occupation, Participation and Health, 27,* 13–22. http://dx.doi.org/10.1177/153944920702700103

Whiteneck, G. G., Charlifue, S. W., Gerhart, K. A., Overholser, J. D., & Richardson, G. N. (1992). Quantifying handicap: A new measure of long-term rehabilitation outcomes. *Archives of Physical Medicine and Rehabilitation, 73,* 519–526.

Whiteneck, G. G., Dijkers, M. P., Heinemann, A. W., Bogner, J. A., Bushnik, T., Cicerone, K. D., . . . Millis, S. R. (2011). Development of the Participation Assessment With Recombined Tools–Objective for use after traumatic brain injury. *Archives of Physical Medicine and Rehabilitation, 92,* 542–551. http://dx.doi.org/10.1016/j.apmr.2010.08.002

Whiteneck, G. G., Harrison-Felix, C. L., Mellick, D. C., Brooks, C. A., Charlifue, S. B., & Gerhart, K. A. (2004). Quantifying environmental factors: A measure of physical, attitudinal, service, productivity, and policy barriers. *Archives of Physical Medicine and Rehabilitation, 85,* 1324–1335. http://dx.doi.org/10.1016/j.apmr.2003.09.027

Willer, B., & Corrigan, J. (1994). Whatever It Takes: A model for community-based services. *Brain Injury, 8,* 647–659. http://dx.doi.org/10.3109/02699059409151017

Willer, B., Ottenbacher, K. J., & Coad, M. L. (1994). The Community Integration Questionnaire: A comparative examination. *American Journal of Physical Medicine and Rehabilitation, 73,* 103–111. http://dx.doi.org/10.1097/00002060-199404000-00006

Wise, E. K., Hoffman, J. M., Powell, J. M., Bombardier, C. H., & Bell, K. R. (2012). Benefits of exercise maintenance after traumatic brain injury. *Archives of Physical Medicine and Rehabilitation, 93,* 1319–1323. http://dx.doi.org/10.1016/j.apmr.2012.05.009

Wood, R. L., & Doughty, C. (2013). Alexithymia and avoidance coping following traumatic brain injury. *Journal of Head Trauma Rehabilitation, 28,* 98–105. http://dx.doi.org/10.1097/HTR.0b013e3182426029

Wood, R. L., & Rutterford, N. A. (2006). Psychosocial adjustment 17 years after severe brain injury. *Journal of Neurology, Neurosurgery, and Psychiatry, 77,* 71–73. http://dx.doi.org/10.1136/jnnp.2005.065540

World Health Organization. (2001). *International classification of functioning, disability and health.* Geneva: Author.

Wressle, E., Eeg-Olofsson, A. M., Marcusson, J., & Henriksson, C. (2002). Improved client participation in the rehabilitation process using a client-centered goal formulation structure. *Journal of Rehabilitation Medicine, 34,* 5–11. http://dx.doi.org/10.1080/165019702317242640

Yalom, I. (1995). *The theory and practice of group psychotherapy.* New York: Basic Books.

Ylvisaker, M. (2003). Context-sensitive cognitive rehabilitation after traumatic brain injury: Theory and practice. *Brain Impairment, 4,* 1–16. http://dx.doi.org/10.1375/brim.4.1.1.27031

Ylvisaker, M., & Feeney, T. (1998). Everyday people as supports: Developing competencies through collaboration. In M. Ylvisaker (Ed.), *Traumatic brain injury rehabilitation: Children and adolescents* (pp. 429–464). Boston: Butterworth-Heinemann.

Zoltan, B. (2007). *Vision, perception, and cognition: A manual for the evaluation and treatment of the adult with acquired brain injury* (4th ed.). Thorofare, NJ: Slack.

CHAPTER 8

Special Considerations for Traumatic Brain Injury in Military Personnel

Jenny Owens, OTD, OTR/L

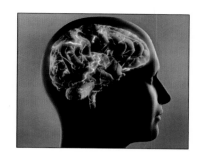

Learning Objectives

After completion of this chapter, readers will be able to
- Identify the incidence and significance of mild traumatic brain injury (mTBI) in the military population;
- Identify signs, symptoms, and functional implications of mTBI in military personnel;
- Select appropriate evaluation measures for mTBI in military personnel;
- Identify appropriate interventions for mTBI in military personnel; and
- Delineate the challenges to recovery and reintegration that are unique to the combat-injured population.

Introduction

The occupational therapy profession was birthed during a time of war. During and after World War I, wounded military personnel were found to have improved rehabilitative outcomes when engaged in functional activities including arts, crafts, and constructional tasks. Consequently, the medical community's understanding of recovery was altered by the recognition that the healing process can be expedited through meaningful and purposeful activity (Newton, 2007). Building on the foundations of the post–World War I reconstruction aides, today's occupational therapists continue to make vital contributions to help wounded military service personnel heal in body, mind, and spirit. The wars in Iraq and Afghanistan have further developed occupational therapists' expertise in the rehabilitative care of **polytrauma** injuries, including mild traumatic brain injury (mTBI; see Chapter 1) and **posttraumatic stress disorder** (PTSD). This chapter aims to help occupational therapists understand and respond to the unique challenges faced by combat-wounded military personnel.

Key Words

- **blast injury**
- **community reintegration**
- **executive function**
- **exertional testing**
- **functional assessment**
- **metacognition**
- **military mind-set**
- **multidisciplinary treatment approach**
- **personal and situational factors**
- **polytrauma**
- **postconcussion syndrome**
- **PTSD**
- **relaxation training**
- **return to duty**
- **visual disturbances**

Building on the foundations of the post–World War I reconstruction aides, today's occupational therapists continue to make vital contributions to help wounded military service personnel heal in body, mind, and spirit.

Since the onset of Operation Enduring Freedom (OEF) and Operation Iraqi Freedom (OIF), service members have sustained **traumatic brain injuries** (TBIs) at an unprecedented rate. Since 2000, 333,169 cases of TBI have been diagnosed in U.S. military personnel (Armed Forces Health Surveillance Center, 2015). This number includes both combat- and non–combat-related injuries (e.g., motor vehicle accidents, falls, recreational and training accidents). Approximately 274,568 cases of mTBI have been reported, compared with 28,192 cases of moderate, 3,463 cases of severe, and 4,904 cases of penetrating TBI. Some have estimated that at least 22% of Army service members who have deployed have sustained a TBI (Okie, 2005). The use of explosives (e.g., rocket-propelled grenades [RPGs] and improvised explosive devices [IEDs]) as primary weapons in modern warfare has contributed to the prevalence of TBI on the battlefield (Gawande, 2004). Estimates are that approximately 60% of blasts in combat result in TBI (Okie, 2005). Advances in body armor, combat medicine, and vehicle design have allowed service members to survive explosions that might otherwise have resulted in serious injury or death because of widespread damage to the brain, body, or both.

Unlike the neurotrauma seen in civilian acceleration–deceleration mechanical deformation injury, blast injuries occur when an invisible shock wave enters the body with a concussive force. Multiple types of injuries caused by blast waves have been documented in the literature. *Primary blast injury* describes direct trauma to bodily organs caused by overpressure from the blast itself. *Secondary blast injury* refers to injury caused by shrapnel or debris that is flung through the air after a blast. *Tertiary blast injury* occurs when a person is thrown to the ground or into another stationary object in the wake of a blast. *Quaternary blast injury* is characterized by thermal damage to organs induced by the intense heat of the explosion (Hicks, Fertig, Desrocher, Koroshetz, & Pancrazio, 2010). Blast exposure can lead to **contusion, cerebral edema, diffuse axonal injury,** and **hemorrhage** (Levi et al., 1990; Schwartz et al., 2008). Depending on the circumstances of the blast, service members can sustain any or all types of blast injury, resulting in mild to severe TBI.

Presentation of Mild Traumatic Brain Injury in Service Members

Common symptoms of mTBI include headache, nausea or vomiting, dizziness, blurred vision, irritability, sleep disturbances, and **memory** and **attention** problems (Defense and Veterans Brain Injury Center, n.d.-a). For most people (70%–90%), these symptoms resolve during the first 3 months of recovery (Levin, Goldstein, & MacKenzie, 1997). Service members whose symptoms do not resolve in the anticipated time frame may receive treatment from the U.S. Department of Defense (DoD), the Veterans Health Administration (VHA), or community health care systems. Persistent postconcussive symptoms can be cognitive, somatic, and behavioral and may affect a service member's ability to perform his or her job in deployed and nondeployed settings. For many service members, the headaches, nausea, and dizziness induced by exertion render them unable to maintain physical training standards. Others report memory problems that disrupt daily task completion, and sleep disturbances that affect their ability to adhere to punctuality standards.

A recent RAND study estimated a PTSD prevalence of 13.8% among OIF–OEF veterans (Tanielian & Jaycox, 2008). The presence of PTSD and related mental health disorders can complicate the clinical presentation of mTBI because many symptoms of these diagnoses resemble those of mTBI, and PTSD and mental health symptoms may actually mask the severity of the underlying **impairments** and residual capabilities. In fact, people with depression and PTSD have been shown to present with postconcussion-like symptoms (Foa, Cashman, Jaycox, & Perry, 1997; Iverson, 2006). Civilian studies have shown that nearly 30% of people with poly-trauma injuries develop a diagnosable mental health condition within the 1st year after injury (Bryant et al., 2010).

Additionally, OIF–OEF studies have shown that 30% to 39% of service members with mTBI also have concomitant PTSD (Carlson et al., 2011; Polusny et al., 2011). PTSD and depression have been identified as influencing the course and outcome of mTBI recovery, illustrating that these factors are associated with persistent physical health problems 3 to 4 months after mTBI (Hoge et al., 2008). Occupational therapists working with veterans should be familiar with the mTBI–PTSD symptom cluster to make appropriate referrals. Correctly identifying underlying contributors to the symptoms will also help occupational therapists select appropriate assessment and intervention methods.

Performance Implications

The symptoms of mTBI and PTSD can lead to widespread functional decline involving many occupational performance areas. **Activities of daily living, instrumental activities of daily living,** rest and sleep, education, work, **leisure,** and **social participation** are all vulnerable to dysfunction in the wounded military population. Sensory (i.e., visual, auditory, vestibular) and cognitive (i.e., attention, memory, **executive function**) client factors and emotional regulation performance skills are frequently affected. As a result, service members affected by mTBI and PTSD often experience difficulty reintegrating into previously held occupational, community, and family roles (Institute of Medicine, 2010). For example, service members might report losing their train of thought when briefing other soldiers, a worsening in shooting accuracy because of blurred vision, or being unable to complete certain physical training exercises because of dizziness.

Cognitive Dysfunction

Decreased memory for daily tasks is a very common complaint. Service members report difficulty remembering basic steps in their routines such as shaving or remembering to bring their wallet with them when leaving the house. Daily memory failures are particularly frustrating because they involve little details that can add up to create big problems, such as locking one's keys in the car while it is still running. Executive dysfunction is also frequently observed, resulting in difficulty with initiation, organization, prioritization, and completion of daily tasks. Cognitive problems affect one's ability to follow instructions at work; accomplish errands; and recall conversations shared with friends, family, and medical providers.

Perceived repeated failures can greatly diminish one's sense of **self-efficacy** and role fulfillment over time. Service members with mTBI–PTSD symptoms may become hyperaware of their difficulties and develop performance anxiety related to completion of daily responsibilities. A task once performed automatically, such as calling in a specific report over the radio, now requires cognitive control. These symptoms can result in inefficiency and frustration on the part of the service member and can impact his or her effectiveness within the unit.

Social Dysfunction

Service members with the mTBI–PTSD symptom cluster often experience activity limitations affecting social and community participation. Service members recovering from mTBI–PTSD often avoid activities that take place in crowded community environments. Many service members experience a feeling of overstimulation brought on by loud noises, bright lights, and constant movement that can lead to an increase in **postconcussion syndrome** symptoms including headache, nausea, dizziness, and cognitive slowing. Other service members experience increased **anxiety** and discomfort in environments in which they feel a loss of control.

Many service members also experience decreased emotional regulation skills. They may demonstrate difficulty managing frustration and irritability in the context of community-based activities such as waiting in line at the post office, making a return at a department store, or negotiating the correction of an erroneous order at a restaurant. These reactions may lead to decreased participation in many community and social activities including dining out; shopping; visiting with friends; and attending amusement parks, sporting events, movies, festivals, concerts, and religious services. Additionally, many service members express a lack of interest in building social relationships, especially with people who do not share their combat experiences, which can swiftly lead to social isolation when a service member becomes geographically separated from combat comrades because of a permanent change of duty station or service termination.

Mood changes, including irritability, depression, and emotional numbness, can disrupt relationships in service members recovering from mTBI–PTSD. Service members may disengage from particular parenting roles because they recognize a tendency to lose patience with young children. They may also exhibit decreased open communication with spouses and family members (Monson, Taft, & Fredman, 2009). Decreased sexual interest, intimacy, or sexual performance are other common issues among service members with mTBI and PTSD.

> Many service members express a lack of interest in building social relationships, especially with people who do not share their combat experiences, which can swiftly lead to social isolation.

Recovery Process

Acute management of TBI in the combat zone varies on the basis of injury severity and the presence of polytrauma. The term *polytrauma,* as defined by VHA clinical directives, refers to "two or more injuries, one of which may be life threatening, sustained in the same incident that affect multiple body parts or organ systems and result in physical, cognitive, psychological, or psychosocial impairments and functional disabilities" (VHA, 2013, p. 1). People with polytrauma and severe or penetrating TBI are medically evacuated from the combat zone to receive advanced medical and rehabilitative care at DoD and VHA polytrauma sites.

People with mTBI are typically treated in the combat zone and returned to duty. Service members who are within 50 meters of a blast are required to complete a TBI evaluation, which involves taking the Military Acute Concussion Evaluation (French, McCrea, & Baggett, 2008). When indicated, deployed service members may be temporarily relieved of their duties to rest and recover in one of several Concussion Care Centers established in places such as Afghanistan. Active-duty occupational therapists are assigned to these sites to provide acute **concussion** care as well as unit education on early identification and prevention of mTBI. Initial acute concussion treatment emphasizes sleep, with gradual addition of activities including self-care, home management, and leisure tasks as well as cognitive, visual, and vestibular rehabilitation.

Finally, service members undergo **exertional testing** and functional assessment of relevant military activities to determine their readiness to return to duty. *Exertional testing* involves having the service member exercise to 65% to 85% of his or her maximum heart rate and then assessing for resurgence of postconcussion syndrome symptoms such as dizziness, headache, or visual changes (Bazarian et al., 2008; Kennedy & Moore, 2010). The average length of stay at a Concussion Care Center ranges from 3 to 15 days.

Military Culture

The military culture adds another layer to the complexity of combat-related mTBI–PTSD. From a civilian perspective, it is difficult to understand the pressures faced by service members and their families over the course of a military career. However, it is imperative that occupational therapists treating veterans make a concerted effort to become educated on the military mentality, combat-related **stress,** reintegration challenges faced by service members as they return from deployment, available resources for veterans (see Box 8.1), and the warrior-to-civilian transition process that takes place when service members exit the military. In doing so, occupational therapists will be poised to enter into sound therapeutic alliances with veteran service members and help them to overcome the unique challenges they face.

Box 8.1. Online Resources for Veterans

Website	Organization and Description
http://www.brainline.org	**Brainline.org** provides TBI education, links to other resources, personal testimonies, multimedia training, opportunities to ask questions, and research updates for clients, friends and family, and professionals. The website has a special military-specific portal at http://www.brainlinemilitary.org.
http://www.braintrauma.org/tbi-faqs/military-tbi/	The **Brain Trauma Foundation** summarizes current research, defines terms related to TBI, provides educational materials for service members and families, and directs professionals to relevant conferences and workshops.
http://dvbic.dcoe.mil/	The **Defense and Veterans Brain Injury Center's** mission is to serve active-duty military, their beneficiaries, and veterans with TBI through state-of-the-art clinical care, innovative clinical research initiatives and educational programs, and support for force health protection services. The website includes educational materials, fact sheets, crisis intervention information, and a collection of current research publications.
http://www.dcoe.health.mil	The **Defense Centers of Excellence** integrates knowledge and identifies, evaluates, and disseminates evidence-based practices and standards for the treatment of psychological health and TBI within the Defense Department. The website provides educational and research-based resources for service members, families, news media, and professionals.
http://www.realwarriors.net	**Real Warriors** is a multimedia campaign to encourage help-seeking behavior and resilience among service members, veterans, and military families coping with invisible wounds such as posttraumatic stress. The website includes crisis support, message boards, podcasts, and educational materials for service members, veterans, families, and professionals.

Note. TBI = traumatic brain injury.

The military mind-set is cultivated from the 1st day of basic training. Service members are trained to put the needs of the unit before their own. They are admonished never to be the weakest link. They grow to possess a certain level of distrust of people and systems, which keeps them on guard, ready to defend at any moment. They are taught to be decisive, in control, and powerful. No task is too great; they are willing to push their minds, bodies, and spirits to the point of collapse to complete the mission. Similar, in many ways, are military families. They shoulder the burdens of home and family life while sacrificing time spent with loved ones, stability, social relationships, and peace of mind for the good of the country. Consequently, many military family members also present with mental health needs, which can be addressed by occupational therapists (Cogan, 2014).

The military mind-set is highly adaptive in training and combat scenarios. It can, however, pose barriers to function once a service member returns home.

The military mind-set is highly adaptive in training and combat scenarios. It can, however, pose barriers to function once a service member returns home. Difficulty turning off the military mind-set may negatively affect social, community, and family relationships as well as self-perception and self-efficacy. The military mind-set, coupled with combat exposure, may lead service members to engage in high-risk behaviors such as extreme sports, racing, skydiving, and ultimate fighting (Killgore et al., 2008). It may also cause them to underreport mTBI–PTSD symptoms, because doing so would be a sign of weakness, and to have difficulty trusting medical providers. Service members may never be able to completely turn off the military mind-set. However, occupational therapists can assist service members by identifying where it is disrupting function and by providing strategies to regulate maladaptive responses.

Role of the Occupational Therapist

In the following sections, I discuss occupational therapy services in two settings with three goals: (1) the combat zone, in which the goal is rapid return to the deployment mission, and (2) the rehabilitation center, in which the goal is either return to active-duty military or transition to the civilian community.

The Combat Zone

Occupational therapy in the combat zone consists primarily of providing a safe, structured environment in which service members exposed to blasts can rest and recuperate. Therapeutic activities are graded on the basis of cognitive and physical demand as service members gradually resume normal daily function. The goal of intervention in this setting is for service members to be able to successfully complete required daily tasks while remaining free of postconcussive symptoms (e.g., headache, nausea, vision problems, dizziness). To determine a service member's readiness to return to his or her deployment mission, occupational therapists observe the service member completing military-relevant and physically demanding tasks while monitoring performance and symptoms. Because of the austere nature of the combat environment, the pace of operations, and variations in training and experience across deployed occupational therapists, few standardized assessments for mTBI are used by occupational therapists in the combat zone.

Rehabilitation Center

The multifaceted nature of the mTBI–PTSD symptom complex lends itself to a multidisciplinary treatment approach (Hoge et al., 2008). Additionally, it is not enough simply to offer concurrent therapies to address isolated areas of dysfunction; rather, an integrated, coherent treatment approach is preferred (Batten & Pollack, 2008). The occupational therapist's role on the treatment team centers on global functional performance with a particular emphasis on reintegration, either to the unit or to the community. Because mTBI–PTSD symptoms are numerous and widespread, occupational therapists working with this population may address anything from driving and sleep hygiene to memory supports and strategies for coping with anxiety. Occupational therapists working with active-duty service members will likely engage in **vocational rehabilitation** and work hardening to assist service members in returning to duty, a common goal of many injured military personnel.

Evaluation

Evaluation consists of obtaining a thorough history including prior interests; career goals; perceived strengths; and previously held vocational, family, and social roles. It is also important for the occupational therapist to be familiar with any behavioral health history or psychological trauma because these factors will influence treatment progression. It may be helpful to administer a PTSD screening tool, such as the PTSD Checklist–Military Version (PCL–M), to assess the type and intensity of the service member's PTSD symptoms (see Exhibit 8.1). When PTSD symptoms are observed, the occupational therapist should adapt his or her approach and the clinic environment to help the service member feel most comfortable. For example, using incandescent (vs. fluorescent) lights, allowing the service member to view the exits, explaining the source of any alarms or unanticipated noises, and maintaining a calm, respectful demeanor can help establish trust with a veteran who has combat-related stress.

An assessment of occupational performance using a tool such as the Canadian Occupational Performance Measure (COPM; Law et al., 2014) has great utility in this practice area. It serves to help clinicians and service members identify goals that are intrinsically motivating and will likely have the greatest effect on functional performance and **quality of life.** The COPM can be administered in 25 to 35 minutes and can be used in many different practice settings.

Service members with blast-induced mTBI are at risk for visual dysfunction (Brahm et al., 2009; Capó-Aponte, Urosevich, Temme, Tarbett, & Sanghera, 2012). Occupational therapists should perform a vision screen to identify the functional implications of vision changes and to determine whether a referral to **behavioral optometry** or neuro-ophthalmology is indicated (Weisser-Pike, 2014). A vision screen may consist of a questionnaire; functional observation; and acuity, **visual fields, pursuits, saccades, convergence,** and **accommodation** testing (Radomski, Finkelstein, Llanos, Scheiman, & Wagener, 2014). The occupational therapist's role is then to provide education to the service member, family, and team on the functional impact of the visual disturbances and to provide training in compensatory strategies and modifications for improved function. Remedial vision training may also be indicated and can be carried out by the occupational therapist under the supervision of a behavioral optometrist.

Cognitive performance testing is a key component of the evaluation of service members with mTBI and PTSD. Occupational therapists incorporate results of standardized testing and real-world observations of functional performance and

Exhibit 8.1. PTSD Checklist–Military Version (PCL–M)

Instruction to patient: Below is a list of problems and complaints that veterans sometimes have in response to stressful military experiences. Please read each one carefully, fill in the circle to indicate how much you have been bothered by that problem in the last month.

1 = Not at all	2 = A little bit	3 = Moderately	4 = Quite a bit	5 = Extremely

RESPONSE					
1. Repeated, disturbing memories, thoughts or images of a stressful military experience?	1	2	3	4	5
2. Repeated, disturbing dreams of a stressful military experience?	1	2	3	4	5
3. Suddenly acting or feeling as if a stressful military experience were happening again (as if you were reliving it)?	1	2	3	4	5
4. Feeling very upset when something reminded you of a stressful military experience?	1	2	3	4	5
5. Having physical reactions, e.g., heart pounding, trouble breathing, or sweating, when something reminded you of a stressful military experience?	1	2	3	4	5
6. Avoid thinking about or talking about a stressful military experience or avoid having feelings related to it?	1	2	3	4	5
7. Avoid activities or situations because they remind you of a stressful military experience?	1	2	3	4	5
8. Trouble remembering important parts of a stressful military experience?	1	2	3	4	5
9. Loss of interest in things you used to enjoy?	1	2	3	4	5
10. Feeling distant or cut off from other people?	1	2	3	4	5
11. Feeling emotionally numb or being unable to have loving feelings for those close to you?	1	2	3	4	5
12. Feeling as if your future will somehow be cut short?	1	2	3	4	5
13. Trouble falling or staying asleep?	1	2	3	4	5
14. Feeling irritable or having angry outbursts?	1	2	3	4	5
15. Having difficulty concentrating?	1	2	3	4	5
16. Being "super alert" or watchful on guard?	1	2	3	4	5
17. Feeling jumpy or easily startled?	1	2	3	4	5

Scoring: The PCL is a self-report measure that takes approximately 5–10 minutes to complete. Interpretation of the PCL should be completed by a clinician. A total symptom severity score (range = 17–85) can be obtained by summing the scores from each of the 17 items. A diagnosis can be made by: 1) Determining whether an individual meets DSM–IV symptom criteria, i.e., at least one B item (questions 1–5), 3 C items (questions 6–12), and at least 2 D items (questions 13–17). Symptoms rated as "Moderately" or above (responses 3 through 5) are counted as present. 2) Determining whether the total severity score exceeds a given cutpoint. 3) Combining methods (1) and (2) to ensure that an individual has sufficient severity as well as the necessary pattern of symptoms required by the DSM.

Source. From *Mild Traumatic Brain Injury Pocket Guide*, by Defense and Veterans Brain Injury Center, n.d.-b. In the public domain.

Note. DSM–IV = *Diagnostic and Statistical Manual of Mental Disorders* (4th ed.; American Psychiatric Association, 1994); PTSD = posttraumatic stress disorder.

identification of personal and situational factors that affect performance. Occupational therapists may choose from among several assessments, depending on the specific needs of the service member being evaluated. Assessments should be sensitive enough to detect mild changes and incorporate cognitive domains such as attention, memory, and executive function. The Mild Traumatic Brain Injury Rehabilitation Toolkit (Weightman, Radomski, Mashima, & Roth, 2014) suggests several cognitive assessments that may be used with this population. It identifies the Behavioural Assessment of the Dysexecutive Syndrome, Cognistat, Contextual Memory Test, Mortera–Cognitive Screening Measure, Rivermead Behavioural Memory Test, and the Test of Everyday Attention as practice options.

Functional assessments are also important in the occupational therapy evaluation process. Driving assessments may be indicated for service members exhibiting difficulties managing the cognitive, sensory, and emotional demands of driving (Lew, Amick, Kraft, Stein, & Cifu, 2010). An initial driving screen measures visual, perceptual, cognitive, motor, and coordination skills in addition to investigating the effects of pain and **fatigue** on driving performance (Defense and Veterans Brain

Injury Center, n.d.-b). When indicated, service members may undergo a comprehensive driving assessment, which typically consists of an in-depth clinical assessment and an on-the-road evaluation. Comprehensive driving assessments are performed by clinicians who have adequate driver rehabilitation experience and training. DoD and VHA facilities often have driver rehabilitation specialists on staff or may be able to refer to community-based clinicians offering these services. Although there is great variability among models, driving simulators may also have some utility in the driver screening and rehabilitative processes.

The Assessment of Military Multitasking Performance (AMMP) is a performance-based assessment that is currently under development (Radomski et al., 2013). It incorporates measurements similar to those of the Multiple Errands Test (Shallice & Burgess, 1991) and consists of several tasks measuring executive functions and dual-task performance in the context of military-relevant activities. The AMMP is used to assist clinicians in making decisions regarding service members' readiness to return to duty.

Intervention

In 2007, expert clinical recommendations for the treatment of mTBI in the military population were published in *Clinical Practice Guidance: Occupational Therapy and Physical Therapy for Mild Traumatic Brain Injury* (Radomski, Weightman, Davidson, Rodgers, & Bolgla, 2010). In 2009, this lengthy document was summarized and condensed to meet the educational needs of civilian occupational therapists working with service members and veterans. The resulting article, published in the *American Journal of Occupational Therapy,* outlined recommended occupational therapy practices for mTBI care (Radomski, Davidson, Voydetich, & Erickson, 2009).

Education is a critical foundation for mTBI–PTSD recovery. Service members benefit from education that normalizes their experience and helps them to understand that they are not alone. It is also advised that mTBI–PTSD education focus on setting a positive expectation for recovery (Ponsford, 2005). As service members are made aware that many of their symptoms will resolve over time, they begin to focus on their capabilities and potentials rather than on their limitations. It may be helpful to explain typical human **information processing** and how memory is affected by the availability of attentional resources at the time when new information is presented. The occupational therapist can examine and explain to service members how personal and situational factors present demands on attention that can disrupt the flow of information processing throughout their day. Service members and occupational therapists can collaborate on strategies to effectively manage personal and situational factors to improve attention and memory.

Education and strategy development are grounded in ***metacognition*** (i.e., higher level thinking skills). Occupational therapists facilitate metacognition and anticipatory awareness by training service members to identify cognitive vulnerabilities and potential strategies to compensate for them before engaging in a given task. This approach uses the Dynamic Interactional Model for cognitive rehabilitation (Toglia, 2011). It is recommended that family members participate in the education and strategy development process so as to assist service members in generalizing and implementing recommended strategies. Involving the family in rehabilitation can also help improve psychological distress (Erbes, Polusny, MacDermid, & Compton, 2008).

As service members are made aware that many of their symptoms will resolve over time, they begin to focus on their capabilities and potentials rather than on their limitations.

Remedial cognitive training is often helpful to those with mTBI. In a recent review of the literature, Cicerone et al. (2011) asserted that sufficient evidence is now available to support cognitive rehabilitation to address problems with attention, memory, social communication, and executive function in people with TBI. A recent military-focused consensus panel on cognitive rehabilitation suggested the following interventions on the basis of the civilian mTBI literature:

> direct attention training; selection and training of external memory/organizational aids; training in internal memory strategies; metacognitive strategy training; social pragmatics training (targeting self-perception, self-awareness, and social skills); environmental modification (more organized and less distracting environments); brain injury education for patients, family, and employers; and aggressive support but gradual reentry into community and vocational/educational activities. (Batten et al., 2009, p. 8)

Remedial cognitive exercises are tailored to meet the needs of each service member and build toward strategy implementation and skill transfer to more functional activities.

Occupational therapists work with service members to establish daily routines. Many service members returning from combat struggle to develop an individual routine because they have grown accustomed to functioning within the routine of their units while overseas. They may need assistance with structuring daily activities for enhanced productivity, work–life balance, energy conservation, pacing, or sleep hygiene. They may also benefit from using environmental cues such as calendars, alarms, or checklists to assist with routine maintenance.

After a deployment, service members often have difficulty reintegrating into previously held family roles. It is important that the occupational therapist work with the service member and his or her family to identify roles that the service member is able to resume. Graded treatment activities that simulate these roles, including realistic environmental distractions and inherent multitasking demands, are helpful for skill development and strategy transfer. For example, a service member might prepare a meal while washing a load of laundry and paying bills. This activity provides an opportunity for enhanced self-monitoring and behavioral management while challenging attention, memory, and executive skills.

In some cases, **vision rehabilitation** may be warranted. Under the supervision of an optometrist, the occupational therapist may address common visual disturbances associated with mTBI, including convergence insufficiency, accommodative dysfunction, and oculomotor problems. Vision rehabilitation programs are fairly intensive and will require advanced training as well as strong collaboration between the occupational therapist and the optometrist. In addition to vision rehabilitation, occupational therapists provide education to the service member, family, and health care team on the functional implications of visual disturbances. If permanent visual deficits are present, compensatory strategies may be developed to maximize safety and function.

Socialization may be addressed through group treatment. Groups focusing on leisure and sports engagement are highly motivating for service members. A preliminary study on a community-based, sports-oriented occupational therapy has shown the potential for such programs to aid in the treatment of veterans with PTSD and depression (Rogers, Mallinson, & Peppers, 2014). Groups designed around cognitive strategy training are also effective in fostering socialization. Because of the military structure, service members are very familiar with operating in teams and may find groups a relevant and accessible avenue for treatment.

Relaxation training is foundational when addressing mTBI–PTSD symptom clusters. Because of the prevalence of emotional and behavioral changes in this population, it is critical that service members learn to regulate their overall state of **arousal** to effectively manage daily stressors. Service members benefit from developing individual strategies such as **diaphragmatic breathing, progressive muscle relaxation,** and **guided imagery** as well as engaging in group-based interventions such as yoga or tai chi.

A systematic approach to community reintegration is recommended. Occupational therapists assist service members with identifying goals related to community engagement and use task analysis and activity grading to provide appropriate challenges for enhanced function. Service members incorporate cognitive and relaxation techniques during community reintegration activities to manage emotional and behavioral symptoms in real time. Successful experiences serve to enhance self-confidence and self-efficacy in real-life situations.

Return to Duty and Transition to Civilian Life

Returning to duty is a primary goal of many wounded service members. In some settings, occupational therapists play a major role in the return-to-duty decision-making process. Therefore, it is critical for occupational therapists to understand the skill sets required for various military job roles. For occupational therapists working with the Army, the *Soldier's Manual of Common Tasks* (Headquarters, Department of the Army, 2009) is a helpful tool that breaks down basic soldiering tasks by outlining conditions, standards, performance steps, and performance measures for each task.

Occupational therapy intervention for return to duty embodies two complementary approaches:

1. Instruction in compensatory cognitive strategies that is functionally compatible with the service member's job requirements and
2. Completion of simulated work tasks of increasing realism to evoke an adaptive response to challenges. Simulated work tasks may incorporate implementation, rehearsal, and refinement of compensatory strategies (Weightman et al., 2014, p. 375).

Before returning to duty, service members may complete a functional assessment in which they perform tasks representative of the physical, cognitive, and emotional demands of their actual jobs. The functional assessment serves to inform the return-to-duty decision-making process by providing clinicians with the opportunity to observe the functional implications of residual symptoms as well as the service member's adaptability to realistic situations. Several DoD military treatment facilities have developed functional assessment programs to assist with safely returning service members to duty (Kelley et al., 2013). Additionally, several research initiatives are under way to advance this effort. Focus areas include the creation of a validated assessment tool and the appropriate grading of activity levels after acute concussion or mTBI.

Because of the military structure, service members are very familiar with operating in teams and may find groups a relevant and accessible avenue for treatment.

Service members transitioning out of the military face another challenge: successfully integrating into the civilian workforce or education system. Many service members will be working outside of the military or pursuing higher education for the first time. Service members experience a distinct cultural shift from military to civilian environments, procedures, and social interactions. Some may require occupational therapy intervention to help with résumé writing, job search and interview skills, professional correspondence training, and basic finance. Others will benefit from education and training in the use of adaptive equipment and strategies for classroom use. Occupational therapists may also direct service members to existing resources designed to help ease this transition. Many universities offer resources specifically for student veterans. The DoD offers the Soldier for Life–Transition Assistance Program to all soldiers separating from the Army. The VHA Vocational Rehabilitation program is another valuable resource. Community-based organizations such as the Wounded Warrior Project, Operation We Are Here, and Real Warriors also provide resources and guidance for transitioning veterans.

Case Study: Sgt. Bravo

Sgt. Bravo was an exceptional soldier. He quickly progressed through the ranks, scoring at the top of his class in numerous elite Army schools. He was the go-to guy, a leader of and mentor to the lower ranking soldiers in his platoon. At the age of 27, he was a sergeant and on his third deployment. The first two had been to Iraq, where he had been involved in countless explosions caused by IEDs, mortar attacks, and RPGs. Once or twice he had been knocked out, but each time he had just dismissed it and soldiered on. His third deployment was to Afghanistan. The terrain there was different; barren desert was replaced by jagged mountain peaks that necessitated that the majority of transportation be done on foot or by air.

Sgt. Bravo was out on a night mission, crammed in the back of a Chinook helicopter as it descended to land in a remote mountain pass. He was the last man on the ramp when the helicopter took a direct hit from an RPG. Flames immediately engulfed the interior of the aircraft, and Sgt. Bravo was knocked unconscious. He came to in less than a minute and was then able to move to safety.

Sgt. Bravo sustained partial-thickness burns to his face, neck, back, and wrists as well as inhalation burns and shrapnel to the lower extremities. He was medically evacuated from the theater to Landstuhl Regional Medical Center in Germany and then on to Brooke Army Medical Center in San Antonio, Texas. There, he underwent several months of rehabilitation for his burns. During the course of his recovery, he began to show signs of psychological trauma when he was informed that several of the other soldiers on the mission had been killed. He was enrolled in prolonged exposure therapy for several weeks that included education, breathing techniques for relaxation, real-world practice dealing with stress-provoking situations, and talking through the trauma with a psychologist. Sgt. Bravo was unable to complete the program because of a strong desire to avoid processing his trauma.

He returned to his assigned duty post and to his wife and two children, but he was different. He had trouble remembering to complete daily tasks, frequently misplaced things, and forgot conversations with his wife. He was referred to the Traumatic Brain Injury Clinic for evaluation. He received evaluations by personnel from primary care; physical, occupational, and speech therapy; behavioral health;

and neurology. The occupational therapy evaluation revealed a significant decrease in engagement in several occupational performance areas. Sgt. Bravo was no longer in his unit but was placed in the Warrior Transition Battalion, where his main responsibility was to attend medical appointments. He was not engaged in any productive activities outside the home, including leisure, social, or community-based activities.

Within the home, he reported decreased energy and follow-through, disrupting completion of home management tasks. He reported difficulty transitioning back into his husband and father roles and stated that he spent most of his time "zoned out" on the couch unless given a specific task to do by his wife. His wife told him that she felt like he had become another child for whom she had to care. He expressed increased irritability and anxiety, especially in community settings, and reported several outbursts leading to being escorted out of community venues. He also reported headaches with decreased sleep quality and frequent middle-of-the-night awakening. Standardized cognitive testing revealed moderate impairments in attention, memory, and executive function. His vision screen was notable for subjective reports of light sensitivity, intermittent double or blurred vision, and skipping lines and missing words when reading.

Sgt. Bravo's case was discussed in the weekly team meeting with the other clinicians who would provide his care. It was noted that he had been diagnosed with PTSD and depression. Sgt. Bravo was recommended to receive occupational, physical, and speech therapy. He was then assigned a case manager and followed by a primary care physician.

Occupational therapy began with collaborative goal setting with Sgt. Bravo. The COPM was used to identify the most important areas to be addressed. Treatment began with patient and family education about how the brain processes information, to help Sgt. Bravo and his family understand the connection between his injury and his cognitive symptoms. Sgt. Bravo worked with the occupational therapist on identifying personal and situational factors that had a potential negative impact on his **cognition,** including pain, medication, fatigue, anxiety, depression, and environmental distractions. An emphasis was placed on helping Sgt. Bravo and his family understand that his cognitive and behavioral symptoms are common for an injury such as his and educating them about the typical sequence of recovery.

In the next phase of intervention, Sgt. Bravo and his occupational therapist generated compensatory strategies to assist with the completion of daily tasks such as keeping his keys, wallet, and phone in a consistent location at home and entering all appointments into his smartphone. Sgt. Bravo and his wife worked to identify a list of home management tasks he would complete and posted a weekly calendar on the refrigerator outlining these tasks. Initially, Sgt. Bravo was resistant to a compensatory approach because he felt that he should not need external supports to complete basic tasks. Several sessions focused on helping Sgt. Bravo to understand the benefit of these strategies as well as when and how to use the devices and memory aids to support his functional independence.

Sgt. Bravo benefited from education about his body's response to prolonged stress that had accumulated over numerous combat tours. He began to realize that what he described as "being edgy" was really his body being in a constant protective fight-or-flight mode. His occupational therapist explained how this stress response also affected his ability to use his cognitive skills effectively. Sgt. Bravo agreed that he needed to relearn how to relax effectively to reintegrate into a civilian environment. With the support of his occupational therapist, he learned several relaxation techniques and grounding strategies including diaphragmatic breathing, progressive muscle relaxation, and guided imagery. He was encouraged to use these strategies throughout the day, under both stressful and nonstressful circumstances. He found that they were helpful for preparing to fall asleep and for use in stressful community environments.

The final phase of treatment consisted of putting the cognitive and behavioral strategies together in real-world scenarios. Sgt. Bravo planned a meal preparation activity and completed the necessary grocery shopping with his occupational therapist. The Subjective Units of Discomfort Scale (Kaplan & Smith, 1995) was used to measure his discomfort before, during, and after the activity. Although he did experience a spike in anxiety, Sgt. Bravo was able to complete the shopping activity using **coping** strategies as needed. His occupational therapist was able to make observations about the effectiveness of his memory, visual scanning, and problem solving as well as his social interactions. Motivational interviewing techniques were helpful in debriefing after the outing. Sgt. Bravo gained additional insight into the interactions among his behavioral symptoms, cognition, and functional performance. Strategies were modified and reinforced in the context of a highly relevant activity.

Throughout treatment, Sgt. Bravo's progress was affected by several factors. First, Sgt. Bravo was resistant to intensive PTSD treatment. He expressed distrust of providers and of the system that made him unwilling to talk about his traumatic experiences. Because of his negative experience with prolonged exposure therapy, he did not believe other psychotherapeutic techniques would be effective. He was extremely socially isolated because most of his friends from his old unit had either left the Army or moved to other posts. He struggled with the shift in his identity from the go-to guy to the injured guy who was no longer a leader and decision maker and was no longer a part of a team. He was informed he was being medically discharged from the Army because he was not retainable as a result of the severity of his injuries. He faced the uncertainty of returning to civilian life, where he would have to begin a job search with a limited support structure.

Sgt. Bravo was encouraged to become involved in classes to prepare for the transition to the civilian workforce. He began taking a basic electrician course at a local community college and found it rewarding. He stated that it structured his week and gave him something to look forward to. He completed a new résumé and participated in several job fairs. He was also directed to local volunteer opportunities and community support groups.

When Sgt. Bravo was discharged from occupational therapy services, he was strongly encouraged to continue working with his social worker on addressing his PTSD. In collaboration with his occupational therapist, he created a summary sheet highlighting his strategies for memory, attention, sleep, and behavioral symptoms. He was instructed to post it in a prominent place in his home to continue implementing the strategies in real-world situations. Sgt. Bravo went on to receive primary care, case management, and behavioral health services through the Warrior Transition Battalion until he was medically separated from the Army.

Conclusion

Service members face challenges to health and wellness both on and off the battlefield. Occupational therapists play a vital role in the rehabilitative process by assisting service men and women with recovery and reintegration into meaningful roles and occupations. Occupational therapists are uniquely poised to address the complex physical, cognitive, and psychosocial sequelae associated with combat-induced mTBI and related psychological disorders. As in World War I, today's occupational therapists are shaping modern rehabilitation through innovation and client-centered care. In the wake of the wars in Iraq and Afghanistan, occupational therapists in all practice areas must be prepared to effectively evaluate and treat a growing population of veterans and their families.

Occupational therapists are uniquely poised to address the complex physical, cognitive, and psychosocial sequelae associated with combat-induced mTBI and related psychological disorders.

References

American Psychiatric Association. (1994). *Diagnostic and statistical manual of mental disorders* (4th ed.). Arlington, VA: Author.

Armed Forces Health Surveillance Center. (2015). *DoD worldwide numbers for TBI.* Retrieved from http://dvbic.dcoe.mil/dod-worldwide-numbers-tbi

Batten, S., Beal, S., Bleiberg, J., Boccio, P., Boyd, T., Cicerone, K., . . . Comper, P. (2009). *Proceedings from Defense Centers of Excellence for Psychological Health and Traumatic Brain Injury and Defense and Veterans Brain Injury Center Consensus Conference on Cognitive Rehabilitation for Mild Traumatic Brain Injury.* Washington, DC: Defense Centers of Excellence.

Batten, S., & Pollack, S. J. (2008). Integrative outpatient treatment for returning service members. *Journal of Clinical Psychology, 64,* 928–939. http://dx.doi.org/10.1002/jclp.20513

Bazarian, J., Boerman, H., Bolenbacher, R., Dalton, D., De John, M., Doncevic, S., . . . Williams, C. (2008). *Proceedings from Defense and Veterans Brain Injury Center Consensus Conference on the Acute Management of Concussion/Mild Traumatic Brain Injury (mTBI) in the Deployed Setting.* Washington, DC: Defense and Veterans Brain Injury Center.

Brahm, K. D., Wilgenburg, H. M., Kirby, J., Ingalla, S., Chang, C. Y., & Goodrich, G. L. (2009). Visual impairment and dysfunction in combat-injured servicemembers with traumatic brain injury. *Optometry and Vision Science, 86,* 817–825. http://dx.doi.org/10.1097/OPX.0b013e3181adff2d

Bryant, R. A., O'Donnell, M. L., Creamer, M., McFarlane, A. C., Clark, C. R., & Silove, D. (2010). The psychiatric sequelae of traumatic injury. *American Journal of Psychiatry, 167,* 312–320. http://dx.doi.org/10.1176/appi.ajp.2009.09050617

Capó-Aponte, J. E., Urosevich, T. G., Temme, L. A., Tarbett, A. K., & Sanghera, N. K. (2012). Visual dysfunctions and symptoms during the subacute stage of blast-induced mild traumatic brain injury. *Military Medicine, 177,* 804–813. http://dx.doi.org/10.7205/MILMED-D-12-00061

Carlson, K. F., Kehle, S. M., Meis, L. A., Greer, N., MacDonald, R., Rutks, I., . . . Wilt, T. J. (2011). Prevalence, assessment, and treatment of mild traumatic brain injury and posttraumatic stress disorder: A systematic review of the evidence. *Journal of Head Trauma Rehabilitation, 26,* 103–115. http://dx.doi.org/10.1097/HTR.0b013e3181e50ef1

Cicerone, K. D., Langenbahn, D. M., Braden, C., Malec, J. F., Kalmar, K., Fraas, M., . . . Ashman, T. (2011). Evidence-based cognitive rehabilitation: Updated review of the literature from 2003 through 2008. *Archives of Physical Medicine and Rehabilitation, 92,* 519–530. http://dx.doi.org/10.1016/j.apmr.2010.11.015

Cogan, A. M. (2014). Supporting our military families: A case for a larger role for occupational therapy in prevention and mental health care. *American Journal of Occupational Therapy, 68,* 478–483. http://dx.doi.org/10.5014/ajot.2014.009712

Defense and Veterans Brain Injury Center. (n.d.-a). *Concussion/mTBI information: Signs and symptoms.* Retrieved from https://dvbic.dcoe.mil/sites/default/files/2013_SS_Mild_08.06.13.pdf

Defense and Veterans Brain Injury Center. (n.d.-b). *Mild traumatic brain injury pocket guide.* Retrieved from https://dvbic.dcoe.mil/sites/default/files/DCoE_mTBI-Pocket-Guide.pdf

Erbes, C. R., Polusny, M. A., MacDermid, S., & Compton, J. S. (2008). Couple therapy with combat veterans and their partners. *Journal of Clinical Psychology, 64*, 972–983. http://dx.doi.org/10.1002/jclp.20521

Foa, E. B., Cashman, L., Jaycox, L., & Perry, K. (1997). The validation of a self-report measure of posttraumatic stress disorder: The Posttraumatic Diagnostic Scale. *Psychological Assessment, 9*, 445–451. http://dx.doi.org/10.1037/1040-3590.9.4.445

French, L., McCrea, M., & Baggett, M. (2008). The Military Acute Concussion Evaluation (MACE). *Journal of Special Operations Medicine, 8*, 68–77. Retrieved from https://www.jsomonline.org/Publications/2008168French.pdf

Gawande, A. (2004). Casualties of war: Military care for the wounded from Iraq and Afghanistan. *New England Journal of Medicine, 351*, 2471–2475. http://dx.doi.org/10.1056/NEJMp048317

Headquarters, Department of the Army. (2009). *Soldier's manual of common tasks: Warrior skills Level 1.* Retrieved from http://www.milsci.ucsb.edu/sites/secure.lsit.ucsb.edu.mili.d7/files/sitefiles/resources/STP%2021-1-SMCT,%20Warrior%20Skills,%20Level%201.pdf

Hicks, R. R., Fertig, S. J., Desrocher, R. E., Koroshetz, W. J., & Pancrazio, J. J. (2010). Neurological effects of blast injury. *Journal of Trauma, 68*, 1257–1263. http://dx.doi.org/10.1097/TA.0b013e3181d8956d

Hoge, C. W., McGurk, D., Thomas, J. L., Cox, A. L., Engel, C. C., & Castro, C. A. (2008). Mild traumatic brain injury in U.S. soldiers returning from Iraq. *New England Journal of Medicine, 358*, 453–463. http://dx.doi.org/10.1056/NEJMoa072972

Institute of Medicine. (2010). *Returning home from Iraq and Afghanistan: Preliminary assessment of readjustment needs of veterans, service members, and their families.* Washington, DC: National Academies Press.

Iverson, G. L. (2006). Misdiagnosis of the persistent postconcussion syndrome in patients with depression. *Archives of Clinical Neuropsychology, 21*, 303–310. http://dx.doi.org/10.1016/j.acn.2005.12.008

Kaplan, D., & Smith, T. (1995). A validity study of the Subjective Units of Discomfort (SUD) score. *Measurement and Evaluation in Counseling and Development, 27*, 195–199.

Kelley, A. M., Ranes, B. M., Estrada, A., Webb, C. M., Milam, L., & Chiaramonte, J. (2013). *Evaluation of the Military Functional Assessment Program: Preliminary assessment of the construct validity using an archived database of clinical data* (USAARL Report No. 2013-19). Retrieved from http://www.dtic.mil/dtic/tr/fulltext/u2/a587286.pdf

Kennedy, C. H., & Moore, J. L. (2010). *Military neuropsychology.* New York: Springer.

Killgore, W. D., Cotting, D. I., Thomas, J. L., Cox, A. L., McGurk, D., Vo, A. H., . . . Hoge, C. W. (2008). Post-combat invincibility: Violent combat experiences are associated with increased risk-taking propensity following deployment. *Journal of Psychiatric Research, 42*, 1112–1121. http://dx.doi.org/10.1016/j.jpsychires.2008.01.001

Law, M., Baptiste, S., Carswell, A., McColl, M. A., Polatajko, H., & Pollock, N. (2014). *The Canadian Occupational Performance Measure* (5th ed.). Ottawa, Ontario: CAOT Publications.

Levi, L., Borovich, B., Guilburd, J. N., Grushkiewicz, I., Lemberger, A., Linn, S., . . . Feinsod, M. (1990). Wartime neurosurgical experience in Lebanon, 1982–85. II: Closed craniocerebral injuries. *Israel Journal of Medical Sciences, 26*, 555–558.

Levin, H. S., Goldstein, F. C., & MacKenzie, E. J. (1997). Depression as a secondary condition following mild and moderate traumatic brain injury. *Seminars in Clinical Neuropsychology, 2*, 207–215.

Lew, H. L., Amick, M. M., Kraft, M., Stein, M. B., & Cifu, D. X. (2010). Potential driving issues in combat returnees. *NeuroRehabilitation, 26*, 271–278.

Monson, C. M., Taft, C. T., & Fredman, S. J. (2009). Military-related PTSD and intimate relationships: From description to theory-driven research and intervention development. *Clinical Psychology Review, 29*, 707–714. http://dx.doi.org/10.1016/j.cpr.2009.09.002

Newton, S. (2007, Jan.–Mar.). The growth of the profession of occupational therapy. *U.S. Army Medical Department Journal*, pp. 51–58.

Okie, S. (2005). Traumatic brain injury in the war zone. *New England Journal of Medicine, 352*, 2043–2047. http://dx.doi.org/10.1056/NEJMp058102

Polusny, M. A., Kehle, S. M., Nelson, N. W., Erbes, C. R., Arbisi, P. A., & Thuras, P. (2011). Longitudinal effects of mild traumatic brain injury and posttraumatic stress disorder comorbidity on postdeployment outcomes in National Guard soldiers deployed to Iraq. *Archives of General Psychiatry, 68*, 79–89. http://dx.doi.org/10.1001/archgenpsychiatry.2010.172

Ponsford, J. (2005). Rehabilitation interventions after mild head injury. *Current Opinion in Neurology, 18,* 692–697. http://dx.doi.org/10.1097/01.wco.0000186840.61431.44

Radomski, M. V., Davidson, L., Voydetich, D., & Erickson, M. W. (2009). Occupational therapy for service members with mild traumatic brain injury. *American Journal of Occupational Therapy, 63,* 646–655. http://dx.doi.org/10.5014/ajot.63.5.646

Radomski, M. V., Finkelstein, M., Llanos, I., Scheiman, M., & Wagener, S. G. (2014). Composition of a vision screen for service members with traumatic brain injury: Consensus using a modified nominal group technique. *American Journal of Occupational Therapy, 68,* 422–429. http://dx.doi.org/10.5014/ajot.2014.011445

Radomski, M. V., Weightman, M. M., Davidson, L., Finkelstein, M., Goldman, S., McCulloch, K., . . . Stern, E. B. (2013). Development of a measure to inform return-to-duty decision making after mild traumatic brain injury. *Military Medicine, 178,* 246–253. http://dx.doi.org/10.7205/MILMED-D-12-00144

Radomski, M. V., Weightman, M. M., Davidson, L., Rodgers, M., & Bolgla, R. (2010). *Clinical practice guidance: Occupational therapy and physical therapy for mild traumatic brain injury.* Falls Church, VA: U.S. Army Office of the Surgeon General.

Rogers, C. M., Mallinson, T., & Peppers, D. (2014). High-intensity sports for posttraumatic stress disorder and depression: Feasibility study of ocean therapy with veterans of Operation Enduring Freedom and Operation Iraqi Freedom. *American Journal of Occupational Therapy, 68,* 395–404. http://dx.doi.org/10.5014/ajot.2014.011221

Schwartz, I., Tuchner, M., Tsenter, J., Shochina, M., Shoshan, Y., Katz-Leurer, M., & Meiner, Z. (2008). Cognitive and functional outcomes of terror victims who suffered from traumatic brain injury. *Brain Injury, 22,* 255–263. http://dx.doi.org/10.1080/02699050801941763

Shallice, T., & Burgess, P. W. (1991). Deficits in strategy application following frontal lobe damage in man. *Brain, 114,* 727–741. http://dx.doi.org/10.1093/brain/114.2.727

Tanielian, T., & Jaycox, L. H. (Eds.). (2008). *Invisible wounds of war: Psychological and cognitive injuries, their consequences, and services to assist recovery.* Santa Monica, CA: RAND Corporation.

Toglia, J. P. (2011). A Dynamic Interactional Model of cognition in cognitive rehabilitation. In N. Katz (Ed.), *Cognition, occupation, and participation across the life span: Neuroscience, neurorehabilitation, and models of intervention in occupational therapy* (3rd ed., pp. 161–202). Bethesda, MD: AOTA Press.

Veterans Health Administration. (2013). *VHA handbook 1172.01: Polytrauma system of care.* Washington, DC: U.S. Department of Veterans Affairs. Retrieved from http://www.va.gov/optometry/docs/VHA_Handbook_1172_01_Polytrauma_System_of_Care.pdf

Weightman, M. M., Radomski, M. V., Mashima, P. A., & Roth, C. R. (2014). *Mild Traumatic Brain Injury Rehabilitation Toolkit.* Fort Sam Houston, TX: U.S. Army, Borden Institute.

Weisser-Pike, O. (2014). Assessing abilities and capacities: Vision and visual processing. In M. V. Radomski & C. A. Trombly Latham (Eds.), *Occupational therapy for physical dysfunction* (7th ed., pp. 105–122). Baltimore: Lippincott Williams & Wilkins.

Glossary

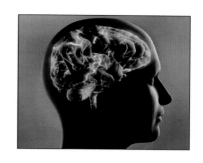

accommodation—The ability to change the focus of the eye so that objects at different distances can be seen clearly (Scheiman, 2002).

acetylcholine—A neurotransmitter involved in both the peripheral and the central nervous systems (Stahl, 2008).

acquired brain injury—Injury to the brain that is not congenital or degenerative and that incorporates traumatic brain injuries and nontraumatic brain injuries (such as stroke, hypoxia, and tumor; Fleming & Nalder, 2011).

activities of daily living—Activities related to taking care of one's own body, such as self-feeding, bathing, grooming, dressing, sexual activity, toilet use, and hygiene (American Occupational Therapy Association [AOTA], 2014).

afferent—(*a* = to; *ferre* = to carry) A nerve fiber that conducts action potentials from the periphery toward the central nervous system (i.e., sensory neurons; Purves et al., 2012).

agnosia—Failure to recognize a visual or other sensory stimulus (e.g., sound) or specific stimulus types (e.g., faces; see *prosopagnosia*). Agnosia affects one sensory system, but the person may retain the ability to recognize the stimulus using other sensory systems (Lezak, Howieson, Bigler, & Tranel, 2012; Milner & Teuber, 1968).

allocortex—Areas of cerebral cortex with fewer than six distinct layers of neurons ("other cortex"). Examples include the three-layered *archicortex* ("original cortex") of the hippocampal formation, the *paleocortex* ("old cortex") of the olfactory area, and the transitional or *mesocortex* ("middle cortex") of the limbic cortex (Blumenfeld, 2010; Nolte, 2009; Purves et al., 2012).

amygdala—Collection of nuclei in the anteromedial part of the temporal lobe that forms part of the limbic system; the major functions of the amygdala include autonomic, emotional, and sexual behavior (Blumenfeld, 2010; Nolte, 2009; Purves et al., 2012).

anger—An emotional reaction that may include outbursts, decreased impulse control, increased irritability, hostility, and insult (Scarpa & Raine, 1997).

anosognosia—Explicit verbal denial of the presence of impairment or disease (Ergh, Rapport, Coleman, & Hanks, 2002); also called *denial of deficit* (Lezak et al., 2012).

anoxia—Lack of oxygen to the brain. Death of neurons may occur if the absence of circulatory oxygen lasts longer than 4 minutes, and severe diffuse ischemic anoxia lasting 10 minutes or more leads to irreversible damage absent unusual circumstances (e.g., rapid temperature reduction, as in some cases of drowning; Posner, Saper, Schiff, & Plum, 2007).

antecedent—A precursor or cue; an event that precedes and increases or decreases the likelihood that a behavior will occur (Giles, 2011).

anterior cerebral artery—Major paired artery that sweeps across the medial surface of each hemisphere in the longitudinal fissure, supplying the medial surface of the frontal and anterior parietal lobes (Purves et al., 2012).

anterior cingulate gyrus—Area of cerebral cortex in the prefrontal lobe that is hypothesized to have executive control over information processing, especially target detection, and is linked to frontal lobe regions involved in working memory and to posterior regions for visual orienting and feature identification (Blumenfeld, 2010; Nolte, 2009; Purves et al., 2012).

anterior nucleus of the thalamus—Relay nucleus of the thalamus that primarily functions in the limbic system; receives inputs from the mammillary bodies and other limbic structures and sends outputs to the cingulate gyrus (Blumenfeld, 2010; Nolte, 2009; Purves et al., 2012).

anxiety—An overwhelming sense of worry or fear that may involve physical changes such as decreased energy and concentration, tachycardia, nausea, tense muscles, shortness of breath, and headache (National Stroke Association, 2006).

apathy—A reduction in motivation or a lack of initiative (Starkstein, Fedoroff, Price, Leiguarda, & Robinson, 1993).

aphasia—Impaired production or comprehension of speech or ability to communicate because of brain pathology (Lezak et al., 2012).

apraxia—Inability to organize and skillfully execute purposeful movements (Lezak et al., 2012).

arousal—State of being awake and responsive that forms the basis for attention and purposeful responses (Edlow et al., 2012).

aspiration—Entry of food, fluid, or a foreign body below the vocal cords and into the lungs (Avery, 2010).

association cortex—Portions of the cerebral cortex that receive and integrate sensory or motor information. This higher order information processing can involve single (*unimodal*) or multiple (*heteromodal*) sensory or motor modalities (Blumenfeld, 2010; Martini, 2009; Nolte, 2009; Purves et al., 2012).

astrocytes—One of the major types of glial cells in the central nervous system. Astrocytes have numerous cellular extensions that contact most of the surface area of neuronal dendrites and cell bodies and are thought to play a major role in preserving the ionic balance of the neuronal environment. Other cellular extensions terminate in flattened expansions called *end-feet* which completely encase vessels within the central nervous system contributing to formation of the blood–brain barrier (Purves et al., 2012).

ataxia—A movement disorder related to uncoordinated movements and postural instability (Armutlu, 2013).

attention—Focused awareness—a necessary precondition for most activities; ability to detect and orient to stimuli (Lezak et al., 2012).

automaticity—Characteristic of a behavior whereby it is initiated and executed with minimal conscious decision making (Giles, 2011).

axon—Neuronal process that conducts the action potential away from the cell body (*soma*) and toward the target (most frequently, the axon terminals that make synaptic connections with other neurons; Hall, 2011; Martini, 2009; Purves et al., 2012; Rhoades & Bell, 2009; Widmaier, Raff, & Strang, 2006).

basal nuclei—Group of subcortical nuclei (historically referred to as *basal ganglia*), most prominently including the striatum, globus pallidus, substantia nigra, and subthalamic nucleus. The basal nuclei collectively organize motor behavior. Damage to these nuclei has traditionally been considered to cause disorders characterized by involuntary movements, difficulty initiating movement, and alterations in muscle tone. Damage to certain parts of the basal nuclei can also cause disturbances of cognition and motivation (Blumenfeld, 2010; Nolte, 2009; Purves et al., 2012).

basilar artery—Large vessel formed by the union of the two vertebral arteries that runs upward along the anterior median surface of the pons, giving rise to many penetrating branches that supply the pons and caudal midbrain (Blumenfeld, 2010; Moore, Dalley, & Agur, 2010; Nolte, 2009; Purves et al., 2012).

basilar skull fracture—A linear fracture at the base of the skull that is usually associated with a dural tear and leakage of cerebrospinal fluid from the nose (*rhinorrhea*) or ear (*otorrhea*). Patient may present with bruising over the mastoids (i.e., battle sign) or bruising around the eyes (i.e., raccoon eyes). Cranial nerve function may also be disrupted (Kumar, Abbas, Fausto, & Aster, 2010; Moore, Dalley, & Agur, 2010).

behavioral optometry—An extension of traditional optometric practice that requires its practitioners to take a holistic approach to the treatment of visual disorders (Barrett, 2008).

blob cells—The color-processing cells of the primary visual cortex (Purves et al., 2012).

blood–brain barrier—The anatomical and transport barriers that collectively isolate the extracellular fluids of the central nervous system from those of the general circulation. The blood–brain barrier controls the entry and rates of transport of substances into the brain's extracellular space from the capillary blood, primarily as the result of astrocytes and capillary permeability (Martini, 2009; Purves et al., 2012).

bottom-up approach—An approach to rehabilitation that focuses on improving thinking skills via the repetitive practice of fundamental cognitive processes, such as structured practice in attention skills (Robertson & Murre, 1999).

botulinum toxin—A potent neuromuscular blocking agent that may be used for the treatment of spasticity (Borg-Stein & Stein, 1993).

brainstem—Region of the brain that lies between the diencephalon and the spinal cord consisting of the midbrain, pons, and medulla (Blumenfeld, 2010; Nolte, 2009; Purves et al., 2012).

Brodmann's areas—Fifty-two regions of the cortex, described and numbered by Korbinian Brodmann (a German neurologist) in 1909 on the basis of observed structural differences. Many of the numbers continue to be used in reference to cortical areas because they correlate with functional divisions of the cortex (Purves et al., 2012).

calcarine sulcus (or fissure)—A major groove or furrow within the cerebral cortex on the medial aspect of the occipital lobe and the location of the primary visual cortex. The calcarine sulcus originates anteriorly in the temporal lobe near the splenium of the corpus callosum and continues posteriorly into the occipital lobe (Moore et al., 2010; Nolte, 2009).

caudate nucleus—One of the nuclei that compose the basal nuclei (together with the putamen, globus pallidus, subthalamic nucleus, and substantia nigra); forms the most medial part of the striatum. It receives input from widespread association areas of the cerebral cortex and is therefore thought to be more involved in cognitive functions and less directly in movement (Blumenfeld, 2010; Nolte, 2009; Purves et al., 2012).

central nervous system—Brain and spinal cord (Posner et al., 2007).

central sulcus (of Rolando)—A major groove or furrow on the lateral aspect of the cerebral hemispheres that forms the boundary between the frontal and parietal lobes. The central sulcus is also the transition zone between primary motor and primary somatosensory cortex. The anterior bank (*precentral gyrus*) contains the primary motor cortex, and the posterior bank (*postcentral gyrus*) contains the primary sensory cortex (Moore et al., 2010; Nolte, 2009).

cerebellum—Large, highly convoluted subdivision of the brain ("little brain") that lies behind the forebrain and above the brainstem. It receives inputs from sensory systems, the cerebral cortex, and other sites and participates in the planning and coordination of movement and cognitive functions (Moore et al., 2010; Nolte, 2009).

cerebral cortex—Extensive, superficial gray matter layer covering the surfaces of the cerebral hemispheres. The majority of the cerebral cortex is composed of neocortex, which has six cell layers (I–VI) designated from the surface inward (Nolte, 2009).

cerebral edema—The excess accumulation of water in the intracellular or extracellular spaces of the brain (Pollay, 1996).

cerebral hemisphere—Right or left half of the cerebral cortex as divided by the longitudinal fissure (Moore et al., 2010; Nolte, 2009).

cerebrospinal fluid—The fluid that permeates the ventricles and cavities of the brain and spinal cord (Posner et al., 2007).

cerebrovascular accident—Brain cell death resulting from lack of oxygen when the blood flow to the brain is impaired by blockage or rupture of an artery to the brain (MedicineNet.com, 2013).

cerebrum—Largest and most *rostral* (i.e., near the front or nose) part of the brain composed of two cerebral hemispheres. Together with the diencephalon, it forms the forebrain (Moore et al., 2010; Nolte, 2009).

chronic traumatic encephalopathy—A condition characterized by cognitive and functional decline and emotional disturbance associated with multiple blows to the head, years or decades before, during sports or military activity; previously termed *punch drunk syndrome* or *dementia pugilistica* (Baugh, Robbins, Stern, & McKee, 2014; Baugh et al., 2012; Gavtt, Stern, & McKee, 2011).

cingulate gyrus—Prominent gyrus on the medial aspect of the cerebral hemisphere, partially surrounding the corpus callosum and considered part of the limbic system; involved in emotional processing, learning and memory, reward anticipation, decision making, and impulse control (i.e., executive functions; Blumenfeld, 2010; Nolte, 2009).

Circle of Willis—The arterial anastomosis at the base of the brain, connecting the anterior and posterior cerebral circulations and supplying arterial blood to the brain. Components include the internal carotid arteries and the anterior and posterior cerebral arteries, interconnected by the anterior and posterior communicating arteries. The anatomy of the Circle of Willis allows for redundancies such that should one part of the circle become blocked or narrowed, perfusion may continue (Moore et al., 2010; Nolte, 2009).

cognition—Information-processing functions of the brain, including attention, memory, and executive functions (e.g., problem solving, planning, self-awareness, self-monitoring; AOTA, 2013).

coma—State of unconsciousness and unarousability (even with vigorous stimuli) in which the patient lies with eyes closed (Posner et al., 2007).

commissural fibers—Bundles of axons (white matter) that interconnect and permit communication between the two cerebral hemispheres by crossing over from one hemisphere and into the other. Commissural fibers are predominantly located in the corpus callosum (Martini, 2009; Purves et al., 2012).

community integration—A multidimensional concept involving various aspects of human functioning including independence and social integration, satisfaction and quality of life, productivity, and community mobility (McCabe et al., 2007).

community mobility—Planning and moving around in the community and using public or private transportation, such as driving, walking, bicycling, or accessing and riding in buses, taxicabs, or other transportation systems (AOTA, 2014).

concentration—Direction of thoughts and actions toward a given stimulus and suppression of awareness of competing distractions (Lezak et al., 2012).

concussion—Any physical trauma to the head that results in neurological sequelae; may or may not meet the minimum criteria for mild traumatic brain injury (De Kruijk, Twijnstra, & Leffers, 2001).

consciousness—State of full awareness of the self and the environment (Posner et al., 2007).

constraint-induced movement therapy—The forced use of the affected limb in functional activities via restraint of the unaffected limb; used to encourage return of motor function and control of the affected limb (Hayner, Gibson, & Giles, 2010; Taub, Uswatte, & Pidikiti, 1999).

contracture—Loss of muscle-group tissue length (shortening) limiting range of motion (Gillen, 2013a).

contralateral—On the opposite side (e.g., each hemisphere controls the contralateral extremities; Purves et al., 2012).

contusion—A bruise on the brain resulting from direct impact to the head (Brain Injury Association of America, 2012).

convergence—The eyes' ability to turn inward to focus on a near object (Scheiman, 2002).

coping—Sum of attempts, regardless of success, by which a person endeavors to manage a stressful situation (Lazarus & Folkman, 1984).

corona radiata—Bundles of fibers entering or leaving the internal capsule (Blumenfeld, 2010; Nolte, 2009; Purves et al., 2012).

corpus callosum—A massive curvilinear bundle of commissural fibers that bridges most cortical areas of the two cerebral hemispheres and serves to join them functionally, allowing for a unitary consciousness (Blumenfeld, 2010; Nolte, 2009; Purves et al., 2012).

cortical column—Functional unit of the cerebral cortex at the microscopic level that receives inputs from and sends signals within and outside the cortex; layers of neurons within a column all share a specific aspect of a neurological task (e.g., a column in the visual cortex may be responsible for detecting an edge at a certain angle at a small spot of the retina; Purves et al., 2012).

corticothalamic fibers—Axons of neurons located in the cerebral cortex (usually Layer VI) that project to the thalamus (Purves et al., 2012).

coup–contrecoup injury—Bruising of brain tissue directly opposite the site of impact to the head (e.g., bruising in occipital lobes after frontal lobes strike the skull); results from linear violent collisions of the brain with the skull, such as in acceleration–deceleration injuries (Posner et al., 2007).

covert visual orienting network—One of the brain's attentional systems that is active in shifting attention from one focus to another in the external environment without shifting visual orientation (Purves et al., 2012).

day treatment program—Postacute outpatient program for medically stable clients in need of rehabilitation. Services have a holistic focus and address cognitive or neurobehavioral impairments, awareness, emotional functioning, interpersonal skills, and independent living. Clients may reside at home or be in a 24-hour residential treatment program (Malec, 2001; Seel, Wright, Wallace, Newman, & Dennis, 2007).

decerebrate posture—Abnormal posturing of limbs in rigid extension, backward arching of the head, arms in adduction and extension, and wrists fully pronated and downward pointing of the toes indicating severe injury to the brain at the level of the upper brainstem (Posner et al., 2007).

decorticate posture—Abnormal posturing of arms, wrists, and fingers in flexion and abduction with extension, internal rotation of the legs, and plantar flexion at the ankles (Posner et al., 2007).

deep vein thrombosis—Occlusion of a major vein caused by the formation of a clot (*thrombus*) most often occurring in the lower extremity, abdomen, or pelvic area (Atkins, 2014).

defense mechanisms—Mostly involuntary, unconscious strategies a person uses to protect the self from excessive anxiety and negative emotions associated with the emergence of unconscious material (Freud, 1992).

dendrite—Neuronal process (fiber) that receives sensory information through synaptic input and transmits these electrical signals toward the cell body (Martini, 2009; Purves et al., 2012; Rhoades & Bell, 2009; Widmaier et al., 2006).

denial—Refusal to acknowledge the accuracy of information about the self or one's own feelings regarding that information (Freud, 1992).

detection—Conscious recognition that an object is present, along with recognition of the object's identity and its significance; detection plays a special role in selecting a target from many alternatives, a process known as *target detection* (Posner & Petersen, 1990).

diaphragmatic breathing—A relaxation technique that involves taking deep abdominal breaths and exhaling them in a slow, measured manner (Rakal, 2010).

diaschisis—Transient suppression of brain activity outside the brain region that is the immediate site of damage (Lezak et al., 2012).

diencephalon ("in-between brain")—The caudal subdivision of the embryonic forebrain, lying just rostral to the midbrain. The diencephalon includes the epithalamus, thalamus, and hypothalamus (Blumenfeld, 2010; Nolte, 2009; Purves et al., 2012).

diffuse axonal injury—Mechanical injury to white brain matter caused by stretching, shearing, and rotational forces (Smith, Meaney, & Shull, 2003).

diplopia—Double vision (Gillen, 2011).

discrepancy score—The standard method of rating lack of awareness as a difference between the client and either the caregiver or the clinician (Visser-Keizer, Meyboom-de Jong, Deelman, Berg, & Gerritsen, 2002).

diurnal rhythms—Cyclic repetition (intensification and weakening) of biological phenomena or processes that occurs at daily intervals (Purves et al., 2012).

divided attentional deficit—An attentional system breakdown in which a person fails to process information necessary for optimal task performance (Schneider, Dumais, & Shiffrin, 1984).

dysarthria—Impaired articulation attributable to paralysis, incoordination, or spasticity of the muscles used for speaking (Lezak et al., 2012).

dysmetria—A condition in which a movement either overshoots the target (*hypermetria*) or fails to reach the target (*hypometria;* Preston, 2013).

dysphagia—Disorder of swallowing (Avery, 2010).

efferent—(*e* = out or away; *ferre* = to carry) A nerve fiber that conducts action potentials away from the central nervous system to the periphery (i.e., motor neurons; Purves et al., 2012).

embolism—The obstruction of a blood vessel by a mass, which may be a blood clot, a colony of bacteria, a foreign body, or air (Gillen, 2013a).

emotion—A short-term affective state triggered by an event or object that causes global change in the brain, body, and behavior (Dalgleish, 2000; Dalgleish & Power, 1999).

emotional lability—A neurological syndrome that is characterized by uncontrollable emotional expressions of excessive or spontaneous crying or laughing; common after stroke or traumatic brain injury (House, Dennis, Molyneux, Warlow, & Hawton, 1989; Work, Colamonico, Bradley, & Kaye, 2011).

end feel—The quality of movement felt by the therapist during passive range of motion at the end of the available range of motion. End feel will vary depending on the joint under consideration and the type of structure that constrains the range of motion. A variety of terms are used to describe the variability in end feel from hard to soft (Reese & Bandy, 2009).

end-feet—Cellular extensions terminate in flattened expansions that completely encase vessels within the central nervous system, contributing to formation of the blood–brain barrier, and surround synapses to modulate synaptic action by controlling uptake of neurotransmitter at or near the synaptic cleft (Purves et al., 2012).

enteral feeding—Tube feeding directed into the stomach or duodenum (Avery, 2010).

episodic memory—Memory of discrete events with perceptual and temporal correlates still attached to them (Tulving, 1983, 2002).

errorless learning—Method of learning in which client errors are prevented by providing sufficient cueing to enable the client to achieve correct performance (Kessels & de Haan, 2003).

executive attention network—Detection network that provides conscious recognition that an object is present, along with its identity and significance, playing a special role in selecting a target from alternatives (Purves et al., 2012).

executive function—Higher level mental processing that includes initiation, organization, sequencing, and problem solving (Stuss, 1991).

exertional testing—An assessment used to help determine whether a service member is fit to return to duty after sustaining a concussion; it involves having the service member exercise to 65% to 85% of maximum heart rate and then assessing for resurgence of postconcussion syndrome symptoms such as dizziness, headache, or visual changes (Bazarian et al., 2008; Kennedy & Moore, 2010).

expanding-retrieval technique—Strategy for increasing a client's ability to learn information by recalling material at spaced intervals; often used with clients exhibiting memory disorders (Clare et al., 2000).

explicit memory—Memory that is available to awareness and involves a conscious and intentional recollection process (Tulving, 2002).

extracellular fluid—Liquid containing proteins and electrolytes found between the cells of the body that provides much of the liquid environment of the body (Hall, 2011; Martini, 2009; Rhoades & Bell, 2009; Widmaier et al., 2006).

extrastriate visual cortex—Areas of the occipital, temporal, and parietal lobes involved in processing visual information after initial reception in the striate (or primary visual) cortex (Purves et al., 2012).

fatigue—Awareness of a decreased capacity for physical or mental activity resulting from an imbalance in the availability, utilization, or restoration of resources needed to perform an activity (Aaronson et al., 1999).

feeling—The internal, subjective mental representation of the emotion (Dalgleish, 2000; Dalgleish & Power, 1999).

FIM™—Assessment measure (Hamilton, Granger, Sherwin, Zielezny, & Tashman, 1987) consisting of 18 items that grades the level of cognitive and physical assistance necessary for function. Item scores range from 1 (*completely dependent*) to 7 (*completely independent*), and total scores range from 18 to 126 (Uniform Data System for Medical Rehabilitation, 1997).

focal brain injury—A contusion or bruising of brain tissue, most often at the poles of the frontal and temporal lobes, resulting from impact of the brain against the skull during an acceleration–deceleration injury in closed brain injury, blood clot, or localized damage in penetrating injury. A focal lesion is a localized and abnormal state of brain tissue (Lezak et al., 2012).

foramen magnum—The inferior aperture of the skull through which the spinal cord passes (Moore et al., 2010).

fovea (of the macula lutea)—The portion (of the macula lutea) of the retina that provides the sharpest vision because it has a high density of cones (Martini, 2009; Purves et al., 2012).

frame of reference—A set of guidelines for practice that provides descriptive and prescriptive treatment principles for how to set up the human and nonhuman environment so that activities may be used as the means to facilitate change in underlying impairments and functional performance (Mosey, 1986, 1996).

frontal lobe—The most anterior region of the brain; controls motor, cognitive, and executive functions (Blumenfeld, 2010; Moore et al., 2010; Nolte, 2009).

functional impairment—Interference with independence in everyday activity (Ganguli et al., 2011).

ganglia—Collection of neuronal cell bodies located in the peripheral nervous system that are anatomically discrete and typically serve a specific function (Blumenfeld, 2010; Purves et al., 2012).

gastrostomy tube—Tube placed through the abdominal wall and into the stomach that may be used for enteral feeding; also called *percutaneous endoscopic gastrostomy* or *gastric tube* (Avery, 2010).

genome—The complete DNA sequence of an organism containing its entire genetic information (Nussbaum, McInnes, & Willard, 2007).

Glasgow Coma Scale—Used to assess, on the basis of eye opening, verbal response, and motor response, the level of consciousness and reaction to stimuli in a neurologically impaired patient (Teasdale & Jennett, 1974).

glia—Diverse collection of nonneuronal cell types in the peripheral and central nervous systems that perform a wide variety of metabolic, electrical, and mechanical functions to support and protect the neurons; also called *neuroglia* or *glial cells* (Hall, 2011; Martini, 2009; Purves et al., 2012).

globus pallidus—One of the nuclei that compose the basal nuclei (together with the caudate, putamen, subthalamic nucleus, and substantia nigra), lying medial to the putamen. It is named "pale globe" because of the many myelinated fibers passing through it. Together with the putamen, it composes the lenticular nucleus. The globus pallidus has two segments, the internal (GPi) and external (GPe) segments (Blumenfeld, 2010; Nolte, 2009; Purves et al., 2012).

Goal Attainment Scaling—An individualized criterion-referenced measure of progress in achieving targeted goals (Ottenbacher & Cusick, 1993).

goniometric measurement—The measurement of angles and range of motion of a joint (Killingsworth, Pedretti, & Pendleton, 2013).

gray matter—Regions of the central nervous system composed of neuronal cell bodies, neuroglia, and unmyelinated axons, including the cerebral and cerebellar cortices, as well as the various nuclei of the brain (Purves et al., 2012).

group interventions—Use of distinct knowledge and leadership techniques to facilitate learning and skill acquisition across the lifespan through the dynamics of group and social interaction. Groups may be used as a method of service delivery (AOTA, 2014).

guided imagery—A complementary therapy that uses visualization to induce a state of deep relaxation (Shamini et al., 2012).

gyrus—Ridge or complex convolution; gyri are of varying widths and form the surface of the cerebral hemisphere, separated by grooves called *sulci*. Some gyri are consistently located from person to person and others are not, but nonetheless the gyri often form the basis for the division of the hemispheres into lobes (Blumenfeld, 2010; Nolte, 2009; Purves et al., 2012).

habit—Consistent response to stimuli that develops through repetition (AOTA, 2014).

hematoma—A local collection of blood outside blood vessels. When related to the brain it is a collection of blood in or around the brain that may be epidural, subdural, subarachnoid, or intraventricular. In *epidural hematoma*, bleeding occurs in the area between the skull and the dura mater; in *subdural hematoma*, bleeding occurs between the dura and the arachnoid mater; and in *subarachnoid hematoma*, bleeding occurs in what is typically a potential space between the arachnoid membrane and the pia mater. *Intraventricular hematoma* involves bleeding in the ventricles of the brain (Purves et al., 2012).

hemiplegia—Paralysis of one side of the body (Lezak et al., 2012).

hemorrhage—Bleeding from a ruptured blood vessel.

heteromodal association areas—Sensory processing areas of the brain that receive input from several unimodal sensory areas (Purves et al., 2012).

heterotopic ossification—Abnormal (ectopic) deposition of bone tissue in the soft tissue at abnormal locations, usually surrounding joints (Adler, 2013).

heterotypic isocortex—Areas of cortex that do not display the prototypical six layers of cells present in isocortex (Nolte, 2009; Purves et al., 2012).

home-based rehabilitation—Programs in which services are delivered in a home that is rented or owned by the client, not established or rented out by the program (Glenn, Rotman, Goldstein, & Selleck, 2005).

homonymous hemianopsia—A visual deficit in which the same (right or left) half of the visual field of both eyes is lost as a result of destruction of the right or left primary visual cortex or destruction or interruption of the fibers leading to it (Lezak et al., 2012; Moore et al., 2010; Purves et al., 2012).

homotypic isocortex—Cortical areas that display the prototypical six layers of varying thickness and differing proportions of neurons (Nolte, 2009).

hydrocephalus—The accumulation of cerebrospinal fluid in the brain, contributing to increased intracranial pressure and resulting from impaired reabsorption or obstruction of the flow of cerebrospinal fluid (Lezak et al., 2012).

hypertension—Blood pressure in the arterial system that is persistently at or above 140 mm Hg systolic or 90 mm Hg diastolic. The heart must work harder than normal to circulate blood through the constricted artery system (American Heart Association, 2014).

hypertonicity—A state of increased muscle tension (Preston, 2013).

hypoxic brain damage—Damage to the brain attributable to lack of oxygen caused either by decreased oxygenation of the blood (e.g., carbon monoxide poisoning) or by decreased blood flow to the brain (Posner et al., 2007).

immediate memory—Automatic learning and retrieval system of sensory information (also called *sensory memory*) that serves to mentally maintain how a stimulus looked (*iconic* or *visual sensory memory*) or sounded (*echoic* or *auditory sensory information*) for only a very short period of time (i.e., seconds) and is dependent on the visual and auditory cortices, respectively (Cohen & Conway, 2008).

impairment—Problems in body functions or structures such as significant deviation or loss (World Health Organization, 2001).

implicit memory—Knowledge that is expressed in performance without one's awareness that one possesses it (Giles, 2011).

information processing—The mental capacity to perceive and react to the environment (Unsworth, 1999).

instrumental activities of daily living—Activities that relate to independent living in the home and community, such as care of others, community mobility, meal preparation, and shopping (AOTA, 2014).

insular lobe—Central lobelike portion of the cerebral cortex that lies deep to the lateral fissure; its functions are not well understood but are known to include gustatory and autonomic areas (also called *insula*; Nolte, 2009).

ischemia—A lack of blood supply that may result from a clot or a narrowing of blood vessels either globally, as after a cardiac arrest, or locally, as after vascular occlusion (Posner et al., 2007).

isocortex—Area of the brain consisting of a huge number of columnar functional modules organized into primary sensory and motor areas, unimodal association areas, multimodal association areas, and limbic areas (Blumenfeld, 2010; Nolte, 2009; Purves et al., 2012).

job performance—Performing the requirements of a job, including work skills and patterns; time management; relationships with coworkers; leadership and supervision; creation, production, and distribution of products and services; initiation, sustainment, and completion of work; and compliance with work norms and procedures (AOTA, 2014).

lateral geniculate nucleus—One of the major thalamic relay nuclei, the role of which is to relay visual information from the retina via the optic tract to the primary visual cortex. The lateral geniculate nucleus is located within, above, and below the calcarine sulcus (Blumenfeld, 2010; Nolte, 2009; Purves et al., 2012).

lateral sulcus (Sylvian fissure)—A long, deep groove or furrow on the lateral aspect of each cerebral hemisphere arising during fetal development; it separates the frontal lobes from the temporal lobes inferiorly and laterally. The insula lies hidden within the depths of this sulcus (Blumenfeld, 2010; Moore et al., 2010; Nolte, 2009; Purves et al., 2012).

lateral ventricles—The first and second ventricles (right and left lateral ventricles); the largest cavities of each cerebral hemisphere, following a *C*-shaped course and containing cerebrospinal fluid (Moore et al., 2010; Nolte, 2009).

learned nonuse—The inability to use reemerging motor activation as a result of the extinction of use when the central nervous system was in shock or other processes made movement impossible (Taub et al., 1999).

leisure—Nonobligatory activity that is intrinsically motivating and takes place during time not committed to other occupations (AOTA, 2014).

leisure participation—Planning and participating in appropriate leisure activities; maintaining a balance of leisure activities with other occupations; and obtaining, using, and maintaining equipment and supplies as appropriate (AOTA, 2014).

life satisfaction—A cognitively oriented, subjective judgment of one's current life situation in relation to one's expectations (Corrigan, Bogner, Mysiw, Clinchot, & Fugate, 2001).

limbic lobe—Region of the cortex that lies superior to the corpus callosum on the medial aspect of the cerebral hemispheres and forms the cortical component of the limbic system (Nolte, 2009; Purves et al., 2012).

locus coeruleus—A column of pigmented, blue-black neurons near the floor of the fourth ventricle, extending through the rostral pons. Neurons in this region provide most of the noradrenergic innervation of the cerebrum (Purves et al., 2012).

long and short association fibers—Axons that interconnect various sites within the same cerebral hemisphere (Martini, 2009).

longitudinal fissure—Extensive, sagittally oriented vertical cleft separating the two cerebral hemispheres (Blumenfeld, 2010; Moore et al., 2010; Nolte, 2009).

macula lutea—The central region of the retina that contains the fovea and is specialized for very sharp color vision (Martini, 2009; Purves et al., 2012).

major neurocognitive disorder—Significant decline in cognitive functioning in two or more higher order cognitive domains (i.e., complex attention, executive ability, learning and memory, language, visuoconstructional–perceptual ability, social cognition; Ganguli et al., 2011).

mammillary bodies—Small, paired prominences that form the posterior portion of the hypothalamus and the ventral aspect of the diencephalon. The mammillary bodies are functionally part of the caudal hypothalamus and play a role in memory (Blumenfeld, 2010; Nolte, 2009).

mediodorsal nucleus—A thalamic relay nucleus that receives its main inputs from the amygdala, olfactory cortex, and basal nuclei. The mediodorsal nucleus sends its main outputs to frontal cortex, and its main roles are in the limbic pathways and as a major relay to frontal cortex (Blumenfeld, 2010; Nolte, 2009; Purves et al., 2012).

medulla oblongata—The most caudal portion of the brainstem, extending from the pons to the spinal cord. The medulla is crucial to many vital functions (respiratory, cardiovascular, visceral activity) and integrative activities and also transmits signals from most sensory and motor tracts of the central nervous system (Blumenfeld, 2010; Nolte, 2009; Purves et al., 2012).

memory—Acquisition, storage, and retrieval of knowledge (Cohen & Conway, 2008).

mesocortex—Transitional region of the cerebral cortex ("middle cortex") that is three to six cell layers deep and is found in the limbic cortex of the parahippocampal gyrus and the anterior inferior insula (Blumenfeld, 2010).

metacognition—A higher level cognitive function; the capacity to understand one's own cognition. Also described as "thinking about thinking" (Unsworth, 1999).

microglia—One of the major types of glial cells in the central nervous system. Microglial cells are specialized macrophages, which are phagocytic and engulf waste material and debris, especially that associated with repairing damage following neuronal injury (Purves et al., 2012).

middle cerebral artery—Major paired artery that arises from the carotid artery and turns laterally and enters the lateral sulcus (Sylvian fissure), where it bifurcates into a *superior division,* which provides blood to the lateral surface of the frontal and anterior parietal lobes, and an *inferior division,* which supplies the superior part of the temporal lobe. Branches of the middle cerebral artery known as *lenticulostriate arteries* supply the basal nuclei and internal capsule and are the most common sites for a stroke (Purves et al., 2012).

mild neurocognitive disorder—Mild cognitive deficits in one or more higher cognitive domains (i.e., complex attention, executive ability, learning and memory, language, visuoconstructional–perceptual ability, social cognition); the person can function independently, often through increased effort or compensatory strategies (Ganguli et al., 2011). The generally accepted criteria for mild neurocognitive disorder are presence of a memory or other cognitive limitation, objective deficits on standardized objective cognitive tests, intact general intellectual function, and lack of significant deficits in social or occupational function (Brooks & Loewenstein, 2010).

minimally conscious state—Inconsistent awareness of self, the environment, and people in the environment marked by following simple commands, communication of *yes–no* responses, intelligible verbalization, and clearly purposeful responses (Giacino et al., 2002).

Mini-Mental State Examination—Widely used assessment of global cognition (Folstein, Folstein, & McHugh, 1975).

mood—A general state of lesser intensity and of longer duration that can be caused by an emotion (Dalgleish, 2000; Dalgleish & Power, 1999).

motor association cortex (primary motor cortex)—The area of frontal lobe that is involved in motor planning of intended movements (Blumenfeld, 2010; Nolte, 2009; Purves et al., 2012).

muscle paresis—The partial or incomplete paralysis of a muscle (Lezak et al., 2012).

myelin—Fatty, membranous, multilayered axonal sheath produced by either Schwann cells (in the peripheral nervous system) or oligodendrocytes (in the central nervous system) interrupted periodically by nodes of Ranvier. Myelination increases the conduction velocity of the axon it surrounds by insulating it and enabling saltatory conduction (Hall, 2011; Martini, 2009; Purves et al., 2012).

nasogastric tube—Tube introduced through the nose and guided into the stomach; may be used for enteral feeding (Avery, 2010).

neural network—Group of neurons that share a similar function and therefore are organized into specific groups (Nolte, 2009).

neuromodulation—Physiological adjustment of some chemical neurotransmitters to the sensitivities of multiple neurons, thereby either facilitating or inhibiting signaling, synaptic transmission, or growth of the neuron. Neuromodulators are secreted by a small group of neurons but diffuse through large areas of the nervous system and therefore are more systemic and slower acting than classical synaptic transmission, in which a presynaptic neuron directly influences a postsynaptic neuron (Hall, 2011; Martini, 2009; Rhoades & Bell, 2009).

neuron—Excitable cell of the nervous system that is electrically active and specialized for intercellular communication. Most typically, motor neurons are *multipolar,* with numerous dendrites and a single axon emerging from an axon hillock, whereas sensory neurons are *unipolar* (i.e., only one protoplasmic process extends from the cell body), and special sensory neurons are *bipolar* (i.e., only two protoplasmic processes extend from the cell body; Blumenfeld, 2010; Nolte, 2009; Purves et al., 2012).

neuroplasticity—The brain's ability to structurally and functionally adapt in response to damage as a result of its history of activation; includes the processes of neurogenesis and rerouting of connections (Lezak et al., 2012; Nolte, 2009; Purves et al., 2012).

neurotransmitter—Chemical compound synthesized and released by neurons into the synaptic cleft that affects the transmembrane potential of another nearby neuron. The purpose is to transmit information from one neuron to another, and the result may lead to neuronal excitation or inhibition depending on the type of neurotransmitter and the magnitude of its activity. Most neurotransmitters are small amine molecules, amino acids, or neuropeptides, but some are gases that simply diffuse across neuronal membranes (Hall, 2011; Martini, 2009; Rhoades & Bell, 2009; Widmaier et al., 2006).

nonsynaptic diffusion neurotransmission—Diffusion through the extracellular fluid of neurotransmitters and other neuroactive substances released at sites that may be remote from the target cells, with the resulting activation of extra-synaptic receptors (Purves et al., 2012).

nuclei—Collection of neuronal cell bodies located in the central nervous system that are anatomically discrete and typically serve a specific function (Blumenfeld, 2010; Purves et al., 2012).

nystagmus—Rapid, repetitive, and rhythmic saccadic eye movements that may also be associated with a slow drift of the eyes in the opposite direction (Posner et al., 2007).

object relations—An eclectic theoretical approach that views people, media, and activities as objects invested with psychic energy. Interaction with these objects is necessary to satisfy personal needs and promote psychological growth and ultimately leads to self-actualization (Bruce & Borg, 1987).

occipital lobe—Most posterior lobe of the cerebral hemisphere; includes the primary visual cortex. The occipital lobe is specifically located within the borders of the calcarine sulcus and adjoining areas of visual association cortex (Blumenfeld, 2010; Moore et al., 2010; Nolte, 2009).

olfaction—Sense of smell (Hall, 2011; Purves et al., 2012).

oligodendrocytes—One of the major types of glial cells in the central nervous system that produces myelin. Oligodendrocytes have numerous cytoplasmic extensions that wrap several turns around an axon, and the multiple layers of cell membranes are converted into myelin. A single oligodendrocyte may myelinate from a few to up to 40 axons (Purves et al., 2012).

orientation—Ability to identify person, place, and time (see also *spatial orientation;* Lezak et al., 2012).

overlearning—Practice of a skill beyond the point at which mastery has been achieved to make the skill less susceptible to forgetting (Rohrer, Taylor, Pashler, Wixted, & Cepeda, 2005).

parietal lobe—A central lobe of the brain that is bounded by the frontal lobe anteriorly, the temporal lobe laterally, and the occipital lobe posteriorly (Blumenfeld, 2010; Moore et al., 2010; Nolte, 2009).

passive range of motion—Maximum amount of motion at a given joint achieved when the joint is moved by an outside force (e.g., the therapist; Killingsworth et al., 2013).

perfusion (cerebral perfusion)—The dispersion of blood to brain tissue; the degree to which blood suffuses brain tissue. Cerebral perfusion pressure is the blood pressure minus intracranial pressure (Posner et al., 2007).

peripheral nervous system—Anatomically, the collection of neurons and nervous tissue that lies outside of the brain and spinal cord; physiologically, the neurons that carry information toward and away from the central nervous system (Nolte, 2009; Purves et al., 2012).

perseveration—Continuation or repetition of a response once it is no longer appropriate (Lezak et al., 2012).

persistent vegetative state—Remaining in a vegetative state for at least 30 days (see *vegetative state;* Posner et al., 2007).

petechial hemorrhage (intraparenchymal hemorrhage)—Pinpoint hemorrhage resulting from broken capillaries in gray matter of the brain, typically as a result of shearing forces at the time of traumatic brain injury and not always visible using current imaging techniques (Lezak et al., 2012; Posner et al., 2007).

plasticity—See *neuroplasticity.*

polytrauma—Concurrent injury to the brain and several body areas or organ systems that results in physical, cognitive, and psychosocial impairments (Veterans Health Administration, 2005).

postconcussion syndrome—The typical pattern of deficits after mild traumatic brain injury, including headache, fatigue, attention deficit, intolerances, and irritability (Posner et al., 2007).

posterior cerebral artery—Major paired artery and terminal branch arising from the bifurcation of the basilar artery at the level of the midbrain and forming the posterior part of the Circle of Willis. The posterior cerebral artery supplies the inferior surface of the brain and the occipital pole (Moore et al., 2010; Nolte, 2009).

posterior inferior cerebellar artery—A long, circumferential branch of the vertebral artery, supplying much of the inferior surface of the cerebellum (Moore et al., 2010; Nolte, 2009).

postsynaptic—A term of reference designating a neuron downstream to a synapse (Hall, 2011; Martini, 2009; Rhoades & Bell, 2009; Widmaier et al., 2006).

posttraumatic amnesia—The period after trauma in which the acquisition of new declarative knowledge is severely impaired. It is said to be resolved when continuous memory for ongoing events is restored (Lezak et al., 2012).

posttraumatic stress disorder—A mental health condition brought on by experiencing or witnessing a terrifying event followed by persistent symptoms of avoidance, reexperiencing, or hyperarousal (Mayo Health Clinic, 2014).

postural hypotension—Hypotension potentially leading to loss of balance or syncope that occurs with positional changes, especially when transitioning from sitting to standing (Johnston, Harper, & Landefeld, 2013).

prefrontal cortex—Most anterior region of the cerebrum and the part of the frontal lobe immediately anterior to the primary and supplementary (association) motor cortices; important for working memory, planning, expression of personality, and choice of appropriate social behavior (Blumenfeld, 2010; Purves et al., 2012).

premotor cortex—Cortical areas on the lateral surface of the frontal lobe immediately anterior to the primary motor cortex. Premotor cortex is important for the planning of voluntary movements (Blumenfeld, 2010; Purves et al., 2012).

presynaptic—A term of reference designating a neuron upstream to a synapse (Hall, 2011; Martini, 2009; Rhoades & Bell, 2009; Widmaier et al., 2006).

primary blast injury—Direct trauma to bodily organs caused by overpressure from the blast itself (Hicks, Fertig, Desrocher, Koroshetz, & Pancrazio, 2010).

primary visual cortex (striate cortex)—Cortical region in the occipital lobe (Brodmann's area 17) that lies on the banks of the calcarine fissure. The role of primary visual cortex is to sort visual information and distribute it to other cortical areas (Purves et al., 2012).

priming (cognitive or perceptual)—Process in which memory recall is facilitated by means of prior exposure to the stimulus that elicits it (Squire & Schacter, 2002).

progressive muscle relaxation—A relaxation technique that involves progressive tensing and relaxation of major skeletal muscle groups with the goal of reducing stress and muscle tension (Bernstein, Borkovec, & Hazlett-Stevens, 2000).

projection fibers—Axons (white matter) that carry information from the thalamus to the cerebral cortex (Martini, 2009; Purves et al., 2012).

proprioception—Awareness of joint position in space, independent of vision (Cooper & Canyock, 2013).

prosody—The expressive intonations of speech including variation in pitch, stress, and duration of speech sounds. Loss of appreciation and production of speech prosody is particularly associated with right-hemisphere damage (Lezak et al., 2012).

prosopagnosia—Difficulty in identifying familiar faces and impairment in learning new faces (Lezak et al., 2012).

prospective memory—The ability to remember to do things in the future, to carry out future intentions (Gillen, 2013b).

psychoeducation—Professionally delivered educational modality that integrates and synergizes psychotherapeutic and educational interventions. It reflects a shift from traditional medical models to a more holistic and competence-based approach, stressing health, collaboration, coping, and empowerment (Lukens & McFarland, 2004).

psychoeducational interventions—Interventions that focus on the structured presentation of information about dementia and caregiving-related issues; may include an active role by participants. Support may be part of a psychoeducational group but is secondary to the educational content (Pinquart & Sörensen, 2006).

pursuits—Tracking movements of the eyes designed to keep a moving stimulus on the fovea (Purves et al., 2001).

putamen—One of the major nuclei that compose the basal nuclei; the part of the striatum that is involved most prominently in the motor functions of the basal nuclei and that receives its inputs from the cerebral cortex (Blumenfeld, 2010; Nolte, 2009; Purves et al., 2012).

quality of life—Dynamic appraisal of the client's life satisfaction (perceptions of progress toward goals), hope (real or perceived belief that one can move forward toward a goal through selected pathways), self-concept (the composite of beliefs and feelings about oneself), health and functioning (e.g., health status, self-care capabilities), and socioeconomic factors (e.g., vocational, educational, and income; AOTA, 2014; Radomski, 1995).

quaternary blast injury—Blast injury characterized by thermal damage to organs induced by the intense heat of the explosion (Hicks et al., 2010).

range of motion—Maximum amount (arc) of motion at a given joint (Killingsworth et al., 2013).

rating of perceived exertion—Method of measuring the intensity of physical activity based on a total feeling of exertion and fatigue. It is a behavior-anchored scale used to describe exertion levels, ranging from 6 (*no exertion at all*) to 20 (*maximal exertion*; Borg, 1998).

rehabilitation—Services provided to people with physical or cognitive deficits that limit their participation in daily life activities and important social roles. Interventions are designed to assist people to resume these life activities and roles (AOTA, 2014).

residential rehabilitation—Program in which clients live in a home owned or rented by the program or its parent organization. Programs may be termed *community based, community reentry, congregate living, day treatment, independent living, transitional living, supervised living,* or *vocational* (Glenn et al., 2005).

saccades—Rapid small eye movements that allow one to rapidly shift fixation points (Scheiman, 2002).

secondary blast injury—Injury caused by shrapnel or debris flung through the air after a blast (Hicks et al., 2010).

self-efficacy—A person's belief in his or her functional capability to perform as required to influence how events affect his or her life (Bandura, 1977).

self-esteem—A person's appraisal of his or her self-worth, typically containing beliefs about himself or herself (Fox, 2008; Heatherton & Polivy, 1991).

self-management of chronic conditions—Active participation in efforts to protect and promote one's own health through various activities and to organize daily life (Coleman & Newton, 2005).

semantic memory—Memory of general knowledge without acquisition context (Tulving, 2002).

short-term memory—Processing and temporary storage of information needed to carry out activities as diverse as understanding, learning, and reasoning for a limited amount of material to be readily accessible for a brief period of time (i.e., several seconds); also called *active* or *primary memory* (Cohen & Conway, 2008).

social environment—Presence of, relationships with, and expectations of people, groups, or populations with whom clients have contact. The social environment includes availability and expectation of significant others such as spouse, friends, and caregivers; relationships with individuals, groups, or populations; and relationships with systems (e.g., political, legal, economic, institutional) that influence norms, role expectations, and social routines (AOTA, 2014).

social participation—Activities associated with organized patterns of behavior in interaction with others (AOTA, 2014).

somatic sensation—Sensations and perceptions arising from skin, muscle, and bones (sense of the body; Hall, 2011; Purves et al., 2012).

somatosensory cortex—The region of the cerebral cortex in the parietal lobe in which nerve fibers transmitting somatic sensory information synapse (Purves et al., 2012).

spaced-retrieval technique—Strategy for maximizing recall of relatively limited amounts of information (e.g., face–name associations) in people with severe memory disorder by recalling material at spaced intervals of increasing duration (Cermak, Verfaellie, Lanzoni, Mather, & Chase, 1996; Davis, Massman, & Doody, 2001; Schacter, Rich, & Stampp, 1985).

spasticity—A state of hypertonicity with velocity-dependent increase in tonic stretch reflexes (Preston, 2013).

spatial orientation—Ability to sense the location or direction of movement of objects or of points in space in relation to one another or to oneself (Lezak et al., 2012).

stereognosis—The identification of an object through touch (Lezak et al., 2012).

stereopsis (astereopsis)—Stereoscopic vision (or its absence); important in depth perception (Lezak et al., 2012).

stress—Negative emotional states (e.g., fear, sadness, anxiety, frustration, anger, depression) evoked by a situation (Taylor, 2006).

striate cortex—Primary visual cortex in the occipital lobe (Brodmann's area 17), named for its striped appearance when observed with the naked eye that results from the prominence of Layer IV in myelinated sections (Purves et al., 2012).

striatum—An inclusive term referring to the caudate nucleus and putamen of the basal nuclei. The striatum is the major point of entry into the basal nuclei circuitry, receiving inputs from large cortical areas and projecting inhibitory outputs to the globus pallidus and substantia nigra (Blumenfeld, 2010; Nolte, 2009).

Structured Functional Cognitive Assessment—A performance-based assessment that provides the structured documentation of operationally defined perceptual and cognitive–behavioral observations during performance of activities of daily living and allows for the establishment of appropriate burden of care (Mortera, 2004, 2012).

subarachnoid hemorrhage—A bleed adjacent to the brain; an acute medical emergency often the result of an aneurysm and often preceded by severe headache and leading to alteration in consciousness, coma, or death (Posner et al., 2007).

subcortical—Pertaining to the portion of the brain that lies below the cerebral cortex; this region is responsible for the fast, unconscious activities involving structures of the diencephalon and brainstem (Nolte, 2009; Purves et al., 2012).

subluxation—Incomplete dislocation in which contact remains between joint surfaces, often of the glenohumeral joint after cerebrovascular accident (Gillen, 2013a).

substantia nigra—Large nucleus at the base of the midbrain positioned between the red nucleus and cerebral peduncle that receives input from several cortical and subcortical structures. The *substantia nigra pars compacta* contains closely packed, pigmented dopaminergic neurons that send their output to the striatum, and the *substantia nigra pars reticulata* contains more loosely arranged GABAergic neurons that receive inputs from the striatum and send their output to the thalamus (Blumenfeld, 2010; Purves et al., 2012).

subthalamic nucleus—Large nucleus at the base of the midbrain, medial and superior to the junction of the internal capsule and cerebral peduncle; the basis of the indirect route through the basal nuclei, receiving input from the striatum and participating in the modulation of motor control (Blumenfeld, 2010; Purves et al., 2012).

sulcus—A groove or furrow of varying depth along the surface of the cerebral hemisphere. Some sulci are consistently located and others are not, but they often form the basis for the division of the hemispheres into lobes (Moore et al., 2010; Nolte, 2009).

superior colliculus—A large, rounded mass of gray matter that forms the roof of the midbrain. It receives input from the retina and visual cortex, sends outputs to the pulvinar and other structures, and plays an important role in orienting movements of the head and eyes (Nolte, 2009; Purves et al., 2012).

supported employment—Paid work in real work settings for people with severe disabilities who would be unable to work without permanent support at the job site (Wehman et al., 1988).

suprachiasmatic nucleus—A rice grain–sized hypothalamic nucleus that lies above the optic chiasm and receives direct input from the retina. Suprachiasmatic nucleus neurons are sensitive to light via the retina and serve as the "master clock" of circadian rhythms (Blumenfeld, 2010; Purves et al., 2012).

supratentorial herniation—Imbalance in pressure in different compartments of the brain caused by an expanding mass lesion; if severe, it can cause displacement of brain tissue of various types (e.g., tonsillar, uncal, falcine, central). In central transtentorial herniation, increased pressure leads to herniation through the tentorial opening, an early sign of which is alteration of consciousness (Posner et al., 2007).

sympathetic nervous system—Division of the visceral motor (autonomic) nervous system in which the visceral effectors engage mostly adrenergic synapses. This division is often referred to as the "flight, fright, or fight" system because its activity is engaged during periods of stress and when survivability is challenged (Purves et al., 2012).

synapse—Point of contact between neurons at which one neuron is able to influence the other (electrically or, most often, chemically; Hall, 2011; Martini, 2009; Rhoades & Bell, 2009; Widmaier et al., 2006).

temporal lobe—Most inferior lobe of each cerebral hemisphere, lying inferior to the lateral sulcus (Sylvian fissure) and anterior to the occipital lobe. The temporal lobe contains auditory sensory and association cortex, part of the posterior language cortex, visual and higher order association cortex, primary and association olfactory cortex, the amygdala, and the hippocampus (Blumenfeld, 2010; Moore et al., 2010; Nolte, 2009).

tertiary blast injury—Injury that occurs when a person is thrown to the ground or into another stationary object in the wake of a blast (Hicks et al., 2010).

thalamus—Collection of nuclei that form the majority of the diencephalon. The thalamus has numerous functions, but its primary role is to relay sensory information from lower centers of the central nervous system to the various regions of the cerebral cortex (Blumenfeld, 2010; Nolte, 2009; Purves et al., 2012).

third ventricle—One of four spaces in the brain that are formed as the lumen from the embryonic neural tube. The third ventricle is a vertically oriented cavity within the diencephalon separating the thalamus and hypothalamus and is confluent anteriorly with both lateral ventricles via the interventricular foramina and posteriorly with the fourth ventricle through the aqueduct (Moore et al., 2010; Nolte, 2009).

tone—The resting state of muscle (mild contraction), ready for movement (Preston, 2013).

top-down approach—An approach to rehabilitation that involves the engagement of higher processes to regulate lower processes as in training in self-awareness or metacognitive control strategies (Robertson & Murre, 1999).

traumatic brain injury—An insult to the brain resulting from external impact or acceleration–deceleration force exerted on the brain (Lezak et al., 2012).

unilateral neglect—A condition in which a person fails to report, respond to, or orient to novel stimuli or maintain attention to stimuli presented unilaterally (Lezak et al., 2012).

unimodal association cortices—Areas of sensory cortex specialized for processing information from one specialized primary sensory receptive area (Purves et al., 2012).

vegetative state—A state that may follow coma (usually appearing in 10–30 days) in which a cyclical pattern of arousal states resumes and that includes eye opening in a patient who shows no other indication of awareness of self or of the environment (Posner et al., 2007).

vertebral artery—One of the two major arteries that supplies the brainstem, cerebellum, and occipital lobe of the cerebrum. The vertebral artery originates as the first branch of the subclavian artery, courses cranially via the transverse foramina of cervical vertebrae, enters the base of the skull through the foramen magnum, and finally ascends along the medulla and pons where the two vertebral arteries join to form the basilar artery (Moore et al., 2010; Nolte, 2009).

vestibular function—Sensation related to position, balance, and secure movement against gravity (AOTA, 2014).

vigilance network—Network of the brain involving the right frontal and parietal regions that enables the maintenance of a sustained state of alertness (Purves et al., 2012).

vision rehabilitation—The combined implementation of vision therapy (an organized therapeutic regimen to treat several neuromuscular, neuropsychological, and neurosensory conditions that interfere with visual function) and patient education on the functional implications of visual dysfunction. Vision rehabilitation requires a collaborative relationship between the occupational therapist and the optometrist or ophthalmologist and often requires advanced preparation on the part of the occupational therapist (Scheiman, 2002).

visual field—The area visible to one eye. Because the optics of the eye reverse and invert the image on the retina, the temporal field is seen by the nasal retina, the superior part of the field is seen by the inferior retina, and the blind spot (corresponding to the optic disk) is temporal to the fovea in the visual field (Moore et al., 2010; Nolte, 2009; Purves et al., 2012).

vocational rehabilitation (traumatic brain injury [TBI] specific)—A rehabilitation approach designed to serve survivors of TBI, with the main goal of achieving a rehabilitation outcome (i.e., return to work, employment, job retention; Fadyl & McPherson, 2009).

volunteer participation—Performing unpaid work activities for the benefit of selected causes, organizations, or facilities (AOTA, 2014).

white matter—Regions of the central nervous system that contain mostly myelinated axons and therefore appear white (Purves et al., 2012).

working memory—Knowledge briefly held in awareness while a mental operation (e.g., planning, organizing, problem solving, paying attention) is performed (Cohen & Conway, 2008).

References

Aaronson, L., Teel, C., Cassmeyer, V., Pallikkathayll, L., Pierce, J., Press, A., . . . Wingate, A. (1999). Defining and measuring fatigue. *Image: The Journal of Nursing Scholarship, 31,* 45–50.

Adler, C. (2013). Spinal cord injury. In H. M. Pendleton & W. Schultz-Krohn (Eds.), *Pedretti's occupational therapy: Practice skills for physical dysfunction* (7th ed., pp. 954–982). St. Louis: Mosby.

American Heart Association. (2014). *What is high blood pressure?* Retrieved from http://www.heart.org/HEARTORG/Conditions/HighBloodPressure/AboutHighBloodPressure/What-is-High-Blood-Pressure_UCM_301759_Article.jsp

American Occupational Therapy Association. (2013). Cognition, cognitive rehabilitation, and occupational performance. *American Journal of Occupational Therapy, 67*(Suppl.), S9–S31. http://dx.doi.org/10.5014/ajot.2013.67S9

American Occupational Therapy Association. (2014). Occupational therapy practice framework: Domain and process (3rd ed.). *American Journal of Occupational Therapy, 68*(Suppl.), S1–S48. http://dx.doi.org/10.5014/ajot.2014.682006

Armutlu, K. (2013). Ataxia: Physical therapy and rehabilitation applications for ataxic patients. In J. H. Stone & M. Blouin (Eds.), *International encyclopedia of rehabilitation.* Buffalo, NY: Center for International Rehabilitation Research Information and Exchange. Retrieved from http://cirrie.buffalo.edu/encyclopedia/en/article/112

Atkins, M. S. (2014). Spinal cord injury. In M. V. Radomski & C. A. Trombly Latham (Eds.), *Occupational therapy for physical dysfunction* (7th ed., pp. 1168–1214). Philadelphia: Wolters Kluwer.

Avery, W. (2010). *Dysphagia care and related feeding concerns for adults* (Self-Paced Clinical Course, 2nd ed.). Bethesda, MD: American Occupational Therapy Association.

Bandura, A. (1977). Self-efficacy: Toward a unifying theory of behavioral change. *Psychological Review, 84,* 191–215. http://dx.doi.org/10.1037/0033-295X.84.2.191

Barrett, B. (2008). A critical evaluation of the evidence supporting the practice of behavioural vision therapy. *Ophthalmic and Physiological Optics, 29,* 4–25. http://dx.doi.org/10.1111/j.1475-1313.2008.00607.x

Baugh, C. M., Robbins, C. A., Stern, R. A., & McKee, A. C. (2014). Current understanding of chronic traumatic encephalopathy. *Current Treatment Options in Neurology, 16,* 306. http://dx.doi.org/10.1007/s11940-014-0306-5

Baugh, C. M., Stamm, J. M., Riley, D. O., Gavett, B. E., Shenton, M. E., Lin, A., . . . Stern, R. A. (2012). Chronic traumatic encephalopathy: Neurodegeneration following repetitive concussive and subconcussive brain trauma. *Brain Imaging and Behavior, 6,* 244–254. http://dx.doi.org/10.1007/s11682-012-9164-5

Bazarian, J., Boerman, H., Bolenbacher, R., Dalton, D., De John, M., Doncevic, S., . . . Williams, C. (2008, July 31–August 1). *Proceedings from Defense and Veterans Brain Injury Center Consensus Conference on the Acute Management of Concussion/Mild Traumatic Brain Injury (mTBI) in the Deployed Setting.* Washington, DC: Defense and Veterans Brain Injury Center. Retrieved from http://www.pdhealth.mil/downloads/clinical_practice_guideline_recommendationsJuly_Aug08.pdf

Bernstein, D. A., Borkovec, T. D., & Hazlett-Stevens, H. (2000). *New directions in progressive relaxation training: A guidebook for helping professionals.* Santa Barbara, CA: Greenwood Publishing.

Blumenfeld, H. (2010). *Neuroanatomy through clinical cases* (2nd ed.). Sunderland, MA: Sinauer Associates.

Borg, G. (1998). *Borg's Perceived Exertion and Pain Scales.* Champaign, IL: Human Kinetics.

Borg-Stein, J., & Stein, J. (1993). Pharmacology of botulinum toxin and implications for use in disorders of muscle tone. *Journal of Head Trauma Rehabilitation, 8,* 103–106.

Brain Injury Association of America. (2012). *About brain injury.* Retrieved from http://www.biausa.org/about-brain-injury.htm

Brooks, L. G., & Loewenstein, D. A. (2010). Assessing the progression of mild cognitive impairment to Alzheimer's disease: Current trends and future directions. *Alzheimer's Research and Therapy, 2,* 28. http://dx.doi.org/10.1186/alzrt52

Bruce, M., & Borg, B. (1987). *Frames of reference in psychosocial occupational therapy.* Thorofare, NJ: Slack.

Cermak, L. S., Verfaellie, M., Lanzoni, S., Mather, M., & Chase, K. A. (1996). Effects of spaced repetitions on amnesia patients' recall and recognition performance. *Neuropsychology, 10,* 219–227. http://dx.doi.org/10.1037/0894-4105.10.2.219

Clare, L., Wilson, B. A., Carter, G., Breen, K., Gosses, A., & Hodges, J. R. (2000). Intervening with everyday memory problems in dementia of Alzheimer type: An errorless learning approach. *Journal of Clinical and Experimental Neuropsychology, 22,* 132–146. http://dx.doi.org/10.1076/1380-3395(200002)22:1;1-8;FT132

Cohen, G., & Conway, M. A. (2008). *Memory in the real world* (3rd ed.). Hove, England: Psychology Press.

Coleman, M. T., & Newton, K. S. (2005). Supporting self-management in patients with chronic illness. *American Family Physician, 72,* 1503–1510.

Cooper, C., & Canyock, J. D. (2013). Evaluation of sensation and intervention for sensory dysfunction. In H. M. Pendleton & W. Schultz-Krohn (Eds.), *Pedretti's occupational therapy: Practice skills for physical dysfunction* (7th ed., pp. 575–589). St. Louis: Mosby.

Corrigan, J., Bogner, J., Mysiw, W., Clinchot, D., & Fugate, L. (2001). Life satisfaction after traumatic brain injury. *Journal of Head Trauma Rehabilitation, 16,* 543–555.

Dalgleish, T. (2000). Roads not taken: The case for multiple functional-level routes to emotion. *Behavioral and Brain Sciences, 23,* 196–197. http://dx.doi.org/10.1017/S0140525X00272427

Dalgleish, T., & Power, M. J. (1999). *Handbook of cognition and emotion.* Chichester, England: Wiley.

Davis, N. R., Massman, P. J., & Doody, R. S. (2001). Cognitive intervention in Alzheimer disease: A randomized placebo-controlled study. *Alzheimer Disease and Associated Disorders, 15,* 1–9.

De Kruijk, J. R., Twijnstra, A., & Leffers, P. (2001). Diagnostic criteria and differential diagnosis of mild traumatic brain injury. *Brain Injury, 15,* 99–106. http://dx.doi.org/10.1080/026990501458335

Edlow, B. L., Takahashi, E., Wu, O., Benner, T., Dai, G., Bu, L., . . . Folkerth, R. D. (2012). Neuroanatomic connectivity of the human ascending arousal system critical to consciousness and its disorders. *Journal of Neuropathology and Experimental Neurology, 71,* 531–546. http://dx.doi.org/10.1097/NEN.0b013e3182588293

Ergh, T. C., Rapport, L. J., Coleman, R. D., & Hanks, R. A. (2002). Predictors of caregiver and family functioning following traumatic brain injury: Social support moderates caregiver distress. *Journal of Head Trauma Rehabilitation, 17,* 155–174. http://dx.doi.org/10.1097/00001199-200204000-00006

Fadyl, J., & McPherson, K. (2009). Approaches to vocational rehabilitation after traumatic brain injury: A review of the evidence. *Journal of Head Trauma Rehabilitation, 24,* 195–212. http://dx.doi.org/10.1097/HTR.0b013e3181a0d458

Fleming, J., & Nalder, E. (2011). Transition to community integration for persons with acquired brain injury. In N. Katz (Ed.), *Cognition, occupation, and participation across the life span: Neuroscience, neurorehabilitation, and models of intervention in occupational therapy* (3rd ed., pp. 51–70). Bethesda, MD: AOTA Press.

Folstein, M. F., Folstein, S. E., & McHugh, P. R. (1975). "Mini-Mental State": A practical method for grading the cognitive state of patients for the clinician. *Journal of Psychiatric Research, 12,* 189–198. http://dx.doi.org/10.1016/0022-3956(75)90026-6

Fox, E. (2008). *Emotion science: Cognitive and neuroscientific approaches to understanding human emotions.* Basingstoke, England: Palgrave Macmillan.

Freud, A. (1992). *The ego and the mechanisms of defence.* London: Karnac Books.

Ganguli, M., Blacker, D., Blazer, D. G., Grant, I., Jeste, D. V., Paulsen, J. S., . . . Sachdev, P. S.; Neurocognitive Disorders Work Group of the American Psychiatric Association *DSM–5* Task Force. (2011). Classification of neurocognitive disorders in *DSM–5:* A work in progress. *American Journal of Geriatric Psychiatry, 19,* 205–210. http://dx.doi.org/10.1097/JGP.0b013e3182051ab4

Gavtt, B. E., Stern, R. A., & McKee, A. C. (2011). Chronic traumatic encephalopathy: A potential late effect of sport-related concussive and subconcussive head trauma. *Clinical Sports Medicine, 30,* 179–188. http://dx.doi.org/10.1016/j.csm.2010.09.007

Giacino, J. T, Ashwal, S., Childs, N., Cranford, R., Jennett, B., Katz, D. I., . . . Zasler, N. D. (2002). The minimally conscious state: Definition and diagnostic criteria. *Neurology, 58,* 349–353. http://dx.doi.org/10.1212/WNL.58.3.349

Giles, G. M. (2011). A neurofunctional approach to rehabilitation following brain injury. In N. Katz (Ed.), *Cognition, occupation, and participation across the life span: Neuroscience, neurorehabilitation, and models of intervention in occupational therapy* (3rd ed., pp. 351–381). Bethesda, MD: AOTA Press.

Gillen, G. (2011). *Stroke rehabilitation: A function-based approach* (3rd ed.). St. Louis: Mosby.

Gillen, G. (2013a). Cerebrovascular accident/stroke. In H. M. Pendleton & W. Schultz-Krohn (Eds.), *Occupational therapy: Practice skills for physical dysfunction* (7th ed., pp. 844–880). St. Louis: Mosby.

Gillen, G. (2013b). Evaluation and treatment of limited occupational performance secondary to cognitive dysfunction. In H. M. Pendleton & W. Schultz-Krohn (Eds.), *Occupational therapy: Practice skills for physical dysfunction* (7th ed., pp. 648–677). St. Louis: Mosby.

Glenn, M., Rotman, M., Goldstein, R., & Selleck, E. (2005). Characteristics of residential community integration programs for adults with brain injury. *Journal of Head Trauma Rehabilitation, 20,* 393–401.

Hall, J. E. (2011). *Guyton and Hall textbook of medical physiology* (12th ed.). Philadelphia: Saunders/Elsevier.

Hamilton, B. B., Granger, C. V., Sherwin, F. S., Zielezny, M., & Tashman, J. S. (1987). A uniform national data system for medical rehabilitation. In M. J. Fuhrer (Ed.), *Rehabilitation outcomes: Analysis and measurement* (pp. 137–147). Baltimore: Paul H. Brookes.

Hayner, K., Gibson, G., & Giles, G. M. (2010). Comparison of constraint-induced movement therapy and bilateral treatment of equal intensity in people with chronic upper-extremity dysfunction after cerebrovascular accident. *American Journal of Occupational Therapy, 64,* 528–539. http://dx.doi.org/10.5014/ajot.2010.08027

Heatherton, T., & Polivy, J. (1991). Development and validation of a scale for measuring state self-esteem. *Journal of Personality and Social Psychology, 60,* 895–910. http://dx.doi.org/10.1037/0022-3514.60.6.895

Hicks, R. R., Fertig, S. J., Desrocher, R. E., Koroshetz, W. J., & Pancrazio, J. J. (2010). Neurological effects of blast injury. *Journal of Trauma, 68,* 1257–1263. http://dx.doi.org/10.1097/TA.0b013e3181d8956d

House, A., Dennis, M., Molyneux, A., Warlow, C., & Hawton, K. (1989). Emotionalism after stroke. *British Medical Journal, 298,* 991–994. http://dx.doi.org/10.1136/bmj.298.6679.991

Johnston, C. B., Harper, G. M., & Landefeld, C. S. (2013). Geriatric disorders. In M. A. Papadakis, S. J. McPhee, & M. W. Rabow (Eds.), *Current medical diagnosis and treatment* (52nd ed., pp. 57–73). New York: McGraw-Hill Medical.

Kennedy, C. H., & Moore, J. L. (2010). *Military neuropsychology.* New York: Springer.

Kessels, R. P. C., & de Haan, E. H. F. (2003). Mnemonic strategies in older people: A comparison of errorless and errorful learning. *Age and Ageing, 32,* 529–533. http://dx.doi.org/10.1093/ageing/afg068

Killingsworth, A. P., Pedretti, L. W., & Pendleton, H. M. (2013). Joint range of motion. In H. M. Pendleton & W. Schultz-Krohn (Eds.), *Pedretti's occupational therapy: Practice skills for physical dysfunction* (7th ed., pp. 529–574). St. Louis: Mosby.

Kumar, V., Abbas, A. K., Fausto, N., & Aster, J. (2010). *Robbins and Cotran pathologic basis of disease* (8th ed.). Philadelphia: Saunders/Elsevier.

Lazarus, R. S., & Folkman, S. (1984). *Stress, appraisal, and coping.* New York: Springer.

Lezak, M. D., Howieson, D. B., Bigler, E. D., & Tranel, D. (2012). *Neuropsychological assessment* (5th ed.). New York: Oxford University Press.

Lukens, E. P., & McFarland, W. R. (2004). Psychoeducation as evidence-based practice: Considerations for practice, research, and policy. *Brief Treatment and Crisis Intervention, 4,* 205–225. http://dx.doi.org/10.1093/brief-treatment/mhh019

Malec, J. (2001). Impact of comprehensive day treatment on societal participation for persons with acquired brain injury. *Archives of Physical Medicine and Rehabilitation, 82,* 885–895. http://dx.doi.org/10.1053/apmr.2001.23895

Martini, N. (2009). *Fundamentals of anatomy and physiology* (8th ed.). San Francisco: Pearson Benjamin Cummings.

Mayo Health Clinic. (2014). *Post-traumatic stress disorder (PTSD).* Retrieved from http://www.mayoclinic.org/diseases-conditions/post-traumatic-stress-disorder/basics/definition/con-20022540

McCabe, P., Lippert, C., Weiser, M., Hilditch, M., Hartridge, C., & Villamere, J.; ERABI Group. (2007). Community reintegration following acquired brain injury. *Brain Injury, 21,* 231–257. http://dx.doi.org/10.1080/02699050701201631

MedicineNet.com. (2013). *Definition of cerebrovascular accident.* Retrieved from http://www.medterms.com/script/main/art.asp?articlekey=2676

Milner, B., & Teuber, H.-L. (1968). Alteration of perception and memory in man. In L. Weiskrantz (Ed.), *Analysis of behavioral change* (pp. 268–375). New York: Harper & Row.

Moore, K. L., Dalley, A. F., & Agur, A. M. R. (2010). *Clinically oriented anatomy* (6th ed.). Baltimore: Lippincott Williams & Wilkins.

Mortera, M. H. (2004). The development of the Cognitive Screening Measure for individuals with brain injury: Initial examination of content validity and interrater reliability. *Dissertation Abstracts International: Section A. Humanities and Social Sciences, 65,* 906.

Mortera, M. H. (2012). International Brain Injury Association's 9th World Congress on Brain Injury: Meeting the Need for Ecologically Valid Instrument Development: Innovation in Structured Functional Cognitive Assessment (SFCA) for individuals with traumatic brain injury. *Brain Injury, 26,* 318.

Mosey, A. C. (1986). *Psychosocial components of occupational therapy.* New York: Raven Press.

Mosey, A. C. (1996). *Applied scientific inquiry in the health professions: An epistemological orientation* (2nd ed.). Bethesda, MD: American Occupational Therapy Association.

National Stroke Association. (2006). *Recovery after stroke: Coping with emotions.* Retrieved from http://www.stroke.org/site/DocServer/NSAFactSheet_Emotions.pdf?docID=990

Nolte, J. (2009). *The human brain: An introduction to its functional anatomy* (6th ed.). Philadelphia: Elsevier.

Nussbaum, R., McInnes, R. R., & Willard, H. F. (2007). *Thompson and Thompson genetics in medicine* (7th ed.). Philadelphia: Saunders/Elsevier.

Ottenbacher, K., & Cusick, A. (1993). Discriminative versus evaluative assessment: Some observations on Goal Attainment Scaling. *American Journal of Occupational Therapy, 47,* 349–354.

Pinquart, M., & Sörensen, S. (2006). Helping caregivers of persons with dementia: Which interventions work and how large are their effects? *International Psychogeriatrics, 18,* 577–595. http://dx.doi.org/10.1017/S1041610206003462

Pollay, M. (1996). Blood–brain barrier, cerebral edema. In R. H. Wilkins & S. S. Rengachary (Eds.), *Neurosurgery* (2nd ed., pp. 335–344). New York: McGraw-Hill.

Posner, J. B., Saper, C. B., Schiff, N. D., & Plum, F. (2007). *Plum and Posner's diagnosis of stupor and coma* (4th ed.). Oxford, England: Oxford University Press.

Posner, M. I., & Petersen, S. E. (1990). The attention system of the human brain. *Annual Review of Neuroscience, 13,* 25–42. http://dx.doi.org/10.1146/annurev.ne.13.030190.000325

Preston, L. A. (2013). Evaluation of motor control. In H. M. Pendleton & W. Schultz-Krohn (Eds.), *Occupational therapy: Practice skills for physical dysfunction* (7th ed., pp. 461–488). St. Louis: Mosby.

Purves, D., Augustine, G. J., Fitzpatrick, D., Hall, W. C., LaMantia, A. S., & White, L. E. (2012). *Neuroscience* (5th ed.). Sunderland, MA: Sinauer Associates.

Purves, D., Augustine, G. J., Fitzpatrick, D., Katz, L. C., LaMantia, A., McNamara, J. O., & Williams, S. M. (Eds.). (2001). Types of eye movements and their functions. In *Neuroscience* (2nd ed.). Sunderland, MA: Sinauer Associates. Retrieved from http://www.ncbi.nlm.nih.gov/books/NBK10991/

Radomski, M. (1995). There is more to life than putting on your pants. *American Journal of Occupational Therapy, 49,* 487–490. http://dx.doi.org/10.5014/ajot.49.6.487

Rakal, D. (2010). *Learning deep breathing.* Retrieved from http://psychcentral.com/lib/learning-deep-breathing/0003203

Reese, N. B., & Bandy, W. D. (2009). *Joint range of motion and muscle length testing* (2nd ed.). St. Louis: Saunders/Elsevier.

Rhoades, R. A., & Bell, D. R. (2009). *Medical physiology: Principles for clinical medicine* (3rd ed.). Baltimore: Lippincott Williams & Wilkins.

Robertson, I. H., & Murre, J. M. J. (1999). Rehabilitation of brain damage: Brain plasticity and principles of guided recovery. *Psychological Bulletin, 125,* 544–575. http://dx.doi.org/10.1037/0033-2909.125.5.544

Rohrer, D., Taylor, K., Pashler, H., Wixted, J. T., & Cepeda, N. J. (2005). The effect of overlearning on long-term retention. *Applied Cognitive Psychology, 19,* 361–374. http://dx.doi.org/10.1002/acp.1083

Scarpa, A., & Raine, A. (1997). Psychophysiology of anger and violent behavior. *Psychiatric Clinics of North America, 20,* 375–394. http://dx.doi.org/10.1016/S0193-953X(05)70318-X

Schacter, D. L., Rich, S. A., & Stampp, M. S. (1985). Remediation of memory disorders: Experimental evaluation of the spaced-retrieval technique. *Journal of Clinical and Experimental Neuropsychology, 7,* 79–96. http://dx.doi.org/10.1080/01688638508401243

Scheiman, M. (2002). *Understanding and managing vision deficits: A guide for occupational therapists* (2nd ed.). Thorofare, NJ: Slack.

Schneider, W., Dumais, S. T., & Shiffrin, R. M. (1984). Automatic and control processing and attention. In R. Parasuraman & D. R. Davis (Eds.), *Varieties of attention* (pp. 1–27). London: Academic Press.

Seel, R., Wright, G., Wallace, T., Newman, S., & Dennis, L. (2007). The utility of the FIM+FAM for assessing traumatic brain injury day program outcomes. *Journal of Head Trauma Rehabilitation, 22,* 267–277. http://dx.doi.org/10.1097/01.HTR.0000290971.56130.c8

Shamini, J., McMahon, G. F., Hasen, P., Kozub, M. P., Porter, V., King, R., & Guarneri, E. M. (2012). Healing touch with guided imagery for PTSD in returning active duty military: A randomized controlled trial. *Military Medicine, 177,* 1015–1021.

Smith, D. H., Meaney, D. F., & Shull, W. H. (2003). Diffuse axonal injury in head trauma. *Journal of Head Trauma Rehabilitation, 18,* 307–316.

Squire, L. R., & Schacter, D. L. (Eds.). (2002). *Neuropsychology of memory* (3rd ed.). New York: Guilford.

Stahl, S. M. (2008). *Stahl's essential psychopharmacology* (3rd ed.). Cambridge, England: Cambridge University Press.

Starkstein, S. E., Fedoroff, J. P., Price, T. R., Leiguarda, R., & Robinson, R. G. (1993). Apathy following cerebrovascular lesions. *Stroke, 24,* 1625–1630. http://dx.doi.org/10.1161/01.STR.24.11.1625

Stuss, D. T. (1991). Self-awareness and the frontal lobes: A neuropsychological perspective. In J. Strauss & G. R. Goethals (Eds.), *The self: Interdisciplinary approaches* (pp. 255–278). New York: Springer-Verlag.

Taub, E., Uswatte, G., & Pidikiti, R. (1999). Constraint-induced movement therapy: A new family of techniques with broad application to physical rehabilitation—A clinical review. *Journal of Rehabilitation Research and Development, 36,* 237–251.

Taylor, S. E. (2006). *Health psychology* (6th ed.). Boston: McGraw-Hill.

Teasdale, G., & Jennett, B. (1974). Assessment of coma and impaired consciousness: A practical scale. *Lancet, 2,* 81–84.

Tulving, E. (1983). *Elements of episodic memory.* Oxford, England: Clarendon Press.

Tulving, E. (2002). Episodic memory: From mind to brain. *Annual Review of Psychology, 53,* 1–25. http://dx.doi.org/10.1146/annurev.psych.53.100901.135114

Uniform Data System for Medical Rehabilitation. (1997). *Guide for the Uniform Data Set for Medical Rehabilitation (including the FIM™ instrument), version 5.1.* Buffalo, NY: Author.

Unsworth, C. (1999). *Cognitive and perceptual dysfunction.* Philadelphia: F. A. Davis.

Veterans Health Administration. (2005). *VHA Directive 2005-024: Polytrauma Rehabilitation Centers.* Washington, DC: U.S. Department of Veterans Affairs.

Visser-Keizer, A. C., Meyboom-de Jong, B., Deelman, B. G., Berg, I. J., & Gerritsen, M. J. (2002). Subjective changes in emotion, cognition, and behaviour after stroke: Factors affecting the perception of patients and partners. *Journal of Clinical and Experimental Neuropsychology, 24,* 1032–1045. http://dx.doi.org/10.1076/jcen.24.8.1032.8383

Wehman, P., Kreutzer, J., Stonnington, H., Wood, W., Sherron, P., Diambra, J., . . . Groah, C. (1988). Supported employment for persons with traumatic brain injury: A preliminary report. *Journal of Head Trauma Rehabilitation, 3,* 82–94.

Widmaier, E. P., Raff, H., & Strang, K. T. (2006). *Vander's human physiology: The mechanisms of body function* (11th ed.). New York: McGraw-Hill.

Work, S. S., Colamonico, J. A., Bradley, W. G., & Kaye, R. E. (2011). Pseudobulbar affect: An under-recognized and under-treated neurological disorder. *Advances in Therapy, 28,* 586–601. http://dx.doi.org/10.1007/s12325-011-0031-3

World Health Organization. (2001). *International classification of functioning, disability and health.* Geneva: Author.

Subject Index

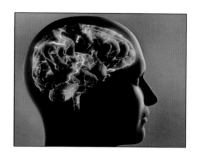

Boxes, case studies, exhibits, figures, and tables are indicated by "b," "cs," "e," "f," and "t," respectively, following page numbers.

Process-specific approaches to rehabilitation, 96, 97
Program-based vocational rehabilitation, 255
Progressive muscle relaxation, 311
Projection fibers, 47, 48*f*
PROM. *See* Passive range of motion
Prophylactic antibiotics, 9
Proprioception, 18*t*, 60*t*, 185*t*, 191, 202
Prosody, 46*t*
Prosopagnosia, 47, 189*t*
Prospective memory, 107, 108, 109, 110, 187–188, 260
Protein-based neurotransmitters, 39
Psychoeducation, 22, 274
Psychological denial, 252
Psychological functioning, 236–238
Psychosocial functioning, 237
PTA. *See* Posttraumatic amnesia
PTSD. *See* Posttraumatic stress disorder
PTSD Checklist–Military Version (PCL–M), 307, 308*e*
Pulvinar region, 57
Punch-drunk syndrome. *See* Chronic traumatic encephalopathy (CTE)
Punishment, in behavior management programs, 181
Pupillary constriction, 186, 187
Pursuits, visual, 307
Putamen, 64, 65, 65*t*
Pyramidal neurons, 41, 42, 42–43*f*, 43

Q

Quality of life
assessment of, 21, 307
community integration and, 232, 239
employment and, 247, 254
holistic rehabilitation programs and, 118
impairments and, 91, 183, 233
occupational therapy programs and, 162
suicidal ideation and, 237
Quality of Life After Brain Injury scale, 17*t*, 21
Quaternary blast injuries, 302

R

Racial differences, in incidence of TBI, 5, 7
Rancho Los Amigos Levels of Cognitive Functioning (RLA LCF) Scale
at community phase of rehabilitation, 233
development and use of, 142, 143
level I, 140, 140*t*, 153
level II, 140*t*, 141, 153
level III, 140*t*, 141, 152, 158, 167*cs*, 178
level IV, 178, 179–182, 179*b*, 183, 190, 194, 198, 201–202
level V, 178, 181–182, 183, 190, 208
level VI, 178–179, 183, 208
structure of, 16–20, 18–19*t*
Random practice, 111
Range of motion (ROM)
assessment of, 183, 190
casting for, 153–154, 205
of eyes, 187

intracranial pressure and, 10
joint injury and, 152
neuromuscular function impairment and, 151
passive. *See* Passive range of motion (PROM)
restrictions on, 156–157
surgical interventions for, 235
RAVLT (Rey Auditory Verbal Learning Test), 105
RBMT. *See* Rivermead Behavioural Memory Test
Reality orientation therapy, 209
Real Warriors program, 305*b*, 312
Receptive fields, 51, 55
Rehabilitation. *See also* Interventions; Occupational therapy
acute care. *See* Acute care settings
for blast-related TBI, 304–305, 306–312
for cognitive impairments, 95–98, 98*t*
community phase of. *See* Community phase of rehabilitation
complications during, 11–12, 14–15
costs of, 4
day treatment programs, 245*f*, 246, 274, 276–279*cs*
discharge planning, 161, 176, 177–178
family and caregivers in, 176–177
goals of, 139
holistic approaches, 96–97, 117–119
home-based programs, 245*f*, 249
inpatient. *See* Inpatient rehabilitation settings
length of stay, factors influencing, 16
measurement of, 15–22, 17–19*t*
for mTBI, 94*b*
outpatient programs, 213–215, 245–246, 245*f*, 279–280*cs*
residential programs, 244, 246–247
school reentry programs, 248–249, 256–257
subacute care. *See* Subacute rehabilitation settings
telerehabilitation, 249
transitional living programs, 246–247
vision, 186, 207, 310
vocational, 245*f*, 247–248, 255, 307
Rehabilitation Institute of Chicago–Functional Assessment Scale (RIC–FA), 17*t*, 20
Rehospitalizations, 275
Relaxation training, 311, 314*cs*
Residential rehabilitation programs, 244, 246–247
Resilience, functional, 100
Resource facilitation, 255
Restitution models of rehabilitation, 96
Retinas, 36, 44–45, 50–52, 53*f*, 186
Retinotopic organization, 51
Retrograde neurotransmission, 38
Return-to-play laws, 4
Return-to-work interventions, 254–256, 270
Revised Westmead PTA Scale, 105
Rey Auditory Verbal Learning Test (RAVLT), 105

RIC–FA (Rehabilitation Institute of Chicago–Functional Assessment Scale), 17*t*, 20
Rigidity, 206
Risperidone, 213
Rivermead Behavioural Memory Test (RBMT), 102, 107, 188, 221*cs*
Rivermead Post-Concussion Symptoms Questionnaire, 13
RLA LCF Scale. *See* Rancho Los Amigos Levels of Cognitive Functioning Scale
ROM. *See* Range of motion

S

Saccades, 187, 307
Salience network, 84
Satisfaction With Life Scale, 17*t*, 21
Scanning therapy, 207
SCAT–2 (Sports Concussion Assessment Tool–2), 93*b*
School, reentry into, 248–249, 256–257
Screening tools. *See* Assessments
Seat belts, 5, 6
Secondary blast injuries, 302
Secondary brain injuries, 8, 84, 87
Second-impact syndrome, 4
Second messengers, 39
Seizures, 11, 12
Selective attention, 103
Self-awareness
assessment of, 107, 113, 189–190, 263–265, 264*t*
of attentional drift, 116
community participation and, 244
deficits in, 21, 113–114, 189–190, 259
executive functions and, 115
hierarchy of, 264
interventions for, 211
relationship with recovery, 233–234
social competence and, 271
training in, 96, 97, 267
Self-Awareness of Deficits Interview, 113
Self-care tasks, 158, 178, 179
Self-efficacy, 22, 115, 118, 264–265, 303
Self-esteem, 112, 237–238, 254, 257
Self-managed memory aids, 109–110
Self-management skills, 119
Self-propelled manual wheelchairs, 155
Self-report measures, 114–115
Semantic memory, 61*t*, 63, 64
Seniors. *See* Older adults
Sensory cortex, 43, 43*f*
Sensory (immediate) memory, 59, 60*t*
Sensory processing, 148–151
Sensory regulation approach, 149
Sensory stimulation programs, 149–151
Serial casting and splinting, 10, 152–154, 167*cs*, 205
Serotonin, 38
Service Obstacles Scale, 253
Sexual arousal, 250–251
SFCA (Structured Functional Cognitive Assessment), 189, 194–195
Short association fibers, 47, 48, 48*f*
Short-term memory, 59, 60*t*, 179*b*

primary prevention programs for, 4–5
recovery and complications, 11–12. *See also* Rehabilitation
sports-related, 4, 6–7, 6*b*, 14, 87, 94*b*
unconsciousness resulting from, 139–173. *See also* Disorders of consciousness
Traumatic Brain Injury Model Systems program, 4, 21, 22
Treatment principles, 197–203. *See also* Occupational therapy; Pharmacological interventions; Rehabilitation; Surgical interventions
Trial-and-error learning, 112

U

Uncal herniation, 10
Unconsciousness. *See* Disorders of consciousness
Unilateral neglect, 189
Unimodal association cortices, 44
Unresponsive wakefulness syndrome, 141

V

Validity of assessments, 102, 115, 142–143, 188, 194
Valproic acid, 213
Vanishing cues, 108
Vasogenic cerebral edema, 9
Vegetative state
assessment of, 143, 147
characteristics of, 140, 140*t*, 141
pharmacological management of, 212
sensory processing and stimulation in, 148–149
wheelchair positioning in, 155
Vehicular injuries. *See* Motor vehicle–related TBI
Ventral visual pathway (ventral/what stream), 54–55, 55*f*, 56
Verbal memory, 106, 109
Vermis, 79, 80*t*
Vestibular function, 80, 149, 202, 235
Veterans. *See* Military personnel
VHA Vocational Rehabilitation program, 312
Vigilance network, 58, 59*f*
Visceral motor fibers, 70
Visceral sensory fibers, 70
Vision impairments, 185–187, 206–207, 307
Vision rehabilitation programs, 186, 207, 310
Visual acuity tests, 186
Visual association cortex, 53–54, 54*f*
Visual fields, 50–51, 50*f*, 185–186, 207, 208, 307
Visual fixation, 187
Visual imagery techniques, 108–109, 311
Visual networks, 49–56, 50*f*, 52–55*f*
Visual pathways, 186, 187
Visual scanning, 187
Visual sensory memory, 59
Visuospatial sketchpad, 63

Vocational rehabilitation, 245*f*, 247–248, 255, 307. *See also* Employment
Volitional movement, 152
Volunteer work, 254–255, 256, 279*cs*

W

War injuries. *See* Blast-related TBI
Watershed areas of brain, 10
Western Neuro Sensory Stimulation Profile, 100
Whatever It Takes approach, 267–268
Wheelchairs, 154–156, 167–168*cs*, 203–204
Whiplash, 49, 82
White matter
basal nuclei in, 64
of cerebellum, 79
of cerebrum, 40, 47–48, 64
composition of, 47–48
CSF leakage into, 9
in diffuse axonal injuries, 7–8, 40
hematomas in, 11
injury severity and loss of, 105
Work. *See* Employment
Working memory, 59, 60*t*, 63, 105, 106
Wounded Warrior Project, 312

X

X rays, 11

Y

Youth. *See* Children and adolescents

Citation Index

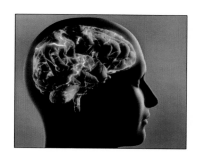

Boxes, case studies, exhibits, figures, and tables are indicated by "b," "cs," "e," "f," and "t," respectively, following page numbers.